Recent Results
in Cancer Research

152

Managing Editors
P.M. Schlag, Berlin · H.-J. Senn, St. Gallen

Associate Editors
V. Diehl, Cologne · D.M. Parkin, Lyon
M.F. Rajewsky, Essen · R. Rubens, London
M. Wannenmacher, Heidelberg

Founding Editor
P. Rentchnik, Geneva

Springer
Berlin
Heidelberg
New York
Barcelona
Hong Kong
London
Milan
Paris
Singapore
Tokyo

H.-J. Senn   R. Gelber   A. Goldhirsch
B. Thürlimann   (Eds.)

Adjuvant Therapy
of Primary Breast Cancer VI

With 58 Figures and 60 Tables

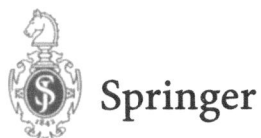 Springer

Prof. Dr. med. Hans-Jörg Senn
Zentrum für Tumordiagnostik und Prävention
Rorschacherstrasse 150
CH-9006 St. Gallen, Switzerland

Richard D. Gelber, Ph. D.
Dana Farber Cancer Institute
Biostatistics
44 Binney Street
Boston, 02115, USA

Prof. Dr. med. Aron Goldhirsch
Ospedale Civico
CH-6900 Lugano, Switzerland

Priv.-Doz. Dr. med. Beat Thürlimann
Kantonsspital St. Gallen
Klinik C für Innere Medizin
Abteilung für Onkologie und Hämatologie
CH-9007 St. Gallen, Switzerland

ISBN-13: 978-3-642-45771-5   e-ISBN-13: 978-3-642-45769-2
DOI: 10.1007/978-3-642-45769-2

Library of Congress Cataloging-in-Publication Data
Adjuvant therapy of primary breast cancer VI / H.-J. Senn ... [et al.] (eds.). p. cm. –
(Recent results in cancer research, ISSN 0080-0015; 152) Based on the lectures presented
at the 6th International Conference on Adjuvant Therapy of Primary Breast Cancer, held in
St. Gallen, Switzerland. Includes bibliographical references and index. ISBN 3-540-64085-1
(hardcover: alk. paper). 1. Breast-Cancer-Adjuvant treatment – Congresses. I. Senn, Hans-
jörg. II. International Conference on "Adjuvant Therapy of Primary Breast Cancer" (6th:
1998: Saint Gall, Switzerland). III. Series. [DNLM: 1. Breast Neoplasms – drug therapy
congresses. 2. Breast Neoplasms – diagnosis congresses. 3. Adjuvants, Pharmaceutic congresses. 4. Adjuvants, Immunologic congresses. W1RE106P v. 152 1998]. RC261.R35 vol.
152 [RC280.B8] 616.99'4 s – dc21 [616.99'44906] DNLM/DLC for Library of Congress.

© Springer-Verlag Berlin · Heidelberg 1998

Softcover reprint of the hardcover 1st edition 1998

The use of general descriptive names, registered names, trademarks, etc. in this publication
does not imply, even in the absence of a specific statement, that such names are exempt
from the relevant protective laws and regulations and therefore free for general use.

Product liability: The publisher cannot guarantee the accuracy of any information about
dosage and application contained in this book. In every individual case the user must
check such information by consulting the relevant literature.

Production: PRO EDIT GmbH, D-69126 Heidelberg
Typesetting: K+V Fotosatz GmbH, D-64743 Beerfelden

SPIN 10667008   19/3133-5 4 3 2 1 0 – Printed on acid-free paper

Preface

This RRCR-conference-volume marks "number six" in a 20-year evolution of international conferences on the adjuvant therapy of primary breast cancer. Starting in 1978, a handful of some 80 enthusiastic breast cancer surgeons and oncologists, met in a secluded mountain resort near St. Gallen in Eastern Switzerland, to exchange their early data of some pioneer trials on adjuvant systemic therapy of early breast cancer, and to correlate their future research efforts to overcome the frustrating prognostic stagnation of this dominant neoplastic disease in Western females during the past decades. Repeated every 3–4 years, these St. Gallen International Conferences on Adjuvant Therapy of Primary Breast Cancer have continuously grown in numbers of participants and in normative, therapeutic influence by being published in major oncology journals [1–3], the last (6th) conference having taken place from February 25–28, 1998 with more than 1800 attendees from over 50 countries worldwide.

What is the fascination of adjuvant therapy in primary (early) breast cancer, and what has changed·during the last 3 years since March 1995, to justify another international gathering of this size, and of the world's leading experts in the field?

There is no question, that providing even more effective care and designing appropriate recommendations for the multitudes of patients with so-called early breast cancer or at high risk of developing the disease, remain highly important public health goals. While the prevailing theme at earlier conferences was to distinguish the role of prognostic and predictive factors, used for the proper selection of adjuvant treatment regimens [3], the conference reported in this volume had to set slightly different goals, since several important developments have occurred in recent years. These include the following:

– The discovery of 2 major breast cancer susceptibility genes (BRCA 1 and 2) and the availability of genetic testing of women at high risk.

- The emerging possibilities of chemo/endocrine-prevention of breast cancer in well defined categories of high-risk women.
- The advent of minimal invasive surgery for diagnostic as well as therapeutic interventions, at the level of the primary tumor (image-guided stereotactic biopsy, or within the axilla (introduction of sentinel-node-biopsy versus traditional axillary dissection).
- The concept of primary (pre-operative) chemotherapy, in order to facilitate breast-conserving surgery and hopefully to improve prognostic results.

Following the traditional pattern of the St. Gallen adjuvant breast cancer conferences, an invited consensus panel of international experts was again confronted with the whole set of scientific presentations by representatives of major breast cancer trial groups worldwide, and had to develop practicable future guidelines for the selection of specific adjuvant treatments in defined patient populations. The panel carefully reviewed its earlier 1995 recommendations [3] and tried to modify these on the basis of new emerging evidence from recent clinical research. This volume contains the majority of the invited lectures as well as the respective consensus recommendations for 1998 ff. It offers a more or less complete surview of the various aspects of diagnosing and treating early breast cancer, with proper emphasis on new entities such as DCIS (ductal carcinoma in situ), becoming more and more prevalent in countries and areas with effective mammographic screening. The volume and its closing consensus panel also highlight the emerging role of combined adjuvant hemo-endocrine therapies, leading to substantial clinical benefit in most patient subgroups of women with early, operable breast cancer.

It is the hope of the editors as well as of the large number of authors of this volume, that their recommendations may be constructively transmitted to the patient level, in research as well as in private or hospital practice. While the consensus panel issued its recommendations at the end of this volume especially for the many patients, treated outside of clinical prospective trials, it made it clear to the medical public, that its primary recommendation to breast patients and their home physicians and surgeons still is: to participate as much as possible in well designed, prospective clinical trials, in order to finally develop more appropriate and better tolerable treatment guidelines for primary (early) breast cancer with more clinical impact and in more reasonable time than before!

In this respect we want to thank all the panelists, moderators, speakers, discussants and conference participants, who again transformed this past 6th Conference on the Adjuvant Treatment of Primary Breast Cancer into another major success, both scientifically and socially. The stage is already set for "ABC-01" on February 21–24, 2001.

St. Gallen, Switzerland   *Hans-Jörg Senn*
                                                            Beat Thürlimann
Lugano, Switzerland and Milano, Italy   *Aron Goldhirsch*
Boston, MA, USA   *Richard Gelber*
October 1998

References

1. Senn HJ, Goldhirsch A, Gelber RD, Osterwalder B (1989) Adjuvant therapy of primary breast cancer. Recent Results in Cancer Research 115:1–296
2. Glick JH, Gelber RD, Goldhirsch A, Senn HJ (1992) Meeting Highlights: Adjuvant therapy for primary breast cancer. J Natl Cancer Inst 84:1476–1485
3. Goldhirsch A, Wood WC, Senn HJ, Glick JH, Gelber RD (1995) Meeting Highlights: International consensus panel on the treatment of primary breast cancer. J Natl Cancer Inst 87:1441–1447

Contents

IV. In Situ Breast Cancer

V. Controversies About the Axilla

VI. Integrated Therapy: Changing Surgical Procedures for Breast Cancer

VII. Integrated Therapy: Primary Adjuvant Systemic Therapy

VIII. Integrated Therapy: Radiation Therapy / Endocrine Treatment

XII. Clinical Research Around the World: Review of Cooperative Group Trials

XIII. International Consensus Conference on Primary Treatment of the Breast: Update 1998

Subject Index

List of Contributors*

Abrams, J. S.[417]
Agostara, B.[453]
Amoroso, D.[453]
Anderson, E.[227]
Asselain, B.[217]
Ausili Cefaro, G. P.[453]
Bass, S. S.[170]
Basser, R. L.[355]
Bellantone, R.[453]
Bergh, J.[328]
Berman, C.[170]
Bernhard, J.[390]
Beuzeboc, P.[217]
Blamey, R.[227]
Blichert-Toft, M.[149]
Boccardo, F.[453]
Bolognesi, A.[453]
Bonadonna, G.[314]
Bonanni, B.[11]
Bonetti, M.[373]
Capri, G.[314]
Clarke, R. B.[227]
Coates, A.[390, 412, 429]
Cole, B. F.[373]
Come, S.[247]
Conte, P. F.[305]
Coombes, R. C.[277]
Costa, A.[11]
Cox, C. E.[170]

Crook, T.[35]
Davidson, N. E.[368]
Decensi, A.[11]
Del Mastro, L.[305]
Desmond, K. A.[396]
Diéras, V.[217]
Dixon, J. M.[227]
Dorval, T.[217]
Dowsett, M.[227]
Dubey, A. K.[247]
Fallowfield, L.[412]
Farris, A.[453]
Fentiman, I. S.[135]
Gallo, L.[453]
Ganz, P.[396]
Garusi, C.[202]
Gelber, R. D.[373, 481]
Gelber, S.[373]
Genta, F.[453]
Giai, M.[453]
Gianni, L.[314]
Glick, J. H.[481]
Goldhirsch, A.[373, 481]
Greuze, M.[202]
Guerrieri Gonzaga, A.[11]
Gusterson, B. A.[35]
Harder, F.[180]
Harris, A. L.[217, 341]
Harris, J.[247]

---

* The address of the principal author is given on the first page
of each contribution.
[1] Page on which contribution begins.

Hayes, D. F.[71]
Howell, A.[227]
Hürny, C.[390]
Jäger, D.[94]
Jäger, E.[94]
Johnston, S. R. D.[227]
Jordan, V. C.[265]
Jouve, M.[217]
Kaufmann, M.[471]
Kinne, D. W.[161]
Knuth, A.[94]
Kocher, T.[180]
Ku, N. N.[170]
Kurtz, J. M.[143]
Lu, Y. J.[35]
Manetti, L.[11]
Margolese, R. G.[193]
Masetti, R.[105]
Mesiti, M.[453]
Meyerowitz, B. E.[396]
Miller, W. R.[227]
Mouridsen, H. T.[298, 441]
Mustacchi, G.[453]
Nicholson, R.[227]
Osin, P.[35]
Pacini, P.[453]
Palangié, T.[216]
Patrone, F.[453]
Perry, C.[202]
Petit, J.-Y.[202]
Piccart, M. J.[447]
Pierga, J. Y.[217]
Pollak, M.[63]

Pouillart, P.[217]
Pritchard, K. I.[22, 285]
Ravdin, P. M.[86]
Recht, A.[247]
Reintgen, D. S.[170]
Rietjens, M.[202]
Robertson, J. F. R.[227]
Rowland, J. H.[396]
Rubagotti, A.[453]
Rutqvist, L. E.[255]
Sassi, M.[453]
Schieppati, G.[453]
Scholl, S. M.[217]
Senn, H.-J.[481]
Shipley, J.[35]
Shons, A. R.[170]
Shulman, L.[247]
Silverstein, M. J.[105]
Sismondi, P.[453]
Smith, I. E.[323]
Snyderwine, E. G.[3]
Torhorst, J.[180]
Torrisi, R.[11]
Valagussa, P.[314, 368]
Van de Velde, C. J. H.[447]
Van de Vijver, M. J.[123]
Villa, A.[453]
Wallgren, A.[298]
Weber, B. L.[49]
Wood, W. C.[212]
Yeatman, T. J.[170]
Zuber, M.[180]

I. Epidemiology and Its Lessons

Diet and Mammary Gland Carcinogenesis

E. G. Snyderwine

Laboratory of Experimental Carcinogenesis, National Cancer Institute, Building 37, Room 3C28, Bethesda, MD 20892-4255, USA

Introduction

The etiology of human breast cancer is largely unknown. However, there are three broad determinants of breast cancer risk. One determinant is heredity, such as carrying a germline mutation in the BRCA1 or BRCA2 gene. Another is hormonal and reproductive factors. Women have a 180-fold higher risk of breast cancer than men, and among women, the age at menarche, age at menopause, age at first childbirth, and parity influence breast cancer risk. A third determinant is environment, which includes the country where a woman was born and raised, lifestyle habits, and diet. It appears likely that these three broad factors are not mutually exclusive but are interactive, thereby adding to the complexity in the etiology of breast cancer.

The strong influence of environment on human breast cancer risk is illustrated by the finding that age-adjusted breast cancer incidence rates vary widely among women living in different countries (Kelsey and Horn-Ross 1993; Willett 1997 a,b). Breast cancer incidence rates are relatively high among women living in North America and parts of Europe. Roughly five-fold lower rates are observed in Asian countries including Japan, China, and Thailand. Offspring of populations that migrate from a low- to a high-incidence country develop breast cancer rates approximating those of the new host country. However, the pace of change in the incidence rate varies with populations. Breast cancer rates among Japanese immigrants to the United States approach those of the general US population after the second or third generation (Buell 1973), a delay that may in part be associated with the rate of acculturation (Willett 1997a).

The difference in breast cancer risk between high-incidence and low-incidence countries, such as the US and Japan, respectively, is largely due to the difference in the incidence of postmenopausal breast cancer (Kelsey and Horn-Ross 1993). Prior to age 50, or roughly the age of menopause, the difference between the countries is slight, but after age 50, the difference progressively increases with increasing age. Postmenopausal breast cancer, or sporadic breast cancer, is more likely to be linked to environmental and lifestyle factors such as dietary habits. Dietary habits are very different between people in the US and Japanese consuming a traditional diet. Whereas in US diet is rich in calories, cooked meat, and dietary fat (comprising approximately 35% of calories), the traditional Japanese diet is largely carbohydrate-based (derived from rice), with some protein from fish, and a level of dietary fat comprising on the order of 15% of calories. The breast cancer incidence rates have been steadily increasing in Japan over the last 25–30 years, and the increase may partly be associated with changes in lifestyle factors, including a westernization of the Japanese diet (Wynder et al. 1997).

Dietary Components

Overview

Many dietary components have been evaluated in epidemiological or animal studies for their influence on breast cancer risk (Hunter and Willett 1996; World Cancer Research Fund/American Institute for Cancer Research 1997). Components that have been examined include macroconstituents such as total calories, dietary fat, alcohol, and dietary fiber. Of these components, alcohol is currently the most well-established dietary risk factor in human breast cancer (Longnecker et al. 1995). Studies with alcohol have shown that moderate consumption increases a woman's breast cancer risk approximately 10%. In addition, recent studies demonstrating that alcohol intake alters estrogen metabolism provide a potential mechanism for the association of alcohol with breast cancer. In contrast, dietary fiber may be a protective factor in diet because of its capacity to lower serum estrogen levels via a reduction in the deconjugation and reabsorption of estrogens excreted via the biliary system. Several microconstituents in the diet that have been studied for their potential role in breast cancer include nutritive components such as vitamins and minerals, nonnutritive phytochemicals, and mutagens/carcinogens in foodstuffs (Block et al. 1992; Hunter and Willet 1996; World Cancer Research Fund/American Institute for Cancer Research 1997). Fruits and vegetables in the human diet are rich in phytochemicals several of which have protective action against breast cancer. The importance of specific phytochemicals including isothiocyanates (e.g., sulforaphane), phytoestrogens (e.g., genistein and daidzein), indoles (indole-3-carbinol), and carotenoids (β-carotene) is supported by animal studies showing a protective effect of these compounds in experimental models of mammary gland carcinogenesis (for example see Zhang et al. 1994). Epidemiological studies also support a weak protective effect of carotenoids on breast cancer. However, it is not yet known whether carotenoids per se or other components in carotenoid-rich foods are responsible for the protective effect (Hunter and Willett 1996; World Cancer Research Fund/American Institute for Cancer Research 1997). Although the protective effect of fruits and vegetables is thought to be largely due to specific components such as vitamins, minerals, fiber, and anticarcinogenic phytochemicals present in the foodstuff, high fruit and vegetable intake rather than intake of any specific component is most strongly and consistently correlated with a lower breast cancer risk.

In addition to potentially beneficial components, diet also contains carcinogens, several of which have been shown to induce mammary gland cancer in rats, and dietary fat, a strong promoter of mammary gland carcinogenesis in rodent models. The topics of dietary carcinogens and dietary fat are discussed more fully below.

Dietary Fat

One of the first dietary components to be implicated in the high incidence of breast cancer in the US and other high-risk countries was dietary fat. Ecological studies showed a linear correlation between per capita consumption of dietary fat and the incidence and mortality of breast cancer, with countries showing the highest intake of dietary fat experiencing the highest incidence and mortality from the disease and vice versa (Carroll et al. 1986). Animal studies have strongly supported the role of dietary fat intake, especially linoleic acid, in mammary gland cancer promotion (Rogers 1997; Wynder et al. 1997). Nevertheless, the hypothesis that dietary fat plays a role in breast cancer is a subject of considerable controversy and debate (Hunter and Willett 1996; Wynder et al. 1997). Ten prospective studies addressing the role of dietary fat in breast cancer have not shown an association between dietary fat intake and breast cancer (World Cancer Research Fund/American Institute for Cancer Research 1997). The Nurses Health Study (Willett et al. 1992) reported a relative risk of 1.0 (0.7–1.3) for women consuming more than 49% of calories from fat versus women consuming 29% of calories from fat. In a recent pooled analysis of seven prospective studies involving over 300 000 women and approximately 5 000 breast cancer cases, there was no association between breast cancer and fat intake over a range of less than 20% to more than 45% of energy from dietary fat (Hunter et al. 1996). In contrast, case control studies are generally more supportive of an association between fat intake and breast cancer risk (World Cancer Research Fund/American Institute for Cancer Research 1997). In a meta-analysis of twelve case-control studies, Howe et al. (1990) reported a significant increase in risk of breast cancer for a higher intake of dietary fat (odds ratio 1.35 for a 100 g increase in daily fat intake).

There are several unresolved issues regarding the role of dietary fat in breast cancer. Food frequency questionnaires used in prospective epidemiology studies may not adequately reflect dietary fat intake (Wynder et al. 1997). In addition, prospective epidemiology studies have largely addressed dietary fat intake over a relatively short duration during adulthood. It is not yet known if dietary fat intake during childhood and adolescence affects risk in later life (Wynder et al. 1997). Different kinds of dietary fatty acids may also pose different risks. The role of high levels of dietary linoleic acid, a relatively recent dietary modification, in human breast cancer risk is still unresolved (Willett 1997 a,b). Finally, animal and experimental studies support the thesis that dietary fat is not carcinogenic but serves as a promoter of mammary carcinogenesis (Ghoshal et al. 1994; Rogers 1997; Wynder et al. 1997). By definition, promotion by dietary fat would require that initiation by other factors also occur in order to affect the carcinogenic process. Speculatively, variation in the exposure to initiating agents in the environment may partly obscure the role of dietary fat as a promotional factor.

Mutagens and Carcinogens

Diet is a rich source of natural and cooking-derived mutagens and carcinogens (National Research Council 1982). Of the mutagen/carcinogens found in the diet, two cooking-derived classes of carcinogens induce mammary gland cancer in animal models (El-Bayoumy 1992; Snyderwine 1994). The first class is the polycyclic aromatic hydrocarbons associated with barbecued meats. These compounds are formed from the pyrolysis of fats that occurs when fat drips from the meat onto the coals, forming smoke that is redeposited on the meat surface. Another class of compounds are the heterocyclic amines (HCAs). Amino acid and creatine precursors in meat react chemically to produce these carcinogens during high-temperature cooking by a variety of methods such as broiling, frying, barbecuing, and baking. 2-Amino-1-methyl-6-phenylimidazo[4,5-b]pyridine (PhIP), the major carcinogenic HCA found in the Western diet, has been shown to induce cancer in the mammary gland, colon, and prostate gland of rats, three organ sites that show a relatively high incidence of cancer in the Western world (Layton et al. 1995; Sugimura 1995; Weisburger et al. 1995). Studies have shown that PhIP forms DNA adducts in the mammary gland of rats that may contribute to the initiation of carcinogenesis (Ghoshal et al. 1995; Snyderwine 1994). Although the levels of the HCAs in the diet of individuals consuming cooked meat are in the part-per-billion range – significantly lower than the levels shown to induce cancer in laboratory animals – HCAs are regarded as possible human carcinogens (Sugimura 1995).

Carcinogens plus Promotional Factors

Experimental studies have shown that the carcinogenicity of PhIP is potentially modulated by other dietary factors such as a high fat diet, as well as various protective factors including indole-3-carbinol, chlorophyllin, and tea polyphenols (Guo et al. 1995; Weisburger et al. 1995). In the rat mammary gland carcinogenicity model, a high fat diet containing linoleic acid (and fed ad libitum) is a strong promotional factor for carcinogenesis (Ghoshal et al. 1994; Snyderwine, unpublished observations). The incidence, growth rate, and invasiveness of carcinomas were higher in rats on a high fat diet than in rats on a low fat diet. No tumors were detected in rats on either a high fat or low fat diet that were not given PhIP. These findings support the notion that PhIP, a carcinogen found in the human diet, would be more likely to be a risk factor for breast cancer when the gland is under strong promotional influences such as occurs with ad libitum consumption of a high fat diet. PhIP exposure concomitant with a high fat diet is typical of the Western diet.

Energy Balance and Body Weight Gain

Several epidemiology studies have shown that body weight gain is a risk factor for postmenopausal breast cancer (Brinton and Swanson 1992; Trentham-Dietz et al. 1997; World Cancer Research Fund/American Institute for Cancer Research 1997; Ziegler et al. 1996). Ziegler et al. (1996) reported a two- to three-fold increase in relative risk with a recent weight gain of over 11 lb (5 kg) for women in their early 50s. The results from experimental studies in rats are parallel to the findings in humans, further supporting the notion that weight gain is a strong promotional factor for breast cancer. In the rat mammary gland carcinogenicity model for PhIP described above, the enhancement of mammary carcinogenesis by a high fat diet was associated with a significantly higher body weight gain in rats on the high fat diet than in rats on the low fat diet (Ghoshal et al. 1994; Snyderwine, unpublished observations). Previous studies using the rat model and the experimental mammary gland carcinogen 7,12-dimethylbenz[a]anthracene reported that the enhancement of mammary gland carcinogenesis by a high fat diet was largely associated with ad libitum feeding (Welsch et al. 1990). Restricted feeding of the high fat diet did not promote mammary gland carcinogenesis. In addition, ad libitum feeding, but not restricted feeding, of a high fat diet was associated with a significantly higher body weight than that seen in the low fat diet group.

There has been a long-standing dispute over whether dietary fat per se or increased caloric consumption is associated with the promotional effects of a high fat diet (Welsch et al. 1990). While studies have begun to provide a mechanistic basis for the effects of high levels of dietary fat (i.e., increased consumption of specific fatty acids, especially linoleic acid) on mammary gland cancer promotion (Rogers 1997; Rose 1996; Wynder et al. 1997), the current epidemiological evidence supports the supposition that the predominant effect of high dietary fat intake in women is likely to be linked to an increase in energy intake leading to weight gain, which is in turn associated with promotion of mammary gland cancer (Hunter and Willett 1996; Willett 1997a). Energy balance, i.e., energy intake and expenditure, currently appears to be a stronger determinant of breast cancer risk in women than either dietary fat intake or caloric consumption per se (World Cancer Research Fund/American Institute for Cancer Research 1997). Caloric consumption can be offset by increased physical activity or caloric expenditure, and studies have shown that physical activity or energy expenditure is associated with a lower risk of breast cancer (Mittendorf et al. 1995; World Cancer Research Fund/American

Institute for Cancer Research 1997). The energy balance concept (Willett 1997a) appears to provide a unifying hypothesis for the experimental and epidemiological observations regarding the effects of dietary fat intake, caloric consumption, body weight, and physical activity on breast cancer risk.

There is cogent evidence to further support the energy balance hypothesis from results describing the effect of energy intake/expenditure on hormone levels, especially estrogens, that play an important role in mammary gland carcinogenesis (World Cancer Research Fund/American Institute for Cancer Research 1997). A diet rich in calories and energy, such as a Western diet, is associated with earlier childhood growth and development that can result in an earlier age of menses (Sherman et al. 1981; World Cancer Research Fund/American Institute for Cancer Research 1997). Whereas the average age of menses in the US is 12–13, in rural China, the age is roughly 17. Thus, exposure of the mammary gland to ovarian hormones begins at a younger age in the higher risk population. The Western diet (and lifestyle) appears also be associated with adult weight gain which can lead to adiposity. Adipose tissue contributes significantly to the production of estrogen in postmenopausal women (World Cancer Research Fund/American Institute for Cancer Research 1997). Adiposity has also been associated with a later on-set of menopause and consequently an increased lifetime exposure of the mammary gland to estrogen (World Cancer Research Fund/American Institute for Cancer Research 1997).

Dietary Recommendations for Breast Cancer Prevention

There is substantial scientific evidence that modifying caloric intake in order to avoid adult weight gain, avoiding alcohol, and increasing consumption of fruits and vegetables are likely to help lower breast cancer risk. (The general recommendation by the National Cancer Institute is five servings of fruits and vegetables per day.) There is a moderate amount of scientific evidence to support minimizing the consumption of cooked meat and adhering to a low fat diet to help lower breast cancer risk. These practices are also likely to help with weight maintenance as well as to have potential benefits for offsetting cardiovascular disease. At the present time there appears to be little scientific evidence to support the use of dietary supplements, such as vitamin supplements, over increasing fruits and vegetable consumption and adhering to a sound nutritional program as outlined by the well-known Food Pyramid Guide. Practical approaches to dietary modification, combined with increased physical activity, are likely to be of potential overall benefit in minimizing the risk of breast cancer.

Summary

The variation in human breast cancer incidence rates worldwide suggests that lifestyle factors, especially diet, influence breast cancer risk. There is convincing evidence that diets associated with rapid growth and greater adult height increase breast cancer risk. In addition, diet and other lifestyle factors which lead to high body mass, especially during postmenopausal years, also appear to increase risk. Several dietary components have been evaluated in epidemiological and animal studies for their role in breast cancer. Dietary fat was once implicated in the high incidence of breast cancer in the Western world, but its role in breast cancer is now controversial. In contrast, alcohol consumption is currently recognized as the best-established dietary risk factor in this disease. Carcinogens that cause mammary gland cancer in rats such as heterocyclic amines and polycyclic aromatic hydrocarbons are found in cooked meat, but it is not yet known if these carcinogens are etiological factors in human breast cancer. Fruits and vegetables are rich in potential chemopreventive factors that may lower breast cancer risk. Practical approaches to dietary modification that include increasing fruit and vegetable consumption, eating a low fat diet, reducing cooked meat consumption, and avoiding alcohol are likely to be of potential overall benefit in lowering the risk of human breast cancer.

References

Block G, Patterson B, Subar A (1992) Fruit, vegetables, and cancer prevention: a review of the epidemiological evidence. Nutr Cancer 18:1–29

Brinton LA, Swanson CA (1992) Height and weight and various ages and risk of breast cancer. Ann Epidemiol 2:597–609

Buell P (1973) Changing incidence of breast cancer in Japanese-American women. J Natl Cancer Inst 51:1479–1483

Carroll KK, Braden LM, Bell JA, Kalamegham R (1986) Fat and cancer. Cancer 58:1818–1825

El-Bayoumy K (1992) Environmental carcinogens that may be involved in human breast cancer etiology. Chem Res Toxicol 5:585–590

Ghoshal A, Preisegger K-H, Takayama S, Thorgeirsson SS, Snyderwine EG (1994) Induction of mammary tumors in female Sprague-Dawley rats by the food mutagen 2-amino-1-methyl-6-phenylimidazo[4,5-*b*]pyridine and effect of dietary fat. Carcinogenesis 15:2429–2433

Ghoshal A, Davis CD, Schut HAJ, Snyderwine EG (1995) Possible mechanisms for PhIP-DNA adduct formation in the mammary gland of female Sprague-Dawley rats. Carcinogenesis 16:2725–2731

Guo D, Schut HA, Davis CD, Snyderwine EG, Bailey GS, Dashwood RH (1995) Protection by chlorophyllin and indole-3-carbinol against 2-amino-1-methyl-6-phenylimidazo[4,5-*b*]pyridine (PhIP)-induced DNA adducts and colonic aberrant crypts in the F344 rat. Carcinogenesis 16:2931–2937

Howe GR, Hirohata T, Hislop TG, Iscovich JM, Yuan JM et al (1990) Dietary factors and risk of breast cancer: combined analysis of 12 case-control studies. J Natl Cancer Inst 82:561–569

Hunter DJ, Willett WC (1996) Nutrition and breast cancer. Cancer Causes Control 7:56–68

Hunter DJ, Spiegelman D, Adami H-O, Beeson L, van den Brandt PA et al (1996) Cohort studies of fat intake and risk of breast cancer: a pooled analysis. N Engl J Med 334:356–361

Kelsey JL, Horn-Ross PL (1993) Breast cancer: magnitude of the problem and descriptive epidemiology. Epidemiol Rev 15:7–16

Layton DW, Bogen KT, Knize MG, Hatch FT, Johnson VM, Felton JS (1995) Cancer risk of heterocyclic amines in cooked foods: an analysis and implications for research. Carcinogenesis 16:39–52

Longnecker MP, Newcomb PA, Mittendorf R, Greenberg ER, Clapp RW et al (1995) Risk of breast cancer in relation to lifetime alcohol consumption. J Natl Cancer Inst 87:923–929

Mittendorf R, Longnecker MP, Newcomb PA, Dietz AT, Greenberg R et al (1995) Strenuous physical activity in young adulthood and risk of breast cancer (United States). Cancer Causes Control 6:347–353

National Research Council (1982) Diet, nutrition, and cancer. National Academy Press, Washington, DC

Rogers AE (1997) Diet and breast cancer: studies in laboratory animals. J Nutr 127:933S–935S

Rose DP (1996) The mechanistic rationale in support of dietary cancer prevention. Prev Med 25:34–37

Sherman B, Wallace R, Bean J, Schlabaugh L (1981) Relationship of body weight to menarcheal and menopausal age: implications for breast cancer risk. J Clin Endocrinol Metab 52:488–493

Snyderwine EG (1994) Some perspectives on the nutritional aspects of breast cancer research. Cancer 74 Suppl:1070–1077

Sugimura T (1995) History, present, and future, of heterocyclic amines, cooked food mutagens. In: Adamson RH, Gustafsson JA, Ito N, Sugimura T, Wakabayashi K, Yamazoe Y (eds) Heterocyclic amines in cooked foods: possible human carcinogens. Princeton Scientific Publishing, Princeton, NJ, pp 214–231

Trentham-Dietz A, Newcomb PA, Storer BE, Longnecker MP, Baron J et al (1997) Body size and risk of breast cancer. Am J Epidemiol 145:1011–1019

Weisburger JH, Rivenson A, Kingston DGI, Wilkins TD, van Tassell RL et al (1995) Dietary modulation of the carcinogenicity of the heterocyclic amines. In: Adamson RH, Gustafsson JA, Ito N, Sugimura T, Wakabayashi K, Yamazoe Y (eds) Heterocyclic amines in cooked foods: possible human carcinogens. Princeton Scientific Publishing, Princeton, NJ, pp 240–250

Welsch CW, House JL, Herr BL, Eliasberg SJ, Welsh MA (1990) Enhancement of mammary carcinogenesis by high levels of dietary fat: a phenomenon dependent on ad libitum feeding. J Natl Cancer Inst 82:1615–1620

Willett WC (1997a) Fat, energy and breast cancer. J Nutr 127:921S–923S

Willett WC (1997b) Specific fatty acids and risk of breast and prostate cancer: dietary intake. Am J Clin Nutr 66 Suppl:1557S–1563S

Willett WC, Hunter DJ, Stampfer MJ, Colditz G, Manson JE, Spiegelman D et al (1992) Dietary fat and fiber in relation to the risk of breast cancer. An 8-year follow-up. JAMA 268:2037–2044

World Cancer Research Fund/American Institute for Cancer Research (1997) Food, nutrition and the prevention of cancer: a global perspective. American Institute for Cancer Research, Washington, DC

Wynder EL, Cohen LA, Muscat JE, Winters B, Dwyer JT, Blackburn G (1997) Breast cancer: weighing the evidence for a promoting role of dietary fat. J Natl Cancer Inst 89:766–775

Zhang Y, Kensler TW, Cho C-G, Posner GH, Talalay P (1994) Anticarcinogenic activities of sulforaphane and structurally related synthetic norbornyl isothiocyanates. Proc Natl Acad Sci USA 91:3147–3150

Ziegler RG, Hoover RN, Nomura AMY, West DW, Wu AH et al (1996) Relative weight, weight change, height, and breast cancer risk in Asian-American women. J Natl Cancer Inst 88:650–660

Prevention of Breast Cancer: Focus on Chemoprevention

A. Costa, B. Bonanni, L. Manetti, A. Guerrieri Gonzaga, R. Torrisi, and A. Decensi

FIRC Chemoprevention Unit, European Institute of Oncology, Via Riparnonti 435, 20141 Milan, Italy

Introduction

Breast cancer remains one of the "big killers" worldwide, even when the slight reduction in mortality figures of these last few years is taken into account. Given the current results of conventional cancer treatment, there are good reasons for improving the available preventive strategies and thus for exploring new ways in this direction. At present, prospects for breast cancer prevention are being developed in three main areas: (a) lifestyle, to study various risk factors, including delayed first pregnancy and number of pregnancies; (b) genetics, to understand the real importance of familial breast cancer and of genetic testing; and (c) chemoprevention, to identify agents potentially able to inhibit the development of invasive cancer.

Lifestyle

Among the risk factors for breast cancer there is strong evidence that ovarian hormones play an important role. Subsequent to ovarian ablation, breast cancer may be reduced up to 75%, depending on parity, weight, and age at the time of artificial menopause. Other events associated with hormonal changes have similarly been found to influence breast cancer risk, among them age at menarche, age at first childbirth, and age at menopause. The role of reproductive risk factors may be different for women with or without a family history: a recent study (Colditz et al. 1996) reported that among women with a family history of breast cancer there is little protection from later age at menarche, no protection from multiple births, nor from early age at first birth, and, particularly, first pregnancy has an adverse effect.

Other breast cancer risk factors correlated to the above hormonal factors are high-fat diet and sedentary lifestyle. There is some evidence, based on epidemiological observation, that breast cancer may be prevented in certain women by changing their endogenous hormonal profile through a change to a low-fat diet or increased levels of exercise (Prentice et al. 1990; Bernstein et al. 1987).

Genetics

It is now more evident that the susceptibility of an individual also influences the role of carcinogens and growth factors in accelerating the carcinogenic process. Known genetic syndromes and abnormalities linked to a high lifetime probability of developing breast cancer are estimated to occur in 5%–10% of the general population, thus contributing only to the minority of breast cancers. The study of high-risk genes is very important not only for the identification of high-risk populations who are at increased need for a preventive intervention, but also to better understand the etiology and biology of breast cancer.

Among the growing list of these genes are BRCA1 and BRCA2. An inherited mutation on BRCA1 and BRCA2 increases the lifetime risk of breast and ovarian cancer, and possibly colon cancer. Male mutation carriers (predominantly BRCA2) are at increased risk of prostate cancer and breast cancer. Importantly, breast cancers among women with BRCA1 or BRCA2 mutations tend to occur at younger ages than in other women.

Women with mutations predisposing them to breast or ovarian cancer may consider prophylactic mastectomy and/or oophorectomy. In a simulation study for decision analysis (Schrag et al. 1997), it was recently suggested that prophylactic mastectomy and, to a lesser extent, oophorectomy might provide substantial gains in life expectancy for young women. However, neither approach completely protects against breast cancer, and a number of psychological, sexual, reproductive, and financial aspects must be considered too. Moreover, women at higher genetic risk may wish a less invasive preventive approach, opting for inclusion in chemoprevention clinical trials.

Chemoprevention

Cancer chemoprevention is a specific pharmacological intervention, potentially able to inhibit invasive cancer development either by blocking the DNA damage that initiates carcinogenesis, or by arresting or reversing the progression of premalignant cells. According to Sporn's (1991) concept, this approach assumes that "carcinogenesis" is a disease, the end result of which is cancer. Therefore, chemoprevention is comparable to drug therapy for cardiovascular disease precursors, such as hypertension and hyperlipidemia.

Different target populations for breast cancer chemoprevention may be recognized. Primary chemoprevention may involve a wide population of healthy women with a moderate risk due to reproductive factors or nonpenetrant genetic factors (e.g., one first-degree relative with breast cancer) or because of exposure to known promoting agents (e.g., hormone replacement therapy). A second level of primary chemoprevention may involve a limited population at very high risk because of penetrating genetic predisposition to cancer (e.g., BRCA1 mutation carriers). Secondary chemoprevention may involve subjects with premalignant or early malignant lesions (e.g., breast atypical hyperplasia and carcinoma in situ or microinvasive disease, and long-term survivors from invasive disease).

Rationale and Selection of Biomarkers

Prevention trials using clinical endpoints are subject to high costs since a very high number of participants and years of follow-up are necessary. Detecting a 15% reduction in the risk of breast cancer with a given agent in a 2-year trial with a 3-year follow-up would require in excess of 10000 patients even in a high-risk population with a rate of second primary breast cancers of approximately 3% per year (e.g., premenopausal women with previous breast cancer). New large trials cannot be justified at present, and preliminary information can be gathered only from a smaller study of surrogate endpoints. Should this be successful, there would be a stronger case to justify a larger trial. Also, the risk of unexpected detrimental effects has recently been highlighted and much emphasis put on the search for intermediate, surrogate endpoints. Surrogate endpoints are biological markers or events that may be assessed or observed prior to the clinical appearance of the disease, and that bear some relationship to the development of that disease. They are referred to as intermediate since they occur some time between a given intervention affecting the disease process and the time of the clinical diagnosis of the disease. The use of surrogate endpoint biomarkers in pivotal cancer chemoprevention trials may lead to a rational choice of agents which are likely to affect cancer incidence in subsequent phase III trials. In the study of surrogate endpoints, our group focused on insulin-like growth factors and on mammographic density.

The insulin-like growth factor (IGF) family of structurally related ligands (including IGF-I, IGF-II, and insulin at supraphysiological concentrations) and their receptors and binding proteins are important for normal human growth and development, and are involved in the specialized functions of most physiologic systems. While the major role of insulin is to control metabolic homeostasis, the IGF system plays a pivotal permissive role in cell proliferation of both epithelial and mesenchymal tissues in at least three different ways: (1) it is highly mitogenic; (2) it protects normal and tumor cells from apoptosis, as shown by both in vitro and in vivo studies; and (3) it is required by several types of cells for the establishment and maintenance of the transformed phenotype and for tumorigenesis.

Importantly, higher plasma IGF-I levels have recently been associated with a four-fold higher risk of premenopausal breast cancer. Unlike with other hormonal factors, there is wide variability between subjects in IGF-I levels. Thus, this biomarker appears a significant candidate for an intermediate endpoint (Baserga 1995; Pollack and Hankinson 1998).

Since tamoxifen and fenretinide decrease plasma IGF-I levels (Pollack et al. 1990; Torrisi et al. 1993), IGF-I is likely to be extensively studied as a surrogate endpoint biomarker in breast cancer prevention trials.

Current Experience with Chemopreventive Agents

Two agents are currently being tested as breast cancer preventive agents in phase III trials, namely tamoxifen and the synthetic retinoid N-4-(hydroxyphenyl)retinamide (fenretinide or 4-HPR).

Tamoxifen

Experimental studies on the possibility of pharmacological cancer-prevention with tamoxifen (Jordan et al. 1991; Maltoni et al. 1988) and the clinical results relating to adjuvant tamoxifen in breast cancer patients over the past years (Cancer Research Campaign Breast Cancer Trials Group 1992; Fisher et al. 1989) have emphasized that tamoxifen is currently the drug which best meets the requirements of efficacy and tolerability in potentially preventing breast cancer. Myocardial infarction and bone fractures are less frequent in tamoxifen-treated women, showing a beneficial effect on bone density and in the prevention of cardiovascular illnesses through the use of this drug (Costantino et al. 1997; Powles et al. 1996).

Such observations have led researchers to consider tamoxifen as a possible agent to prevent or delay the development of breast cancer and to increase the control of cardiovascular diseases and osteoporosis in postmenopausal women. Based on the reduction of contralateral breast cancer observed in the meta-analysis of adjuvant studies, tamoxifen's preventive efficacy is being assessed in three large intervention studies, including the ongoing Italian trial on hysterectomized women which had recruited 5408 women as of December 31, 1997. In these three randomized, double-blind, placebo-controlled trials (UK, USA, Italy), breast cancer chemoprevention with tamoxifen represents a major effort involving the participation of more than 20000 healthy women so far, who committed themselves to taking a placebo or 20 mg/day of tamoxifen for 5 years. While the UK and US studies include high-risk subjects, in the Italian study only hysterectomized, non-high-risk women are randomized, age being the only risk factor for breast cancer in the Italian cohort (Veronesi 1995).

The major end-point of the Italian trial is the reduction of breast cancer incidence. Secondary endpoints are the effects on bone metabolism and related fractures, those on the cardiovascular system and thromboembolic events, and treatment toxicity. Since approximately 20% of all women in the trial are undergoing hormone replacement therapy (HRT), the trial will also test the joint effect of tamoxifen and HRT, a combined treatment which may potentially minimize their adverse effects (e.g., the increase of breast cancer associated with HRT, the vasomotor and urogenital symptoms given by tamoxifen).

The major concern remains the increased risk of endometrial cancer associated with tamoxifen administration. Indeed, the NSABP B-14 trial on 2661 women with stage I breast cancer who received tamoxifen for 5 years as adjuvant treatment has shown respectively a seven-fold and a two-fold increased risk of contracting endometrial cancer compared to the risk of subjects on placebo and to population-based rates (Fisher et al. 1994).

One possible way to minimize the risk might be the addition of an anti-proliferative or differentiating agent (Friedman et al. 1994). Interestingly, the inhibitory effect of 4-HPR observed on the IGF-I system both in vitro and in vivo (Torrisi et al. 1993) might be a mechanism counteracting the critical effect played by IGF-I on tamoxifen-induced endometrial carcinogenesis.

Moreover, there is good evidence that the risk of endometrial cancer induced by tamoxifen is both time- and dose-dependent, the higher relative risk being observed with daily doses of 40 or 30 mg/day of tamoxifen (Rutqvist et al. 1995). This dose-response relationship is likely to reflect an interaction between a tamoxifen genotoxic effect and its estrogen agonistic effect (Jordan 1995; Stearns and Gelmann 1998). Thus, another plausible way to lower the risk is a reduction of the dose.

For this reason we have recently tested the effect of three doses of tamoxifen on the change in estrogen receptor-regulated biomarkers – known to reflect tamoxifen biological activity including total cholesterol as the primary endpoint. A comparable potency of a lower dose of tamoxifen would provide strong support for the assessment of the preventive efficacy and safety of low dose tamoxifen in a larger trial. After adjustment for baseline values, there were no significant changes in subjects' total cholesterol among the three doses (Table 1). A similar pattern was observed also for LDL-cholesterol (Fig. 1) and on IGF-I levels (data not shown). Interestingly, the higher the baseline, the greater was the reduction in total cholesterol levels during tamoxifen, without any difference among doses; no effect was observed in the placebo group.

In conclusion, the conventional 20 mg/day dose seems to exceed the dose required for a full biological activity of tamoxifen. As modulation of several biomarkers through tamoxifen and similar compounds is mostly related to the binding of the estrogen receptor, the equivalent activity of the lower doses might also reflect an equivalent potency against breast cancer formation (Coezy et al. 1982). Thus, the equivalent biological activity of 5 mg/day tamoxifen provides strong support for the assessment of the efficacy and toxicity of low doses of tamoxifen in both the preventive and the therapeutic setting.

Table 1. Changes in subjects' total cholesterol levels after 2 months of treatment with tamoxifen at different dosages (mean and 95% CI)[a]

Variable	Placebo (n = 26)	Tamoxifen 5 mg (n = 27)	Tamoxifen 10 mg (n = 23)	Tamoxifen 20 mg (n = 27)	p for baseline by treatment interaction
Total cholesterol (mg/dl)	3.4 (−7.2 , 14.0)	−27.8 (−38.2 , −17.3)	−25.3 (−36.5 , −14.1)	−15.3 (−25.3 , −5.3)	0.01

[a] Levels are expressed as least square means.

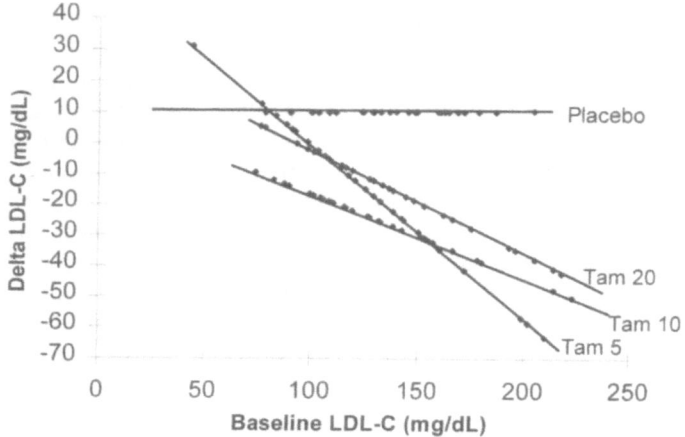

Fig. 1. Effects of 2 months of tamoxifen treatment on the change in LDL-cholesterol according to baseline values. The interaction term between treatment (each tamoxifen dose versus placebo) and baseline value on the change in LDL-cholesterol level has borderline significance ($p=0.08$). Lines represent the estimated change in LDL-cholesterol in each group (respectively receiving tamoxifen 5 mg/day, 10 mg/day, or 20 mg/ day)

The Synthetic Retinoid 4-HPR

Natural retinoids play a crucial role in cellular proliferation and differentiation, but their poor clinical tolerability prevented the use of these compounds as cancer preventive agents (Sporn and Newton 1979). One of the less toxic vitamin A analogs studied for breast cancer chemoprevention is fenretinide or 4-HPR, a synthetic amide derivative of all-trans retinoic acid (Costa et al. 1994). The inhibition of chemically induced mammary carcinoma in rats with 4-HPR was first described by Moon et al. (1979). A phase I–II study led to the identification of 200 mg/day administration with a monthly 3-day interruption as the best tolerated schedule to allow partial retinol recovery and storage in the retina (Costa et al. 1989). In contrast to retinoic acid, it was demonstrated that blood 4-HPR levels remain constant during administration for as long as 5 years (Formelli et al. 1993), that the drug selectively accumulates in the human breast (Metha et al. 1991), and, finally, that a significant decline of plasma retinol levels is responsible for the increased rod thresholds occurring in a certain proportion of subjects (Decensi et al. 1994). Although 4-HPR was synthesized nearly 20 years ago, its mechanism of action has only recently been partially elucidated. This retinoid appears to be the prototype of a new class of selective ligands of retinoic acid receptors (Fanjul et al. 1994). Its selective binding to nuclear receptors is likely to be the basis of its specific biological activities and its favorable pharmaceutical properties. In recent years, 4-HPR has been shown to be active in vitro and in vivo against mammary, bladder, lung, ovary, cervix, neuroblastoma, leukemia, and prostate preclinical models (Lotan 1995).

On the basis of the selective accumulation of 4-HPR in the human breast (Metha et al. 1991) and its good tolerability in humans (Costa et al. 1989), we started a phase III trial aimed at reducing contralateral breast cancer in 1987. Overall, 2 972 women with a history of stage I breast cancer were randomized to receive 4-HPR or no intervention for 5 years. The primary endpoint of the study was the occurrence of contralateral breast cancer as the first malignant event. The eligible women were diagnosed with stage I invasive breast cancer or DCIS within the previous 10 years and underwent definitive surgery without adjuvant chemotherapy. These women were randomized to receive 200 mg/day 4-HPR vs no intervention. The limitations of toxicity evaluation without a placebo group were realized, but having a placebo group was considered disadvantageous due to the long duration of intervention, the large size of the placebo capsule, and the likelihood that non-specific effects of an intervention are generally early events. The women are followed with a complete medical examination and blood tests every 6 months, a mammogram and chest-X ray every year, and a bone scan every 18 months.

An exploratory analysis of the study was performed after a median of 75 months or two-thirds of the person-years of total follow-up (Decensi et al. 1997). The analysis shows a reduction in contralateral breast cancer in premenopausal women who received 4-HPR: the risk of contralateral breast cancer was reduced by approximately 40% (of borderline statistical significance). In contrast, a nonsignificant trend to an increase in contralateral tumours was observed in postmenopausal women. Interestingly, a similar pattern was observed in the change in circulating IGF-I in a subset of 78 consecutive women from the phase III trial.

The joint effect of menopausal status, treatment, and their interaction on the change in IGF-I is reported in Table 2. The data indicate the occurrence of a qualitative interaction between treatment and menopausal status, i.e., both variables modify each other's effect on Δ IGF-I with a cross-over pattern (Fig. 2). This effect was more evident when menopause was replaced by age either as a continuous or a categorical predictor ($p = 0.008$ or $p = 0.03$ for the interaction term, respectively). Specifically, the IGF-I levels in untreated controls declined with age as expected. In contrast, a reverse effect is observed during fenretinide (4-HPR) treatment.

Table 2. Effect of treatment and menopause on Δ IGF-I (1 year-baseline) (ng/ml)[a]

	Premenopause	Postmenopause ≤7 years	Postmenopause >7 years
4-HPR group	-24 ± 39 ($n = 13$)	-16 ± 22 ($n = 12$)	-6 ± 18 ($n = 14$)
Control group	9 ± 35 ($n = 13$)	1 ± 25 ($n = 14$)	-12 ± 32 ($n = 12$)

[a] Mean ± SD; F-test for the interaction term = 2.77, $p = 0.069$.

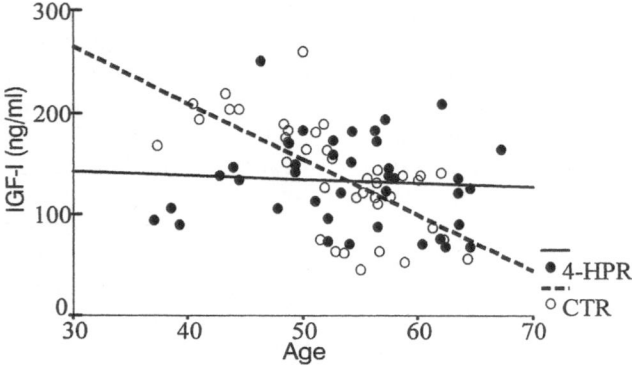

Fig. 2. Effect of fenretinide (4-HPR) as a function of age on plasma IGF-I concentrations measured after 1 year of treatment. Levels of IGF-I are adjusted for baseline values. *CTR* control group

New Compounds

Together with tamoxifen and fenretinide, there is a long list of chemoprevention agents that may be used in breast cancer prevention.

Micronutrients that are considered to have protective potential against breast cancer are vitamin E and selenium (Knekt 1991; Osborne and Telang 1991). Use of nonsteroid anti-inflammatory drugs (such as sulindac), indole-3-carbinol and aromatase inhibitors (such as vorozole) have been reported to be associated with reduced risk of breast cancer (He and Shut 1997; Lubet et al. 1997).

Perhaps more importantly, new drugs are currently under evaluation which mimic the positive effects of estrogens on both bone and cardiovascular system without increasing the cancer risk for breast and uterus: these are the selective estrogen receptor modulators (SERMs). A promising SERM is raloxifene. This drug proved to increase bone mineral density, to lower serum concentrations of total and LDL-cholesterol, and not to stimulate the endometrium (Delmas et al. 1997). Finally, the new SERM LY353381·HCI has been reported to be a potent estrogen antagonist in breast and uterus, an estrogen agonist in bone and cardiovascular tissues, and to be very effective in inhibiting mammary carcinogenesis in rats (Sporn et al. 1997).

Conclusions

Prevention is clearly one of the doors we have to go through in order to arrive to the unfolding and solving of the cancer problem. Today we know much more about the various aspects of the long and complex carcinogenic process leading to that final entity which is breast cancer. Thus, we can try and manipulate some of the events that have an important role along this process.

Something can be already done on a practical basis, e.g., reducing fats in the diet or changing a sedentary lifestyle by increasing physical exercise. A big effort should be put into studying high-risk genes and their applicability in genetic testing and counseling, which is growingly demanded by a currently much more aware population.

Chemoprevention is another important strategy against breast cancer which can and must be implemented, adopting a similar attitude to that which has been employed for a long time with encouraging results by cardiologists in their own field. The efficacy of the chemopreventive approach is based on a remarkably large host of solid data from the last 20 years. Along this line of research, studies on tamoxifen and fenretinide have lately provided encouraging results. Moreover, the combination of these two agents – already demonstrated to be effective in preventing experimental breast cancer – looks quite promising, and a clinical trial is currently underway.

In addition, new selective estrogen receptor modulators (SERMs) with potentially improved safety profiles may become available. Importantly, the recent demonstration that estrogen receptor overexpression in normal breast tissue may increase breast cancer risk (Khan et al. 1998) provides further rationale for the use of SERMs in at-risk subjects, including HRT users.

Summary

Present prospects of breast cancer prevention are being developed in three main areas: (a) genetics, to understand the real importance of familial breast cancer and genetic testing; (b) lifestyle, to study various risk factors, including delayed first pregnancies and smaller number of pregnancies, and months of breast feeding; (c) chemoprevention, to identify chemical agents potentially able to inhibit the development of invasive cancer either by blocking the DNA damage that initiates carcinogenesis or by arresting or reversing the progression of premalignant cells. Different target populations for breast cancer chemoprevention may be recognized. Primary chemoprevention may involve a wide population of healthy women with a moderate risk due to nonpenetrant genetic factors (e.g., one first-degree relative with breast cancer) or exposure to known promoting agents (e.g., hormone replacement therapy). A second level of primary chemoprevention may involve a limited population at very high risk because of highly penetrating genetic predisposition to cancer (e.g., BRCA1 mutation carriers). Secondary chemoprevention may involve subjects with premalignant or early malignant lesions, e.g., breast atypical hyperplasia and carcinoma in situ or microinvasive disease. Prevention trials using clinical endpoints are always subject to high costs. Also, the risk of unexpected detrimental effects has recently been highlighted, and much emphasis has been put on the search for intermediate, surrogate endpoints. Surrogate endpoints are biological markers that may be assessed or observed prior to the clinical appearance of the disease, bearing some relationship to the development of that disease. They are referred to as

Estrogen/Hormone Replacement Therapy and the Etiology of Breast Cancer

K. I. Pritchard

Department of Medical Oncology, Sunnybrook Health Science Center,
Bayview Regional Cancer Center, 2075 Bayview Avenue, Toronto M4N 3M5, Canada

There have been many analyses of the association between the use of estrogen/hormone replacement therapy (ERT/HRT) and the development of breast cancer. Most data are derived from observational studies, however, and although interventional studies are underway, no data from them are as yet available. As ERT/HRT is increasingly studied, some issues are becoming quite clear while others remain more difficult to elucidate. In this paper, the term *estrogen replacement therapy* (ERT) is used to refer to estrogen used alone, while *combined therapy or hormone replacement therapy* (HRT) refers to an estrogen given together with a progestational.

The aims of ERT/HRT for women in the general population relate to relief of short- and long-term symptoms. The short-term symptoms include vasomotor effects and the quality of life changes associated with them, as well as urogenital effects, dyspareunia, frequency, urgency, and stress incontinence. Indeed, these latter effects impinge into the area of long-term symptomatology. The major long-term problems that have been addressed by the use of ERT/HRT, however, remain those of cardiac disease and of osteoporosis. In addition, it is becoming increasingly apparent that ERT/HRT reduces the risk of other diseases such as colon cancer (Calle et al. 1995), and may improve long-term cognitive function (Kawas et al. 1997; Tang et al. 1996; Paganini-Hill and Henderson 1996). While the major subject of this review is the effect of ERT/HRT on the incidence of and mortality from breast cancer, it is impossible to properly consider the role of ERT/HRT in the absence of its other effects.

It has now been clearly demonstrated that ERT/HRT, given either at the time of menopause or later, is associated with a reduction in loss of bone density and a reduction in fracture rates as long as its use is continued. Once discontinued, however, its effects appear to dissipate rapidly with time, so that past users do not show the same benefit from ERT/HRT even if they have previously used it for long periods of time. Important data in this area include a prospective cohort study of 10 000 postmenopausal nonblack women, in which current estrogen use was associated with a relative risk (RR) of 0.30 for wrist fracture, RR of 0.66 for nonspine fractures, and RR of 0.60 for

Khan SA, Rogers MAM, Khurama KK et al (1998) Estrogen receptor expression in benign breast epithelium and breast cancer risk. J Natl Cancer Inst 90:1

Knekt P (1991) Role of vitamin E in the prophylaxis of cancer. Ann Med 23:3–12

Lotan R (1995) Retinoids and apoptosis: implications for cancer chemoprevention and therapy. J Natl Cancer Inst 87:1655–1657

Lubet RA, Bowden C, De Coster R et al (1997) Vorozole: effects on MNU-induced rat mammary tumors. Am Assoc Cancer Res Proc 38:372

Maltoni C, Pinto G, Paladini G (1988) Project of experimental bioassays on chemoprevention agents performed at the Bologna Institute of Oncology; report on tamoxifen control of spontaneous mammary tumours on Sprague-Dawley rats. Cancer Invest 6:643–658

Metha RG, Moon RC, Hawthorne M et al (1991) Distribution of fenretinide in the mammary gland of breast cancer patients. Eur J Cancer 27:138–141

Moon RC, Thompson HJ, Becci PJ et al (1979) N-(4-hydroxyphenyl) retinamide, a new retinoid for prevention of breast cancer in the rat. Cancer Res 39:1339–1346

Osborne MP, Telang NT (1991) Primary prevention of breast cancer. In: Bland KI, Copeland EM (eds) The breast: comprehensive management of benign and malignant diseases. Saunders, Philadelphia, pp 246–261

Pollack M, Hankinson S (1998) Biology of breast cancer risk and prognosis. Eur J Cancer Suppl 1:4

Pollack M, Costantino J, Polychronacos C et al (1990) Effect of tamoxifen on serum insulin-like growth factor I levels in stage I breast cancer patients. J Natl Cancer Inst 82:1693–1697

Powles TJ, Hickish T, Kanis JA et al (1996) Effect of tamoxifen on bone mineral density measured by dual-energy X-ray absorptiometry in healthy premenopausal and postmenopausal women. J Clin Oncol 14:78–84

Prentice R, Thompson D, Clifford C et al (1990) Dietary fat reduction and plasma estradiol concentration in healthy postmenopausal women. J Natl Cancer Inst 82:129–134

Rutqvist LE, Johansson H, Signomklao T et al (1995) Adjuvant tamoxifen therapy for early stage breast cancer and second primary malignancies. J Natl Cancer Inst 87:645–651

Schrag D, Kuntz KM, Garber JE et al (1997) Decision analysis – effects of prophylactic mastectomy and oophorectomy on life expectancy among women with BRCA1 or BRCA2 mutations. N Engl J Med 336:1465–1471

Sporn MB (1991) Carcinogenesis and cancer: different perspectives of the same disease. Cancer Res 51:6215–6218

Sporn MB, Newton DL (1979) Chemoprevention of cancer with retinoids. Fed Proc 38:2528–2534

Sporn MB, Suh N, Peer C et al (1997) LY353381·HCI, a new benzothiophene for chemoprevention of brast cancer. Am Assoc Cancer Res Proc 38:500

Stearns V, Gelmann EP (1998) Does tamoxifen cause cancer in humans? J Clin Oncol 16:719–722

Torrisi R, Pensa F, Orengo MA et al (1993) The synthetic retinoid fenretinide lowers plasma IGF-I levels in breast cancer patients. Cancer Res 53:4769–4771

Veronesi U, for the Italian Tamoxifen Prevention Study (1995) Prevention of breast cancer with tamoxifen: the Italian study in hysterectomized women. Breast 4:267–272

Estrogen/Hormone Replacement Therapy and the Etiology of Breast Cancer

K. I. Pritchard

Department of Medical Oncology, Sunnybrook Health Science Center, Bayview Regional Cancer Center, 2075 Bayview Avenue, Toronto M4N 3M5, Canada

There have been many analyses of the association between the use of estrogen/hormone replacement therapy (ERT/HRT) and the development of breast cancer. Most data are derived from observational studies, however, and although interventional studies are underway, no data from them are as yet available. As ERT/HRT is increasingly studied, some issues are becoming quite clear while others remain more difficult to elucidate. In this paper, the term *estrogen replacement therapy* (ERT) is used to refer to estrogen used alone, while *combined therapy or hormone replacement therapy* (HRT) refers to an estrogen given together with a progestational.

The aims of ERT/HRT for women in the general population relate to relief of short- and long-term symptoms. The short-term symptoms include vasomotor effects and the quality of life changes associated with them, as well as urogenital effects, dyspareunia, frequency, urgency, and stress incontinence. Indeed, these latter effects impinge into the area of long-term symptomatology. The major long-term problems that have been addressed by the use of ERT/HRT, however, remain those of cardiac disease and of osteoporosis. In addition, it is becoming increasingly apparent that ERT/HRT reduces the risk of other diseases such as colon cancer (Calle et al. 1995), and may improve long-term cognitive function (Kawas et al. 1997; Tang et al. 1996; Paganini-Hill and Henderson 1996). While the major subject of this review is the effect of ERT/HRT on the incidence of and mortality from breast cancer, it is impossible to properly consider the role of ERT/HRT in the absence of its other effects.

It has now been clearly demonstrated that ERT/HRT, given either at the time of menopause or later, is associated with a reduction in loss of bone density and a reduction in fracture rates as long as its use is continued. Once discontinued, however, its effects appear to dissipate rapidly with time, so that past users do not show the same benefit from ERT/HRT even if they have previously used it for long periods of time. Important data in this area include a prospective cohort study of 10 000 postmenopausal nonblack women, in which current estrogen use was associated with a relative risk (RR) of 0.30 for wrist fracture, RR of 0.66 for nonspine fractures, and RR of 0.60 for hip fractures. Women who had previously used estrogen showed no benefit even if they had used it for more than 10 years and even if use was begun soon after menopause. This study also showed that the results were similar for ERT versus HRT (combined), for women over or under 75 years of age, for smokers and nonsmokers, and regardless of initial bone mass at the time estrogen was begun (Cauley et al. 1995). Interventional studies of the use of ERT in postmenopausal women have also been carried out. A study, published in the *New England Journal of Medicine* (*NEJM*), showed that estrogen use begun shortly after menopause resulted in a reduction of fractures by 50% (Weiss et al. 1980). Additional studies have now shown that estrogen can be associated with this effect even when it is begun in women with established osteoporosis and a median age of over 65 years (Lufkin et al. 1992). In all studies the effect of ERT/HRT seems confined to current users.

There are now a number of alternatives for the treatment of osteoporosis including the bisphosphonates and the so-called selective estrogen receptor modulators (SERMs). Can they replace ERT/HRT in this setting? A recent report in the *NEJM* showed that in a randomized study comparing (1) placebo, (2) alendronate 2.5 mg, (3) alendronate 5 mg, and (4) HRT, alendronate proved better than placebo, but not quite as good as HRT in preventing the usual bone loss in postmenopausal women which is clearly seen in the placebo arm of this study (Fig. 1). Interestingly, alendronate appeared somewhat more effective in increasing bone mass in the hip (Fig. 2) than in the distal forearm (Fig. 3). In the distal forearm as well, even HRT was able only to maintain bone mass while, in the hip, both doses of alendronate and HRT resulted in increased bone density (Hosking et al. 1998). Raloxifene as well has been shown to prevent and to some degree reverse osteoporosis, but like alendronate is somewhat less effective than ERT in this setting (Delmas et al. 1997).

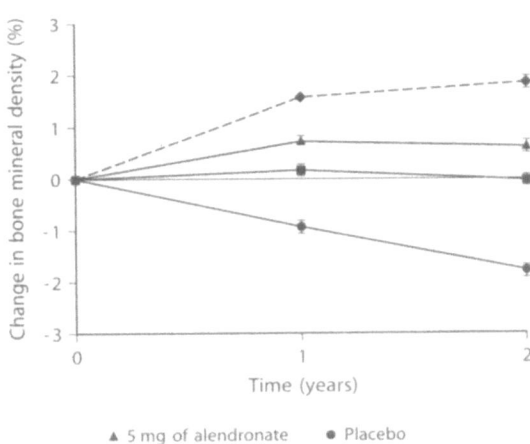

Fig. 1. Percent changes in total body bone density (mean ± SE) in patients in a randomized trial of two different dosages of alendronate versus estrogen-progestin versus placebo

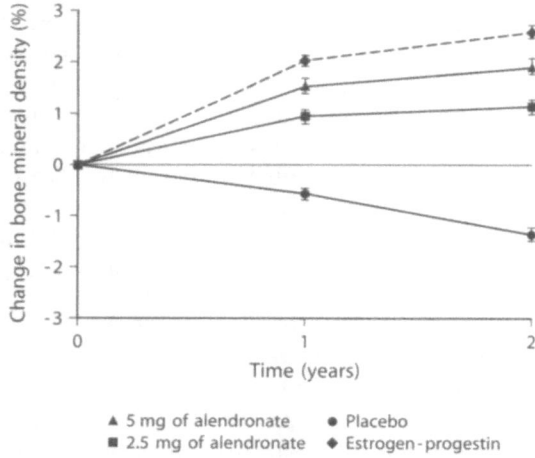

Fig. 2. Percent changes in bone density of the hip (mean ± SE) in patients in a randomized trial of two different dosages of alendronate versus estrogen-progestin versus placebo

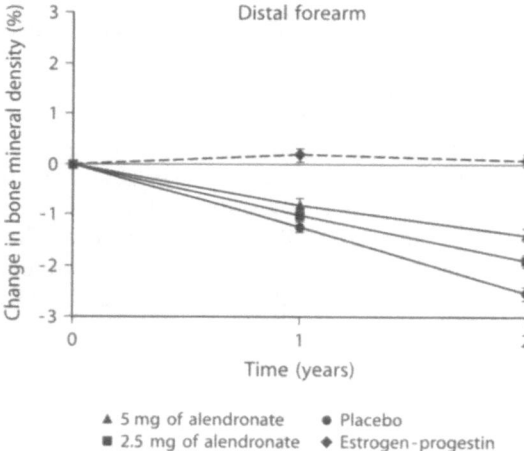

Fig. 3. Percent changes in bone density of the distal forearm (mean ± SE) in patients in a randomized trial of two different dosages of alendronate versus estrogen-progestin versus placebo

There are many studies in the literature suggesting that ERT, and perhaps HRT as well, reduce the risk of cardiac events and of death from cardiac disease in postmenopausal women. A population-based study of postmenopausal women published in the *NEJM* showed that both estrogen and combined therapy increased HDL and decreased LDL in postmenopausal women (Nabulsi et al. 1993). Fibrinogen levels were also decreased by both therapies. Eden and others have shown that the addition of a progestational to estrogen in postmenopausal women tends to lessen the increase in HDL and the decrease in LDL in comparison to estrogen given alone (Eden 1991). In many observational studies, however, combined therapy appears similarly efficacious in preventing cardiac disease to estrogen use alone (Psaty et al. 1994; Falkeborn et al. 1992).

Others have pointed out that estrogen use in postmenopausal women effects not just lipid levels. It is estimated by modeling studies that only about 40% of the beneficial effect of estrogen on cardiovascular outcome may be related to changes in lipid levels. Estrogen also has direct effects on vessel walls, on myocardium, and of course on platelets (Lobo 1991). Thus, drugs such as the various lipid-lowering agents, which presumably act on lipids alone, may not be able to replace ERT/HRT in producing this effect. In addition to studies of lipid levels, there are a variety of population-based case-control studies (Psaty et al. 1994) (Table 1) and prospective cohort studies (Falkeborn et al. 1992) (Table 2) showing that ERT and HRT are associated with a reduced rate of myocardial infarction (MI) (Psaty et al. 1994) and of hospitalization for first MI (Falkeborn et al. 1992).

The only available interventional study of ERT/HRT is the PEPI trial, a five-arm study in which women were randomized to receive for 3 years premarin 0.625 mg daily versus premarin plus progestationals given in three different forms versus placebo (PEPI Trial 1995). Early results of this study have shown that all four of the ERT/HRT preparations increased HDL, decreased LDL, and reduced fibrinogen levels. The most dramatic positive effects were seen with premarin used alone, but the effects of premarin plus a cyclic micronized progestin were not significantly different from those of premarin alone in comparison to placebo. The PEPI trial was not significantly powered to measure actual cardiovascular endpoints.

On the negative side, it is well known that ERT given alone is associated with an increased risk of endometrial cancer. Ever use of estrogen is associated with a relative risk of 2.31, while more than 8 years of use is associated with a relative risk of 8. More than 5-year use of 0.625 mg premarin is associated with a relative risk of 4.8 (Grady et al. 1992a). It is clear from observational studies that the risk of developing endometrial cancer increases

Table 1. Relative risk (RR) of myocardial infarction between 1986 and 1990 in postmenopausal women in a health cooperative (Psaty et al. 1994) (*CI* 95% confidence interval)

	RR	CI
Nonusers	1	1
Estrogen users	0.69	0.47–1.00
Estrogen-progestin users	0.68	0.38–1.22

Table 2. Relative risk of hospital admission for first myocardial infarction in all women in uppsala county, Sweden (Falkeborn et al. 1992)

	RR	CI
Nonusers	1	1
Estrogen users	0.69	0.54–0.86
Estrogen-progestin users	0.53	0.30–0.87

with the dose and duration of estrogen replacement. It is less clear that the mortality from endometrial cancer increases with ERT, but it probably does, although to a lesser degree. It is believed that when progestins are given together with estrogen for at least 12 of the 28 days of the cycle, the risk of increased incidence of endometrial cancer is totally abrogated (Pike et al. 1997; Grady and Ernster 1997). Interestingly, the PEPI trial investigators discontinued the premarin alone arm after the first year because of a 34% incidence of endometrial hyperplasia in comparison to 1% in all of the HRT (combined) arms. In the premarin-alone arm, there was also a 6% incidence of hysterectomy in comparison to a 1% incidence in each of the other arms. No endometrial cancer was found in any study patient.

It has long been appreciated that the development of breast cancer is related to estrogen and to hormonal cycling. A vast body of epidemiologic and animal model data exist to support this hypothesis. Epidemiologic data clearly show that early menarche and late menopause are associated with an increased incidence of breast cancer, while premature ovarian ablation results in a considerable reduction in incidence.

A wide variety of observational studies of the use of ERT/HRT have also been carried out. The results of these are, or at least have been in the past, somewhat less clear. There have been more than 40 case-control and cohort studies and at least six meta-analyses completed in this area, but as yet, interventional studies have not produced mature data. The meta-analyses show that for ever users of ERT/HRT, there is no significant increase in the risk of developing breast cancer in comparison to never users. There is, however, a small but significant increase in risk for current users of ERT/HRT. This has been variously reported at 1.23 [95% confidence intervals (CI) = 1.12 – 1.6] and at 1.40 (95% CI = 1.20 – 1.63) (Colditz et al. 1993; Sillero-Arenas et al. 1992). The increased incidence becomes more clear when one looks at women who are current users and have used ERT/HRT for more than 15 years. Here the relative risk is estimated at 1.30 in two meta-analyses (95% CI = 1.12–1.6 and 95% CI = 1.04–1.14) (Colditz et al. 1993; Steinberg et al. 1991). A more updated meta-analysis shows that women who have taken ERT for more than 20 years have a RR = 1.35. What is somewhat unclear from these data, however, is whether there is a threshold of time after which use of ERT/HRT is associated with an increased risk of breast cancer, or whether indeed there is a steady increase in risk with ERT/HRT which only becomes clearly visible after 10 – 20 years because it is relatively small.

The most recent publication from the Nurses Health Study, once again, reflects the phenomenon of current versus ever use, in which past users of ERT/HRT have no increased risk of developing breast cancer or of dying from it. In current users, however, the authors estimate that 1 year of ERT increases the risk of developing breast cancer by 4%, whereas 1 year of HRT increases the risk by 9%. This study shows that, because of the overall effects on other diseases, in women who have taken ERT for 10 years there is a 20% decrease in the risk of death. After ERT is used for more than 10 years, however, this decrease in the risk of death, while maintained, becomes smaller, in large part because of the increase in incidence of breast cancer and because of an increased mortality from breast cancer. While many other studies have reported an increased incidence of breast cancer in women taking ERT/HRT (at least long-term), the Nurses Health Study is one of the first to report an increased mortality from breast cancer in such women (Grodstein et al. 1997).

There is some reason to believe that, as in endometrial cancer, the risk of developing breast cancer associated with ERT may be higher than the actual risk of dying from it. In breast cancer, possible explanations for this have been suggested by several authors who have shown that breast cancers developing in women on ERT/HRT may be smaller or have a better grade or better differentiation (Harding et al. 1996; Bonnier et al. 1995). Paradoxically, however, it has been suggested that there are also fewer ER+ tumors in this setting (Harding et al. 1996; Bonnier et al. 1995). Overall, the suggestion is that in women who develop breast cancer while on ERT/HRT, mortality may be lower than in women who develop breast cancer while not receiving ERT/HRT. Norlock et al. (1998) have recently shown interesting data suggesting that women developing breast cancer while receiving ERT/HRT have the same proportion of ER+ tumors as do those not receiving ERT/HRT, but that in women with ER+ tumors which developed while they were receiving ERT/HRT, progesterone receptor (PgR) levels are higher and S-phase levels are also higher. It may be that when estrogen is withdrawn from these women, their tumors are controlled, resulting in a better outcome.

With regard to the Nurses Health Study and other observational cohort studies of this type, it seems important to remember that one is still dealing with fairly small relative risks (less than 2) and that any such small relative risks can, in observational studies such as this, be due to bias. That is, it is clear that women who take ERT/HRT are different in many ways from women who do not, and that their underlying risks of developing breast cancer or of dying of it or of other causes may be different.

There is even more controversy about women with a family history of breast cancer. There are few good data concerning the risk of ERT/HRT in this setting. It seems that in most studies the RR is the same for women with and without a family history, so that the proportionate increase in risk would be the same (Colditz et al. 1996). Because these women may be at higher underlying risk, however, the absolute increase in risk may be greater. This is an extrapolation, however, and the direct data that clarify this matter are sparse and controversial (Steinberg et al. 1991, 1994).

There have also been recent data showing that women receiving ERT/HRT have denser mammograms and that there may be more false negatives on mammography than in women not receiving ERT/HRT (Laya et al. 1996). In addition, as mentioned above, the risk of gallbladder disease is increased in women receiving ERT/HRT, but the risk of colon cancer and of cognitive dysfunction may be lower (Calle et al. 1995).

In summary, overall, for the average woman the lifetime mortality risk from breast cancer is about 3.3% if she does not take ERT, and about 4.2% if she does take it. For the same average woman, the lifetime risk of dying of heart disease is 22% if she does not take ERT and 15.7% if she does. Thus, for the average woman, there is a 6.3% reduction in cardiac mortality associated with ERT and a 0.9% increase in breast cancer mortality. Examined in another way, the average woman taking ERT/HRT will have a 1.1 year prolongation in her life overall, while a woman with high cardiovascular risk factors may have a prolongation of about 1.6 years. Grady's projections for the 50-year-old woman with various risk factors are shown in Table 3. She suggests that for women with no risk factors, the increased life expectancy associated with ERT is 0.9 years, while for women with no other risk factor and a hysterectomy, the increase in life expectancy is 1.1 years. For women with cardiac risk factors the increase in life expectancy is 1.6 years, while for women with a high risk of breast cancer, although the increase in life expectancy is only 0.6 years, it is still better with ERT/HRT than without (Grady et al. 1992b).

From all of these data, one can make some definite conclusions and some which are probable or possible. It seems now relatively clearly demonstrated that ERT/HRT is associated with an increased risk of developing breast cancer. It seems equally apparent that, for whatever reason, only current users display this increased risk and that this increased risk becomes much more visible when use has been long-term. In addition, it seems clear that the use of ERT/HRT decreases overall mortality. There is at least one study suggesting that after periods of 10 years or more it also increases breast cancer mortality. In this study, however, ERT/HRT continues to provide overall mortality benefits even after 10 years of use. It also seems that although absolute mortality benefits vary with underlying risk profiles, ERT/HRT provides some overall increase in life expectancy even for a woman with a very high risk of developing breast cancer.

There are suggestions that combined therapy (HRT) is associated with a greater increase than ERT in terms of breast cancer development. It also seems probable that the increased risk seen in long-term users is not a threshold effect, but likely occurs steadily over time and is simply difficult to measure with shorter term use because the effect is relatively small. There is some suggestion at present that women with a family history of breast cancer have a similar RR of developing breast cancer in association with the use of

Table 3. Lifetime probabilities of selected conditions for a 50-year-old woman treated with long-term ERT/HRT (Grady et al. 1992b)

	Lifetime probaility		Odds ratio	
	Incidence (%)	Mortality (%)	ERT	HRT
Heart disease	46	31	0.65	0.80
Stroke	20	8	0.96	0.96
Hip fracture	15	1.5	0.75	0.75
Breast cancer	10	3	1.25	1.25

ERT/HRT; however, if this proportional risk increase is the same, the absolute risk increase for these women will be greater because of their increased underlying risk. It remains to be clearly established (1) what the meaning of the *ever* versus *current use* phenomenon is, (2) whether the risk of ERT/HRT over time is constant or whether there is a threshold risk, and (3) what the role of ERT/HRT is in women with a family history of breast cancer. Now that we better understand the genetics and are using new definitions of family history in breast cancer, we may see that there are more consistent differences in the risks of developing breast cancer in association with ERT/HRT in groups with certain family histories or genes. In addition, there remains a paucity of data concerning the relative roles of combined HRT versus ERT and the risks of developing or dying of breast cancer.

Summary

ERT/HRT is clearly of use in relieving menopausal symptoms such as hot flashes and genitourinary changes. ERT/HRT also clearly reduces the risks of osteoporotic fracture, of cardiovascular events and deaths, and of developing colon cancer. ERT and, perhaps even more, HRT are, however, associated with an increased risk of developing breast cancer. This effect becomes more marked with long-term use (≥ 10 years); ERT/HRT use for more than 10 years is also associated with an increase in deaths from breast cancer. Because the underlying mortality risk for the average woman is, however, much greater from cardiovascular disease ($\sim 22\%$) than from breast cancer ($\sim 3.3\%$), the reduction in risk of cardiovascular death associated with ERT/HRT (from 22% to 15%) much outweighs the increase in risk of death from breast cancer (from 3.3% to 4.1%). Thus, overall, the average woman will gain more year(s) of life than she will lose by taking ERT/HRT. Even for a woman with a high risk of breast cancer and a low risk of cardiovascular disease, there will still be a net, although lower, gain in year(s) of life. Thus, the use of ERT/HRT would seem well worth considering for a well woman at the time of menopause.

References

Bonnier P, Romain S, Giacalone PL (1995) Clinical and biologic prognostic factors in breast cancer diagnosed during postmenopausal hormone replacement therapy. Obstet Gynecol 85:11–17

Calle EE, Miracle-McMahill HL, Thun MJ, Heath CW (1995) Estrogen replacement therapy and risk of fatal colon cancer in a prospective cohort of postmenopausal women. J Natl Cancer Inst 87:517–523

Cauley JA, Seeley DG, Ensrud K, Ettinger B, Black D, Cummings SR (1995) Estrogen replacement therapy and fractures in older women. Ann Inter Med 122:9–16

Colditz GA, Egan KM, Stampfer MJ (1993) Hormone replacement therapy and risk of breast cancer: results from epidemiologic studies. Am J Obstet Gynecol 168:1473–1480

Colditz GA, Rosner B, Speizer FE (1996).Risk factors for breast cancer according to family history of breast cancer. For the Nurses Health Study Research Group. J Natl Cancer Inst 99:365–371

Delmas PD, Bjarnason NH, Mitlak BH, Ravoux AC, Shah AS, Huster, WJ, Draper M, Christiansen C (1997) Effects of raloxifene on bone mineral density, serum cholesterol concentrations, and uterine endometrium in postmenopausal women. N Engl J Med 337:1641–1647

Eden JA (1991) Progestogens: an occasional review. J Obstet Gynecol 17:289–295

Falkeborn M, Persson I, Adami HO, Bergstrom R, Eaker E, Lithell H, Mohsen R, Naessen T (1992) The risk of acute myocardial infarction after estrogen and estrogen-progestogen replacement. Br J Obstet Gynaecol 99:821–828

Grady D, Ernster VL (1997) Hormone replacement therapy and endometrial cancer: are current regimens safe? J Natl Cancer Inst 89:1088–1089

Grady D, Cummings SR, Petitti D, Rubin SM, Audet AM (1992a) Guidelines for counselling postmenopausal women about preventive hormone therapy. Ann Intern Med 117:1038–1041

Grady D, Rubin SM, Petitti DB, Fox CS, Black D, Ettinger B, Ernster VL, Cummings SR (1992b) Hormone therapy to prevent disease and prolong life in postmenopausal women. Ann Intern Med 117:1016–1037

Grodstein F, Stampfer M., Colditz GA, Willett WC, Manson JE, Joffe M, Rosner B, Fuchs C, Hankinson SE, Hunter DJ, Hennekens CH, Speizer FE (1997) Postmenopausal hormone therapy and mortality. N Eng J Med 336:1769–1775

Harding C, Knox WF, Faragher EB (1996) Hormone replacement therapy and tumour grade in breast cancer: prospective study in a screening unit. Br Med J 312:1646–1647

Hosking D, Chilvers CED, Christiansen C, Ravn P, Wasnich R, Ross P, McClung M, Balske A, Thompson D, Daley M, Yates AJ (1998) Prevention of bone loss with alendronate in postmenopausal women under 60 years of age. N Engl J Med 338:485–492

Kawas C, Resnick S, Morrison A, Brookmeyer R, Corrada M, Zonderman A, Bacal C, Lingle DD, Metter E (1997) A prospective study of estrogen replacement therapy and the risk of developing Alzheimer's disease: the Baltimore Longitudinal Study of Aging. Neurology 48:1517–1521

Laya MB, Larson EB, Taplin SH, White E (1996) Effect of estrogen replacement therapy on the specificity and sensitivity of screening mammography. Natl Cancer Inst 88:643–649

Lobo BA (1991) Effects of hormonal replacement on lipids and lipoproteins in postmenopausal women. J Clin Endocrinol Metab 73:925–931

Lufkin EG, Wahner HW, O'Fallon WM, Hodgson SF, Kotowicz MA, Lane AW, Judd HL, Caplan RH, Riggs BL (1992) Treatment of postmenopausal osteoporosis with transdermal estrogen. Ann Intern Med 117:1–9

Nabulsi MB, Folsom AR, White A, Patsch W, Heiss G, Wu KK, Szklo M (1993) Association of hormone-replacement therapy with various cardiovascular risk factors in postmenopausal women. N Engl J Med 328:1069–1075

Norlock FE, Oleske DM, Cobleigh MA (1998) Hormone replacement therapy use correlates with high S-phase in estrogen-receptor-positive primary human breast cancer. Proc Am Soc Clin Oncol 17:109a

Paganini-Hill A, Henderson VW (1996) Estrogen replacement therapy and risk of Alzheimer disease. Arch Intern Med 156:2213–2217

PEPI Trial (1995) Effects of estrogen or estrogen/progestin regimes on heart disease risk factors in postmenopausal women. The Postmenopausal Estrogen/Progestin Interventions (PEPI) trial. JAMA 273:199–208

Pike MC, Peters RK, Cozen W, Probst-Hensch NM (1997) Estrogen-progestin replacement therapy and endometrial cancer. J Natl Cancer Inst 89:1110–1116

Psaty BM, Heckbert SR, Atkins D, Lemaitre R, Koepsell TD, Wahl PW, Siscovick DS, Wagner EH (1994) The risk of myocardial infarction associated with the combined use of estrogen and progestins in postmenopausal women. Arch Intern Med 154:1333–1339

Sillero-Arenas M, Delgado-Rodriguez M, Rodigues-Canteras R, Bueno-Cavanillas A, Galvez-Vargas R (1992) Menopausal hormone replacement therapy and breast cancer: a meta-analysis. Obstet Gynecol 79:286–294

Steinberg KK, Thacker SB, Smith SJ, Stroup DF, Zack MM, Flanders D, Berkelman RL (1991) A meta-analysis of the effect of estrogen replacement therapy on the risk of breast cancer. JAMA 265:1985–1990

Steinberg KK, Smith SJ, Thacker SB, Stroup DF (1994) Breast cancer risk and duration of estrogen use: the role of study design in meta-analysis. Epidemiology 5:415–421

Tang MX, Jacobs D, Stern Y, Marder K, Schofield P, Gurland P, Andrews H, Mayeux R (1996) Effect of estrogen during menopause on risk and age at onset of Alzheimer's disease. Lancet 348:429–432

Weiss NS, Ure CL, Ballard SH, Williams AR, Daling SR (1980) Decreased risk of fractures of the hip and lower forearm with postmenopausal use of estrogen. N Engl J Med 303:1195–1198

II. Genetics of Breast Cancer

Experimental Pathology and Breast Cancer Genetics: New Technologies

P. Osin*, J. Shipley, Y. J. Lu*, T. Crook*, and B. A. Gusterson*

Section of Cell Biology and Experimental Pathology, Institute of Cancer Research, Haddow Laboratories, Sutton, Surrey, SM2 5NG, UK

Introduction

A silent revolution is taking place that has the potential to have an enormous impact on medicine, but it requires a high investment in technology and research before it can be of practical use. The reason for the silence is the high cost of the technology involved, putting it out of the reach of most academic centres. With the realisation that all of the human genes will be known and sequenced in the next few years, the next objective is to harness this information to identify new drug targets, to improve methods of diagnosis and to identify inherited genetic differences that increase the risk of developing particular diseases (Karp and Broder 1995). This will also facilitate analysis of the interaction of environmental factors and genetics. The way is being led by biotechnology and pharmaceutical companies and the larger institutes such as the National Cancer Institute (NCI). At the NCI, part of Klausner's strategic planning was to establish the 'genome anatomy project' (see website http://inhouse.ncbi.nlm.nih.gov/ncicgap/). Such strategic planning was anathema to many scientists, but it must be the way forward in some areas of science where number crunching is the order of the day. Even though most doctors are not aware of the future applications, investors are clamouring to have a slice of the action, as indicated by a recent issue of *Business Week* that was devoted entirely to 'The Biotech Century'. For academics wishing to be involved there is the difficulty that alone they cannot afford the capital costs, while by collaborating with industry it is difficult to get a deal that enables the information gained to go directly into the public domain. The NCI initiative is very important, as everything is being released over their website, including detailed protocols, and most of the current technology is being directed at diagnosing mutations in known genes or looking at mRNAs that are expressed in different disease states to obtain a profile or 'index' of the tissue or tumour involved (Brown and Hartwell 1998). The limitations are related to sensitivity and representation of the RNAs isolated from small numbers of cells where an amplifica-

---

* *Current address:* Institute of Cancer Research, The Breakthrough Toby Robins Breast Cancer Research Centre, 237 Fulham Road, London, SW3 6JB, UK

tion procedure is required. In addition, RNA levels do not directly relate to protein expression, and studies of RNA will not identify mutations or subtle changes in proteins that may be of more importance, such as phosphorylation and glycosylation. Many companies in the last 2 years have therefore started to direct their attention to expression profiling at the protein level, and if the difficulties of sensitivity can be overcome, this may prove to be the best way forward for some applications (Strachan et al. 1997).

Whilst these developments are taking place, there are simpler ways that are already available to study tumours, including screening for loss of heterozygosity, mutation analysis, comparative genomic hybridisation and spectral karyotyping. The future is very exciting, but the explosion of data for any particular tumour would indicate that there will be a need to invest in as many people analysing the data as those generating it, especially if we are hoping to be able to identify which combination of expressed genes are markers of the elements of tumour progression.

Molecular Diversity in Breast Cancer

Cancer arises through an accumulation of specific mutations which alter the phenotype and proliferation of cells. Cytogenetics and molecular analysis have revealed an array of aberrations and genes which can be implicated in a proportion of breast cancer cases. When considering breast cancer there are clear situations where there is a family history of predisposition. This is seen classically in BRCA1 and BRCA2 carriers, which are the most common, but other predisposition genes such as the ATM gene in ataxia-telangiectasia and the *p53* gene in Li-Fraumeni syndrome are other examples. What is becoming clear is that there is variable penetrance of the genes, and thus in the case of BRCA1 and BRCA2 there may be different risks depending upon the specific mutations involved and the effects of other potentially modifying genes. In addition, there is very good evidence to suggest that there are other genes involved, which are part of the 'normal' polymorphic diversity of gene structure in the population. If we consider breast cancer in general, the risk of contralateral breast cancer in a woman with breast cancer is higher than the risk of breast cancer in an unaffected individual. This is particularly true in the case of lobular carcinoma in situ, where the risk of multifocality and bilaterality is as high as 60%. If bilateral breast cancer and multifocal disease is common, the explanations are either field changes due to a systemic carcinogenic insult or an inherited predisposition. If we assume that these 'predisposition' genes are of variable penetrance, it would be possible to propose that all breast cancers are due to predisposition genes that have variable effects but act to predispose the normal breast epithelium to environmental carcinogens and to DNA damage. It is also to be predicted that these predisposing genes act through disturbances of DNA repair mechanisms or indirectly affect the ability of the cell to undergo DNA repair through disturbance of the G1/S checkpoint.

We have to explain the key effect of estrogen and the protective effect of estrogen withdrawal in premenopausal women. The likely explanation is that the majority of the key carcinogens are only active on dividing cells, and by withdrawing the estrogen drive the number of target cells is reduced; this is also the explanation of the association of increased breast cancer risk with the other endocrine risk factors. Once there is a second hit in a DNA repair defect gene or in a mutation molecule such as *p53*, which predisposes to genomic instability, the stage is set for rapid accumulation of genetic change which is manifest as mutations, loss of heterozygosity and gene amplification. As there are many molecules involved in abnormal proliferation, loss of cell-cell contact, loss of cell-matrix contact, motility and invasion, it is not surprising that tumours have such immense diversity, since the majority of genes that are mutated are random hits (Kerangueven et al. 1997). In the case of BRCA1 there is evidence that mutations in this gene are associated with *p53* mutations (Crook et al. 1997), and some tissues seem to be more prone to certain genetic changes, but many are common to the majority of tumours.

The initial event that 'predisposes' the breast cell to the secondary changes may well be a predetermining event for subsequent change. Thus, in lobular carcinomas there is a higher incidence of microsatellite instability (Aldaz et al. 1995) and absence of *p53* mutations or c-erbB-2 amplification (Fisher et al. 1996). This contrasts with ductal carcinoma in situ (DCIS), where there is a high incidence of *p53* mutation and c-erbB-2 amplification (Steeg et al. 1996).

Two recent observations were made that may be critical to our understanding of breast cancer. Firstly in familial gastric cancer there is an E-cadherin mutation in the germline (Guildford et al. 1998). This indicates that in some cases the predisposing gene is one which is generally considered to be mutated late in tumour progression. When looking at comedo DCIS it is clear that cytologically the tumour cells have all the appearances of a highly aggressive lesion. At the loss of heterozygosity level they are indistinguishable from invasive carcinomas. This raises the distinct possibility that these in situ components already have the genotype of a metastatic tumour. Future studies of DCIS will be critical in testing this hypothesis once markers are available for those proteins that are necessary for the invasive and metastatic process. It is to be hoped that this possibility is disproved, as future diagnosis will be increasingly on the basis of fine-needle aspiration cytology where it is essential that DCIS and invasive cancer can be distinguished prior to neoadjuvant chemotherapy.

Another critical observation was the recent publication by Cahill et al. (1998) on mutations in mitotic checkpoint genes that can lead to chromosomal instability and aneuploidy. It would be of interest to see if in the breast there is a reciprocal relationship between those tumours with microsatellite instability and mismatch repair defects (possibly lobular carcinomas) and those with aneuploidy and possible chromosomal instability through mutations in mitotic checkpoint genes (possibly DCIS). Both would result in genetic instability.

The identification of genetic events characteristic for different stages of the carcinogenesis could have implications for new approaches to the diagnosis, prevention and treatment of breast cancer, but how will we define these events and relate them to the particular stages of tumour progression? The use of in vitro and in vivo assays to detect individual mutations and proteins involved in invasion and angiogenesis is the well-trodden path, but it is becoming clear that it is not one molecule, but the combination of a number of molecules working in concert that are responsible for the malignant phenotype (Gusterson 1993). Thus, although five to eight events may be critical, many other changes assist the progression of the tumour.

The discovery and cloning of breast cancer-predisposing genes BRCA1 and BRCA2 enables identification of an individual carrying a susceptibility gene with confidence before the onset of the disease. Direct mutation analysis can not only confirm the mutation, but also reveal a predisposition to the development of a specific tumour, by site and type of mutation. The mutation in the so-called ovarian cancer cluster region in BRCA2 gene has a higher affinity to the development of ovarian cancer, whilst mutations outside this region predispose to breast cancer (Gauther et al. 1997). A mutation analysis by sequencing is a labour-intensive process and very expensive (currently over US$2000 for BRCA1 and BRCA2). Rapid and cheaper throughput assays are being developed using microarray technology.

The molecular genetic profile of the tumour has prognostic value, but more importantly it can be used to predict tumour behaviour and response to therapy. Thus, cancers with *p53* gene mutation have been shown to have a worse prognosis and are resistant to DNA-damaging chemotherapeutic agents. It is essential that in the future we can profile all the abnormalities in a tumour and know their functional significance. This is a long way off, but it is the aim for the future. By profiling tumours and checking their profile against clinical follow-up in large clinical trials we will be able to identify the key combinations responsible for the clinical phenotype.

Modern Technology

Recent advances in technology mean that small numbers of cells can be screened for alterations in genes and changes of expression of RNAs in ways not previously possible.

Laser Microdissection

Modern methods of molecular biology enable genetic changes to be identified in single cells from fresh, frozen or paraffin-embedded tissue. It is important that the cells are collected in a way that prevents contamination by other cell types and without contact with RNA- and DNA-degrading enzymes. The microdissected tissues, from in situ disease for example, can be used for a number of purposes including the production of cDNA libraries that will have representation of all of the RNA species in a particular cell type or in a lesion. Similarly, protein or DNA can be extracted for analysis. Laser capture microdissection (LCM) enables the removal of cells in a field as small as 30 μm in diameter. A transparent film is placed upon a tissue section on a slide. A pathologist selects a sector containing cells appropriate for the study and activates the laser. The laser beam causes adhesion of tissue within the chosen field to the film. The cells removed with the film are suitable for molecular studies. The tissue can be either paraffin-embedded or frozen and the section can be stained with a standard histochemical or immunocytochemical stain. It is important to emphasise that the laser energy is absorbed by the film and does not damage either nucleic acid or protein, so LCM-produced material could be used for practically any molecular study (Emmert-Buck et al. 1996). The limitation is the amount and the quality of the RNA available. Thus, libraries are PCR-based and it is difficult to obtain libraries that represent the quantitative values of the individual species in the starting material. In addition, the size of the RNA under optimal conditions is only 1 KB and thus separate libraries from optimally collected tissues have to be made for full-length cDNA clones. Details on LCM and its application can be found under the Human Genome Anatomy Project on the NCI website (http://www.nci.nih.gov).

Comparative Genomic Hybridisation and FISH

Fluorescence in situ hybridisation (FISH) has been extensively used in the past decade as a way of studying chromosomal abnormalities. Recently, through the production of chromosome-specific paints labelled with a combination of fluorochromes and false colour representation, it has been possible to identify complex chromosome abnormalities using the technique of spectral karyotyping (Veldman et al. 1997).

The approach of comparative genomic hybridisation (CGH) will screen the whole genome for gains, losses and amplification of genomic material. CGH was originally described using high molecular weight DNA from cell lines and fresh material (James et al. 1997). Combining this approach with the PCR using degenerate oligonucleotide primers (DOP-PCR), sufficient representative DNA can be generated to enable analysis of archival material and small regions of specimens in a way not previously possible (Telenius et al. 1992). The DNA produced and normal reference DNA are differentially labelled with fluorochromes and hybridised to normal metaphase chromosomes under suppression conditions with unlabelled Cot1 DNA. A fluorescence ratio outside the normal range at a particular chromosome location is indicative of a copy number change in that region. The major advantage of CGH is the possibility of a whole genome screen in one experiment. During the last 5 years more than 1500 tumours have been studied using CGH (http://nhgri.nih.gov/DIR/LCG/CGH).

Applications of CGH in Research and Practice

Creating a Database of the Genetic Profile Characteristic of Different Tumours

An analysis of large series of histologically identical tumours enables the identification of non-random genomic changes. For example: 91% of breast tumours have genomic abnormalities in one of three chromosomal regions: gains 1 q, 8 q, loss of 13 q (Tirkkonen et al. 1998). These data could be used in search and identification of novel oncogenes (gains, amplifications) and tumour suppressor genes (losses of chromosomal material) (Chen et al. 1996 b; Courjal and Theiller 1997). Investigating a genomic profile of familial tumour syndromes would be very helpful in the search of hereditary cancer predisposition genes.

Models of Tumour Progression and Evolution

Comparison of patterns of chromosomal copy number changes in tumours in different stages of progression (in situ and invasive, original tumour and metastasis) provides information about the genetic relationship between these groups (James et al. 1997). Also, the location of genes involved in different steps of tumour progression (invasiveness, metastasising) may be identified. Using CGH on microdissected glands (Fig. 1) we have recently shown that the genetic profile of lobular carcinoma in situ and atypical lobular hyperplasia suggests that these lesions represent a single entity (Osin et al. 1998). A difference in genomic changes characteristic for in situ and invasive carcinomas of breast both lobular and ductal type has also been demonstrated (Kuukasjärvi et al. 1997; Nishizaki et al. 1997). These data will facilitate our understanding of the relationship between intra-epithelial lesions in the breast and their malignant potential.

Possible Clinical Use of CGH

Creation of a genomic profile database could have significant diagnostic applications. However, use of traditional CGH methods in routine tumour diagnostics is limited because of the length of the procedure. Nevertheless, CGH could be of great value in identifying the origin of histologically unclassifiable tumours and revealing their relationship to known entities. Combining CGH data with follow-up studies and clinical trial information could associate patterns of genomic changes with different clinical outcome. These data might be very helpful in predicting the prognosis of an individual patient and choosing the most effective therapies. The main limitation with CGH is its inability to reveal reciprocal translocations. The resolution of CGH is poor, with the region of chromosome copy number change generally being limited to 5–10 Mb. These restrictions force CGH to be used in combination with other methods such as multicolor chromosome painting strategies (M-FISH), spectral karyotyping and loss of heterozygosity.

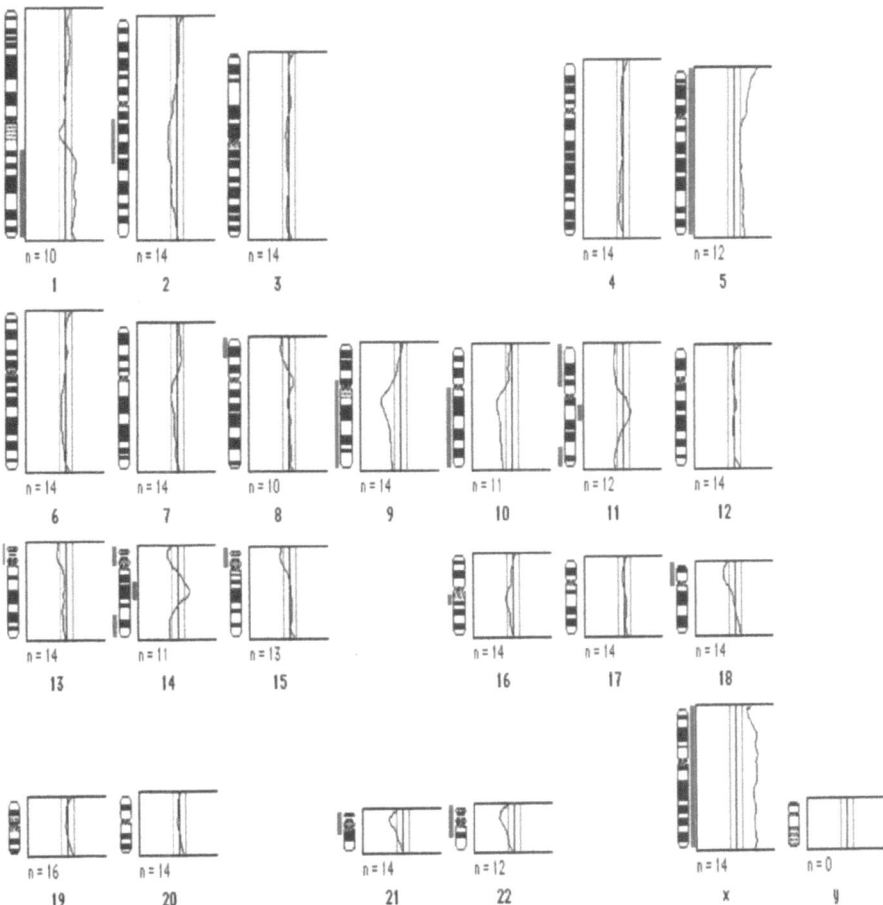

Fig. 1. Example of CGH analysis of microdissected paraffin-embedded lobular carcinoma in situ of the breast. The figure shows a profile of the average red-to-green fluorescence ratios from analysis of seven metaphase spreads. A ratio outside the limits of 0.2 smaller or greater than 1 indicated by the *red* and *green* vertical lines, respectively, is indicative of a copy number change. The heterochromatic regions adjacent to the centromeres are not informative. Gain of material from chromosome 1,5,11,14 and X and loss of regions from chromosomes 2,8,9,10,11,14 and 18 is indicated by this analysis. *Note:* Computer profile shows *gains* in *green* and *loss* in *red*

Loss of Heterozygosity

CGH is a powerful method for elucidation of chromosomal imbalance in a whole genome, despite its poor resolution. Loss of heterozygosity (LOH) analysis is a method based on PCR using oligonucleotide repeats from genomic regions of interest as primers. The products of PCR are analysed by electrophoresis in polyacrylamide gels. Reduction from two bands in normal tissue from an individual to one in the tumour sample suggests that the corresponding part of the chromosome has been lost during oncogenesis. The phenomenon of LOH is related to the mechanism of inactivation of tumour suppressor genes, when one allele is aberrant in the germline or somatically, usually by point mutation or small deletion. Loss of the second allele during oncogenesis in most cases involves loss of a large part of the chromosome, thus producing homozygous loss. Identification of areas of LOH will suggest a possible location of novel genes involved in the evolution of cancer. LOH data for breast cancer indicate non-random loss at 1p, 1q, 3p, 6q, 8p, 11p, 15q, 16q, 17p and 18q. Detection of similar areas of LOH in high-grade DCIS and invasive ductal carcinoma suggests that they have a common genetic background [1, 6]. Recent studies of LOH in pre-invasive breast lesions have demonstrated the clonal character of lobular carcinoma in situ, atypical ductal hyperplasia and also some forms of ductal hyperplasia without atypia (Lakhani et al. 1995 a,b, 1996; Nayar et al. 1997). Consistent areas of LOH in these lesions indicate the possible presence of genes involved in the earliest stages of breast cancer development.

Advantages of LOH assessment are increased resolution (compared with CGH) and speed. The limitation of LOH is the availability of suitable markers and the dependence on large amounts of DNA; from microdissected lesions only a few markers (4–6) can be studied, making a genome-wide search in individual lesions impossible. More recently, the application of DOP-PCR technique to LOH analysis has been shown to generate sufficient DNA for using more markers without loss of accuracy (Chen et al. 1996 a).

Array and 'Chip' Technology

The building of a complete molecular profile (index) of normal cells and of cells in different stages of tumour progression will require a comprehensive database of all the genomic, RNA and protein expression changes that define each normal cell type and the changes that occur in malignant progression. Once that has been achieved it will be possible to look for the clinical correlations of these changes to define new diagnostics and therapeutic targets. This is an enormous task and will require considerable input into relational databases to analyse the many thousands of pieces of information that will come from the analyses of an individual cell.

Methods are being developed that can be considered as 'open' or 'closed', but they all depend on the ability to array either cDNA or oligonucleotides on glass slides, filters or microchips at high density (Marshall and Hodgson 1998; Schafer and Hawkins 1998). In an open system the objective is to identify new genes that are expressed, so a cDNA library from a tissue is gridded out and is then interrogated using RNA extracted from two different tissues, for example normal versus tumour. A good example of this is seen in the work of Trent in the identification of genes involved in tumour progression (De Risi et al. 1996). The 'closed' systems are where arrays are produced of the full sequence of a specific gene such as BRCA1 to identify point mutations in a patient's DNA sample or the gridding of ESTs from known genes. Such an array can then be interrogated with the extracted RNA from a tissue or cell to assess which of the genes are expressed in a particular situation (e.g., before and after hormonal stimulation). The size of the arrays can be from a few spots to many thousands depending upon the question. It may be seen that the method can be used for sequencing and for CGH, where instead of hybridising to normal chromosomes, contigs can be gridded out on arrays representing individual chromosomes and the arrays analysed for areas of loss and gain at high resolution. The methods of analyses are all based on the basic principles of hybridisation and the probes used can be labelled with fluorochromes or radioactivity depending upon the detection system to be used. For example, cloned cDNAs are robotically printed upon a glass slide or oligonucleotides are synthesised in situ on microchips using the principles of photolithography employed in the semiconductor field. The technology allows hundreds of thousands of individual spots to be put discretely in a 1-cm^2 array. cDNA probes are generated after extraction of mRNA from cells that need to be compared (normal and tumour, in situ and invasive, tumour and metastasis, etc.). The probes are differentially fluorescently labelled and hybridised onto cDNA or oligonucleotide arrays. The image is produced by a fluorescent laser system and digital images are computer-analysed. The different fluorescent intensities give quantitative information regarding the relative prevalence of respective cDNA sequences in the sample. The obvious advantage of microarrays is their availability for an automation, simultaneous hybridisation, separate detection of the fluorescent signal and data analysis. Mass production of microarrays keeps cost relatively low.

The exploration of consistent changes in gene expression will have implications for diagnosis and treatment. The expression patterns of genes with known function could be compared in different physiological and pathological conditions (Strachan et al. 1997). The profile of genes with unrevealed function could suggest their possible biological role. Theoretically, with rapid progress of human genome mapping, an expression of most genes in a biological sample could be performed as a single procedure. The effort therefore has to be made to reveal consistent genetic changes that are characteristic of certain stages of tumour progression so as to allow these data to be used in microarray for diagnostic purposes and prognostic assessment.

The first practical applications are likely to be in the fields of diagnostic tests for mutations in susceptibility genes such as BRCA1 (Hacia et al. 1996) and mutations in *p53* as an indicator of resistance to some forms of chemotherapy. Outside the cancer field the opportunities in diagnostics are even more obvious, with the possibility of identifying population polymorphisms that will indicate susceptibility to a range of conditions. A field that will also see immediate application is microbiology, where a single 'chip' could be envisaged that will screen any body fluid for all known pathogens and their antibiotic sensitivity.

Proteomics

Another approach is to investigate proteins within cells directly, for example by high-resolution two-dimensional gel electrophoresis (2-DE). Until recently the use of 2-DE has been restricted by difficulties in the recognition of gel-resolved protein spots and the absence of readily accessed 2-DE databases. Progress in biotechnology and information systems has resolved these problems almost completely and greatly facilitated the capabilities of 2-DE. A combined approach of computer-assisted 2-DE gel analysis, protein N-terminal microsequencing technology and mass spectrometry enables rapid and reliable quantification, assessment of protein patterns and direct sequencing of 2-DE-resolved proteins. The 2-DE-resolved proteins are electrotransferred onto an inert immobilizing matrix. The proteins are then fragmented by proteolysis or extracted by detergent and the peptides generated are separated by reversed phase high performance liquid chromatography (RP-HPLC).

The mass spectrometric estimation of molecular weight of defined peptides is a useful method for protein fingerprinting. A website containing comprehensive updated 2-DE databases for different normal and tumour tissues will allow easy access to the information, leading to unification of the methods and building of a general human protein index (http://www.ludwig.edu.au/www/jpsl/jpslhome.htl 1).

Recently, protein expression has been analysed in different human breast epithelial cell lines. Differential expression of different proteins including cytokeratins has been found to be differentially expressed in different subsets of both normal and malignant cells (Franzen et al. 1997; Rasmussen et al. 1997). This is a good proof of the principle, but the major problem at present is the limited sensitivity of the technique. A major advantage of the 2-DE approach is that differences in the phosphorylation and glycosylation of proteins can be identified, and thus it should be possible to study signalling pathways activated by ligands. Building of complete databases of protein expression in normal tissues and in different tumours is undoubtedly of great significance. Firstly, this database could be used for confirmation of the proposed function of the studied gene. Also, evaluation of abnormalities in protein expression would be useful for diagnostic and screening purposes, especially in cases of tumour-specific proteins. For example, abnormal fusion proteins produced through translocations would be easily identified as abnormal protein products. A further advantage of analysing protein over RNA is that the protein is directly related to function, whereas differences in RNA are not directly correlated with protein levels and are thus poor surrogates of gene function.

Phage Libraries for Antibody Production

Possible clinical applications of tumour-associated antibodies include diagnostics (including biomarkers), imaging and therapeutic purposes. Not only tumour cells, but also tumour vasculature may be a possible target for antibody therapy (Folkman 1971). The antibody can act as an antitumour agent itself due to its direct cytotoxic effect, or can initiate complement-mediated cell lysis. Monoclonal antibodies have been shown to be beneficial in adjuvant therapy of colorectal cancer. An affinity to tumour antigens enables antibodies to be used as a delivery system, and use of radiolabelled antibodies has had promising results in the therapy of radiosensitive tumours. Antibody-directed enzyme prodrug therapy (ADEPT) is based on selective delivery of a specific antibody-enzyme complex to the surface of tumour cells. The enzyme converts a harmless prodrug into a toxic product at the site of activation. Finally, antibodies could be useful in resolving one of the main problems in gene therapy-targeted gene delivery.

The effectiveness of antibody therapy is dependent on antibody specificity, ability to penetrate and affinity (antigen-binding capacity). Modern methods facilitate the identification of antibody-based molecules with preferable features (Chester et al. 1994). Technology using phage libraries is a relatively new method of antibody production. The antibody-variable region genes are amplified from the cDNA of B cells using PCR with specific primers. The amplified fragments are cloned into a phage that displays the gene product on its surface. The complexity of these libraries has now reached 10^{11}, which enables the selection of high specificity and affinity characteristics. The library is used to 'pan' against the antigen or tissue of interest, and thus in principle a complete epitope map of a molecule could be obtained. The problem of obtaining many antibodies to dominant epitopes still remains, as with conventional techniques, but in theory the antibodies can be produced in a few weeks. The library-selected phage can be amplified in bacteria to produce practically unlimited amounts of antibodies. In addition to its clinical applications, this technology has applications in the identification of new biomarkers.

Future Perspectives

It is a reasonable prediction that in 10 years' time all of the genes in the genome will have been identified together with the more common mutations associated with cancer. The translation of this information into benefits for patients will not be immediate, but it will produce the building blocks for future prevention, diagnosis and new therapies.

Summary

The goal is to understand the critical events in tumour development and to apply this understanding to new approaches to diagnosis, prevention and treatment. It is clear that breast cancer is a heterogeneous disease at the molecular level, raising the possibility of a future functional classification based on mechanisms rather than morphology. These molecular phenotypes will also confer predictive value on the potential of the tumour to invade, metastasise and respond to or resist new therapeutic strategies. Studies of the genome in individuals are predicted also to enable the identification of polymorphisms that are associated with increased susceptibility to environmental factors, in addition to possibly explaining de novo variations in responses to drugs and radiation. The difficulty is how to identify which, of the approximately 30000 genes expressed by a typical cancer cell alone or in combination, are the ones involved in these processes. The majority of breast cancers have such a multitude of molecular changes that it is difficult to distinguish between those that are critical to tumour progression and those that are epiphenomena of genetic instability and abnormalities in DNA repair. The identification of the earliest events in carcinogenesis must be the best hope, as it will then be possible to target the events that predispose to other secondary changes before they occur. Genomics and proteomics is the current hope to take us forward. This involves the application of a number of new technologies to facilitate the profiling of individual tumours, including laser-guided microdissection of microscopic lesions, comparative genomic hybridisation and loss of heterozygosity analysis of DNA using microarray technology to study DNA and expressed RNAs and protein profiling using 2D gel mass spectroscopy. With over 100000 mRNAs and proteins to examine in complex tissues and in various combinations, there is obviously going to be a requirement for a large investment in computing power (bioinformatics) to facilitate the analysis of these data in relation to the clinical characteristics of the individual tumour and the patient.

Acknowledgements. We would like to acknowledge support from the US Army, grant DAMD17-94-J-4066. Dr. P. Osin is supported by the Gilbert Fellowship through the Friends of the Hebrew University and Dr. Y.-J. Lu is supported by BreakThrough Breast Cancer.

References

Ahmadian M, Wistuba II, Fong KM, Behrens C, Kodagoda DR, Saboorian MH, Shay J, Tomlinson GE, Blum J, Minna JD, Gazdar AF (1997) Analysis of the FHIT gene and FRA3B region in sporadic breast cancer, preneoplastic lesions, and familial breast cancer probands. Cancer Res 57:3664–3668

Aldaz CM, Chen T, Sahin A, Cunningham D, Bondy M (1995) Comparative allelotype of in situ and invasive human breast cancer: high frequency of microsatellite instability in lobular breast carcinomas. Cancer Res 55:3976–3981

Brown PO, Hartwell L (1998) Genomics and human disease – variations on variation. Nat Genet 18:91–93

Cahill DP, Lengauer C, Yu J, Riggins GJ, Willison JKV, Markowitz SD, Kinzler KW, Vogelstein B (1998) Mutations of mitotic checkpoint genes in human cancers. Nature 392:300–303

Chen T, Dhingra K, Sahin A, Sneige N, Hortobagyi G, Aldaz CM (1996a) Technical approach for the study of the genetic evolution of breast cancer from paraffin-embedded tissue sections. Breast Cancer Res Treat 39:177–185

Chen T, Sahin A, Aldaz CM (1996b) Deletion map of chromosome 16q in ductal carcinoma in situ of the breast: refining a putative tumor suppressor gene region. Cancer Res 56:5605–5609

Chester KA, Begent RHJ, Robson L, Keep P, Pedley RB, Boden JA, Boxer G, Green A, Winter G, Cochet O, Hawkins RE (1994) Phage libraries for generation of clinically useful antibodies. Lancet 343:455–456

Courjal F, Theiller C (1997) Comparative genomic hybridization analysis of breast tumors with predetermined profiles of DNA amplification. Cancer Res 57:4368-4377

Crook T, Crossland S, Crompton MR, Osin P, Gusterson BA (1997) P53 mutations in BRCA1-associated familial breast cancer. Lancet 350:638–639

De Risi J, Penland L, Brown PO, Bittner ML, Meltzer PS, Ray M, Chen Y, Su YA, Trent JM (1996) Use of a cDNA microarray to analyse gene expression patterns in human cancer. Nat Genet 14:457–460

Emmert-Buck MR, Bonner RF, Smith PD, Chuaqui RF, Zhuang Z, Goldstein SR, Weiss RA, Liotta LA (1996) Laser capture microdissection. Science 274:998–1001

Franzen B, Linder S, Alaya AA, Eriksson E, Fujioka K, Bergman AC, Jornvall H, Auer G (1997) Analysis of polypeptide expression in benign and malignant human breast lesions. Electrophoresis 18(3/4):582–587

Folkman J (1971) Tumour angiogenesis: therapeutic implications. N Engl J Med 285:1182–1186

Fisher ER, Constantino J, Fisher B, Palekar AS, Paik SM, Suarez CM, Wolmark N, for the National Surgical Adjuvant Breast and Bowel Collaborating Investigators (1996) Pathologic findings from the National Surgical Adjuvant Breast Project (NSABP) protocol B-17. Five-year observations concerning lobular carcinoma in situ. Cancer 78:1403–1416

Gauther SA, Mangion J, Russel P, Seal S, Barfoot R, Ponder BA, Stratto M, Easton D (1997) Variation of risk of breast and ovarian cancer associated with germline mutations of the BRCA2 gene. Nat Genet 15:103–105

Guildford P, Hopkins J, Harraway J, McLeod M, McLeod N, Harawira P, Taite H, Scoular R, Miller A, Reeve AE (1998) E-cadherin germline mutations in familial gastric cancer. Nature 392:402–405

Gusterson BA (1993) The role of the pathologist in dissecting the biology of breast cancer with special reference to in situ disease. Eur J Cancer 2:51–58

Hacia JG, Brody LC, Chee MS, Fodor SPA, Collins FS (1996) Detection of the heterozygous mutations in BRCA1 using high density oligonucleotide arrays and two-colour fluorescence analysis. Nat Genet 14:441–456

James LA, Mitchell ELD, Menasce L, Varley JM (1997) Comparative genomic hybridisation of ductal carcinoma in situ of the breast: identification of regions of DNA amplification and deletion in common with invasive breast cancer. Oncogene 14:1059–1065

Kallioniemi A, Pekka O, Piper J, Tanner M, Stokke T, Chen L, Smith HS, Pinkel D, Gray JW, Waldman F (1994) Detection and mapping of amplified DNA sequences in breast cancer by comparative genomic hybridization. Proc Natl Acad Sci USA 91:2156–2160

Karp JE, Broder S (1995) Molecular foundations of cancer: new targets for intervention. Nat Med 1:309–320

Kerangueven F, Noguchi T, Coulier F, Allione F, Wargniez V, Simony-Lafontaine J, Longy M, Jacquemier J, Sobol H, Eisinger F, Birnbaum D (1997) Genome-wide search for loss of heterozygosity shows extensive genetic diversity of human breast carcinomas. Cancer Res 57:5469–5474

Kuukasjärvi T, Tanner M, Pennanen S, Karhu R, Kallioniemi OP, Isola J (1997) Genetic changes in intraductal breast cancer detected by comparative genomic hybridization. Am J Pathol 150:1465–1471

Lakhani SR, Collins N, Sloane JP, Stratton MR (1995 a) Loss of heterozygosity in lobular carcinoma in situ of the breast. J Clin Pathol 48:M74–M78

Lakhani SR, Collins N, Stratton MR, Sloane JP (1995 b) Atypical ductal hyperplasia of the breast: clonal proliferation with loss of heterozygosity on chromosomes 16q and 17p. J Clin Pathol 48:611–615

Lakhani SR, Slack DN, Hamoudi RA, Collins N, Stratton MR, Sloane JP (1996) Detection of allelic imbalance indicates that a proportion of mammary hyperplasia of usual type are clonal, neoplastic proliferations. Lab Invest 74:1–7

Marshall A, Hodgson J (1998) DNA chips: an array of possibilities. Nat Biotechnol 16:27–31

Nayar R, Zhuang Z, Merino MJ, Silverberg SG (1997) Loss of heterozygosity on chromosome 11q13 in lobular lesions of the breast using tissue microdissection and polymerase chain reaction. Hum Pathol 28:277–282

Nishizaki T, Chew K, Chu L, Isola J, Kallioniemi A, Wedner N, Waldman FM (1997) Genetic alterations in lobular breast cancer by comparative genomic hybridization. Int J Cancer 74:513–517

Osin P, Lu YJ, Lakhani S, Pilotti S, Gusterson BA, Shipley J (1998) Gains and losses of genomic material in atypical lobular hyperplasia (ALH) and lobular carcinoma in situ (LCIS) of the breast suggest these lesions represent a similar stage of tumour progression. J Pathol Suppl 184:15a

Rasmussen RK, Ji H, Eddes JS, Moritz RL, Reid GE, Simpson RJ, Dorow DS (1997) Two-dimensional electrophoretic analysis of human breast carcinoma proteins: mapping of proteins that bind to the SH3 domain of mixed lineage kinase MLK2. Electrophoresis 18:588–598

Schafer AJ, Hawkins JR (1998) DNA variation and the future of human genetics. Nat Biotechnol 16:33–39

Steeg PS, Clare SE, Lawrence JA, Zhou Q (1996) Molecular analysis of premalignant and carcinoma in situ lesions of the human breast. Am J Pathol 149:733–738

Strachan T, Abitol M, Davidson D, Beckmann JS (1997) A new dimension for the human genome project: towards comprehensive expression maps. Nat Genet 16:126–132

Telenius H, Carter NP, Bebb CE, Nordenskjold M, Ponder BA, Tunnacliffe A (1992) Degenerate oligonucleotide-primed PCR: general amplification of target DNA by a single degenerate primer. Genomics 13:718–725

Tirkkonen M, Tanner M, Kahru R, Kallionemi A, Isola J, Kallionemi OP (1998) Molecular cytogenetics of primary breast cancer by CGH. Genes Chromosomes Cancer 21:177–184

Veldman T, Vignon C, Schröck E, Rowley JD, Ried T (1997) Hidden chromosome abnormalities in haematological malignancies detected by multicolour spectral karyotyping. Nat Genet 15:406–410

Update on Breast Cancer Susceptibility Genes*

B. L. Weber

University of Pennsylvania School of Medicine, Department of Hematology-
Oncology, 1009 Stellar-Chance Laboratories, Philadelphia, PA 19104–6100, USA

Introduction

Approximately 7% of breast cancer and 10% of ovarian cancer in the United
States is thought to be due to the presence of an autosomal dominant susceptibility allele. Two breast cancer susceptibility genes (BRCA1 and BRCA2)
now have been identified (Miki et al. 1994; Wooster et al. 1995; Tavtigian et
al. 1996) and a third (BRCA3) is being actively sought. Breast cancer susceptibility in families with mutations in these genes appears as an autosomal
dominant trait, with breast cancer affecting as many as half of the women in
each generation. Thus, both of these genes are considered high penetrance
genes, as the majority of individuals with these alterations will ultimately develop breast cancer. Mutations in several other high penetrance genes, such
as *p53* (associated with Li-Fraumeni syndrome) and MSH2 (associated with
hereditary non-polyposis colon cancer) also have been identified as causes of
hereditary breast cancer, but are extremely rare in the general population. It
is very likely that many other genes contribute to inherited breast cancer susceptibility in families where the incidence of breast cancer is elevated, but
where the appearance of breast cancer is more scattered, because fewer numbers of carriers will develop breast cancer as a result of these lower penetrance genes. These genetic alterations are complex and what little is known
about candidates for low penetrance cancer susceptibility genes is not yet of
clinical use.

The isolation and study of BRCA1 and BRCA2 (Miki et al. 1994; Hall et al.
1990) have greatly expanded our knowledge of inherited breast cancer. Utilizing direct mutation screening, recent epidemiological studies are providing
increasingly accurate estimates of the fraction of hereditary breast cancer attributable to germline mutations in BRCA1 and BRCA2. These studies also
calculate the penetrance – the disease risk – of inherited mutations more accurately than could be accomplished prior to the isolation of the genes. At
the same time, functional studies are beginning to identify several mecha-

---

* Adapted from Blackwood MA, Weber BL (1998) Breast cancer genetics: past, present and
  future. J Clin Oncol, in press

nisms of cellular growth control with which the breast cancer susceptibility genes interact. Finally, families and individuals can be accurately classified using genetic testing, facilitating studies of tumor type and outcome.

How Much Breast Cancer is Due to BRCA1 and BRCA2?

Early studies estimated that 90% of breast-ovarian cancer families – those with four or more cases of early onset breast cancer and at least one case of ovarian cancer – were linked to the BRCA1 locus. Forty-five percent of site-specific breast cancer families – those characterized by the occurrence of breast cancer alone – were linked to 17q21 (Easton et al. 1993). The second breast cancer susceptibility gene, BRCA2, was linked to chromosome 13 in 1994 (Wooster et al. 1994) and isolated in 1995 (Wooster et al. 1995). Early estimates suggested that BRCA2 might be responsible for 25%–30% of site-specific breast cancer. However, data derived from linkage studies tend to overestimate the true fraction of hereditary breast cancer due to mutations in BRCA1 and BRCA2, as has been shown by more recent studies performed on families that may not be suitable for linkage analysis, but who are more typical of the spectrum of breast cancer families seen by practicing physicians. These studies suggest that BRCA1 mutations account for only 10%–20% of inherited breast cancer, with BRCA2 mutations probably responsible for about half this fraction of families. However, as many as 45% of families with both breast and ovarian cancer may carry BRCA1 mutations (Serova et al. 1997; Shattuck-Eidens et al. 1998; Couch et al. 1997).

Several groups have begun work on models using individual and familial factors to predict the probability of finding germline mutations in BRCA1 (Shattuck-Eidens et al. 1998; Couch et al. 1997; Berry et al. 1997). These studies, despite methodological differences, have identified several factors which predict for increased likelihood of finding a BRCA1 mutation in an individual. These traits include ovarian cancer, particularly in an individual with both breast and ovarian cancer in the family, an early age at breast cancer diagnosis, and Ashkenazi Jewish ancestry (because of the increased mutation frequency in this population). These models, and others under development, were all designed to help guide clinicians in identifying those patients in whom BRCA1 and BRCA2 mutation testing is most likely to be informative.

Do All BRCA1 and BRCA2 Mutation Carriers Develop Cancer?

As noted above, the penetrance of BRCA1 and BRCA2 mutations is high, but like estimates of the contribution of BRCA1 and BRCA2 to inherited breast cancer, the early estimates may be exaggerated due to the peculiarities of the families commonly used for genetic research studies. Female mutation carriers were initially estimated to have an 87% lifetime risk of developing breast cancer and a 40%–60% lifetime risk of developing ovarian cancer (Easton et al. 1994). The cumulative risk of developing a second breast cancer was estimated to be 65% for affected mutation carriers who lived to age 70 (Easton et al. 1994; Ford et al. 1994). The risk profile of BRCA2 was thought to be similar, but with a lower risk of ovarian cancer. Initially, linkage studies estimated the lifetime breast cancer risk to BRCA2 mutation carriers to be 85%, and the lifetime ovarian cancer risk to be 10%–20%.

More recent estimates from a population-based study of ovarian cancer suggest a penetrance of 70%–75% for breast cancer and 25%–30% for ovarian cancer. Using a similar approach, Streuwing and colleagues have recently addressed the question of the penetrance of three common BRCA1 and BRCA2 mutations in a large population-based study of Ashkenazi Jews, suggesting that the estimated lifetime breast cancer risk to carriers of any of the three mutations is 56%, with an ovarian cancer risk of 16.5% (Streuwing et al. 1997). Of additional interest, this study did not support previous suggestions that the location of a mutation within the gene was associated with the variations in the degree of risk for ovarian cancer.

Probable reasons for the discrepancy between recent data and the earlier linkage studies include that: (1) only the most severely affected families were used for linkage studies; (2) even the most sensitive mutation detection techniques fail to identify mutations which do not fall within the region of the gene that encodes the BRCA1 and BRCA2 protein products (estimated to account for over 10%–20% mutations) but linkage analysis will detect these families; and (3) lower sensitivity mutation screening techniques for coding region mutations have been used, again missing families that will be detected by linkage analysis.

Are There Clinical Differences Between Inherited and Sporadic Breast Cancer?

It is well known that inherited breast cancer does have distinctive clinical features – age at onset is considerably younger than in sporadic cases, the prevalence of bilateral breast cancer is higher, and the presence of associated tumors in affected individuals is noted in some families. BRCA1-associated tumors include ovarian, colon, and prostate cancer (Ford et al. 1994), and BRCA2-related tumors include male breast cancer and possibly others (Wooster et al. 1994). The isolation of BRCA1 and BRCA2 now allows careful distinction between inherited and sporadic cancers, and work is ongoing to define the clinical characteristics of related tumors, as these findings will have important implications for the surveillance, diagnosis, and treatment of breast cancer in mutation carriers.

In order to determine whether breast tumors that arise as a result of BRCA1 mutations have clinical and pathologic characteristics that differ from those of sporadic tumors (i.e., those that arise in the absence of a cancer susceptibility gene mutation), two groups have analyzed tumors from breast cancer families. Working prior to the availability of direct mutation testing, Page and colleagues found that, compared to other hereditary breast cancers, breast cancers in women with a high likelihood of carrying BRCA1 mutations are more likely to be aneuploid and to have a high S-phase fraction. This study also suggested that tubular and lobular cancers may be infrequently associated with BRCA1 mutations and more commonly found in BRCA2 mutation carriers (Marcus et al. 1996). Paradoxically, disease-free survival was longer in the women thought likely to carry germline BRCA1 mutations than in matched controls, but this finding remains to be confirmed. A similar finding of improved survival as compared to matched controls has been reported in association with BRCA1-related ovarian cancer (Rubin et al. 1996). Subsequent studies have supported the finding of an increased frequency of high-grade tumors in women with germline BRCA1 mutations (Lakahani et al. 1998; Eisinger et al. 1996), but no other studies included survival data. It also has been suggested that BRCA1 mutations involving the terminal domains, which may have specific functions in inhibiting the cell cycle including protein binding (amino terminus) and transcriptional activation (carboxy terminus), may be associated with more highly proliferative tumors than mutations in other regions of the gene. Taken together, these studies suggest that BRCA1-associated tumors of the breast and ovary are frequently of high grade. The possibility that survival from BRCA1-associated tumors is better than that from sporadic tumors of similar grade remains to be proven, but recent data suggesting that BRCA1- and BRCA2-associated tumors may have increased sensitivity to radiation and to certain chemotherapeutic agents could support this possibility.

BRCA1 and BRCA2 Are Tumor Suppressor Genes

BRCA1 and BRCA2 are thought to be classic tumor suppressor genes, not oncogenes, for several reasons. First, mutations which render BRCA1 and BRCA2 nonfunctional or absent are associated with tumor development, whereas oncogenes are modified in cancer cells in a way that increases, or deregulates, their normal function. Second, approximately half of breast and ovarian tumors from mutation carriers show loss of the normal copy of BRCA1 or BRCA2, leaving behind only the copy of the gene which contains the inherited mutation (Matsushima et al. 1995). Finally, while functional data on BRCA2 are not yet available, several experiments have been done that strengthen the claim that BRCA1 functions as a tumor suppressor. However, recent data linking BRCA1 and BRCA2 to DNA damage repair pathways suggests that at least some of the tumor-suppressive effect of these genes may be due to their ability to assist in the recognition and repair of damaged DNA in addition to direct modulation of cell cycle progression.

BRCA1 and BRCA2 Mutation Spectrum

BRCA1 is a very large gene, making the possible number of mutations enormous and the technical aspects of finding them daunting. Since the identification of BRCA1 in 1994, more than 300 sequence variants have been detected. These variants are distributed along the entire coding region of the gene, and over 50% of them have been identified only once. This means that in most settings, a BRCA1 mutation test must evaluate the entire coding region of the gene. Most mutations described so far generate stop codons, truncating the protein, but others result from mutations in the signals that allow proper splicing of the mRNA, or from single base substitutions that destroy a functional region of the protein.

Controversy exists over whether the location of a mutation within BRCA1 plays a role in the clinical appearance of the family or individual. Two studies (Holt et al. 1996; Gayther et al. 1995) suggested that mutations in the 5′ half of BRCA1 predispose to both breast and ovarian cancer, while mutations closer to the 3′ portion of the gene are predominantly associated with only breast cancer. However, several recent and larger studies have failed to reproduce this finding. As noted previously, it has also been suggested that mutations occurring in the terminal regions of BRCA1 may be associated with a more severe phenotype, as defined by high breast tumor grade (Sobol et al. 1996).

Somewhat surprisingly, all breast cancer-related BRCA1 mutations identified to date are germline mutations (Matsushima et al. 1995), meaning they are present in all cells in the body, including egg or sperm, and therefore can be passed on to the next generation. Acquired mutations – those that occur in a single cell after birth – are not passed on unless that cell happens to be a sperm or egg, but may give rise to cell clones that become cancerous. Acquired (somatic) BRCA1 mutations have not been described in human breast cancers, and only rarely are found in human ovarian cancers (Merajver et al. 1995; Hosking et al. 1995; Takahashi et al. 1995). This finding has led to speculation that BRCA1 may not be an important component of the development of most breast and ovarian cancers, yet it is possible that the function of BRCA1 may be disrupted in other ways in sporadic (noninherited) breast cancer.

BRCA2 is almost twice as large as BRCA1, and thus is even more complex to fully screen for mutations. More than 100 BRCA2 mutations already have been described (Wooster et al. 1995; Tavtigian et al. 1996; Couch et al. 1996; Neuhausen et al. 1996a; Phelan et al. 1996; Lancaster 1996; Miki et al. 1996; Teng et al. 1996; Takahashi et al. 1996), and several similarities with the mutation spectrum of BRCA1 are apparent. First, BRCA2 mutations span the entire coding region of the gene. Second, most mutations reported to date result in premature termination of the protein product. Finally, few mutations have been identified in the BRCA2 gene in sporadic breast or ovarian cancers. These data suggest that, as is the case for BRCA1, BRCA2 mutation testing requires evaluation of the full coding region of the gene. Present BRCA2 mutation testing techniques also fail to identify noncoding mutations, thus false negative mutation test results occur and test results must be interpreted in the context of the predicted probability of finding a mutation.

A few common mutations have been identified in BRCA1 and BRCA2, particularly in specific subpopulations. 185delAG and 5382insC in BRCA1 and the 6174delT in BRCA2 have been identified as common mutations in the Ashkenazi (Eastern European) Jewish population, with a combined frequency of these mutations estimated at 2.0%–2.5% (Tonin et al. 1995, 1996; Streuwing et al. 1995a; Roa et al. 1996). This is strikingly increased compared to the overall mutation frequency in an unselected Caucasian population of about 1 in 1000. This phenomenon is most likely to occur in populations that have historically been geographically or politically isolated from surrounding populations, where reproduction occurs solely within the group. An additional factor is the absence of selection bias before childbearing age, so that most mutation carriers would be expected to reproduce before succumbing to breast or ovarian cancer. The common ancestry of a mutation may be demonstrated by genetic techniques (haplotyping), revealing, in this case, a founder effect in the Ashkenazi Jewish population (Neuhausen et al. 1996b; Berman et al. 1996). Using haplotying, it is estimated that the 185delAG mutation in BRCA1 entered the Eastern European Jewish population in a single individual (the founder) in approximately the twelfth century, and has been propagated throughout that population to the present (Neuhausen et al. 1996). The high frequency of BRCA1 and BRCA2 mutations in this population has a significant impact on clinical estimates of the probability of finding a mutation in certain individuals – recent reports have taken this into consideration and generated separate models for Ashkenazi Jewish families (Couch et al. 1997). One additional consideration that arises when population frequencies are high is the likelihood of finding more than one mutation segregating independently in a family. Several groups have reported individuals who carry mutations in both BRCA1 and BRCA2, and these individuals have relatives that may have either mutation or neither of them. These findings underscore the importance of full pedigree evaluation, of mutation testing for both genes in families with bilineal cancer histories, and the need to evaluate all Ashkenazi Jewish individuals for all three common mutations, even when one of the three mutations has been identified in another family member. Finally, as the effect of population genetics is apparent in the Jewish population, it is important to bear in mind that virtually all of the mutation estimates derive from Caucasians of Northern European ancestry and may not be applicable to African-Americans, Asians, Hispanics or other population groups with differing genetic backgrounds.

In the setting of clinical testing, two categories of mutation test results may be difficult to interpret. First, single base pair changes – missense mutations – do not always result in an altered function of a gene's protein product. Thus missense mutations not located within critical functional domains, or those that make only minimal changes in the surrounding protein structure, are not likely to be disease-associated. For this reason, determination of the functional significance of newly identified missense mutations outside of the RING finger of BRCA1 requires clear correlation with disease status in multiple affected families and individuals. Second, negative test results, particularly from an affected member of a family with a high predicted probability of carrying a breast cancer susceptibility gene mutation, may be difficult to interpret. In interpreting these results, it is important to remember that all routinely available tests fail to identify a minimum of 10% of mutations in both BRCA1 and BRCA2 that occur in non-coding regions, resulting in a false negative test result.

Recommendations for Women with Inherited Susceptibility to Breast Cancer

At present, there is both uncertainty and controversy about management strategies for women in inherited susceptibility to breast cancer. It is not known whether increased surveillance will reduce breast cancer-related mortality in high-risk women. Furthermore, women from high-risk breast cancer families are well aware that mammography and clinical breast exam may not detect premalignant lesions. In the face of a striking family history and close personal losses, these women may be unconvinced that mammography and clinical breast exam offers them the protection they seek. Such women often inquire about prophylactic mastectomy in the absence of other preventive options. While it seems logical that removal of as much "at-risk" tissue as possible will reduce the likelihood of developing a malignancy, there are few data demonstrating the efficacy of prophylactic mastectomy in this setting. Furthermore, there are theoretical considerations calling into question the rationale for prophylactic surgery, as current surgical technique does not allow the complete removal of all breast tissue in prophylactic total mastectomy. Since a germline mutation will be present in all residual breast tissue, individuals may remain at increased risk following surgery. Similarly, prophylactic oophorectomy does not guarantee protection from ovarian carcinoma since tumors may arise spontaneously in the peritoneum. Estimates of the frequency of peritoneal carcinoma in high-risk women range from 2% to 25% (Streuwing et al. 1995b; Piver et al. 1993). Speculation remains over whether these peritoneal malignancies represent metastases from ovarian cancer unrecognized at the time of oophorectomy or whether they are primary lesions arising in the face of a field defect (germline mutations in this instance). The latter possibility seems likely as the cell of origin of epithelial ovarian cancer is the single cell layer of the peritoneal reflection that covers the ovary, not the stromal or germ cell elements of the ovary. Prospective studies with a well-defined population of BRCA1 and BRCA2 mutation carriers are needed to delineate the protective effect of both prophylactic mastectomy and oophorectomy. These uncertainties make it difficult to counsel individuals about the potential benefits of these procedures. Nonetheless, the anxiety faced by women who harbor mutations in a breast cancer susceptibility gene can be overwhelming. Women must be presented with available data and allowed to make decisions which reflect their own needs but do not offer a false sense of security.

Current screening recommendations for women who opt not to undergo prophylactic mastectomy include clinical breast exam and mammography every 6–12 months beginning between age 25 and 35 for women at increased risk of breast cancer determined by direct or indirect molecular demonstration of a breast cancer-related genetic mutation (Hoskins et al. 1995). Although no data exist to determine whether increased frequency of clinical examination and screening mammography in this population reduces mortality, there are preliminary data that BRCA1-related tumors may have a faster growth rate than sporadic tumors (Lakahani et al. 1998). In addition, patient anxiety may be allayed somewhat by offering the option of two mammograms per year. Prophylactic mastectomy may be an option for interested women, who should be provided with information regarding the lack of evidence for *or* against risk reduction by this procedure.

In women with a documented BRCA1 mutation, prophylactic oophorectomy at the completion of child-bearing or at the time of menopause is recommended by the American College of Obstetrics and Gynecology, as no ovarian cancer screening program has been demonstrated to increase the rate of diagnosis of early-stage disease. However, as noted, there is a low but measurable incidence of peritoneal malignancies following oophorectomy which may derive from peritoneal cells which are at similar risk for malignant transformation and are not removed by oophorectomy. It may be prudent for women at increased risk of breast cancer to avoid the use of exogenous estrogens when possible, as no data exist regarding the effect of estrogens on the penetrance of breast cancer susceptibility genes. However, a dilemma arises in that there may be some benefit to taking oral contraceptives to reduce ovarian cancer risk, and that heart disease and osteoporosis are more prevalent in women who do not use estrogen replacement therapy after menopause.

Clinical Implications and Directions for Future Research

While proven preventive interventions specific to the hereditary breast cancer population are still not available, several important clinical questions are currently being investigated. Because of the high rate of second primary breast tumors in BRCA1 and BRCA2 mutation carriers, and because of uncertainty with regard to radiation risks in this population, the appropriateness of breast-conserving therapy in known mutation carriers is being evaluated. Data need to be developed with respect to appropriate breast cancer screening schedules for mutation carriers, and information about the effectiveness of ovarian cancer screening, generally not thought to be effective, will need to be obtained in these mutation carriers. Prophylactic surgery is also controversial, and both families and physicians raise questions about the effectiveness of this aggressive approach in mutation carriers. Although the degree of risk reduction resulting from prophylactic surgery is not presently known, both retrospective and long-term follow-up studies of mutation carriers are underway to address these questions. More specific information about disease penetrance will be an important element in both the development of screening protocols and the evaluation of prophylactic surgical interventions. Finally, additional information about the mechanisms of BRCA1 action is needed in order to identify specific preventive and/or therapeutic strategies. While early BRCA1 gene therapy trials have not yielded significant responses, further definition of disease mechanisms may facilitate the identification of appropriate molecular targets.

Summary

BRCA1 and BRCA2 have now been isolated and a large number of families characterized for the presence of mutations in these breast cancer susceptibility genes. Data from these studies are beginning to provide us with answers to many important questions. It is clear that estimates of attributable risk and penetrance are dependent on the population being studied. For example, studies of large, extensively affected families suggest that 45% of inherited breast cancer is due to BRCA1 mutations, while similar studies in individuals ascertained from breast cancer risk evaluation clinics suggest that the attributable risk is only 15%–20%. Similarly the large families yield penetrance estimates of 87% by age 85, while a more population-based study suggests somewhat lower rates – 60% by age 70. In addition, studies of BRCA1-related tumors suggest that there may be some important molecular differences as compared to sporadic tumors, with a predominance of high grade lesions that are ER negative and an increased rate of *p53* mutations. Controversy remains about the potential for genotype/phenotype correlation, and previous anecdotal reports of improved survival in families with familial breast cancer have yet to be fully evaluated. Finally, clinical recommendations are being formulated, with current recommendations centered on screening for breast cancer risk and prophylactic oophorectomy for presumed reduction of ovarian cancer risk.

References

Abeliovich D, Kaduri L, Lerer I et al (1997) The founder mutations 185delAG and 5382insC in BRCA1 and 6174delT in BRCA2 appear in 60% of ovarian cancer and 30% of early-onset breast cancer patients among Ashkenazi women. Am J Hum Genet 60:505–514

Berman DB, Wagner-Costalas J, Schultz DC et al (1996) Two distinct origins of a common BRCA1 mutation in breast-ovarian cancer families: a genetic study of 15 185delAG mutation kindreds. Am J Hum Genet 58:1166

Berry DA, Parmigiani G, Sanchez J et al (1997) Probability of carrying a mutation of breast-ovarian cancer gene BRCA1 based on family history. J Natl Cancer Inst 89:227–238

Couch FJ, Farid LM, DeShano ML et al (1996) BRCA2 germline mutations in male breast cancer cases and breast cancer families. Nat Genet 13:123–125

Couch FJ, DeShano M, Blackwood MA et al (1997) BRCA1 mutations in women attending clinics that evaluate the risk of breast cancer. N Engl J Med 336:1409–1415

Easton DF, Bishop DT, Ford D et al (1993) Genetic linkage analysis in familial breast and ovarian cancer – results from 214 families. Am J Hum Genet 52:678–701

Easton DF, Bishop DT, Ford D et al (1994) Breast and ovarian cancer incidence in BRCA1 mutation carriers. Lancet 343:962

Eisinger F, Stoppa-Lyonnet D, Longy M et al (1996) Germline mutation at BRCA1 affects the histoprognostic grade in hereditary breast cancer. Cancer Res 56:471

Ford D, Easton DF, Bishop DT et al (1994) Risk of cancer in BRCA1 mutation carriers. Lancet 343:962

Gayther SA, Warren W, Mazoyer S et al (1995) Germline mutations of the BRCA1 gene in breast/ovarian cancer families provide evidence for a genotype/phenotype correlation. Nat Genet 10:208

Hall JM, Lee MK, Newman B et al (1990) Linkage of early onset breast cancer to chromosome 17q21. Science 250:1684

Holt JT, Thompson ME, Szabo C et al (1996) Growth retardation and tumour inhibition by BRCA1. Nat Genet 12:298

Hosking L, Trowsdale J, Nicolai H et al (1995) A somatic BRCA1 mutation in an ovarian tumor. Nat Genet 9:343

Hoskins KF, Stopfer JE, Calzone KA et al (1995) Assessment and counseling for familial cancer risk: a guide for clinicians. JAMA 273:577–585

Lakahani SR, Sloane JP, Gusterson BA et al (1998) The pathology of familial breast cancer: evidence for differences between breast cancers developing in carriers of BRCA1 mutations, BRCA2 mutations, and sporadic cases. Lancet (in press)

Lancaster JM, Wooster R, Mangion J et al (1996) BRCA2 mutations in primary breast and ovarian cancers. Nat Genet 13:238–240

Marcus JN, Watson P, Page DL et al (1996) Hereditary breast cancer: pathobiology, prognosis, and BRCA1 and BRCA2 gene linkage. Cancer 77:697

Matsushima M, Kobayashi K, Erni M et al (1995) Mutation analysis of the BRCA1 gene in 76 Japanese ovarian cancer patients: four germline mutations, but no evidence of somatic mutation. Hum Mol Genet 4:1953

Merajver SD, Pham TM, Caduff RF et al (1995) Somatic mutations in the BRCA1 gene in sporadic ovarian tumors. Nat Genet 9:439

Miki Y, Swensen J, Shattuck-Eidens D et al (1994) A strong candidate for the breast and ovarian cancer susceptibility gene BRCA1. Science 266:66

Miki Y, Katagiri T, Kasumi F et al (1996) Mutation analysis on the BRCA2 gene in primary breast cancers. Nat Genet 13:245–247

Neuhausen SL, Gilewski T, Norton LJ et al (1996a) Recurrent BRCA2 6174delT mutations in Ashkenazi Jewish woman affected by breast cancer. Nat Genet 13:126–128

Neuhausen SL, Mazoyer S, Friedman L et al (1996b) Haplotype and phenotype analysis of six recurrent BRCA1 mutations in 61 families: results of an international study. Am J Hum Genet 58:271–280

Phelan CM, Lancaster JM, Tonin P et al (1996) Mutation analysis of the BRCA2 gene in 49 site-specific breast cancer families. Nat Genet 13:120–122

Piver MS, Jishi MF, Tsukada Y et al (1993) Primary peritoneal carcinoma after prophylactic oophorectomy in women with a family history of ovarian cancer. Cancer 71:2751–2755

Roa BB, Boyd AA, Volcik K et al (1996) Ashkenazi Jewish population frequency for common mutations in BRCA1 and BRCA2. Nat Genet 14:185–190

Rubin SC, Benjamin I, Behbakht K et al (1996) Clinical and pathological features of ovarian cancer in women with germline mutations of BRCA1. N Engl J Med 19:1413–1416

Serova OM, Mazoyer S, Puget N et al (1997) Mutations in BRCA1 and BRCA2 in breast cancer families: are there more breast cancer-susceptibility genes? Am J Hum Genet 60:486–495

Shattuck-Eidens D, Oliphant A, McClure M et al (1998) Complete DNA sequence analysis of BRCA1: 798 woman at high risk for susceptibility mutations. JAMA (in press)

Sobol H, Stoppa-Lyonnet D, Bressac-de-Paillerets B et al (1996) Truncation at conserved terminal regions of BRCA1 protein is associated with highly proliferating hereditary breast cancers. Cancer Res 56:3126

Streuwing JP, Abeliovitch D, Peterz T et al (1995a) The carrier frequency of the BRCA1 185delAG mutation is approximately 1 percent in Ashkenazi Jewish individuals. Nat Genet 11:198

Streuwing JP, Watson P, Easton DF et al (1995b) Prophylactic oophorectomy in inherited breast/ovarian cancer families. J Natl Cancer Inst 17:33–35

Streuwing JP, Hartge P, Wacholder S et al (1997) Cancer risk with 185delAG and 5382insC mutations of BRCA1 and the 6174delT mutation of BRCA2 among Ashkenazi Jews. N Engl J Med 336:1401–1408

Takahashi H, Behbakht K, McGovern PE et al (1995) Mutation analysis of the BRCA1 gene in ovarian cancers. Cancer Res 55:2998

Takahashi H, Chin HC, Bandera CA et al (1996) Mutations of the BRCA2 gene in ovarian carcinomas. Cancer Res 56:2738–2741

Tavtigian SV, Sinard J, Romens J et al (1996) The BRCA2 gene and mutations in chromosome 13q-linked kindreds. Nat Genet 12:333

Teng DHF, Bogden R, Mitchell J et al (1996) Low incidence of BRCA2 in breast carcinoma and other cancers. Nat Genet 13:241–244

Tonin P, Serova O, Lenoir G et al (1995) BRCA1 mutations in Ashkenazi Jewish women. Am J Hum Genet 57:189

Tonin P, Weber B, Offit K et al (1996) Frequency of recurrent BRCA1 and BRCA2 mutations in Ashkenazi Jewish breast cancer families. Nat Med 2:1179–1183

Wooster R, Neuhausen S, Mangion J et al (1994) Localization of a breast cancer susceptibility gene, BRCA2, to chromosome 13q12–13. Science 265:2088

Wooster R, Bignell G, Lancaster J et al (1995) Identification of the breast cancer susceptibility gene BRCA2. Nature 378:789

III. Biology of Breast Cancer: Diagnostic and Prognostic Implications

IGF-I Physiology and Breast Cancer

M. Pollak

Departments of Medicine and Oncology, McGill University
and Jewish General Hospital, Montreal, Quebec, Canada H3T 1E2

Introduction

Knowledge regarding the insulin-like growth factor (IGF) system is increasing rapidly (Jones and Clemmons 1995; Clemmons 1997). Recent research has revealed considerable complexity of the IGF system of mitogens at both the cellular and whole-organism levels. There is evidence to suggest that IGF physiology may be relevant to the pathophysiology of neoplasia in general, and of breast cancer in particular. This review will emphasize recent data of potential interest to clinicians, emphasizing recent results that suggest that IGF-I physiology may be related to risk of breast cancer, and also the rationale for adjuvant breast cancer therapies that target IGF-I.

Insulin-like Growth Factor Physiology and the Breast

Insulin-like growth factors are powerful mitogenic and anti-apoptotic factors that are important members of the network of signals that regulates the proliferative behaviour of cells of many organs, including the breast. Unlike many other growth factors, IGF-I has some properties of both a classic circulating 'endocrine' hormone and of a locally acting tissue growth factor. This means that there is physiological regulation of both IGF levels in the circulation and of IGF bioactivity in tissues. Local factors that influence IGF bioactivity include tissue expression of type I and type II IGF receptors, IGF-I and IGF-II themselves, the various IGF binding proteins, and binding protein proteases. Circulating IGF-I levels, on the other hand, are largely a function of hepatic IGF-I production, which is regulated by a variety of factors, including pituitary growth hormone secretion and nutritional influences (Thissen et al. 1994).

Certain factors that influence circulating IGF-I levels systemically have separate influences on local variables that influence tissue IGF bioactivity. These tend to act in a manner consistent with the direction of change in circulating levels. For example, tamoxifen, which lowers circulating IGF-I levels

(Pollak et al. 1990), also reduces IGF-I receptor number in target tissues for IGF-I action (Huynh et al. 1996a) and upregulates expression of inhibitory IGF binding proteins (Huynh et al. 1996b, c). Conversely, there is evidence that growth hormone, which raises circulating IGF-I level, also upregulates local IGF-I expression (Kleinberg et al. 1990).

IGF-I receptors are present on both normal and neoplastic breast epithelial cells (reviewed in Pollak 1993). The proliferative behaviour of the normal breast is regulated in part by the growth hormone-IGF-I axis, and studies in rhesus monkeys have shown a relationship between IGF-I level and cell proliferation rate in the breast (Ng et al. 1997). There is ample evidence from tissue culture (Yee 1994; Pollak et al. 1988; Arteaga and Osborne 1989) and in vivo (Arteaga et al. 1989; Yang et al. 1996) studies that at least a subset of breast cancer cells retain the IGF responsivity characteristic of the breast epithelial cells from which they are derived.

IGF-I Levels and Breast Cancer Risk

Several lines of investigation support the view that the growth hormone-IGF-I axis plays an important regulatory role in controlling growth and development of glandular structures in the breast (reviewed in Ruan et al. 1992). While it is clear that steroid hormones play key roles in regulating breast development, the fact that the stimulatory actions of estradiol on breast development are greatly attenuated in hypophysectomized animals indicates a role for other pituitary-dependent factors in breast epithelial cells (Nandi 1958). Recent studies have demonstrated that growth hormone is a key pituitary factor required to allow steroid-induced development of the breast to proceed (Kleinberg et al. 1990; Ruan et al. 1992; Feldman et al. 1992). There is evidence that growth hormone acts in this respect not only by raising circulating IGF-I levels, but also by upregulating IGF-I gene expression within the breast (Kleinberg et al. 1990). It is of interest that there is evidence that mice with higher IGF-I levels appear to have advantages in reproduction, as assessed by weight of offspring (Kroonsberg et al. 1989). A variety of factors may underlie this observation, but it is possible that enhanced lactation performance is involved. Thus, there may be selective pressure favouring higher IGF-I levels, notwithstanding the possibility that such selection may predispose to neoplasia later in life. There is evidence that higher IGF-I levels are correlated with higher rates of cellular proliferation in the breast (Ng et al. 1997), and also that higher proliferation rates are associated with increased risk of neoplastic transformation (Cohen and Ellwein 1990, 1991).

Recent laboratory studies provide more direct data compatible with the hypothesis that the growth hormone-IGF-I axis stimulates proliferation of normal breast epithelial cells, and that higher rates of proliferation, over time, increase risk of transformation. For example, it has been shown that transgenic mice that overexpress growth hormone and consequently have high levels of circulating IGF-I exhibit a high incidence of breast cancer (Tornell et al. 1991,

1992), and they also exhibit morphological evidence of mammary gland epithelial cell hyperplasia. Monkeys exposed to exogenously administered growth hormone also show histological evidence of mammary gland epithelial cell hyperplasia (Ng et al. 1997). Such histological changes have been associated with increased breast cancer risk in humans (Marshall et al. 1997). On the other hand, transgenic animals engineered to overexpress a growth hormone antagonist (Chen et al. 1997) show ductal hypoplasia (Ruan et al. 1997). In addition, experiments involving overexpression of IGF-I receptor agonists within the mammary gland showed that such manipulations increased mammary cancer and resulted in incomplete mammary gland involution (Hadsell et al. 1995; Bates et al. 1995). Finally, there is evidence from older studies in mice of a positive correlation between strain-specific evidence of breast cancer and activity of the growth hormone-IGF-I axis (Sinha et al. 1975, 1979). This remains an area of active investigation, and further studies to evaluate the physiological role of the growth hormone-IGF-I axis in the adult breast are required.

In view of the well-documented person-to-person variability in IGF-I levels (Juul et al. 1995a,b) and data suggesting that activity of the growth hormone-IGF-I axis may be a determinant of epithelial cell turnover in the breast, is it possible that individuals with higher levels of IGF-I are at increased risk of breast cancer? Until recently, only circumstantial evidence has been available. In rodent models, energy-restricted diets, which suppress IGF-I (Thissen et al. 1994), are well known to decrease cancer incidence (Ruggeri et al. 1989; Albanes 1987; Welsch 1985). Second, the positive correlation between birthweight and breast cancer risk (Michels et al. 1996) is compatible with the hypothesis if individuals stay true to their birth centile of IGF-I level, as low IGF-I level has been associated with low birthweight (Osorio et al. 1996; Woods et al. 1996). Finally, height, which is positively associated with breast cancer risk in most epidemiologic studies (Hunter and Willett 1993; deWaard et al. 1995; Vatten et al. 1992; Murata et al. 1982; Tretti 1989; Vatten and Kvinnsland 1990; Mondina et al. 1992), is positively correlated with IGF-I levels (Juul et al. 1995a).

The hypothesis that person-to-person variability in function of the growth hormone-IGF-I axis may be related to variability in breast cancer risk has already been studied clinically. Two case-control studies have been carried out to evaluate the possibility that there is a relationship between circulating IGF-I level and breast cancer risk (Bruning et al. 1995; Peyrat et al. 1993). Both found significantly higher IGF-I levels in women with breast cancer than in controls. In the larger of the two studies (with 109 cases) (Bruning et al. 1995), the relationship observed was strongest among premenopausal women.

These studies, while provocative, were potentially limited by their retrospective design. A recent prospective study carried out on the Nurses Health Study cohort (Hankinson et al. 1998) minimizes these concerns. This study, which involved 397 women with breast cancer and 620 age-matched controls, was carried out in a formal blinded fashion, using prospectively acquired blood samples. The study confirmed that there is considerable heterogeneity among women with respect to IGF-I level. No relationship between IGF-I level measured on a sample obtained after menopause and subsequent breast cancer incidence was seen. In contrast, among premenopausal women less than 50 years of age, those in the top tertile of IGF-I level had a relative risk of breast cancer of 4.58 (95% confidence limits 1.75–12) compared to those in the bottom tertile. With adjustment for circulating IGFBP-3 level, which was also measured, the relative risk was 7.28 (95% confidence limits 2.4–22).

These data add substantial direct evidence to support the hypothesis that activity of the growth hormone-IGF-I axis is related to risk of premenopausal breast cancer. If confirmed, they will support the view that reduction of activity of the growth hormone-IGF-I axis deserves study in the context of breast cancer prevention, particularly for women in higher centiles of circulating IGF-I level. However, given the broad confidence limits on the relative risk estimates, studies involving larger numbers of premenopausal women will be needed to provide more precise quantification of the relationship between risk and IGF-I levels. While the data demonstrate the absence of a relationship between postmenopausal IGF-I level and postmenopausal breast cancer risk, the possibility that premenopausal IGF-I level is related to risk of postmenopausal breast cancer deserves investigation, as there is evidence that in general breast cancer risk late in life can be influenced by premenopausal factors. As IGF-I levels decline nonspecifically with increasing age, it is possible that levels in older women are not correlated with levels during adolescence and early adulthood, which may be the critical periods in determination of risk.

If a relationship between IGF-I level and risk is established, somatostatin analogues, growth hormone releasing hormone antagonists, or growth hormone antagonists would deserve evaluation as candidate risk-reducing agents, specifically for those women at increased risk on the basis of their IGF-I level. Furthermore, IGF-I level would deserve evaluation as a candidate intermediate endpoint for prevention studies. Finally, in view of the fact that tamoxifen suppresses IGF-I levels (Pollak et al. 1990), demonstration of an association between IGF-I level and risk would suggest that IGF-I level might be a variable of importance in the interpretation of tamoxifen breast cancer prevention trials. For example, it is possible that risk reduction might be greater in those with highest IGF-I levels prior to chemopreventive intervention. Presently available data from both clinical and laboratory studies are strong enough to justify further research in these areas.

Adjuvant Therapies and IGF-I Physiology

Anti-estrogens are known to have important activity in the adjuvant treatment of breast cancer, and also to lower IGF-I levels and bioactivity (Pollak et al. 1997). Of course, these drugs have multiple other biological actions and it remains unclear to what extent their effects on IGF-I physiology contribute to their therapeutic action. Ongoing clinical trials are evaluating clinical outcomes together with effects of treatment on IGF-I levels and related parameters, and information from these studies will be important in addressing this issue. For example, if it is found that there is a positive relationship between IGF-I level and probability of relapse, we would suspect that effects of antiestrogens on IGF-I physiology are indeed of importance.

There is preclinical evidence that somatostatin analogues have antineoplastic activity in breast cancer models (reviewed in Schally and Pollak 1997), and it has been proposed that these drugs may act in part by lowering IGF-I levels, although direct growth inhibitory actions mediated via somatostatin receptors on neoplastic cells may also contribute to their antiproliferative action (reviewed in Schally and Pollak 1997). No data are available at this time to allow definite conclusions to be drawn regarding the dominant mechanism of action of somatostatin analogues, and it is possible that both IGF-I reduction in the host and direct effects mediated by tumour somatostatin receptors contribute. Studies showing that blockade of IGF-I receptors (Arteaga et al. 1989) or reduction of IGF-I levels (Yang et al. 1996) reduce tumour growth certainly are compatible with the view that somatostatin analogues act in tumour models at least in part by reducing IGF-I levels.

In large-volume metastatic breast cancer, however, early results from clinical trials have not demonstrated clinical activity (Schally and Pollak 1997). It is of interest in this context that preclinical models demonstrate much more significant activity in adjuvant than macrometastatic settings. That is, the compounds show more activity in inhibiting the development of palpable lesions than in causing regression of palpable lesions. Therefore, current major clinical trials are focused on the adjuvant rather than the macrometastatic setting, and compare adjuvant tamoxifen therapy to the combination of tamoxifen and the somatostatin analogue octreotide. The MA14 study run by the National Cancer Institute of Canada and the NSABP B29 study are both designed to examine the hypothesis that combined therapy will result in enhanced IGF-I suppression and in improved outcome.

Summary

Recent studies imply that IGF-I levels vary greatly between normal women, and that premenopausal breast cancer risk is increased among women with higher IGF-I levels. It is known that tamoxifen lowers IGF-I levels, but further research is needed to determine whether antiestrogens will be of particular value in risk reduction for women with high IGF-I levels, and also to determine if IGF-I levels can indeed be used as an intermediate endpoint in risk reduction interventions. With respect to adjuvant therapy, we currently have convincing data that antiestrogens have moderate IGF-I lowering actions, but it remains unclear to what extent these contribute to the therapeutic effect of these compounds. Ongoing trials are addressing this question, as well as the hypothesis that interventions that increase IGF-I suppression will be associated with reduced relapse rates.

References

Albanes D (1987) Total calories, body weight, and tumor incidence in mice. Cancer Res 47:1987–1992

Arteaga CL, Osborne CK (1989) Growth inhibition of human breast cancer cells in vitro with an antibody against the type 1 somatomedin receptor. Cancer Res 49:6237–6241

Arteaga CL, Kitten LJ, Coronado EB, Jacobs S, Kull FC, Allred DC, Osborne CK (1989) Blockade of the type 1 somatomedin receptor inhibits growth of human breast cancer cells in athymic mice. J Clin Invest 84:1418–1423

Bates P, Fisher R, Ward A, Richardson L, Hill DJ, Graham CF (1995) Mammary cancer in transgenic mice expressing insulin-like growth factor II (IGF-II). Br J Cancer 72:1189–1193

Bruning PF, Van Doorn J, Bonfror JMG, Van Noord PAH, Korse CM, Linders TC, Hart AM (1995) Int J Cancer 62:266

Chen NY, Chen WY, Striker LJ, Striker GE, Kopchick JJ (1997) Co-expression of bovine growth hormone (GH) and human GH antagonist genes in transgenic mice. Endocrinology 138:851–854

Clemmons DR (1997) Insulin-like growth factor binding proteins and their role in controlling IGF actions. Cytokine Growth Factor Rev 8:45–62

Cohen SM, Ellwein LB (1990) Cell proliferation in carcinogenesis. Science 249:1007–1011

Cohen SM, Ellwein LB (1991) Genetic errors, cell proliferation, and carcinogenesis. Cancer Res 51:6493–6505

DeWaard F, Cornelis J, Aoki K, Yoshida M (1995) Breast cancer incidence according to weight and height in two cities of the Netherlands and in Aichi prefecture, Japan. Cancer 40:1269–1275

Feldman M, Ruan W, Kleinberg DL (1992) 74th Annual Meeting Program and Abstracts of the Endocrine Society

Hadsell DL, Greenberg NM, Fligger JM, Baumrucker CR, Rosen JM (1995) Targeted expression of des(1–3) human insulin-like growth factor I in transgenic mice influences mammary gland development and IGF-binding protein expression. Endocrinology 137:321–330

Hankinson SE, Willett WC, Colditz GA, Hunter DJ, Michaud D, Deroo B, Rosner B, Speizer FE, Pollak M (1998) Circulating concentrations of insulin-like growth factor I and risk of breast cancer. Lancet (in press)

Hunter DJ, Willett WC (1993) Diet, body size, and breast cancer. Epidemiol Rev 15:110–132

Huynh HT, Nickerson T, Pollak M, Yang XF (1996a) Regulation of insulin-like growth factor I receptor gene expression by the pure antioestrogen ICI 182780. Clin Cancer Res 2:2037–2042

Huynh HT, Yang XF, Pollak M (1996b) A role for insulin-like growth factor binding protein 5 in the antiproliferative action of the antiestrogen ICI 182780. Cell Growth Differ 7:1501–1506

Huynh HT, Yang XF, Pollak M (1996c) Estradiol and antiestrogens regulate a growth inhibitory insulin-like growth factor binding protein 3 autocrine loop in human breast cancer cells. J Biol Chem 271:1016–1021

Jones JI, Clemmons DR (1995) Insulin-like growth factors and their binding proteins: biological actions. Endocr Rev 16:3–34

Juul A, Bang P, Hertel N et al (1995a) Serum insulin-like growth factor I in 1030 healthy children, adolescents, and adults: relation to age, sex, stage of puberty, testicular size, and body mass index. J Clin Endocrinol Metab 78:744–752

Juul A, Dalgaard P, Blum WF, Bang P, Hall K, Michaelsen KF, Muller J, Skakkebaek NE (1995b) Serum levels of insulin-like growth factor (IGF)-binding protein-3 (IGFBP-3) in healthy infants, children, and adolescents: the relation to IGF-I, IGF-II, IGFBP-1, IGFBP-2, age, sex, body mass index, and pubertal maturation. J Clin Endocrinol Metab 80:2534–2542

Kleinberg DL, Ruan W, Catanese V, Newman CB, Feldman F (1990) Non-lactogenic effects of growth hormone on growth and insulin-like growth factor-I messenger ribonucleic acid of rat mammary gland. Endocrinology 126(6):3274–3276

Kroonsberg C, McCutcheon SN, Siddiqui RA, Mackenzie DD, Blair HT, Ormsby JE, Breier BH, Gluckman PD (1989) Reproductive performance and fetal growth in female mice from lines divergently selected on the basis of plasma IGF-1 concentrations. J Reprod Fertil 87:349–353

Marshall LM, Hunter DJ, Connolly JL, Schnitt SJ, Byrne C, London SJ, Colditz GA (1997) Risk of breast cancer associated with atypical hyperplasia of lobular and ductal types. Cancer Epidemiol Biomarkers Prev 6:297–301

Michels KB, Trichopoulos D, Robins JM, Rosner BA, Manson JE, Hunter DJ, Colditz GA, Hankinson SE, Speizer FE, Willett WC (1996) Birthweight as a risk factor for breast cancer. Lancet 348:1542–1546

Mondina R, Borsellino G, Poma S, Baroni M, Di Nubila B, Sacchi P (1992) Breast carcinoma and skeletal formation. Eur J Cancer 28A:1068–1070

Murata M, Kuno K, Sakamoto G (1982) Epidemiology of family predisposition for breast cancer in Japan. J Natl Cancer Inst 69:1229–1234

Nandi S (1958) Pituitary factors required for estradiol actions on mammary tissue. J Natl Cancer Inst 21:1039–1062

Ng S, Zou J, Adesanyn O, Wang J, LeRoith D, Bondy C (1997) GH treatment induces mammary gland hyperplasia in aging primates. Nat Med 3:1141–1144

Osorio M, Torres J, Moya F, Pezzullo J, Salafia C, Baxter R, Schwander J, Fant M (1996) Insulin-like growth factor (IGFs) and IGF binding proteins-1, -2 and -3 in newborn serum: relationships to fetoplacental growth at term. Early Hum Dev 46:15–26

Peyrat JP, Bonneterre J, Hecquet B, Vennin P, Louchez MM, Fournier C, Lefebvre J, Demaille A (1993) Plasma insulin-like growth factor-1 (IGF-1) concentration in human breast cancer. Eur J Cancer 29A:492–497

Pollak M (1993) Effects of adjuvant tamoxifen therapy on growth hormone and insulin-like growth factor I (IGF-I) physiology. In: Salmon SE (ed) Adjuvant therapy of cancer VII. Lippincott, Philadelphia

Pollak M, Polychronakos C, Yousefi S, Richard M (1988) Characterization of insulin-like growth factor (IGF-I) receptors of human breast cancer cells. Biochem Biophys Res Commun 154:326–331

Pollak M, Costantino J, Polychronakos C, Blauer S, Guyda H, Redmond C, Fisher B, Margolese R (1990) Effect of tamoxifen on serum insulin-like growth factor I levels in stage I breast cancer patients. J Natl Cancer Inst 82:1693–1697

Pollak M, Ingle J, Suman V, Kugler J (1997) Rationale for combined antiestrogen-somatostatin analogue therapy of breast cancer. In: Salmon S (ed) Adjuvant therapy of cancer VIII. Lippincott, Philadelphia, pp 145–152

Ruan W, Newman C, Kleinberg D (1992) Intact and amino-terminally shortened forms of insulin-like growth factor I induce mammary gland differentiation and development. Proc Natl Acad Sci USA 89:10872–10876

Ruan W, Knapp J, Chen W, Kopchick JJ, Kleinberg DL (1997) Mammary gland development is impaired in transgenic mice overexpressing a bovine growth hormone antagonist. Proceedings of the Endocrine Society 79th Annual Meeting 79:165

Ruggeri BA, Klurfeld DM, Dritchevsky D, Furlanetto RW (1989) Growth factor binding to DMBA-induced mammary tumors from rats subject to chronic caloric restriction. Cancer Res 49:4135–4141

Schally AV, Pollak M (1997) Mechanisms of antineoplastic action of somatostatin analogues. Proc Soc Exp Biol Med 217:143–152

Sinha YN, Salocks CB, VanderLaan WP (1975) Prolactin and growth hormone levels in different inbred strains of mice: patterns in association with estrous cycle, time of day, and perphenazine stimulation. Endocrinology 1112–1122

Sinha YN, Vlahakis G, VanderLaan WP (1979) Serum, pituitary and urine concentrations for prolactin and growth hormone in eight strains of mice with varying incidence of mammary tumours. Int J Cancer 24:430–437

Thissen JP, Ketelslegers JM, Underwood LE (1994) Nutritional regulation of the insulin-like growth factors. Endocr Rev 15:80–101

Tornell J, Rymo L, Isaakson OGP (1991) Induction of mammary adenocarcinomas in metallothionein promoter-human growth hormone transgenic mice. Int J Cancer 49:114–117

Tornell J, Carlsson B, Pohjanen P, Wennbo H, Rymo L, Isaakson OGP (1992) High frequency of mammary adenocarcinomas in metallothionein promoter-human growth hormone transgenic mice created from two different strains of mice. J Steroid Biochem Mol Biol 43:237–242

Tretli S (1989) Height and weight in relation to breast cancer morbidity and mortality. A prospective study of 570,000 women in Norway. Int J Cancer 44:23–30

Vatten LJ, Kvinnsland S (1990) Body height and risk of breast cancer. A prospective study of 23,831 Norwegian women. Br J Cancer 61:881–885

Vatten LJ, Kvikstad A, Nymoen E (1992) Incidence and mortality of breast cancer related to body height and living conditions during childhood and adolescence. Eur J Cancer 28:128–131

Welsch CW (1985) Host factors affecting the growth of carcinogen-induced rat mammary carcinomas: a review and tribute to Charles Brenton Huggins. Cancer Res 45:3415–3443

Woods KA, Camacho-Hubner C, Savage MO, Clark AJ (1996) Intrauterine growth retardation and postnatal growth failure associated with deletion of the insulin-like growth factor I gene. N Engl J Med 335:1363–1367

Yang XF, Beamer W, Huynh HT, Pollak M (1996) Reduced growth of human breast cancer xenografts in hosts homozygous for the 'lit' mutation. Cancer Res 56:1509–1511

Yee D (1994) The insulin-like growth factor system as a target in breast cancer. Breast Cancer Res Treat 32:85–95

Determination of Clinical Utility of Tumor Markers: A Tumor Marker Utility Grading System

D. F. Hayes

Breast Cancer Center Program, Lombardi Cancer Center,
Georgetown University Medical Center, Washington, DC, USA

Introduction

In the last 20 years, more than 200 papers have been published in the English literature assessing either the prognostic or predictive abilities of several different putative tumor markers. In spite of this plethora of publications, very few factors have been accepted for routine use in clinical practice. In 1995, the American Society of Clinical Oncology convened an Expert Panel to develop evidence-based practice guidelines for the use of tumor markers in breast cancer (ASCO Expert Panel 1996). This panel considered several tissue-based factors, including estrogen receptor (ER), cathepsin D, p53, HER-2/c-neu/erbB-2, and flow cytometrically determined S-phase fraction. After careful deliberation, they concluded that the data were insufficient to recommend the use of any biologically based marker to determine prognosis. Furthermore, the Panel recommended that ER could be used to reliably predict response/benefit from hormone therapy, but that no other predictive factor was sufficiently well-established to be considered for routine clinical use.

In the setting of enormous advances in molecular biology and immunologic techniques, why is ER the only accepted prognostic or predictive factor? Early in their deliberations, the ASCO Expert Panel realized that there has been no framework for performance of tumor marker studies. Unlike clinical investigations of new therapeutic modalities, no consensus has existed for the types of tumor marker studies performed, how to design them, or how to analyze them. Therefore, the general field of tumor marker research has consisted mostly of retrospective studies performed using specimens collected for a variety of reasons and analyzed using many different methods. Therefore, the results of individual studies are usually heterogeneous and conflicting. It has been hard to draw reliable estimates of the clinical utility of any given marker except those that are extraordinarily powerful, such as ER for prediction of response to hormone therapy.

In response to this apparent methodologic deficiency, several members of the Expert Panel co-authored a separate manuscript in which they proposed a framework for reviewing previously performed studies to determine whether the data support recommendation of a given tumor (Hayes et al.

1996). These authors also suggested that this tumor marker utility grading system (TMUGS) could be used to design future tumor marker studies that would result in more reliable data, thus permitting more rapid translation from concept to clinical use. In a second paper, an extension of TMUGS has been proposed, in which methods to reliably estimate the relative strengths of a marker for a particular use are suggested (Hayes and Trock 1998). In this manuscript, we will review TMUGS and its extension, designated "TMUGS plus". The reader is referred to the original publications for more detailed description of TMUGS and "TMUGS plus" (Hayes and Trock 1998; Hayes et al. 1996).

Overview of the Tumor Marker Utility Grading System (TMUGS)

The Tumor Marker Utility Grading Scale (TMUGS) was developed to standardize evaluation of a specific tumor marker. A single-page TMUGS worksheet was proposed that illustrated all of the features of the TMUGS (Fig. 1). The worksheet is divided into two broad sections: the top is used to define the marker being evaluated, and the bottom is used to define the uses, the biological correlation, and the clinical utility of the marker. This system was expressly designed for the purpose of practice guideline development. Therefore, TMUGS will be useful for clinicians and expert clinical reviewers to determine how to use currently available tumor markers. However, TMUGS might also aid clinical and laboratory investigators as they plan studies of new tumor markers.

Definitions and Specifications of Tumor Markers

The first step in evaluating the clinical utility of a tumor marker is a precise definition of the marker. Various designations are often used interchangeably for "tumor marker." By definition, a marker represents an alteration or deviation (qualitatively or quantitatively) from normal of a molecule, substance, or process that can be detected by some type of assay. For the purposes of this proposal, only those alterations that are detected by a special assay, other than routine histopathologic or laboratory evaluations, performed on a body tissue or fluid, will be considered "tumor markers."

The TMUGS worksheet (Fig. 1) is designed to organize the multiple areas of heterogeneity and confusion that have contributed to the lack of a standardized approach to clinical acceptance of specific tumor markers. The top portion of the worksheet includes precise designations and nomenclatures that specifically identify the marker of interest. Many designations may be given to the same family of markers, and one designation may be given to many different types of markers. One marker may acquire different designations when different investigators or commercial interests independently identify and develop a potentially useful marker. Even when investigators de-

DEFINITIONS AND SPECIFICATIONS OF MARKER:

MARKER DESIGNATION/NOMENCLATURE (e.g. ER, P53, CEA, etc.)	MOLECULE/SUBSTANCE ASSAYED & ALTERATION DETECTED (e.g. DNA/mutation, RNA/overexpression, Protein/increased levels, etc.)	ASSAY FORMAT TO DETECT MARKER (e.g. EIA, ICA, SSCP, etc.)
REAGENTS USED (e.g. specific MAb or probe, or commercial assay)	SPECIMEN SOURCE (e.g. frozen or fixed tissue, plasma, urine, circulating cells, etc.)	
DISEASE (e.g. breast cancer, colon cancer, etc.)		

UTILITY:

Marker association with biologic: / Use leads to decision in practice that results in a more favorable clinical outcome:

Uses	Process Utility Score	Process Level of Evidence	Endpoint Utility Score	Endpoint Level of Evidence	Survival Utility Score	Survival Level of Evidence	Disease Free Survival Utility Score	Disease Free Survival Level of Evidence	Quality of Life Utility Score	Quality of Life Level of Evidence	Cost of Care Utility Score	Cost of Care Level of Evidence
Determine risk												
Screening												
Differential diagnosis												
Prognosis: Predict relapse/progression												
Primary												
Metastatic												
Prognosis: Predict response to therapy												
Primary												
Metastatic												
Monitor course												
Detect relapse in patient with no evidence of disease after therapy for primary or recurrent disease												
Follow detectable disease												

Fig. 1. Tumor Marker Utility Grading System (TMUGS) worksheet (Hayes et al. 1996)

scribe the same tumor marker, they may be discussing different molecules or substances, different types of deviations from normal, and different assays to detect these. These ambiguities make it essential to designate precisely what molecule or processes are altered (e.g., DNA, RNA, protein, antibody, cellular response, etc.), and what alteration was detected in that molecule or process (e.g., amplification, mutation, deletion, over-expression, elevated soluble levels, increased cellular activity, etc.) (Fig. 1).

Different assays for the same molecular alteration may not provide equivalent results. Different assay results can be expected to be quite heterogeneous depending on how the assay is constructed and how the results are interpreted. Alternatively, one reagent may be used in different assay formats. For example, a monoclonal antibody may be used for immunohistochemical studies to detect and semiquantify tissue antigen expression, or it might be incorporated into an enzyme-based immunoassay (EIA) to provide a quantitative measure of the same antigen in suspension or solution (Carney et al. 1989). Thus, each claim should be based on independent studies that demonstrate the utility of that marker in the manner in which it was tested, rather than on assumptions that one method provides the same correlation and outcome as another. Moreover, similar assays may provide different results depending on the reagents, conditions, and signal detection systems used in the assay. Additionally, the method of statistical analysis may strongly influence conclusions from a given assay study. For example, changes from normality may be expressed in a continuous or categorical fashion. Many different methods to distinguish an abnormal state from a normal or previous baseline condition have been proposed, and these may be assay-specific (Clark et al. 1989; Simon and Altman 1994; George 1994).

A further source of heterogeneity may be introduced by detecting the tumor marker abnormality in different tissue or specimen types. For example, elevated or overexpressed levels of HER-2/neu protein can be detected in cancer tissue and also in serum (Carney et al. 1989). The biological and clinical significance of a marker detected in association with a cell (for example in the cytosol or membrane) may be very different from those of the same marker when it is detected as a soluble factor in fluid. Furthermore, results obtained from a cellular needle aspirate might be different from those obtained using the same assay on the same cells that are collected by a large biopsy in which tissue architecture is preserved. How these specimens are processed and stored before analysis may also affect results.

Finally, one tumor marker, even if defined precisely and assayed uniformly in one disease, may not have any or may have a completely different clinical utility in another malignancy (see below, Evaluating Clinical Utility of Specific Tumor Markers). Although it is important to designate the disease for which the marker is being evaluated, the TMUGS should be applicable, with minor modifications, to most malignancies.

Evaluating Clinical Utility of Specific Tumor Markers

TMUGS is designed to determine whether knowledge of the marker data in an individual patient can be reliably used to make practice decisions that will improve outcome. Tumor marker data might be useful in at least nine separate clinical situations, designated "uses" for the purpose of the TMUGS (Fig. 1, Utility). These uses include risk assessment, screening, differential diagnosis, prognosis, and monitoring disease course. For each potential use, tumor marker data should be evaluated to determine whether they are reliably associated with the biological process being considered, and whether that association predicts a future endpoint, regardless of whether that knowledge has any clinical therapeutic relevance.

Ultimately, knowledge of tumor marker data should lead to a clinical decision that results in a more favorable clinical outcome than if the marker results were not known. The TMUGS is designed to determine the utility of the marker in helping to reliably make clinical decisions that result in changes in one of four clinical outcomes: overall survival (OS), disease-free survival (DFS), quality of life (QOL), or cost of care (cost).

To rate a marker's utility for each use and each biological process and endpoint, and each clinical outcome, semiquantitative utility scales have been established. The assigned utility score in these scales reflects the reviewer's summary of the state of the art for that marker in each situation. In order to justify the assignment of a specific utility score, the reviewer provides an estimate of the level of evidence to support his/her evaluation, with an associated list of references.

The authors of the TMUGS proposal recognized that, in certain clinical situations, the tumor marker may be closely associated with a biological or clinical endpoint, such as tumor recurrence, yet the treatment options for that disease and use are sufficiently ineffective that knowledge of that endpoint does not lead to a decision that would favorably change the outcome. Therefore, the tumor marker assay's association with a biological process or endpoint was dissociated from assessment of its clinical utility (Fig. 1, Utility, top row). In order to avoid confusion, association between marker results and disease behavior were designated as a "correlation with biological endpoint." In contrast, use of marker results to dictate a clinical decision that is beneficial to the patient were designated as a "favorable clinical outcome." Thus, the term "outcomes" is used only if it specifically refers to a therapeutic decision that leads to a superior clinical result.

Association with a biological process, even if quite good, *does not necessarily imply clinical utility*. If the knowledge of the marker result does not lead to a decision in clinical practice that results in a more favorable clinical outcome (OS, DFS, QOL, cost), then its use in routine clinical practice is discouraged. Nonetheless, on an investigational basis, correlations with biological endpoints are still important to ascertain for the marker in various uses, since these correlations might be extremely valuable if and when therapeutic advances for the disease are made. Subsequent and separate evaluations can then be performed regarding whether tumor marker data have utility in making clinical decisions that result in a favorable clinical outcome.

In summary, the category describing correlation with biological processes and endpoints is intentionally included as the first "utility" to be evaluated for each tumor marker in each use. Association of tumor marker results with a biological process may help set investigational agenda by providing insight for future marker studies that address biological endpoints. Moreover, such studies should also contribute to development of more effective therapies for cancers in which tumor markers are associated with biological endpoints.

Utility Scales to Evaluate Tumor Markers

As a critical component of TMUGS, semiquantitative utility scales were developed to describe the reviewers' interpretation of the current status of a marker for biological and clinical outcomes for each use (Tables 1, 2). In general, the values in these scales reflect the performance characteristics for the assay in relationship to the respective use and the biological process/endpoint and/or favorable clinical outcome.

Two separate scales are used to reflect the distinction between evaluation of a marker's performance characteristics in regard to *biological process and endpoints* (Table 1) and the utility of marker data to produce a more *favorable clinical outcome* (Table 2). Although these scales are similar, they have different functions. As described, good marker correlation with biological process and endpoints does *not* imply clinical utility, although it may. Thus, utility scores from "0" to "++" are assigned for the columns describing biological process and endpoints (Table 2).

A critical evaluation of the marker in the context of existing therapeutic benefits must be made to meet the criteria for a marker to be considered "standard practice." Thus, the scale to evaluate markers for clinical outcomes includes an additional score, "+++" (Table 2). In the favorable clinical outcomes scale (Table 2), only scores "++" and "+++" are sufficient for a mark-

Table 1. Utility scale to evaluate tumor marker for correlation with biological process and endpoint

Utility score	Explanation of score
0	Marker does not correlate with process, or marker does not correlate with expected endpoint
NA	Data are not available regarding marker correlation with process or endpoint for that use
+/–	Preliminary data are suggestive that assay correlates with process, or with endpoint, but substantially more definitive studies are required
+	Assay probably correlates with process or endpoint, but additional confirmatory studies are required
++	Definitive studies demonstrate that assay correlates with process or endpoint

Table 2. Scale to evaluate utility of tumor markers for favorable clinical outcomes (Hayes et al. 1996)

Utility score	Explanation of score
0	Marker has been adequately evaluated for a specific use and the data definitively demonstrate it has *no utility*. The marker should not be ordered for that clinical use
NA	Data are not available for the marker for that use because marker has not been studied for that clinical use
+/−	Data are suggestive that the marker may correlate with biological process and/or endpoint, and preliminary data suggest that use of the marker *may* contribute to favorable clinical outcome, but more definitive studies are required. Thus, the marker is still considered highly investigational and should not be used for standard clinical practice
+	Sufficient data are available to demonstrate that the marker correlates with the biological process and/or endpoint related to the use, and that the marker results might effect favorable clinical outcome for that use. However, the marker is still considered investigational and should not be used for standard clinical practice, for one of three reasons: 1. The marker correlates with another marker or test that has been established to have clinical utility, but the new marker has not been shown clearly to provide any advantage 2. The marker may contribute independent information, but it is unclear whether that information provides clinical utility because treatment options have not been shown to change outcome 3. Preliminary data for the marker are quite encouraging, but the level of evidence (see below) is lacking to document clinical utility
++	Marker supplies information not otherwise available from other measures that is helpful to the clinician in decision making for that use, but the marker cannot be used as sole criterion for decision making. Thus, marker has clinical utility for that use, and it should be considered standard practice in *selected* situations
+++	Marker can be used as the sole criterion for clinical decision making in that use. Thus, marker has clinical utility for that use, and it should be considered standard practice

er to be considered standard clinical practice. In contrast, assignment of a "0" to a marker in a given use implies that sufficient data are available to document that, even if the marker had appeared promising in preliminary studies, it has no utility for that use when critically investigated. A "0" may be assigned because the marker data are so poor that they do not correlate with the biological process or endpoint to be useful (for example, they may have been assigned a "+/−" or "+" in these categories). Alternatively, in the favorable clinical outcomes columns, "0" might be assigned because the therapeutic options available for that disease are insufficient to render tumor marker data of any utility, even if the marker is associated with the biological process/endpoint.

The categories of "+/−" and "+" are assigned during early evaluation of a marker, when results from only a few preliminary studies are available, or when results from several studies conflict. The "+" category implies that the marker is promising but cannot be considered standard clinical practice. The following three scenarios might account for assignment of a "+" score rather than a more definitive "++" for biological correlations or "++" or "+++" for favorable clinical outcomes: (1) the marker correlates with another marker or test that has been established to have clinical utility, but the new marker has not been shown to clearly provide any advantage; (2) the marker may contribute independent information, but it is unclear whether that information provides clinical utility because treatment options have not been shown to change outcome; (3) preliminary data for the marker are quite encouraging, but the level of evidence (see below) is lacking to document clinical utility.

The final two categories "++" and "+++" imply the marker has clinical utility. The "++" category is the one into which many clinically useful markers will be placed. In this setting, the marker complements other information (history, physical, radiography, routine histopathology, other markers) used by the clinician to judge the patient's status and to decide which avenue of practice will be most beneficial to the patient.

Few markers dictate clinical decision-making independently of other clinical features, and therefore most will be assigned "++" or less. Nonetheless, in some situations, changes in clinical practice are indicated based on marker results alone. Markers assigned a "+++" score should be considered standard practice in the evaluation and monitoring of all patients with the disease in question.

Level of Evidence to Assign Utility Score to Marker for Use

Initially, the TMUGS was designed to develop practice guidelines for tumor markers (ASCO Expert Panel 1996). A "Levels of Evidence (LOE) Scale" was modeled for TMUGS based on that proposed by the Canadian Task Force on the Periodic Health Examination (Canadian Task Force on the Periodic Health Examination 1979). The modified Level of Evidence Scale for Tumor Markers is provided in Table 3. As with studies of therapeutic modalities, the design of tumor marker studies will place the obtained results within different levels. The authors of TMUGS agreed that only LOE I or II data are sufficient to reliably assign a TMUGS grade of ++ or +++. These LOE I studies include prospective studies designed specifically to ask a tumor marker question, prospective tumor marker studies that accompany therapeutic clinical trials, and/or overviews of LOE III tumor marker studies (Table 3).

Table 3. Levels of evidence for grading clinical utility of tumor markers (Hayes et al. 1996)

Level	Type of evidence
I	Evidence from a single high-powered prospective study that is specifically designed to test marker or evidence from meta-analysis and/or overview of level II or III studies. In the former case, the study must be designed so that therapy and follow-up are dictated by protocol. Ideally, the study is a prospective randomized trial in which diagnostic and/or therapeutic clinical decisions in one arm are determined based at least in part on marker results, and diagnostic and/or therapeutic clinical decisions in control arm are made independently of marker results. However, may also include prospective but not randomized trials with marker data and clinical outcome as primary objective
II	Evidence from study in which marker data are determined in relationship to prospective therapeutic trial that is performed to test therapeutic hypothesis but not specifically designed to test marker utility (i.e., marker study is secondary objective of protocol). However, specimen collection for marker study and statistical analysis are prospectively determined in protocol as secondary objectives
III	Evidence from large but retrospective studies from which variable numbers of samples are available or selected. Therapeutic aspects and follow-up of patient population may or may not have been prospectively dictated. Statistical analysis for tumor marker was not dictated prospectively at time of therapeutic trial design
IV	Evidence from small retrospective studies which do not have prospectively dictated therapy, follow-up, specimen selection, or statistical analysis. May be matched case controls, etc
V	Evidence from small pilot studies designed to determine or estimate distribution of marker levels in sample population. May include "correlation" with other known or investigational markers of outcome, but not designed to determine clinical utility

Assessment of the Magnitude of Benefit to Justify Assignment of ++ or +++ Grade in TMUGS: TMUGS Plus

Absolute Categories of Prognosis and Relative Strengths of Prognostic Factors

One can select categories of prognosis that are informative for patient decision-making. In a sense, these categories are patterned after the stage I, II, and III categories in the TNM system (American Joint Committee on Cancer 1988). We will assume that patients are willing to risk some measure of undertreatment in order to avoid unnecessary toxicities. Thus, for purposes of TMUGS, three categories are defined. These include "very good" (stage I), in which the odds of dying of breast cancer in the absence of adjuvant systemic therapy (AST) at 10 years is less than 10%, "moderate" (stage II), in which the odds of dying are 10%–50%, and "very poor" (stage III), in which the odds of dying are 50% or more. For purposes of this model, if it is assumed that all patients experience a proportional reduction of 30% in mortality from AST, patients in the very good category would not elect treatment since few would stand to benefit, those in the moderate category probably would elect treatment, and those in the poor category would definitely choose to be treated.

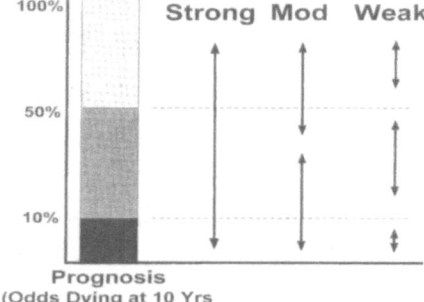

Fig. 2. Conceptual illustration of prognostic factor categories (Hayes and Trock 1998)

Of course, this model rests on two important assumptions: (1) that the impact of AST is moderate, reducing the mortality at 10 years by approximately 30%; and (2) that toxicities and cost of therapy are of concern. If AST reduces mortality by 50% or more, then at least 5% or more of patients in all three categories stand to benefit. Likewise, if AST has no side effects, then even a 1% benefit is justifiable.

One can now place prognostic factors into categories, each of which is defined by this context: strong, moderate, and weak (Fig. 2). They are defined by their relative ability to "move" patients between the three prognostic stages. A strong factor moves a patient across three categories (for example, from very good to very poor). A moderate factor moves a patient across two categories (for example, from very good to moderate, or moderate to poor). A weak factor moves a patient within a category, but is insufficiently powerful to change a patient's prognosis in a clinically important fashion.

Application of These Methods to Prognostic Factor Analysis

Estimation of the prognostic power of a given marker should be performed using LOE I data sets. Few prospective clinical studies have been performed strictly to determine prognosis. Nonetheless, LOE I studies require prospective studies in which accrual is driven by the power required to estimate the prognostic effect, or an overview of lesser evidence studies (LOE III). Companion studies of prognostic factors embedded in prospective therapeutic studies containing an untreated arm constitute LOE II. Most other studies using previously archived specimens from patients not enrolled in prospective studies are considered LOE III. The relative strength of a prognostic factor to move patients between prognostic subgroups, designated a likelihood ratio (LR), can be estimated from overview analyses of LOE III studies. In this case, the confidence limits of the LR will depend, of course, on the available data from the LOE III studies.

We are unaware of any published overview analyses to determine the prognostic power of a tumor marker. The power of such prognostic factors can only be estimated by multivariate analytical methods, including pre-existing, accepted prognostic factors such as TNM staging and histopathology, in the model. Assessment of the prognostic power of a marker is best performed in a population of patients who do not receive AST. Unfortunately, such populations are becoming increasingly uncommon, as widespread application of AST to most patients with invasive breast cancer becomes routine. Assessment of prognostic power in the setting of AST is only reliable if there is no possibility of interaction with therapy, which is of course very difficult to determine. Thus, assessment of new prognostic factors will either have to be performed using archived samples from untreated patients, or in groups of patients for whom prognosis is deemed so favorable by virtue of pre-existing markers (TNM, histopathology) that they are not treated with AST according to current guidelines.

Absolute Categories of Prediction and Relative Strengths of Predictive Factors

A predictive factor is associated with relative benefit (sensitivity or resistance) from a specific therapy. However, as with prognostic factors, the difference in outcomes between a factor-positive and a factor-negative patient depends on the relative strengths of the predictive factor to separate those patients likely to respond (or achieve other endpoints of benefit) from those not likely to. This likelihood ratio (LR) of response (or benefit) is calculated by dividing the beneficial outcome (for example, response) in those patients who are fall into the favorable category by that for those who fall into the unfavorable category. For example, patients whose tumors are ER-rich ("ER-positive") have a substantially higher chance of responding to or benefiting from hormone therapy than those whose tumors are ER-poor ("ER-negative"). For the purposes of TMUGS Plus, we will assume three categories of predictive factors: "weak" factors have LR of 1–2, "moderate" factors have LR of 2–4, and "strong" factors have LR >4 (Table 4).

Table 4. Categories of predictive factors (Hayes and Trock 1998)

Category	Likelihood ratio of patient responding or benefiting if marker positive vs negative
Strong	>4
Moderate	2–4
Weak	1-2

How Should LR for a Predictive Factor be Estimated?

Clearly, the choice of data sets to estimate the LR will determine the reliability and accuracy of the estimate. Ideally, estimates of LR would come from studies that fall into the category of LOE I in TMUGS (Hayes et al. 1996). A second, less optimal, but satisfactory data set could be derived from LOE II studies. The most common tumor marker data sets are from LOE III studies in which specimens were available for testing with a given assay. The predictive value of a marker can only be inferred from LOE III studies, since they do not contain a group of patients treated with a control therapy. Therefore, differences in outcomes may be a result of the prognostic power of the marker, not a predictive effect relative to the specific therapy.

Overview Analyses

Ultimately, the usefulness of a system such as TMUGS, expanded here, rests on the reviewer's assessment of available data. In the original TMUGS manuscript, assignment of a TMUGS grade (0–3+) was left to the discretion of the reviewer (Hayes et al. 1996). Prospective, highly powered tumor markers studies are rare, since most clinical investigators prefer to use limited resources to perform studies of novel therapeutic approaches. Given that most tumor marker studies are LOE III, most available data are so heterogeneous that reliable interpretation is difficult (ASCO Expert Panel 1996). Recently, Trock and his colleagues have published a more objective approach to estimate the relative benefits (LR) of tumor markers using overview or meta-analysis methods (Trock et al. 1997). Such overview methodology was presumed in the original TMUGS proposal, but at the time of the original TMUGS publication (and the ASCO guidelines), few if any overview analyses had been performed for tumor markers. Nonetheless, the authors suggested that if such analyses were performed, they would generate LOE I data (Hayes et al. 1996).

In summary, the relative strengths of putative prognostic and predictive factors should be estimated using LOE I or II data sets. In doing so, the reviewer should be able to reliably estimate the LR for a given marker in untreated patients, and for patients relative to a specific therapy.

A Matrix to Help Decide When to Treat Patients
Based on Prognostic and Predictive Factors

Ultimately, the clinical utility of a marker is based on whether knowledge of the marker influences a clinical decision that results in a better outcome for the patient than if the marker results were not known (Hayes et al. 1996). These outcomes include higher cure rates, prolonged survival, prolonged disease-free survival, improved quality of life, or identical outcomes with lowered cost of care. The marker is only useful if it places the patient into a subgroup that is highly likely to benefit from the therapy (for example, relative to a marker-negative patient) or, alternatively, into a group that can be spared the toxicity of therapy because the therapy is unlikely to work. Using the assumptions and definitions described above, we can place an individual predictive factor into a matrix to assess its clinical utility, as illustrated in Tables 5 and 6.

With these assumptions, patients can be placed into one of three prognostic categories – very good, moderate, and very poor – using clinical and pathologic staging techniques. If no AST is administered, these categories are associated with risks of dying of breast cancer in the ensuing 10 years of 10%, 11%–50%, and >50%, respectively. Let us now assume that, if no predictive factors are used, all patients will experience a proportional reduction in this risk of dying of approximately 30% if they receive both chemotherapy and hormone therapy. However, of course, this means that all patients are exposed to all of the toxicities and long-term complications of these therapies.

In contrast, to optimize benefits/risks, application of prognostic and predictive factors will permit more efficient application of AST. However, as

Table 5. Assumptions of absolute benefit categories relative to treatment decisions (Hayes and Trock 1998)

Recommendations for treatment would be:	If absolute benefit is:
Certain	>10%
Probable	6–9%
Considered, but not strongly recommended	4–5%
Not recommended	0–3%

Table 6. Absolute benefits from adjuvant systemic therapy in context of prognostic factors and predictive factor profiles (Hayes and Trock 1998)

Prognostic category	Absolute mortality in absence of systemic therapy[a]	No. of patients who benefit if no predictive factor[b]	Predictive factors					
			Absolute reduction in mortality due to systemic therapy in patients for whom marker is negative compared to those for whom marker is positive					
			Weak (RR=1.5)		Moderate (RR=3)		Strong (RR=6)	
			Neg.	Pos.	Neg.	Pos.	Neg.	Pos.
Very good	10%	3	1	2	<1	3	<1	3
Moderate	50%	15	6	9	4	11	2	13
Very poor	75%	23	9	14	6	17	3	20

[a] Worst case.
[b] Assuming proportional reduction of 30%.
No shade = no therapy;
Light shade = consider therapy;
Medium shade = probable therapy;
Dark shade = definite therapy.

noted, doing so will result in denial of the benefits of AST for an occasional patient who will otherwise experience recurrence and die. In this regard, we must make an additional set of assumptions. We will assume that there are four categories of absolute benefit for which there is consensus regarding benefits/risks (Table 5). If therapy prevents death due to breast cancer at 10 years in 10% or more of the patients, then therapy is absolutely indicated (recommendation to treat is certain). If the absolute benefit is 6%–9%, then therapy is probably indicated. AST might be considered but is not strongly recommended for those patients in a group with an absolute benefit of 4%–5%. Patients who are in a group for whom the absolute benefit is 3% or less would not be treated. It should be noted that these categories might differ based on the individual preferences of patient and physician. For example, patients might be willing to accept tamoxifen treatment for less absolute benefit, since the toxicities are less, and they might require more absolute benefit before they would consider chemotherapy.

Table 6 illustrates the decision-making process using this model, combining prognostic and predictive factors of relative strengths. In Table 6, the four categories of recommendations for AST are represented by different shading. Cells that represent absolute benefits for which treatment is certain (>10%) are indicated with dark shading. Those cells that represent probable treatment (6%–9%) are indicated by medium shading. Light shading indicates absolute benefits of 4%–5%, and cells with no shading indicate benefits that do not justify AST (1%–3%).

For patients in a very good prognostic category, AST will only prevent death due to breast cancer in 3% at most. Therefore, no matter how powerful the predictive factor used, there is no subgroup into which patients would fall in which the absolute benefit exceeds 3%. In this case, we would not recommend application of a predictive factor, since it would have no clinical utility. In contrast, overall 15% (0.30×50) of moderate-prognosis patients might be helped with AST. In this case, a weak predictive factor does not distinguish one group from another that might be more or less likely to benefit. On the other hand, a moderate predictive factor divides these patients into a factor-negative group in which therapy might be considered, but is not strongly recommended (factor-negative, 4% absolute benefit), versus a factor-positive group in which the therapy is clearly indicated (factor-positive, 11% benefit). A strong predictive factor is even more useful, dividing patients into those in whom therapy is not indicated (factor-negative, 2% benefit) and those in whom it is absolutely indicated (factor-positive, 13% benefit). Finally, for patients with a very poor prognosis, weak and moderate predictive factors divide the patients into those for whom therapy is possibly indicated (6%–9% absolute benefit) versus those for whom therapy is clearly indicated (>10% absolute benefit). However, once again, a strong predictive factor is very useful, dividing patients into those for whom treatment is not indicated versus those for whom treatment is very likely to be beneficial. Thus, prognostic and predictive factors are most helpful if they result in stark contrast between two cells in a given category.

Summary

TMUGS should help make order out of the chaos that exists in evaluation of tumor markers for clinical use. Although it seems cumbersome at first, application of this system by expert reviewers should help separate those markers for which clinical utility clearly exists from those markers for which either more data are necessary or for which further consideration can be discarded. Perhaps as important, this system may serve as a framework in which clinical and translational investigators can design studies prospectively to generate LOE I or II data, and thus hasten the acceptance of new biologic factors into routine clinical practice.

Acknowledgements. The author would like to acknowledge his co-authors on the original manuscripts in which these concepts were first proposed and discussed in greater detail. TMUGS: Drs. Robert Bast, Christopher Desch, Herbert Fritsche, Nancy Kemeny, J. Milburn Jessup, Gershon Locker, John S. Macdonald, Robert Mennel, Larry Norton, Peter Ravdin, Sheila Taube, and Rodger Winn. TMUGS Plus: Dr. Bruce Trock. The author would also like to thank Dr. Gary Clark and Dr. Adrian Harris for helpful discussions.

References

American Joint Committee on Cancer (1988) Breast. In: Beahrs OH, Henson DE, Hutter RVP, Myers MH (eds) Manual for staging of cancer, 3rd edn. Lippincott, Philadelphia, pp 145–150

ASCO Expert Panel (1996) Clinical practice guidelines for the use of tumor markers in breast and colorectal cancer: report of the American Society of Clinical Oncology Expert Panel. J Clin Oncol 14:2843–2877

Canadian Task Force on the Periodic Health Examination (1979) The periodic health examination. Can Med Assoc J 121:1193–1254

Carney W, Petit D, Hamer P, LaVecchio J, McKenzie S, Ng S (1989) Quantitation of *ras* and *neu* oncogene proteins in plasma and carcinoma cells using ELISA formats. Breast Cancer Res Treat 14:187a

Clark GM, Dressler LG, Owens MA, Pounds G, Oldaker T, McGuire WL (1989) Prediction of relapse or survival in patients with node-negative breast cancer by DNA flow cytometry. N Engl J Med 320:627–633

George SL (1994) Statistical considerations and modeling of clinical utility of tumor markers. In: Hayes DF (eds) Hematology/oncology clinics of North America: tumor markers in adult solid malignancies. Saunders, Philadelphia, pp 457–470

Hayes DF, Trock B (1998) Assessing the clinical impact of prognostic factors: statistically significant is not necessarily clinically useful. Breast Cancer Res Treat (in press)

Hayes DF, Bast R, Desch CE, Fritsche H, Kemeny NE, Jessup J, Locker GY, Macdonald J, Mennel RG, Norton L, Ravdin P, Taube S, Winn R (1996) A tumor marker utility grading system (TMUGS): a framework to evaluate clinical utility of tumor markers. J Natl Cancer Inst 88:1456–1466

Simon R, Altman DG (1994) Statistical aspects of prognostic factor studies in oncology. Br J Cancer 69:979–985

Trock B, Leonessa F, Clarke R (1997) Multidrug resistance in breast cancer: a meta-analysis of MDR1/gp170 expression and its possible functional significance. J Natl Cancer Inst 89:917–931

How Can Prognostic and Predictive Factors in Breast Cancer Be Used in a Practical Way Today?

P. M. Ravdin

Division of Oncology, University of Texas Health Sciences Center, San Antonio, Texas, USA

How prognostic and predictive factors might be used in breast cancer is intimately connected to the discussion of the treatment options available to patients today. Adjuvant therapy is only worthwhile if the improvement in outlook is great enough to more than balance the cost and toxicity of therapy. The questions to be addressed are not only whether adjuvant therapy should be given at all, but also which therapy. For example, would the incremental advantages of a given additional therapy justify its use. Basic adjuvant choices for estrogen receptor (ER)-positive and -negative patients are illustrated in Fig. 1.

Is the incremental advantage afforded by systemic adjuvant therapy worth it to an individual patient? To justify the use of systemic adjuvant therapy at all, or chemoendocrine therapy over endocrine therapy alone, the improvement in outcome must justify the cost and toxicity of such therapy. This is well illustrated by the four recent trials comparing tamoxifen to combined chemoendocrine therapy. This choice is the most common one made today since the majority of breast cancer patients are ER-positive and have a prognosis that most clinicians consider justifying some form of systemic adjuvant therapy. The relative advantage of chemoendocrine therapy over endocrine therapy alone is shown in Table 1. The degree of additional benefit conferred by chemotherapy in addition to tamoxifen in postmenopausal ER-positive women is modest, particularly in terms of overall survival. For example, in the SWOG study the overall survival at 5 years was improved from 85% to 86% just 1%, a modest gain for 6 months of CAF (cyclophosphamide, doxorubicin, and 5-fluorouracil). It must be recognized that the follow-up on these trials is short; the long-term overall survival is likely to be greater by about three-fold, but it is clear that even the long-term effects are still modest.

Further, because the overview meta-analysis (Early Breast Cancer Trialists' Collaborative Group 1992) shows that the proportional risk reductions achieved by adjuvant therapy are approximately equal in high- and low-risk patients, we know that in absolute terms patients with low-risk tumors gain much less absolute benefit than the average patient in these trials. Table 2 shows estimated mortality risks at 5 years gathered from the Surveillance, Epidemiology, and End Results (SEER) data base (Carter et al. 1989) (which

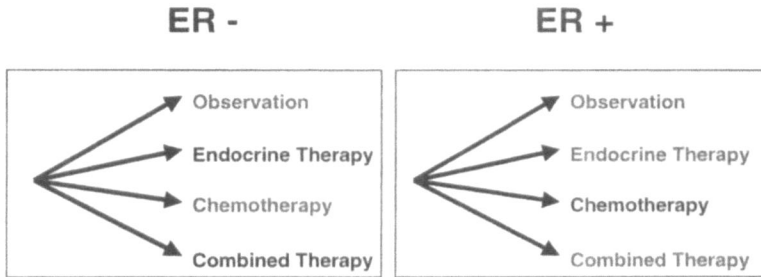

Fig. 1. Basic choices for systemic therapy of breast cancer

Table 1. Magnitude of the benefit of combined chemoendocrine therapy over tamoxifen alone at approximately 5 years' follow-up as shown in four recent clinical trials

	Disease-free survival (%)	Overall survival (%)
SWOG 8814 (Albain et al. 1997)	7	1
MA.4 (Pritchard et al. 1997)	3	2
IBCSG VII (International Breast Cancer Study Group 1997)	7	−2
NSABP B-20 (Fisher et al. 1997)	6	2

Table 2. Estimates of early breast cancer-specific mortality (in %) at 5 years, from the Surveillance, Epideriology, and End Results (SEER) data base (adapted from Carter et al. 1989)

Tumor size (cm)	No. of positive nodes		
	0	1–3	>3
<0.5	1	5	41
0.5–0.9	2	6	46
1.0–1.9	4	13	33
2.0–2.9	8	17	37
3.0–3.9	14	21	43
4.0–4.9	15	30	47
≥5.0	18	27	55

now follows about 14% of the US population) from the late 1970s and early 1980s – an era when few node-negative (NN) patients received adjuvant chemotherapy in the US. Note that NN patients with tumors measuring 1.0–1.9 cm have only a ~ 4% 5-year mortality – only about one quarter of the baseline average risk of patients in the four trials of chemoendocrine therapy mentioned here. Today, many patients in the US with these small NN tumors are treated with combined therapy, and yet the incremental benefit from combined therapy in these patients, at least using present chemotherapy regimens, is very small, often providing less than a 1% survival advantage.

Do patients understand the often modest degree of benefit that they may expect from accepting combined therapy over endocrine therapy alone? A recent survey of American patients found that only about one-quarter recalled being given a quantitative estimate of the net benefit of adjuvant therapy. Most patients had the benefit of therapy discussed in qualitative terms (Ravdin et al. 1988). This study found that even if women are not told of their prognosis they often make their own, often overly pessimistic estimates. Further, they have great faith in present adjuvant therapy, with their median estimate of efficacy that it affords an 80% proportional reduction of the risk of relapse.

Would they accept lower degrees of benefit? Coates and Simes (1992) first asked this question of Australian breast cancer patients who had finished CMF (cyclophosphamide, methotrexate, 5-fluorouracil) chemotherapy and found that, for the average Australian patient, if the chemotherapy had extended their life expectancy by only 6–12 months they would have judged it worthwhile. This result also seems true in American women and, as illustrated in Fig. 2, the average American breast cancer patient who participated in a recent survey would have felt her adjuvant chemotherapy worthwhile if it reduced her risk of breast cancer mortality by a mere 1%! It is, however, important to note that there is almost a bimodal distribution in the degree of benefit that would be felt adequate, with about 25% of the women requiring at least a 5% benefit to feel the therapy worthwhile. Because of differences in the degree of benefit felt worthwhile by different patients, adjuvant treatment guidelines rigidly applied to breast cancer patients would result in many women accepting therapy that they would not choose if they were more fully informed.

There are a number of ways to share with patients quantitative estimates of their prognoses and the absolute benefits of adjuvant therapy options. This can be done simply in the clinic by the clinician with the aid of decision boards (prepared with prognostic estimates based on tumor size and number of nodes) and computer-based tools. An example of such a tool is the program "Adjuvant"! This program makes estimates of patient prognosis primarily on the basis of information from the SEER data base (chiefly tumor size and number of nodes). It uses estimates of the effectiveness of adjuvant therapy on the basis of overview meta-analysis of adjuvant therapy, and

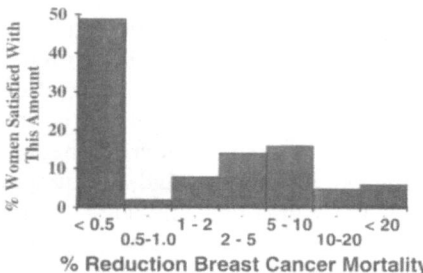

Fig. 2. Reduction in breast cancer mortality that American women regard as making adjuvant therapy worthwhile

uses estimates of national health statistics for adjusting non-breast-cancer-related mortality. The input for making prognosis estimates, illustrated in Fig. 3, is tumor size, number of involved nodes, ER data, age, and menopausal status – coincidentally all the information used in the 1995 St. Gallen adjuvant therapy guidelines.

Figure 4 shows projections for the scenarios with and without endocrine therapy for a patient. This shows projections of overall survival, breast-cancer-specific mortality, and non-breast-cancer mortality at 10 years of followup both with and without different adjuvant therapy options. Such a technique allows patients and their physicians to review the probable benefit in terms of the individual absolute percentage reduction of risk, rather than the relative proportional reduction of risk provided by the Overview analysis. It projects that at 10 years' follow-up this woman has a 57% probability of survival, 35% chance of dying of breast cancer, and an 8% chance of dying of something else. It estimates that adjuvant therapy with tamoxifen can reduce this woman's risk of breast-cancer-related mortality at 10 years by 8%. It can produce estimates for the impact of chemotherapy alone or of combined chemoendocrine therapy. At this time both decision boards' and the program Adjuvant!'s impact on doctor and patient decision making about adjuvant therapy is being evaluated in clinical studies.

A special challenge to the clinician has been which histopathologic and laboratory-based prognostic factors should be used. A major problem is that these tests are not well standardized, with major variations between centers in how the tests are done and how they are interpreted. To have any value a test must confer information that is independent of tumor size and number

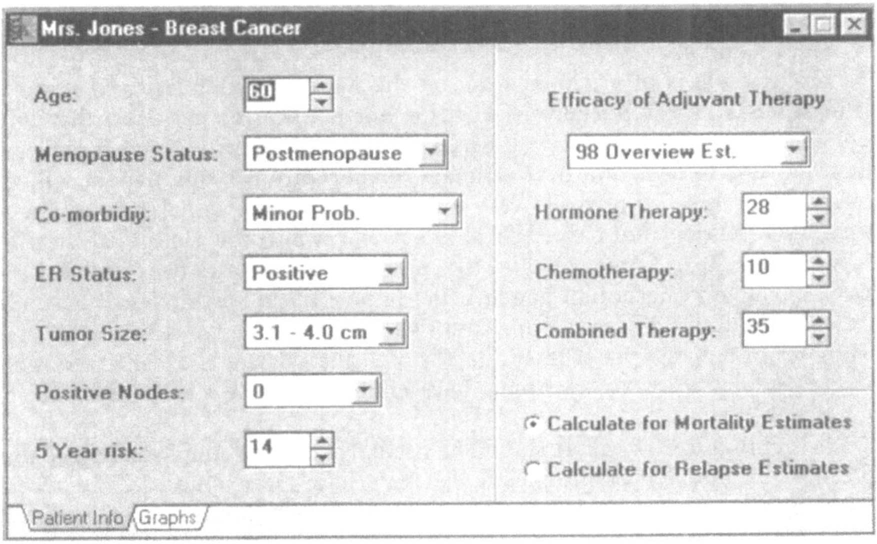

Fig. 3. Data entry for the program "Adjuvant"!

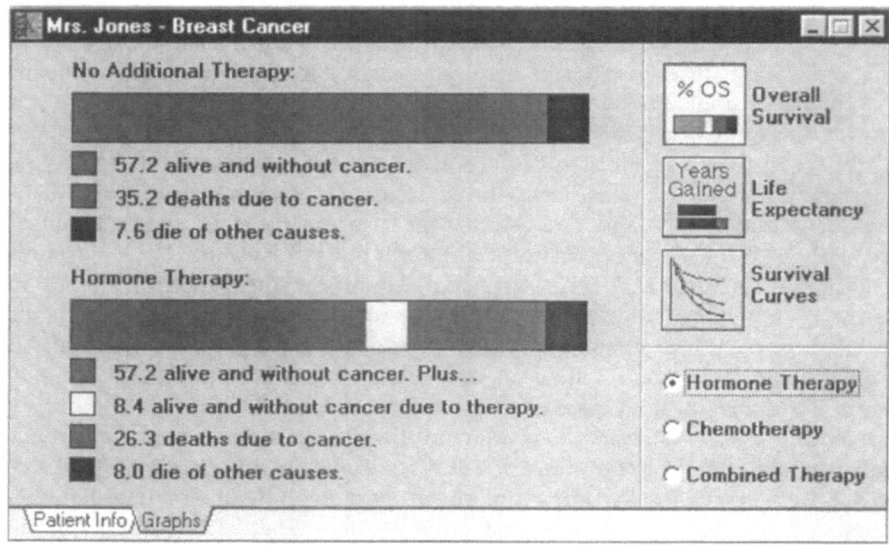

Fig. 4. Adjuvant! screen showing projections of outcome

of nodes, and it must have a big enough impact on outcome to affect clinical decision making. To use prognostic factor information you must know two crucial pieces of information. First, the independent relative risk conferred by the test: does a positive test double the relative risk or perhaps change it a more modest amount? Secondly, you must know the prevalence of a positive test result. Why both these pieces of information are important is shown in Tables 3 and 4.

This example is of a patient who, on the basis of tumor size and number of nodes, has a 10% mortality risk. If for this patient you get a test that confers an independent relative risk of 1.5 and is positive in half of all patients, after the test is done the new estimate of mortality for this patient will be either 8% or 12% – not really very different from the original 10% estimate. Thus, this test does not have clinical relevance, even if the groups are statistically distinct. Even if the relative risk conferred by a test is two-fold, but the test is positive in half of all patients, the impact on the estimates of outcome are only modestly different from 10% (7% versus 14%). For a test to change estimates of outcome by at least a factor of 2, the relative risk conferred must be greater than 2, or the test must have either a high or a low prevalence of positive results.

Which prognostic markers should be used? There is no simple answer to this question. A number of prognostic markers have been studied. The recent guideline recommendations from the 1995 St. Gallen Conference (Goldhirsch et al. 1995) and the American Society of Clinical Oncology (1996) have been remarkably conservative, endorsing no prognostic factors beyond the long-en-

Table 3. Effects of relative risk on estimates of patient outcome, in this example the impact of a prognostic variable conferring different levels of relative risk and prevalences if the variable was in the favorable (F) versus unfavorable range (U), here for patients with a 10% risk of negative outcome. In bold are shown cases with have a risk two-fold different from

Relative risk conferred	Prevalence of variable in unfavorable range (%)		
	25% U/F	50% U/F	75% U/F
1.5	8.8/13.3	8.0/12.0	7.3/10.9
2	8/16	6.7/13.3	5.7/11.4
3	6.7/20.0	5.0/15	4.0/12.0
4	5.7/22.9	4/16	3.1/12.3

Table 4. Net benefit in terms of reduction in risk for a therapy conferring a 30% proportional risk reduction of negative outcome for the patient population in Table 3 (which for the average patient in this 10% risk population would be 3%). In bold are shown cases which have a risk two-fold different from the average

Relative risk conferred	Prevalence of variable in unfavorable range (%)		
	25% U/F	50% U/F	75% U/F
1.5	2.6/4.0	2.4/3.6	2.2/3.3
2	2.4/4.8	2.0/4.0	1.7/3.4
3	2.0/6.0	1.5/4.5	4.0/3.6
4	1.7/6.9	1.2/4.8	0.9/3.7

dorsed ER and progesterone receptor tests. This conservative view is not due to there being no other markers of value, but rather in large part to the nonstandardization of techniques for their measurement and interpretation. Thus it was not possible to give a blanket endorsement to any of the measures.

There are other problems with many of the studies of prognostic factors. The most relevant of these studies evaluate the prognostic impact of various markers in patients with small NN, low-risk tumors, for it is in this population that the benefit of therapy is most marginal, and clinical decisions as to whether to give systemic adjuvant therapy or in particular adjuvant therapy with chemoendocrine are least obvious. Possibly important prognostic markers include both laboratory-based markers and information that can be obtained by light microscopy. Histopathologically determined variables like nodal status, high mitotic rate, histologic grade, and lymphatic vascular invasion represent the integration of very complex processes that are sometimes not well reflected by measuring one or two macromolecules important to those processes. The coming of high-throughput technologies such as the genomic chip may one day completely supersede pathologic variables, but this is still years in the future. Laboratory-based markers do, however, have a very special role, in that it is at the molecular level that resistance to therapy occurs.

At this time there are a number of markers of treatment resistance that have been studied. The estrogen receptor is an example of success, as a predictor of responsiveness to endocrine therapy both as therapy for metastatic disease and also in adjuvant therapy. Endocrine therapies seem at least five times more likely to have an effect if the tumor is ER-positive. We do not have such a powerful predictor for responsiveness to chemotherapy. This literature is as complex and as inconclusive as that for prognostic factors, but one marker, c-erbB-2, has generated the most interest. Even the data for this marker remain inconclusive. For example, c-erbB-2 positivity has been proposed to be a marker of relative resistance to endocrine therapy, specifically tamoxifen. The two strongest studies reach opposite conclusions as to the utility of c-erbB-2 as a predictor of responsiveness to endocrine therapy. The Italian GUN-1 study (Carlomagno et al. 1996) is a randomized trial evaluating the effectiveness of adjuvant tamoxifen in which tamoxifen was an effective adjuvant in c-erbB-2-negative patients while in c-erbB-2-positive patients it was ineffective. In contrast to this, in the largest study of metastatic disease done by the Southwest Oncology Group exclusively in ER-positive patients, c-erbB-2-negative patients were only modestly more responsive to tamoxifen that were c-erbB-2-positive patients: 57% vs 47% (Elledge et al. 1998). This would suggest that c-erbB-2 was a minor modulator of responsiveness of endocrine therapy in ER-positive patients, in many ways similar to the progesterone receptor. Thus the effectiveness of c-erbB-2 for predicting adjuvant therapy remains in doubt. An analysis of one of the very large adjuvant tamoxifen trials such as NSABP B-14 might provide definitive information. At this time denying ER-positive women possibly effective endocrine therapy on the basis of c-erbB-2 information is not supported by the clinical data, which are conflicting.

The use of c-erbB-2 to predict is also a field in which present data, while provocative, are incomplete. The strongest data come from the IBCSG trial 5 and suggest that c-erbB-2 predicts relative treatment resistance to CMF, while a provocative North American trial by the CALGB suggests that c-erbB-2 is a predictor of relative sensitivity to anthracycline-based therapy. In the IBSCG trial multiple cycles of CMF appeared to reduce the hazard of relapse for both c-erbB-2-positive and -negative patients, but more so for c-erbB-2-negative patients, although a formal statistical test between c-erbB-2 and treatment was not done to confirm the results (Gusterson et al. 1992). In the CALGB study the c-erbB-2-negative patients did not benefit from anthracycline dose intensification while c-erbB-2-positive patients did (Muss et al. 1994). However, in a second study the CALGB was unable to replicate this result, perhaps because of insufficient statistical power. Again, new data will clearly be necessary for us to really understand the role of c-erbB-2 in predicting chemosensitivity, and the application of existing results to guide therapy seems premature.

Summary

Since the 1995 St. Gallen conference the standard prognostic and predictive variables have not changed. Good treatment planning (and clinical trial entry and stratification) can be made on the basis of TNM staging, age, and ER and menopausal status. Three years from now, in 2001, this situation will have changed enormously. This will be achieved by better designs for prognostic studies, studies of predictive factors with definitive data from large, statistically powerful cooperative group trials, and perhaps simple computer-based tools to make projections and present data clearly. These advances will lead to still better-individualized selection of adjuvant therapy for breast cancer patients.

References

Albain K, Green S, Osborne K, Cobau C, Levine E, Ingle J, Pritchard K, Schneider D, O'Sullivan J, Hess E, Martino S (1997) Tamoxifen (T) versus cyclophosphamide, adriamycin, and 5-FU plus either concurrent or sequential T in postmenopausal, receptor(+) node(+) breast cancer: a Southwest Oncology Group phase III intergroup trial (SWOG-8814, INT-0100). Proc Am Soc Clin Oncol 16:128a

American Society of Clinical Oncology (1996) Clinical practice guidelines of the use of tumor markers in breast and colorectal cancer. J Clin Oncol 14:2843–2877

Carlomagno C, Perrone F, Gallo C et al. (1996) c-erbB2 overexpression decreases the benefit of tamoxifen in early-stage breast cancer without axillary lymph node metastases. J Clin Oncol 14:2702–2708

Carter CL, Allen C, Henson DE (1989) Relation of tumor size, lymph node status, and survival in 24,740 breast cancer cases. Cancer 63:181–187

Coates AS, Simes RJ (1992) Patients' assessment of adjuvant treatment in operable breast cancer. In: Williams CS (ed) Introducing new treatments for cancer: practical, ethical, and legal problems. Wiley, New York, pp 448–458

Early Breast Cancer Trialists' Collaborative Group (1992) Systemic treatment of early breast cancer by hormonal, cytotoxic, or immune therapy. Lancet 339:1–15, 71–85

Elledge RM, Green S, Ciocca D, Pugh R, Allred DC, Clark GM, Hill J, Ravdin P, O'Sullivan J, Martino S, Osborne CK (1998) HER-2 expression and response to tamoxifen in estrogen receptor-positive breast cancer: a Southwest Oncology Group Study. Clin Cancer Res 4(1):7–12

Goldhirsch A, Wood WC, Senn H-J (1995) International consensus panel on the treatment of primary breast cancer. Eur J Cancer 31A:1754–1759

Gusterson BA, Gelber RD, Goldhirsch A (1992) Prognostic importance of c-erbB-2 expession in breast cancer. International (Ludwig) Breast Cancer Study Group. J Clin Oncol 10:1049–1056

Muss HB, Thor A, Berry DA et al (1994) c-erbB-2 expression and S-phase activity predict response to adjuvant therapy in women with node-positive early breast cancer. N Engl J Med 330:1260–1266

Ravdin PM, Siminoff LA, Harvey JP (1998) What are American women told about their adjuvant therapy? J Clin Oncol 17:211–217

Strategies for the Development of Vaccines to Treat Breast Cancer

E. Jäger, D. Jäger, and A. Knuth

II. Medizinische Klinik, Hämatologie-Onkologie, Krankenhaus Nordwest,
Steinbacher Hohl 2–26, 60488 Frankfurt am Main, Germany

Background

Spontaneous regressions of human tumors have been reported in different types of cancer, especially in melanoma and renal cell carcinoma (Gromet et al. 1978; Balch et al. 1992), but also in other types of cancer such as non-small cell lung cancer, bladder carcinoma, and breast cancer. These observations suggest the interaction of the immune system with antigenic determinants presented by the tumor. Early attempts to activate the immune system against tumor growth were based on observations made in cultured melanoma cells which were shown to be lysed by autologous CD8+T lymphocytes in vitro. The clinical translation of this observation was applied to single patients with metastatic melanoma, who received irradiated autologous tumor cells as a vaccine. Two patients (SK-29 and MZ-2) with recurrent metastatic melanoma have been observed by our group since 1978 and 1982, respectively (Knuth et al. 1984). Both patients received intradermal immunization with irradiated autologous tumor cells for an extended period. Complete regression of tumor manifestations was documented after prolonged immunization with autologous tumor cells. The patients have now remained free of disease for 19 and 14 years, respectively. Based on the favorable clinical evolution in these cases, a systematic search was initiated to identify and characterize the cancer antigens and immune effector mechanisms mediating these tumor regressions in vivo (Knuth et al. 1991, 1992).

Human Tumor Antigens Recognized by the Immune System

Cancer-Testis Antigens

First, cytotoxic T lymphocytes (CTLs) that effectively lyse melanoma cells in vitro were isolated from melanoma patients (Knuth et al. 1991). Antigenic peptides were found to be presented by MHC class I and II molecules. The first antigen recognized by CTLs in an HLA-A1-restricted fashion was isolated from the melanoma tissue of patient MZ-2, designated as MAGE-1 (Van der Bruggen et al. 1991). Later, a family of MAGE-1-related genes (MAGE-1, MAGE-3, BAGE, GAGE) was identified, encoding antigens that are expressed in melanomas and several other tumors, but not in normal tissues except testis (Van der Bruggen et al. 1991; Van den Eynde et al. 1995; Gaugler et al. 1994; Brasseur et al. 1995; Traversari et al. 1992). Therefore, antigens with this pattern of expression were designated "Cancer-testis" (CT) antigens. Most recently, a new CT antigen, NY-ESO-1, was identified from esophageal cancer using a serological approach (SEREX) based on the screening of recombinant tumor cDNA libraries for specific interactions with autologous serum antibodies (Chen et al. 1997). HLA-A2 binding peptides derived from NY-ESO-1 were characterized that elicit strong CTL reactions in vitro (Jäger et al. 1998). Since NY-ESO-1 and other members of the MAGE gene family are frequently expressed in breast cancer, these antigens represent attractive targets for specific immunotherapy in breast cancer patients.

Point Mutations

Another group of potential cancer antigens is created by point mutations. These point mutations may induce strong CTL responses against tumor cells in cancer patients or experimental animals (Coulie et al. 1995; Mandelboim et al. 1994; Wölfel et al. 1995). In breast cancer, mutations of the oncogenic proteins *p53* and Ras have been reported. Spontaneously occurring humoral immune responses to the mutated and wild-type proteins have been detected in patients with breast and gastrointestinal cancer (Disis and Cheever 1996; Schlichtholz et al. 1992). In women with a family history of breast cancer, antibody responses to *p53* occur at a higher incidence than in controls (11% vs 1%) (Disis and Cheever 1996). Since the majority of *p53* antibodies detected are IgG, a preceding CD4+ T cell response to *p53* can be predicted. In a few patients with breast cancer showing accumulation of *p53* in primary tumors, a lymphoproliferative CD4+ T cell response to wild-type *p53* was demonstrated (Tilkin et al. 1995). From these observations made in a limited number of patients it may be concluded that immune responses occur after mutation of oncoproteins. These may be directed against nonmutated portions of the proteins. To date it is unknown whether *p53* as an intracellular protein is available in the extracellular cancer environment to serve as an immunotherapeutic target for humoral and/or cellular effectors to mediate tumor regression.

In animal models, mutant *p53* has been shown to elicit specific CTL responses that mediate lysis of the transformed cells. In a murine sarcoma model, it was demonstrated that vaccination with *p53* peptides combined with IL-12 leads to regression of *p53*-expressing advanced Meth A sarcomas (Noguchi et al. 1995). In many human cancers, including breast cancer, accumulation of wild-type *p53* can be detected in the cytosol. It is assumed that accumulated *p53* is effectively presented by MHC class I molecules in amounts sufficient to elicit specific CTL responses. Therefore, immune responses against wild-type *p53* may be useful in the defense of cancers with *p53* accumulation.

Ras mutations described so far involve single amino acid substitutions, mostly at positions 12 and 61. These are less complex than in *p53* and thus easier to evaluate. CD4+ and CD8+ T cell responses leading to tumor lysis can be elicited by immunization with Ras peptides containing the mutant segment in animal models (Fenton et al. 1995). In humans, it remains to be determined whether wild-type or mutant Ras protein is a useful target for active or passive therapeutic immune interventions. In a limited number of patients with pancreatic cancer, immunization with MHC class I restricted Ras peptides led to proliferative T cell responses (Gjertsen et al. 1995).

Overexpressed Antigens

Some tumor types, including breast cancer, constitutively express normal "self" proteins in abundance. The most extensively studied self antigens that serve as targets for active and passive immunotherapy are Melan A, a melanocyte differentiation antigen present in melanoma and normal melanocytes, and HER-2/neu, a growth factor receptor overexpressed in 30% of breast and ovarian cancers and a variety of other adenocarcinomas (Disis and Cheever 1996). Immune reactions directed against this type of antigen theoretically result in destruction of normal tissues. However, preliminary experiences with peptide immunization in patients with Melan-A-expressing melanomas have not shown prominent toxicity except for the development of vitiligo in a few patients (Jäger et al. 1996a). Patients with HER-2/neu-expressing tumors have been shown to produce spontaneous humoral and cellular immune responses that might be amplified by appropriate routes of immunization into a therapeutic response leading to tumor regression (Disis and Cheever 1996).

Development of Immunotherapeutic Strategies in Breast Cancer

Peptides Derived from CT Antigens as Active Immunogens?

MAGE-1- and MAGE-3-derived peptides have been used as a vaccine in HLA-A1-positive patients with tumors expressing the respective antigens to assess toxicity and immunological responses. Tumor regression responses have been observed in 5/13 melanoma patients after immunization with the MAGE-3-derived, HLA-A1 restricted peptide. CTLs against MAGE-3, however, could not be identified in response to the vaccine in these patients (Marchand et al. 1995). In a subsequent study using systemic granulocyte macrophage colony-stimulating factor (GM-CSF) to improve antigen presentation by enhancement of CD1a+ dermal Langerhans cells followed by intradermal administration of MAGE-1 and MAGE-3 peptides, a partial regression of lung metastases in a melanoma patient was achieved within 3 months of immunization (Jäger et al., unpublished data). Based on these promising results, a phase I study is currently being initiated to evaluate immune reactions to peptide vaccination in patients with MAGE-expressing breast cancer.

CTLs against the HLA-A1-restricted MAGE-1- and MAGE-3-derived peptides were repeatedly isolated from the peripheral blood of patient MZ-2, the patient from whom the MAGE-1 and MAGE-3 genes were cloned (Van der Bruggen et al. 1991; Gaugler et al. 1994). This observation strongly suggests that CTL responses are effective mediators of tumor regression, since this patient experienced a complete regression of MAGE-1- and MAGE-3-positive melanoma metastases after repeated immunization with autologous MAGE-1-/MAGE-3-positive tumor cells. During the course of repeated tumor cell vaccination, an increased incidence of CTLs recognizing autologous tumor cells was detected in the peripheral blood of this patient (Herr et al. 1994). The specificity of CTL responses, however, could not be assessed at that time, since the structure of the autologous tumor-associated antigens was not known. The fact that detection of CTL against MAGE genes in patients with MAGE-positive melanoma is rare may be attributed to either low immunogenicity of MAGE genes or a low incidence of CTL precursors. Different methods for assessing MAGE-specific CTL responses are being evaluated. One of the promising approaches appears to be the ELI spot assay, an ELISA assay that visualizes the direct antigen/T cell receptor interaction by staining the spot-like liberation of γ-interferon by the T cell reacting to a defined antigen.

Lessons from Targeting Differentiation Antigens in Melanoma

Objective tumor responses in a few melanoma patients have been observed after adoptive transfer of tumor-infiltrating lymphocyte (TIL) lines recognizing gp100/Pmel17-, tyrosinase-, and gp75-derived epitopes, suggesting that differentiation antigens can serve as tumor rejection antigens (Kawakami et al. 1994; Bakker et al. 1994; Robbins et al. 1994). To further study the effects of T cell interactions with melanocyte differentiation antigens in vitro and in vivo, we determined (a) the spontaneous CTL reactivity against HLA-A2-restricted peptides derived from the differentiation antigens Melan A/MART-1, tyrosinase, and gp100/Pmel17 in HLA-A2-positive melanoma patients and healthy individuals (Jäger et al. 1996b); (b) cellular immune responses to melanoma-associated peptides administered intradermally as a vaccine to HLA-A2-positive melanoma patients (Jäger et al. 1996a, c); and (c) changes of expression of melanoma-associated antigens and peptide-presenting MHC class I molecules in melanoma tissues showing regression or progression in the presence or absence of antigen-specific CTL responses in vivo (Jäger et al. 1997).

The baseline CTL reactivity against melanoma-associated peptides was determined in melanoma patients and healthy individuals as a basis for the development of active immunotherapeutic strategies using antigenic peptides. Spontaneous CTL reactivity against the differentiation antigens Melan A/ MART-1, tyrosinase, and gp100/Pmel17 is frequently detected in melanoma patients and healthy individuals, without providing differences in intensity and frequency of CTL responses (Jäger et al. 1996b; Rivoltini et al. 1995; Visseren et al. 1995). These findings suggest that CTL responses against self antigens occur spontaneously in individuals and may be amplified by appropriate vaccination.

Antigenic peptides derived from Melan A/MART-1, tyrosinase, or gp100/ Pmel17 were shown to induce delayed-type hypersensitivity (DTH) reactions and specific CD8+ CTL responses after intradermal immunization. The induction of objective clinical responses was associated with measurable CTL responses to the vaccine. Toxic side effects of the vaccine were not observed. Some patients with a favorable clinical development, however, developed reversible vitiligo (Jäger et al. 1996a,c).

Dermal antigen-producing cells, such as dendritic Langerhans' cells, can be stimulated by GM-CSF in vivo (Caux et al. 1992). Combined administration of melanoma-associated peptides and GM-CSF resulted in enhanced DTH reactions and CD8+ CTL responses. Immunohistochemical characterization of DTH-constituting elements showed infiltrates of CD4+ and CD8+ T lymphocytes and strong expression of IL-2 and γ-interferon, suggesting activation of CD4+ Th1 and CD8+ CTL by peptides presented by MHC class I molecules of dermal antigen-producing cells (Jäger et al. 1996c).

Immune Responses to Overexpressed Antigens in Breast Cancer

Immunity to overexpressed antigens – e.g., EGF-R, HER-2/neu – has been detected in patients with breast and gastrointestinal tract cancer (Disis and Cheever 1996; Baselga and Mendelsohn 1994). Since these antigens may also be present in normal tissues, there has been some concern about adverse immune reactions towards normal tissues elicited by immunotherapy. However, the excess expression of antigen in tumor tissues provides an increased therapeutic ratio. Studies employing passive immunotherapy with monoclonal antibodies against HER-2/neu infused into HER-2/neu transgenic mice demonstrated that tumor growth was prevented in these animals (Katsumata et al. 1995). In humans, a phase I clinical trial with a bispecific antibody binding to HER-2/neu and CD16 has demonstrated substantial toxicity and objective tumor responses (Weiner et al. 1995). Immunization trials with MHC class I- and class II-restricted HER-2/neu peptides to induce CD8+ and CD4+ T cell responses in vivo are currently underway. The results will provide further evidence of the therapeutic effect of immune responses against HER-2/neu, and will probably highlight potential adverse effects, e.g., selection of antigen-loss variants and mechanisms of escape from immune recognition.

Perspectives for Active Immunotherapy in Breast Cancer

Breast cancer has been considered only in recent years as a potential target for immunotherapeutic interventions. The growing number of tumor antigens that are expressed in breast cancer and the lessons learned from immunotherapy in malignant melanoma provide a solid base for the development of immunotherapy in breast cancer patients. CT antigens appear to be most promising targets for specific CTL responses induced by peptide or protein vaccines. The detection of spontaneous antibody responses to CT antigens in sera of breast cancer patients also suggest the spontaneous stimulation of CD4+ T cells against peptides presented by MHC class II molecules on the surface of tumor cells. The characterization of these antigens as targets for CD4+ T cell responses will allow concurrent immunization with MHC class I and class II epitopes to potentially mount more effective immune responses.

Future perspectives for tumor vaccine development are focused on more potent strategies of immunization. Vaccination with whole proteins containing multiple possibly relevant antigenic epitopes may increase the chance of multidirectional B and T cell activation. Adjuvants may enhance the immunogenicity of peptides and proteins by activating costimulatory factors and mediating the production of cytokines (Matzinger 1994). Autologous dendritic cells pulsed with peptides/proteins in vitro, or transfected with the relevant genes, may effectively activate both class I and class II restricted T lymphocytes in vivo (Alijagic et al. 1995; Schirmbeck et al. 1995). Cytokines have been identified as playing a key role in T cell activation. GM-CSF has been shown to induce long-lasting Th1 and CD8+ T cell responses by efficient activation of dendritic cells in vivo (Dranoff et al. 1993). Interleukin-12 (IL-12) is a potent activator of Th1 and CD8+ T lymphocytes. At low dose levels it has been shown to mediate complete tumor regressions when used as an adjuvant to immunization with a mutant peptide of *p53* in an animal model (Noguchi et al. 1995). The identification of further tumor antigens will give a broader basis for multidirectional immunization strategies to prevent the escape of antigen-loss variants (Jäger et al. 1996 d). Once the clinical effectiveness of cancer vaccination has become more established, immunotherapy may become another modality for the adjuvant treatment of patients with breast cancer at high risk of recurrence.

Summary

The characterization of tumor-associated antigens recognized by cellular or humoral effectors of the immune system has opened new perspectives for cancer therapy. Several categories of cancer-associated antigens have been described as targets for cytotoxic T lymphocytes (CTLs) in vitro and in vivo: "cancer-testis" (CT) antigens expressed in different tumors and normal testis, melanocyte differentiation antigens, point mutations of normal genes, antigens that are overexpressed in malignant tissues, and viral antigens. Clinical studies using peptides derived from these antigens have been initiated to induce specific CTL responses in vivo. Immunological and clinical parameters for the assessment of peptide-specific reactions have been defined, i.e., induction of delayed-type hypersensitivity (DTH), CTL, autoimmune, and tumor regression responses. Preliminary results demonstrate that tumor-associated peptides alone elicit specific DTH and CTL responses leading to tumor regression after intradermal injection. GM-CSF was proved to be effective in enhancing peptide-specific immune reactions by amplification of dermal peptide-presenting dendritic cells. Long-lasting complete tumor regressions have been observed after induction of CTLs by peptide immunization. However, in a few cases where there was disease progression after initial tumor response, loss of either the tumor antigen targeted by CTLs or of the presenting MHC class I molecule was detected as the mechanism of immune escape under immunization in vivo. Based on these observations, cytokines to enhance antigen and MHC class I expression in vivo are being evaluated to prevent immunoselection. Recently, a strategy utilizing spontaneous antibody responses to tumor-associated antigens (SEREX) has led to the identification of a new CT antigen, NY-ESO-1. In a melanoma patient with high titer antibody against NY-ESO-1, strong HLA-A2-restricted CTL reactivity against the same antigen was also found. Clinical studies involving tumor antigens that induce both antibody and CTL responses will show whether these are better candidates for immunotherapy of cancer.

References

Alijagic S, Müller P, Artuc M, Jurgovsky K, Czarnetzki BM, Schadendorf D (1995) Dendritic cells generated from peripheral blood transfected with human tyrosinase induce specific T cell activation. Eur J Immunol 25:3100–3107

Bakker AB, Schreurs MWJ, deBoer AJ, Kawakami Y, Rosenberg SA, Adema GJ, Figdor CG (1994) Melanocyte lineage-specific antigen gp100 is recognized by melanoma-derived tumor-infiltrating lymphocytes. J Exp Med 179:1005–1009

Balch CM, Houghton AN, Milton GW, Soong SJ (1992) Cutaneous melanoma. Lippincott, Philadelphia

Baselga J, Mendelsohn J (1994) The epidermal growth factor receptor as a target for therapy in breast carcinoma. Breast Cancer Res Treat 29:127–138

Brasseur F, Rimoldi D, Lienard D, Lethe B, Carrel S, Arienti F, Suter L, Vanwijck R, Bourlond A, Humblet Y, Vacca A, Conese M, Lahaye T, Degiovanni G, Deraemaecker R, Beauduin M, Sastre X, Salamon E, Dreno B, Knuth A, Jäger E, Chevreau C, Suciu S, Lachapelle J-M, Pouillart P, Parmiani G, Lejeune F, Cerottini J-C, Boon T, Marchand M (1995) Expression of MAGE genes in primary and metastatic cutaneous melanoma. Int J Cancer 63:375–380

Caux C, Dezutter-Dambuyant C, Schmitt D (1992) GM-CSF and TNFα cooperate in the generation of dendritic Langerhans cells. Nature 360:258–261

Chen Y-T, Scanlan MJ, Sahin U, Türeci Ö, Gure AO, Tsang S, Williamson B, Stockert E, Pfreundschuh M, Old LJ (1997) A testicular antigen aberrantly expressed in human cancers detected by autologous antibody screening. Proc Natl Acad Sci USA 94:1914–1918

Coulie PG, Lehmann F, Lethe B, Herman J, Lurquin C, Andrawiss M, Boon T (1995) A mutated intron sequence codes for an antigenic peptide recognized by cytolytic T lymphocytes on a human melanoma. Proc Natl Acad Sci USA 92:7976–7980

Disis ML, Cheever MA (1996) Oncogenic proteins as tumor antigens. Curr Opin Immunol 8:637–642

Dranoff G, Jaffee E, Lazenbry A, Golumbek P, Levitsky H, Brose K, Jackson V, Hamada H, Pardoll D, Mulligan R (1993) Vaccination with irradiated tumor cells engineered to secrete murine granulocyte-macrophage colony-stimulating factor stimulates potent, specific, and long-lasting anti-tumor immunity. Proc Natl Acad Sci USA 90:3539–3543

Fenton RG, Keller CJ, Hanna N, Taub DD (1995) Induction of T-cell immunity against Ras oncoprotein by soluble protein or Ras-expressing Escherichia coli. J Natl Cancer Inst 87:1853–1861

Gaugler B, Van den Eynde B, Van der Bruggen P, Romero P, Gaforio JJ, DePlaen E, Lethe B, Brasseur F, Boon T (1994) Human gene MAGE-3 codes for an antigen recognized on a melanoma by autologous cytolytic T lymphocytes. J Exp Med 179:921–930

Gjertsen MK, Bakka A, Breivik J, Saeterdal I, Solheim BG, Soreide O, Thorsby E, Gaudernack G (1995) Vaccination with mutant Ras peptides and induction of T-cell responsiveness in pancreatic carcinoma patients carrying the corresponding Ras mutation. Lancet 346:1399–1400

Gromet MA, Epstein WL, Blois MS (1978) The regressing thin malignant melanoma: a distinctive lesion with metastatic potential. Cancer 42:2282–2292

Herr W, Wölfel T, Heike M, Meyer zum Büschenfelde K-H, Knuth A (1994) Frequency analysis of tumor-reactive cytotoxic T lymphocytes in peripheral blood of a melanoma patient vaccinated with autologous tumor cells. Cancer Immunol Immunother 39:93–99

Jäger E, Bernhard H, Romero P, Ringhoffer M, Arand M, Karbach J, Ilsemann C, Hagedorn M, Knuth A (1996a) Generation of cytotoxic T cell responses with synthetic melanoma associated peptides in vivo: implications for tumor vaccines with melanoma associated antigens. Int J Cancer 66:162–169

Jäger E, Ringhoffer M, Arand M, Karbach J, Jäger D, Ilsemann C, Hagedorn M, Oesch F, Knuth A (1996b) Cytolytic T cell reactivity against melanoma associated differentiation antigens in peripheral blood of melanoma patients and healthy individuals. Melanoma Res 6:419–425

Jäger E, Ringhoffer M, Dienes H-P, Arand M, Karbach J, Jäger D, Ilsemann C, Hagedorn M, Oesch F, Knuth A (1996c) Granulocyte macrophage colony-stimulating factor enhances immune responses to melanoma associated peptides in vivo. Int J Cancer 67:54–62

Jäger E, Ringhoffer M, Karbach J, Arand M, Oesch F, Knuth A (1996d) Inverse relationship of melanocyte differentiation antigen expression in melanoma: evidence for immunoselection of antigen-loss variants in vivo. Int J Cancer 66:470–476

Jäger E, Ringhoffer M, Karbach J, Arand M, Oesch F, Jäger D, Knuth A (1997) Immunoselection in vivo: independent loss of MHC class I and melanocyte differentiation antigen expression in metastatic melanoma mediated by antigen-specific CTL. Int J Cancer 71:142–147

Jäger E, Chen Y-T, Drijfhout JW, Karbach J, Ringhoffer M, Jäger D, Arand M, Wada H, Noguchi Y, Stockert E, Old LJ, Knuth A (1998) Simultaneous humoral and cellular immune response against cancer-testis antigen NY-ESO-1: definition of human histocompatibility leucocyte antigen (HLA)-A2-binding peptide epitopes. J Exp Med 187:265–269

Katsumata M, Okudaira T, Samanta A, Clark DP, Drebin JA, Joliceur P, Greene MI (1995) Prevention of breast tumour development in vivo by downregulation of the p185neu receptor. Nat Med 1:644–648

Kawakami Y, Eliyahu S, Delgado CH, Robbins PF, Sakaguchi K, Appella E, Yannelli JR, Adema GJ, Miki T, Rosenberg SA (1994) Identification of a human melanoma antigen recognized by tumor-infiltrating lymphocytes associated with in vivo tumor rejection. Proc Natl Acad Sci USA 91:6458–6462

Knuth A, Danowski B, Oettgen HF, Old LJ (1984) T-cell-mediated cytotoxicity against autologous malignant melanoma: analysis with interleukin-2-dependent T-cell cultures. Proc Natl Acad Sci USA 81:3511–3515

Knuth A, Wölfel T, Meyer zum Büschenfelde K-H (1991) Cellular and humoral responses against cancer: implications for cancer vaccines. Curr Opin Immunol 3:659–664

Knuth A, Wölfel T, Meyer zum Büschenfelde K-H (1992) T cell responses to human malignant tumors. Cancer Surv 13:39–52

Mandelboim O, Berke G, Fridkin M, Feldman M, Eisenstein M, Eisenbach L (1994) CTL induction by a tumour-associated antigen octapeptide derived from a murine lung carcinoma. Nature 369:67–71

Marchand M, Weymants P, Rankin E, Arienti F, Belli F, Parmiani G, Cascinelli N, Bourlond A, Vanwijck R, Humblet Y, Canon J-L, Laurent C, Naeyaert J-M, Plagne R, Deraemaeker R, Knuth A, Jäger E, Brasseur F, Herman J, Coulie PG, Boon T (1995) Tumor regression responses in melanoma patients treated with a peptide encoded by gene MAGE-3. Int J Cancer 63:883–885

Matzinger P (1994) Tolerance, danger, and the extended family. Annu Rev Immunol 12:991–1045

Noguchi Y, Richards EC, Chen YT, Old LJ (1995) Influence of interleukin-12 on p53 peptide vaccination against established Meth A sarcoma. Proc Natl Acad Sci USA 92:2219–2223

Rivoltini L, Kawakami Y, Sakaguchi K, Southwood S, Sette A, Robbins PF, Marincola FM, Salgaller ML, Yannelli JR, Appella E, Rosenberg SA (1995) Induction of tumor-reactive CTL from peripheral blood and tumor-infiltrating lymphocytes of melanoma patients by in vitro stimulation with an immunodominant peptide of the human melanoma antigen MART-1. J Immunol 154:2257–2265

Robbins PF, El-Gamil M, Kawakami Y, Rosenberg SA (1994) Recognition of tyrosinase by tumor-infiltrating lymphocytes from a patient responding to immunotherapy. Cancer Res 54:3124–3126

Schirmbeck R, Melber K, Reimann J (1995) Hepatitis B virus small surface antigen particles are processed in a novel endosomal pathway for major histocompatibility complex class I-restricted epitope presentation. Eur J Immunol 25:1063–1070

Schlichtholz B, Legros Y, Gillet D, Gaillard C, Marthy M, Lane D, Calvo F, Soussi T (1992) Antibodies against p53 in breast cancer patients are directed against immunodominant epitopes unrelated to the mutational hot spot. Cancer Res 52:6380–6384

Tilkin AF, Lubin R, Soussi T, Lazar V, Janin N, Mathieu MC, Lefrere I, Carlu C, Roy M, Kayibanda M (1995) Primary proliferative T cell response to wild-type p53 protein in patients with breast cancer. Eur J Immunol 25:1765–1769

Traversari C, Van der Bruggen P, Luescher IF, Lurquin C, Chomez P, Van Pel A, DePlaen E, Amarcostesec A, Boon T (1992) A nonapeptide encoded by human gene MAGE-1 is recognized on HLA-A1 by cytolytic T-lymphocytes directed against tumor antigen MZ2-E. J Exp Med 176:1453–1457

Van den Eynde B, Peeters O, De Backer O, Gaugler B, Lucas S, Boon T (1995) A new family of genes coding for an antigen recognized by autologous cytolytic T lymphocytes on a human melanoma. J Exp Med 182:689–698

Van der Bruggen P, Traversari C, Chomez P, Lurquin C, De Plaen E, Van den Eynde B, Knuth A, Boon T (1991) A gene encoding an antigen recognized by cytolytic T lymphocytes on a human melanoma. Science 254:1643–1647

Visseren MJW, Van Elsas A, Van der Voort EIH, Ressing ME, Kast WM, Schrier PI, Melief CJM (1995) CTL specific for the tyrosinase autoantigen can be induced from healthy donor blood to lyse melanoma cells. J Immunol 154:3991–3998

Weiner LM, Clark JI, Davey M, Li WS, Garcia-de-Palazzo I, Ring DB, Alpaugh RK (1995) Phase I trial of 2B1, a bispecific monoclonal antibody targeting c-erbB-2 and Fc gamma RIII. Cancer Res 55:4586–4593

Wölfel T, Hauer M, Schneider J, Serrano M, Wölfel C, Klehmann-Hieb E, DePlaen E, Hankeln T, Meyer zum Büschenfelde K-H, Beach D (1995) A p16INK4a-insensitive CDK4 mutant targeted by cytolytic T lymphocytes in a human melanoma. Science 269:1281–1284

IV. In Situ Breast Cancer

Hypothesis and Practice: Are There Several Types of Treatment for Ductal Carcinoma In Situ of the Breast?

M. J. Silverstein[1*] and R. Masetti[2]

[1] The Breast Center, 14624 Sherman Way, Sixth Floor, Van Nuys, CA 91405, USA
[2] Department of Surgery, Catholic University, Largo A. Gemelli 8, 00168 Rome, Italy

The Question

The question is straightforward: Are there several types of treatment for ductal carcinoma in situ (DCIS) of the breast? If that question had been asked 15 or 20 years ago, the answer would have been a simple "no". At that time, the heterogeneity of the disease was not widely appreciated and most patients with DCIS were treated with mastectomy. The answer today is just as simple, but it is now "yes" rather than no.

There are multiple treatments for DCIS and there should be. DCIS is a biologically and histologically heterogeneous group of lesions with diverse malignant potential (Lennington et al. 1994; Patchefsky et al. 1989). There is no reason why a single treatment should be appropriate for all cases. Far more difficult issues arise as one tries to pinpoint the most appropriate treatment for an individual patient, however. For most patients with DCIS today, there will be more than one acceptable treatment, depending on a range of clinical parameters and personal agendas.

Changing Times

Mammography has changed the way DCIS is detected and the nature of the disease found by allowing clinicians to enter the neoplastic continuum at an earlier time. During the same time period, the acceptance of breast-conserving therapy for invasive breast cancer has gradually changed the way DCIS is treated.

Table 1 shows the changing nature of DCIS during the last two decades. Since 1983, the number of new cases of DCIS has increased more than 500% (Ernster et al. 1996) and the presentation has changed. Before mammography became a yearly routine for many women, DCIS was rare, representing less than 1% of all newly diagnosed breast cancers (Nemoto et al. 1980). Today, DCIS is

---

* *Current address:* Department of Surgery, University of Southern California School of Medicine, Los Angeles, CA 90033, USA.

Table 1. Ductal carcinoma in situ: a changing disease

	Before 1985	After 1985
Incidence	Unusual	Common
Presentation	Palpable	Nonpalpable
Diagnosis	Clinical	Mammographic
Classification	Architectural	Biologic
Treatment	Mastectomy	Breast conservation
Reconstruction	None/delayed	Immediate
Confusion	None	Great

common. In 1997, there were more than 36 000 new cases of DCIS in the United States (Parker et al. 1997), representing 17% of all newly diagnosed cases of breast cancer. In centers that rely on mammography, DCIS may represent as much as 20%–40% of all newly diagnosed cases of breast cancer.

Twenty years ago, most patients with DCIS presented with clinical symptoms, such as a breast mass, bloody or serous nipple discharge, or Paget's disease. Today, most lesions are nonpalpable, clinically unapparent, and detected by mammography alone.

Until recently, the treatment for most patients was mastectomy. Today, the majority of patients with DCIS are treated with breast preservation. Fifteen years ago, when mastectomy was common, reconstruction was uncommon and, if performed, it was generally done as a delayed procedure with implants. Today, reconstruction for patients with DCIS treated by mastectomy is common and, when performed, it is generally done immediately, at the time of mastectomy and often with autologous tissue. In the past, when a mastectomy was performed, large amounts of skin were discarded. Today, it is considered safe to perform a skin-sparing mastectomy for DCIS (Jensen et al. 1996; Kroll et al. 1991; Singletary 1995).

In the past, there was no confusion. All breast cancers were generally grouped together and mastectomy was the only treatment. Today, we appreciate that all breast cancers are different. There are multiple treatment choices and, because of this, there may be great confusion. With the appreciation and acceptance of the heterogeneity of DCIS, management has become perplexing for both patients and physicians. Currently, it is not uncommon for DCIS patients to seek multiple opinions and to receive a diverse spectrum of advice ranging from biopsy only to wide excision, segmental resection, quadrant resection to mastectomy. With all treatments other than mastectomy, radiation therapy may be advised.

These changes were brought about by numerous factors, the most important of which were increased use of mammography, the improvement in mammographic technique, and the acceptance of breast conservation therapy for invasive breast cancer.

Pathology of DCIS

In April 1997, a DCIS Pathology Consensus Conference was held at Jefferson Medical College in Philadelphia, Pennsylvania, USA. Agreement was reached regarding a number of basic pathology issues, such as the need to record margin width, tumor extent, nuclear grade, architecture, cell polarization, etc. But there was no consensus on a single unified classification for DCIS (Schwartz et al. 1998).

Pathologists generally divide DCIS into five architectural subtypes (papillary, micropapillary, cribriform, solid, and comedo), often grouping the first four together as noncomedo and contrasting them with comedo. Comedo DCIS is generally associated with high nuclear grade, aneuploidy (Aasmundstad and Haugen 1992), a higher proliferation rate (Meyer 1986), HER2/neu (c-erbB2) gene amplification or protein overexpression (Barnes et al. 1991; Bartkova et al. 1990) and clinically more aggressive behavior (Lagios et al. 1989; Schwartz1994). Noncomedo lesions tend to be the opposite. However, a division by architecture, comedo versus noncomedo, is an oversimplification and is not applicable in all cases. Classification based solely on architecture should not be used for the following reasons.

Any architectural subtype may present with any nuclear grade with or without comedo-type necrosis. It is not uncommon for high nuclear grade noncomedo lesions to express markers similar to high grade comedo lesions and to behave like high grade comedo lesions. Furthermore, mixtures of various architectural subtypes within a single biopsy specimen are common. In the Van Nuys series, approximately 70% of all lesions had significant amounts of two or more different architectural subtypes. Adding to the confusion, there is no uniform agreement among pathologists of exactly how much comedo-type necrosis needs to be present to consider the lesion a comedo DCIS.

To complicate matters further, before a lesion is called a comedo DCIS, many pathologists require the cells to be of high nuclear grade (grade 3) and their growth pattern to be solid. However, some pathologists will allow nuclear grade 2 lesions with significant comedo necrosis to be signed out as comedo DCIS; some may even allow a nuclear grade 1 lesion to be called comedo DCIS. Others will allow a cribriform or micropapillary architectural pattern with significant comedo necrosis to be called comedo DCIS.

The point is clear. Architecture is a poor way to classify DCIS. It is similar to comparing houses by their design. It is not the external architecture that is most important; rather, it is the contents that are key. Current classification systems should be based on factors that reflect the biologic potential of each individual lesion – in other words, the cellular content rather than the arrangement of the cells.

Nuclear grade, comedo-type necrosis, tumor size, and margin width are all important predictors of the probability of local recurrence after breast-conserving treatment (Bellamy et al. 1993; Fisher et al. 1995; Lagios et al. 1989; Silverstein et al. 1995a, b, 1996; Silverstein 1997b; Solin et al. 1993).

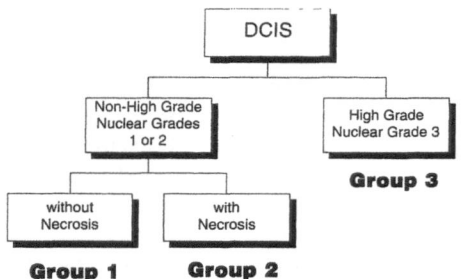

Fig. 1. Van Nuys pathologic classification of ductal carcinoma in situ (DCIS). DCIS patients are sorted into high nuclear grade and non-high nuclear grade. Non-high nuclear grade cases are then sorted by the presence or absence of comedo-type necrosis. Lesions in group 3 (high nuclear grade) may or may not show comedo-type necrosis (Silverstein et al. 1995a)

Two of these factors, nuclear grade and comedo-type necrosis, were used to develop the simple, reproducible (Douglas-Jones et al. 1996) Van Nuys classification (Fig. 1), (Silverstein et al. 1995a). In the Van Nuys classification, high nuclear grade lesions, with or without comedo-type necrosis, are grouped into the worst prognostic category (group 3). Patients with non-high grade lesions (nuclear grade 1 or 2) are then divided according to the presence of necrosis (group 2, an intermediate group) or its absence (group 1, the best prognostic group). This pathologic classification yield three different subgroups of DCIS patients with significantly different rates of local recurrence (Silverstein et al. 1995a). But histologic classification, regardless of which one is used, will never be adequate by itself for determining proper treatment. A small aggressive-appearing lesion may be adequately treated by excision alone if the margins are widely clear, whereas a large although unaggressive-appearing lesion with margin involvement may be better treated by mastectomy with immediate reconstruction. Clearly, factors in addition to morphologic appearance must be considered when planning treatment (Silverstein et al. 1996; Cancer, Silverstein 1997b) (see Van Nuys Prognostic Index below).

Is DCIS Really Breast Cancer?

There is no easy way to tell a patient that she has breast cancer. But is DCIS really breast cancer? When one thinks of cancer, we think of a disease that, if untreated, generally runs an unrelenting course toward death. That is certainly not the natural history of DCIS. The fully expressed malignant phenotype is made up of at least five factors: unlimited growth, genomic elasticity (the ability to change and resist treatment), angiogenesis, invasion, and metastasis (Dickson and Lippman 1995; Lippman 1993). DCIS, to the best of our ability to tell, lacks the latter two factors. In all likelihood, when we understand why some DCIS lesions become invasive and metastasize and others do not, the pathway to far greater understanding of the neoplastic process will have been widened.

When counseling a patient with DCIS, it must be emphasized that she has a borderline lesion, a noninvasive lesion which, at this time, is not a threat to her life. In the Van Nuys series of 733 patients with DCIS, the absolute mortality rate is 0.7%. The 8-year actuarial breast-cancer-specific mortality rate is 0% for mastectomy patients, 1.4% for all patients, and 2.1% for breast-preservation patients (Silverstein et al. 1998b). Numerous other DCIS series (Ashikari et al. 1971; Fisher et al. 1993; Solin et al. 1996) confirm an extremely low mortality rate for DCIS.

One of the most frequent concerns expressed by patients once a diagnosis of cancer has been made is the fear that the cancer has spread. The patient with DCIS whose excision specimens have been completely and sequentially processed can be assured that no invasion was seen microscopically and that the likelihood of systemic spread is minuscule.

The patient needs to be educated that the term "breast cancer" encompasses a wide variety of lesions with a wide range of aggressiveness and lethal potential. The patient with DCIS must be, and needs to be, reassured that she has a minimal lesion and that she may need some additional treatment, which might include further surgery or radiation therapy or both. She needs to know that she will not need chemotherapy, that her hair will not fall out, and that it is highly unlikely that she will die from this lesion. She will, of course, also need careful clinical follow-up.

Treatment of DCIS

For many patients, there will be no single correct treatment approach. There will generally be a choice and the options, although seemingly simple, are not. As the treatment alternatives increase and become more complicated, frustration will increase for both patient and physician.

Numerous ongoing prospective randomized trials are currently in progress (Recht 1997a). Only the one performed by the National Surgical Adjuvant Breast Project (NSABP) (protocol B-17) has been published (Fisher et al. 1993). The results of B-17 were updated in 1995 (Fisher et al. 1995) and 1998 (Fisher et al. 1998). More than 800 patients with DCIS excised with clear surgical margins were randomized into two groups: excision only versus excision plus radiation therapy. The NSABP defines a surgical margin as clear when the tumor has not been transected. In other words, only a few fat cells need be present between DCIS and the inked margins to consider that margin clear. After 8 years of follow-up, there was a statistically significant decrease in local recurrence of both DCIS and invasive breast cancer in patients treated with radiation therapy. The overall local recurrence rate for patients treated by excision only was 27% at 8 years. For patients treated with excision plus irradiation, it was 12% (Fisher et al. 1998). These updated data led the NSABP to stand by their 1993 position and to continue to recommend postoperative radiation therapy for all patients with DCIS who chose to save their breasts. B-17 has been criticized for a number of reasons (Lagios and Page 1993; Page and Lagios 1995), the most important being a lack of pathologic subset analysis in the initial report. Other problems with B-17 include: the lack of size measurements in more than 40% of cases in the original publication, no requirement for mammographic/pathologic correlation or specimen radiography, no uniform guidelines for tissue processing or size estimation, and the NSABP's controversial definition of what constitutes a clear margin. Margins were defined in such a way that outcome differences analyzed by clear versus involved margins could easily be obscured.

In defense of the NSABP, their trial was designed more than 14 years ago, at a time when researchers were asking a single broad question: Does radiation therapy benefit patients with DCIS treated with breast preservation? The NSABP has answered that question and the answer is yes. The NSABP study, however, was not designed to answer the more difficult questions we ask today. For example, exactly which subgroups benefit from radiation therapy and by how much? If the benefit in a defined subgroup is only a few percent, the advantage gained by radiation therapy may be offset by its cost and disadvantages.

Radiation therapy is expensive, time-consuming, and is accompanied by significant side effects in a small percentage of patients (cardiac, pulmonary, etc.) (Recht 1997b). Radiation fibrosis of the breast is a more common side effect, particularly with the type of radiation therapy given during the 1980s. This complication changes the texture of the breast and skin, makes mammographic follow-up more difficult, and may result in delayed diagnosis if there is a local recurrence. The use of radiation therapy for DCIS precludes its use if an invasive recurrence develops at a later date, since the skin and vascular changes that accompany radiation therapy make skin-spearing mastectomy, if needed in the future, more difficult to perform. Clinicians must therefore be secure that the benefits of radiation therapy, in terms of improved recurrence-free survival, will significantly outweigh the side effects, complications, inconvenience, and costs for a given subgroup of patients.

Consider the following two patients, both of whom meet NSABP B-17 criteria and would receive postoperative radiation therapy if treated according to current NSABP recommendations. The first is a woman with a 19-mm low-grade DCIS widely excised with a minimum of 15-mm margins in all directions. Compare her with the second patient, a woman with a 15-mm high-grade lesion in which DCIS approaches to within 0.1 mm of the inked margin but does not involve it. According to the NSABP, both of these patients should be treated with radiation therapy and neither one needs re-excision. At my facility, the first patient would receive no additional therapy. She would be carefully followed with physical examination and mammography every 6 months. The second patient would undergo a wide re-excision before a final treatment decision was made. If significant residual disease approaching the new margins was found, a recommendation for mastectomy and immediate reconstruction would be made; if widely clear new margins with little or no residual DCIS was found, a recommendation for breast conservation would be given. The Van Nuys Prognostic Index, discussed below, explains why I would make those recommendations.

Breast conservation therapy for DCIS ranges from simple excision to various forms of wider excision (segmental resection, quadrant resection, etc.), all of which may or may not be followed by radiation therapy. If breast preservation is not an option, then mastectomy, with or without immediate reconstruction, is generally performed. Since DCIS is a heterogeneous group of lesions rather than a single entity, and because patients have a wide variety of personal needs that must be considered during treatment selection, it is obvious that no single approach will be appropriate for all forms of the disease or for all patients. Methods must be employed to determine the most appropriate treatment for each individual patient.

The most benign-appearing forms of DCIS (for example, low nuclear grade, small-celled without necrosis, estrogen- and progesterone-receptor-positive, c-erbB2-negative, etc.), if untreated, may never cause clinical disease. Less than 50% of low-grade lesions develop into invasive breast cancer over a 25- to 30-year period (Page et al. 1995), leading clinicians to question whether low-grade DCIS should be classified as cancer. Alternatively, the most aggressive-appearing forms of DCIS (high nuclear grade, large-celled with comedo-type necrosis, c-erbB2-positive, etc.), if left untreated, are much more likely to develop into invasive carcinomas in significantly shorter time periods.

The most important question today is which lesions, if untreated, are going to become invasive breast cancer? And how long will it take for this to happen? Are there markers that can be used to predict this? If treated conservatively, which lesions have such high rates of local recurrence, regardless of radiation therapy, that mastectomy is the preferred treatment? When mastectomy is not required, which patients can be treated with excision alone and which ones need postoperative radiation therapy? The questions are simple; the answers are not.

Treatment of the Axilla in Patients with DCIS

There is now general agreement that, for patients with DCIS, the axilla does not need treatment (Hansen and Giuliano 1997; Silverstein et al. 1987). In Van Nuys, the axilla is not treated in patients with DCIS undergoing breast conservation. It is not irradiated and no form of axillary sampling or dissection is performed. (For patients treated with excision plus postoperative radiation therapy, the lower axilla is included in the tangential fields to the breast.)

For patients undergoing mastectomy, our group generally performs a sentinel node biopsy using a vital blue dye, radioactive tracer, or both at the time of mastectomy (Krag et al. 1993; Giuliano et al. 1995; Albertini et al. 1996). This is done in the event that permanent sectioning of the mastecto-

my specimen reveals one or more foci of invasion. If invasion is documented, no matter how small, the lesion is no longer considered DCIS but rather
as an invasive cancer. The sentinel node or nodes are evaluated by hematoxylin and eosin (H&E) staining followed by immunohistochemistry for cytokeratin when routine H&E stains are negative.

The Van Nuys Prognostic Index

As mentioned above, histologic classification by itself yields insufficient information for determining proper treatment. Two additional factors, tumor
size and margin width, are also independent predictors of local recurrence in
patients with conservatively treated DCIS (Silverstein et al. 1995a,b, 1996; Lagios et al. 1989; Solin et al. 1993; Bellamy et al. 1993; Silverstein 1997b; Fisher et al. 1995). It may be possible, by using a combination of these three factors, to select subgroups of patients who do not require irradiation if breast
conservation is elected, or to select patients whose recurrence rate is so high,
even with breast irradiation, that mastectomy is preferable.

As previously discussed, nuclear grade and comedo-type necrosis were
used to develop the Van Nuys Pathologic Classification (Silverstein et al.
1995a). Nuclear grade and comedo-type necrosis reflect the biology of the
DCIS but are inadequate as sole guidelines in the treatment selection process. Tumor size and margin width reflect the distribution of the disease and
the surgeons ability to adequately excise the disease. The Van Nuys Prognostic Index (VNPI) (Silverstein et al. 1996; Silverstein 1997c) was developed by
combining these three factors. Table 2 shows the VNPI scoring system.
Scores from 1 to 3 were given for each of the three different predictors of local breast recurrence (tumor size, margin width, and pathologic classification). The scores for each predictor for each individual patient were totaled
to yield a VNPI score ranging from a low of 3 to a high of 9 for a group of
461 patients with DCIS treated with breast preservation (our series updated

Table 2. Van Nuys Prognostic Index scoring system. One to three points are awarded for each of threedifferent predictors of local breast recurrence (size, margin width, and pathologic classification). Scores for each of the predictors are totaled to yield a VNPI score ranging from a low of 3 to a high of 9 (Silverstein et al. 1996)

	Score		
	1	2	3
Size (mm)	≤15	16–40	≥41
Margins (mm)	≥10	1–9	<1
Pathologic classification	Non-high grade without necrosis (nuclear grades 1, 2)	Non-high grade with necrosis (nuclear grades 1, 2)	High grade with or without necrosis (nuclear grade 3)

through 1997). Figure 2 shows all 461 patients divided into three subgroups by score (3 or 4 versus 5, 6 or 7 versus 8 or 9). The probability of local recurrence is significantly different for each subgroup. More importantly, patients with low VNPI scores (3 or 4) showed no difference in local recurrence-free survival at 8 years regardless of whether or not they received radiation therapy (Fig. 3) and can be considered for treatment with excision only. Patients with intermediate scores (5, 6, or 7) showed a statistically significant decrease in local recurrence rates with radiation therapy (Fig. 4). Conservatively treated patients with VNPI scores of 8 or 9 had unacceptably high local recurrence rates, regardless of irradiation (Fig. 5), and should be considered for mastectomy.

The VNPI is a numerical algorithm based on tumor features and recurrence data from a large series of DCIS patients. It permits quantification of easily measured prognostic factors, in a reproducible fashion, separating DCIS patients into three clearly defined risk groups. It was designed to be usable with the resources of any hospital and to permit a more rational approach to the treatment of DCIS. The VNPI was designed to be used in conjunction with, and not instead of, clinical experience and prospective randomized data. As with all such aids to treatment planning, the VNPI will need to be independently validated.

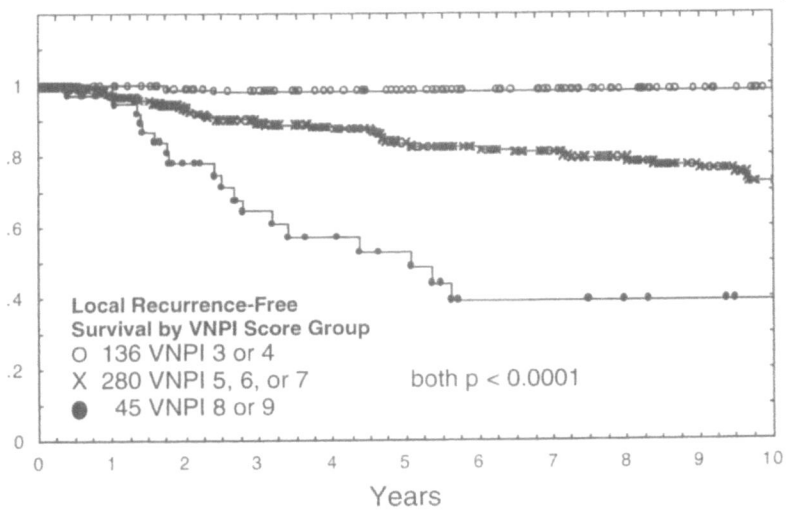

Fig. 2. Probability of local recurrence-free survival for 461 breast conservation patients grouped by Van Nuys Prognostic Index score (3 or 4 versus 5, 6 or 7 versus 8 or 9) (all p <0.0001)

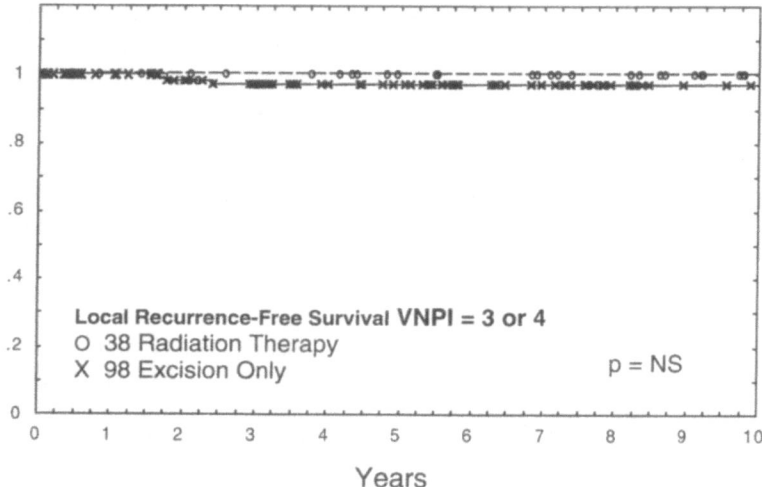

Fig. 3. Probability of local recurrence-free survival for 136 breast conservation patients with Van Nuys Prognostic Index scores of 3 or 4 grouped by treatment (p = NS)

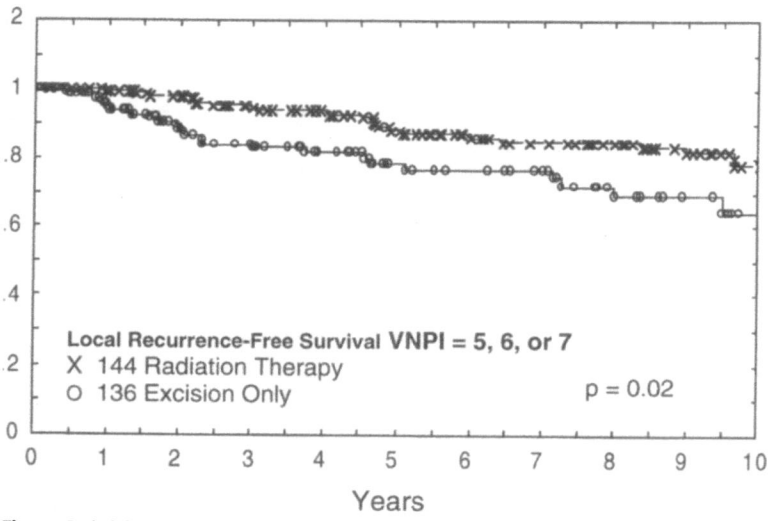

Fig. 4. Probability of local recurrence-free survival for 280 breast conservation patients with Van Nuys Prognostic Index scores of 5, 6 or 7 grouped by treatment ($p = 0.02$)

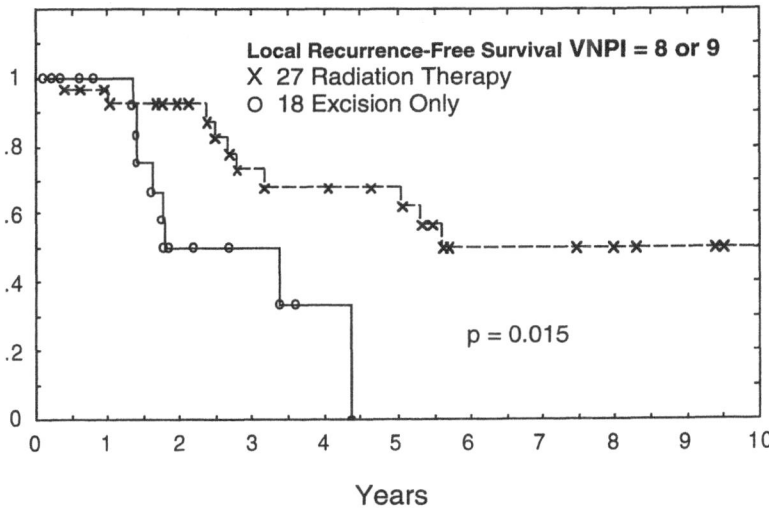

Fig. 5. Probability of local recurrence-free survival for 45 breast conservation patients with Van Nuys Prognostic Index scores of 8 or 9 grouped by treatment (p = 0.015)

Histologic Excision Margins

When the pathologist reports that the inked margins of a specimen are free of disease, what does that mean? Currently, there is no consensus on what constitutes a clear margin; different researchers use different criteria. The reporting pathologist must clearly spell out what is meant by a clear margin.

Does a clear margin mean that the entire lesion has been excised? Not necessarily. Serial subgroup evaluation of the whole breast in patients with DCIS (Holland and Faverly 1997) has revealed that the wider the margin, the lower the likelihood of residual disease. Faverly et al. (1995) suggest that 10 mm would be an excellent choice for clear margins. Using serial subgross technique, they showed that only 8% of DCIS lesions have gaps (skip lesions) greater than 10 mm.

A good solution in describing margins might be to measure margin width in every case rather than to simply report "clear" or "involved". Margin width, the distance between DCIS and the closest inked margin, reflects the completeness of excision. Although the multivariate analysis used to derive the VNPI suggests approximately equal importance for the three significant factors (margin width, tumor size, and histologic classification), the fact that DCIS can be thought of in halstedian terms suggests that margin width should indeed be the single most important factor. In other words, since DCIS is a noninvasive lesion without the ability to invade and metastasize (two critically important components of the fully expressed malignant phenotype), complete excision should cure the lesion. At this point in time, the best way to access complete excision is by margin width.

Table 3. Eight-year probability of local recurrence by treatment and then further subdivided by margin width and additionally by the presence of comedo-type necrosis

	Excision + radiation	Excision only	p value
Number of patients (n=461)	209	252	
Local recurrence rate (all patients)	16%	22%	0.04
Margins≥10 mm (n=131)	4%	5%	NS
Margins=1–9 mm (n=223)	12%	19%	0.05
Margins<1 mm (n=107)	29%	63%	0.002
Eight-year actuarial local recurrence rate by nuclear grade and margin width:			
Nuclear grade 1 (low nuclear grade) (n=100)			
Margins≥10 mm (n=33)	0%	0%	NS
Margins=1–9 mm (n=59)	6%	7%	NS
Margins<1 mm (n=8)	25%	50%	NS
Nuclear grade 2 (intermediate nuclear grade) (n=176)			
Margins≥10 mm (n=42)	10%	0%	NS
Margins=1–9 mm (n=93)	7%	11%	NS
Margins<1 mm (n=41)	23%	44%	NS
Nuclear grade 3 (high nuclear grade) (n=185)			
Margins≥10 mm (n=56)	0%	6%	NS
Margins=1–9 mm (n=71)	25%	39%	NS
Margins<1 mm (n=58)	36%	73%	0.01
Eight-year actuarial local recurrence rate by comedonecrosis and margin width			
Comedonecrosis present (n=286)			
Margins≥10 mm (n=78)	7%	3%	NS
Margins=1–9 mm (n=124)	16%	30%	0.04
Margins<1 mm (n=84)	31%	68%	0.003
Comedonecrosis absent (n=175)			
Margins≥10 mm (n=53)	0%	7%	NS
Margins=1–9 mm (n=99)	9%	10%	NS
Margins<1 mm (n=23)	20%	33%	NS

Data from the Van Nuys Breast Center reveal that there is little benefit from postexcisional radiation therapy if margins are greater than 10 mm, regardless of nuclear grade (Silverstein et al. 1997c) or the presence of comedo-type necrosis (Silverstein et al. 1998a) (Table 3).

Wide margin width increases the probability of complete excision and is an important predictor of local control. DCIS lesions excised with 10 mm or greater margins do not significantly benefit from the addition of radiation therapy, regardless of the presence of comedonecrosis or high nuclear grade. Comedonecrosis and nuclear grade reflect tumor biology and are significant only when there is a high likelihood of residual disease (for example, close or involved margins). Preoperative planning with the use of stereotactic biopsy followed by wide excision with multiple bracketing wires (Silverstein et al. 1997a) is the best way to achieve clear margins and to avoid the need for postoperative radiation therapy.

Why Is Local Recurrence Important?

If all local recurrences were noninvasive (DCIS), there would be little danger and, therefore, little indication for mastectomy as the initial procedure for patients with DCIS. In most reported series approximately half of all local recurrences are invasive (Silverstein et al. 1995b; Solin et al. 1993, 1996). Local recurrences are, therefore, extremely important. When they occur in patients who have struggled to save their breasts, they are both demoralizing and, theoretically, a threat to life. By avoiding mastectomy, we gain both psychological and physical advantages but when there is an invasive recurrence, we have permitted an almost totally curable noninvasive lesion to advance to a potentially less curable form. An invasive recurrence represents a biologic worsening of the stage of disease which may, in turn, ultimately translate into a higher mortality rate for patients initially treated conservatively.

In our experience at Van Nuys, the noninvasive recurrences are diagnosed fairly quickly after initial treatment, whereas the invasive recurrences take more time to develop. The median time to a noninvasive local recurrence was 22 months, most noninvasive recurrences having been seen within the first 5 years after initial treatment. The median time to an invasive local recurrence was 58 months, with multiple invasive recurrences having been seen more than 10 years after initial therapy (Fig. 6).

Similarly, recurrences after radiation therapy were delayed compared with recurrences in patients treated with excision alone. The median time to recurrence after excision alone was 23 months, whereas after radiation therapy it was 56 months (Fig. 7). Again, most recurrences following excision alone were seen within the first 5 years, whereas numerous recurrences after excision plus radiation therapy were not diagnosed until more than 10 years after the original treatment.

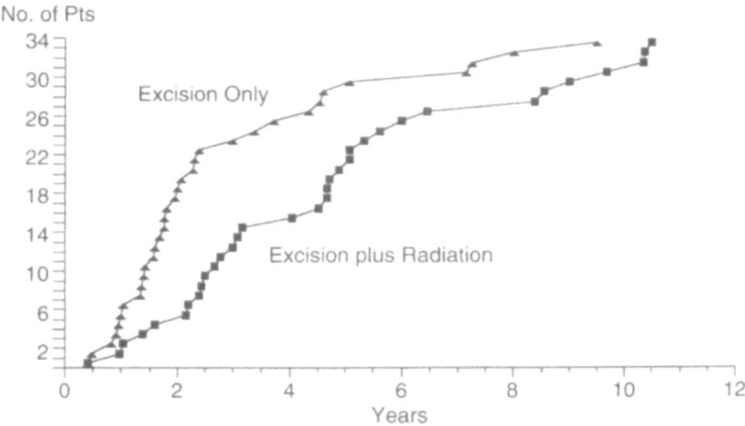

Fig. 6. Number of recurrences (both invasive and noninvasive) grouped according to treatment (excision only versus excision plus radiation therapy), plotted over time. The median time to local recurrence after excision only was 23 months; after excision and radiation therapy, it was 56 months (Silverstein et al. 1998 b)

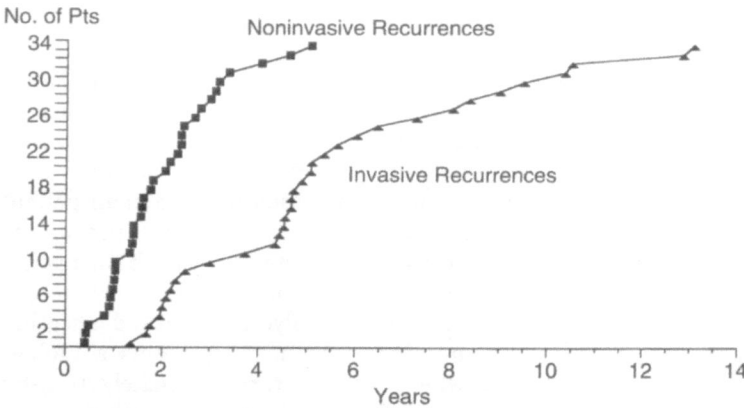

Fig. 7. Number of recurrences grouped according to type of recurrence (invasive versus noninvasive), plotted over time. The median time to a noninvasive recurrence was 22 months; for an invasive recurrence, it was 58 months (Silverstein et al. 1998b)

Outcome After Local Invasive Recurrence Following Conservative Treatment for DCIS

For the last decade, local recurrence (both invasive and noninvasive) has been used as the most important marker of treatment failure for patients with DCIS. As patient accrual increases and follow-up lengthens, more appropriate endpoints might now be invasive local recurrence and breast-cancer-specific mortality caused by invasive local recurrence.

Table 4 updates the outcome after local recurrence for 733 patients accrued from 1979 to 1997. There were a total of 75 recurrences, 35 invasive and 40 noninvasive. All of the patients with noninvasive recurrences did well, without any distant disease and with no (0%) breast cancer mortality (Silverstein et al. 1998b).

Among the 35 patients with invasive recurrences, 51% presented with stage 2A or more disease, 7 developed distant disease, and 5 died of breast cancer. The median follow-up for the 35 patients with invasive recurrences was more than 9 years. The breast cancer mortality rate at 8 years calculated by the Kaplan-Meier method for the subgroup of patients with invasive local recurrences was 14%, the distant disease rate for this subgroup was 27% – rates similar to the ones reported by Solin et al. (1994, 1996). Invasive recurrence after treatment for DCIS is a significant event, converting a patient with previous stage 0 disease to a patient with, on average, stage 2A breast cancer (range stage 1–4).

The treatment for a patient with an invasive recurrence should be based on the stage of the recurrence. Patients initially treated by mastectomy generally require excision of the recurrence followed by radiation therapy to the chest wall and chemotherapy. Patients previously treated by excision and ra-

Table 4. Outcome after local recurrence: 733 patients with DCIS analyzed according to treatment[a]

	Mastectomy	Excision + Radiation	Excision only
Number of patients ($n = 733$)	272	209	252
Total recurrences ($n = 75$)	2	36	37
Invasive recurrences ($n = 35$)	2	18	15
Distant metastases ($n = 7$)	1	5	1
Breast cancer deaths ($n = 5$)	0	4	1
Average DCIS size (mm)	40	18	14
Local recurrence probability (%)	<1	16	21
Distant recurrence probability (%)	<1	3	1
Breast-cancer-specific mortality (%)	0	3	<1
Overall mortality (all causes) (%)	6	7	9

[a] All recurrences and mortality probabilities are Kaplan-Meier estimates at 8 years.

diation therapy generally require mastectomy, followed by chemotherapy, if the invasive recurrence is high grade, greater than 1 cm in diameter, or has poor prognostic markers. Patients previously treated by excision only can undergo re-excision. If clear margins are obtained, they can be considered for breast preservation with radiation therapy. Many, however, will likely opt for mastectomy. The decision to add adjuvant chemotherapy should be based on tumor factors.

In spite of these few fatalities, one must not lose sight of the fact that overall DCIS is a disease with an extremely favorable prognosis. When our entire series of 733 patients is considered through February 1998, the chance of an invasive recurrence at 8 years is 6% and the probability of breast-cancer-specific death is only about 1.4%. It is, however, a tragedy, when a patient with DCIS recurs with invasive breast cancer and then goes on to die of metastatic disease. Patients with DCIS treated with breast preservation should be followed closely. At our center, they are examined physically every 6 months forever. Mammography is performed every 6 months on the ipsilateral breast and on the contralateral breast yearly.

When breast cancer mortality, rather than local recurrence, is the endpoint, patients with DCIS do exceptionally well, regardless of treatment (all $p = NS$). For the 75 patients who suffered recurrence, the 8-year breast-cancer-specific mortality after salvage treatment was 9%. For the 35 patients with invasive recurrences, the 8-year breast-cancer-specific mortality was 14%. These results indicate that most patients who suffer recurrence can be salvaged. For the small subgroup of patients who recur with invasive breast cancer, the mortality rate is similar to that of patients with stage 2A primary breast cancer.

Summary

Currently, we approach DCIS based on its morphology rather than its etiology. However, morphologically normal-appearing tissue surrounding areas of DCIS may reveal losses of heterozygosity similar to the primary tumor (Lakhani et al. 1995; Stratton et al. 1995; Radford et al. 1995; Fujii et al. 1996). In all likelihood, genetic changes precede morphologic evidence of malignant transformation. We in medicine must learn how to recognize these genetic changes, exploit them, and, in the future, prevent them. DCIS is a lesion in which the complete malignant phenotype of unlimited growth, angiogenesis, genomic elasticity, invasion, and metastasis has not been fully expressed. With sufficient time, most noninvasive lesions will learn how to invade and metastasize. We must learn how to prevent this.

References

Aasmundstad TA, Haugen OA (1992) DNA ploidy in intraductal breast carcinomas. Eur J Cancer 26:956–959

Albertini JJ, Lyman GH, Cox C et al (1996) Lymphatic mapping and sentinel node biopsy in the patient with breast cancer. JAMA 276:1818–1822

Ashikari R, Hadju SI, Robbins GF (1971) Intraductal carcinoma of the breast. Cancer 28:1182–1187

Barnes DM, Meyer JS, Gonzalez JG, Gullick WJ, Millis RR (1991) Relationship between c-erbB-2 immunoreactivity and thymidine labelling index in breast carcinoma in situ. Breast Cancer Res Treat 18:11–17

Bartkova J, Barnes DM, Millis RR, Gullick WJ (1990) Immunohistochemical demonstration of c-erbB-2 protein in mammary ductal carcinoma in situ. Hum Pathol 21:1164–1167

Bellamy COC, McDonald C, Salter DM, Chetty U, Anderson TJ (1993) Noninvasive ductal carcinoma of the breast. The relevance of histologic categorization. Hum Pathol 24:16–23

Dickson RB, Lippman ME (1995) Growth factors in breast cancer. Endocr Rev 16(5):559–589

Douglas-Jones AG, Gupta SK, Attanoos RL, Morgan JM, Mansel RE (1996) A critical appraisal of six modern classifications of ductal carcinoma in situ of the breast (DCIS): correlation with grade of associated invasive disease. Histopathology 29:397–409

Ernster VL, Barclay J, Kerlikowske K et al (1996) Incidence of and treatment for ductal carcinoma in situ of the breast. JAMA 275:913–918

Faverly DRG, Burgers L, Bult P, Holland R (1995) Three dimensional imaging of mammary ductal carcinoma in situ: clinical implications. Semin Diagn Pathol 11(3):193–198

Fisher B, Costantino J, Redmond C et al (1993) Lumpectomy compared with lumpectomy and radiation therapy for the treatment of intraductal breast cancer. N Engl J Med 328:1581–1586

Fisher B, Dignam J, Wolmark N et al (1998) Lumpectomy and radiation therapy for the treatment of intraductal breast cancer: findings from National Surgical Adjuvant Breast and Bowel Project B-17. J Clin Oncol 16:441–452

Fisher ER, Costantino J, Fisher B et al (1995) Pathologic finding from the National Surgical Adjuvant Breast Project (NSABP), protocol B-17: intraductal carcinoma (ductal carcinoma in situ). Cancer 75:1310–1319

Fujii H, Marsh C, Cairns P et al (1996) Genetic divergence in the clonal evolution of breast cancer. Cancer Res 56:1493–1497

Giuliano AE, Dale PS, Turner RR, Morton DL, Evans SW, Krasne DL (1995) Improved axillary staging of breast cancer with sentinel lymphadenectomy. Ann Surg 222:394–401

Hansen N, Giuliano A (1997) Axillary dissection for ductal carcinoma in situ. In: Silverstein MJ (ed) Ductal carcinoma in situ of the breast. Williams and Wilkins, Baltimore, pp 577–584

Holland R, Faverly DRG (1997) Whole organ studies. In: Silverstein MJ (ed) Ductal carcinoma in situ of the breast. Williams and Wilkins, Baltimore, pp 233–240

Jensen JA, Handel N, Silverstein MJ (1996) Glandular replacement therapy: an argument for a combined surgical approach in the treatment of noninvasive breast cancer. Breast 2:121–123

Krag DN, Weaver DL, Alex JC, Fairbank JT (1993) Surgical resection and radiolocalization of sentinel lymph node in breast cancer using a gamma probe. Surg Oncol 2:335–340

Kroll SS, Ames F, Singletary SE et al (1991) The oncologic risks of skin preservation at mastectomy when combined with immediate reconstruction of the breast. Surg Gynecol Obstet 172:17–20

Lagios MD, Page DL (1993) Radiation therapy for in situ or localized breast cancer (Letter). N Engl J Med 21:1577–1578

Lagios NM, Margolin FR, Westdahl PR, Rose NM (1989) Mammographically detected duct carcinoma in situ. Frequency of local recurrence following tylectomy and prognostic effect of nuclear grade on local recurrence. Cancer 63:619–624

Lakhani SR, Collins N, Stratton MR, Sloane JP (1995) Atypical ductal hyperplasia: clonal proliferation with loss of heterozygosity on chromosomes 16q and 17p. J Clin Pathol 48:611–615

Lennington WJ, Jensen RA, Dalton LW, Page DL (1994) Ductal carcinoma in situ of the breast. Heterogeneity of individual lesions. Cancer 73:118–124

Lippman ME (1993) The rational development of biological therapies for breast cancer. Science 259:631–632

Meyer J (1986) Cell kinetics of histologic variants of in situ breast carcinoma. Breast Cancer Res Treat 7:171–180

Nemoto T, Vana J, Bedwani RN, Baker HW, McGregor FH, Murphy GP (1980) Management and survival of female breast cancer: results of a national survey by the American College of Surgeons. Cancer 45:2917–2924

Page DL, Lagios MD (1995) Pathologic analysis of the NSABP-B17 trial. Unanswered questions remaining unanswered considering current concepts of ductal carcinoma in situ. Cancer 75:1219–1222

Page DL, Dupont WD, Rogers LW, Jensen RA, Schuyler PA (1995) Continued local recurrence of carcinoma 15-25 years after a diagnosis of low grade ductal carcinoma in situ of the breast treated only by biopsy. Cancer 76:1197–1200

Parker SL, Tong T, Bolden S, Wingo PA (1997) Cancer statistics, 1997. CA Cancer J Clin 47:5–27

Patchefsky AS, Schwartz GF, Finkelstein SD et al (1989) Heterogeneity of intraductal carcinoma of the breast. Cancer 63:731–741

Radford DM, Phillips NJ, Fair KL et al (1995) Allelic loss and the progression of breast cancer. Cancer Res 55:5180–5183

Recht A (1997a) Randomized trial overview. In: Silverstein MJ (ed) Ductal carcinoma in situ of the breast. Williams and Wilkins, Baltimore, pp 463–467

Recht A (1997b) Side effects of radiation therapy. In: Silverstein MJ (ed) Ductal carcinoma in situ of the breast. Williams and Wilkins, Baltimore, pp 347–352

Schwartz GF (1994) The role of excision and surveillance alone in subclinical DCIS of the breast. Oncology 8(2):21–26

Schwartz GF, Lagios MD, Carter D et al (1998) Consensus conference on the classification of ductal carcinoma in situ. Cancer 80:1798–1802

Silverstein MJ (ed) (1997a) Ductal carcinoma in situ of the breast. Williams and Wilkins, Baltimore

Silverstein MJ (1997b) Predicting local recurrence in patients with ductal carcinoma in situ. In: Silverstein MJ (ed) Ductal carcinoma in situ of the breast. Williams and Wilkins, Baltimore, pp 271–284

Silverstein MJ (1997c) Van Nuys prognostic index for DCIS. In: Silverstein MJ (ed) Ductal carcinoma in situ of the breast. Williams and Wilkins, Baltimore, pp 491–504

Silverstein MJ, Rosser RJ, Gierson ED et al (1987) Axillary dissection for intraductal breast carcinoma – is it indicated? Cancer 59:1819–1824

Silverstein MJ, Poller DN, Waisman JR et al (1995a) Prognostic classification of breast ductal carcinoma in situ. Lancet 345:1154–1157

Silverstein MJ, Barth A, Poller DN et al (1995b) Ten-year results comparing mastectomy to excision and radiation therapy for ductal carcinoma in situ of the breast. Eur J Cancer 31:1425–1427

Silverstein MJ, Lagios MD, Craig PH et al (1996) A prognostic index for ductal carcinoma in situ of the breast. Cancer 77:2267–2274

Silverstein MJ, Gamagami P, Colburn WJ (1997a) Coordinated biopsy team: surgical, pathologic and radiologic issues. In: Silverstein MJ (ed) Ductal carcinoma in situ of the breast. Williams and Wilkins, Baltimore, pp 333–342

Silverstein MJ, Lagios MD, Waisman JR et al (1997b) Outcome after local recurrence for patients with ductal carcinoma in situ (DCIS) of the breast. Proc Am Soc Clin Oncol 16:129a

Silverstein MJ, Lagios MD, Lewinsky BS et al (1997c) Breast irradiation is unnecessary for widely excised ductal carcinoma in situ (DCIS) of the breast. Breast Cancer Res Treat 46:23

Silverstein MJ, Lagios MD, Waisman JR et al (1998a) Margin width: a critical determinant of local control in patients with ductal carcinoma in situ (DCIS) of the breast. Proc Am Soc Clin Oncol 17:120a

Silverstein MJ, Lagios MD, Martino S et al (1998b) Outcome after local recurrence in patients with ductal carcinoma in situ of the breast. J Clin Oncol 16:1367–1373

Singletary ES (1995) Skin-sparing mastectomy with immediate breast reconstruction: is it safe? Breast Dis Yearbook Q 6:259–260

Solin LJ, Yet I-T, Kurtz J et al (1993) Ductal carcinoma in situ (intraductal carcinoma) of the breast treated with breast-conserving surgery and definitive irradiation. Correlation of pathologic parameters with outcome of treatment. Cancer 71:2532–2542

Solin LJ, Fourquet A, McCormick B et al (1994) Salvage treatment for local recurrence following breast conserving surgery and definitive irradiation for ductal carcinoma in situ (intraductal carcinoma) of the breast. Int J Radiat Oncol Biol Phys 30:3–9

Solin LJ, Kurtz J, Fourquet A et al (1996) Fifteen year results of breast conserving surgery and definitive breast irradiation for treatment of ductal carcinoma in situ of the breast. J Clin Oncol 14:754–763

Stratton MR, Collins N, Lakhani SR, Sloane JP (1995) Loss of heterozygosity in ductal carcinoma in situ of the breast. J Pathol 175:195–201

Ductal Carcinoma In Situ of the Breast: Histological Classification and Genetic Alterations

M.J. van de Vijver

Department of Pathology, Netherlands Cancer Institute, Plesmanlaan 121, 1066 CX Amsterdam, The Netherlands

Introduction

Ductal carcinoma in situ (DCIS) represents a proliferation of malignant epithelial cells within the ducts and lobules of the breast, without invasion through the basement membrane. It is assumed that most, if not all, invasive carcinomas are preceded by DCIS. It is, however, not known what proportion of DCIS, if left untreated, will progress to invasive carcinoma. Approximately 3% of all breast malignancies are DCIS. Because DCIS grows in pre-existing milk ducts without forming a tumour mass, a lot of cases are clinically asymptomatic. As a result of the formation of microcalcifications in the tumorous areas, many cases of DCIS are detected on the basis of these microcalcifications using mammography. With the increased use of mass population screening using mammography, more cases of DCIS are being detected. In most screening programs, 15%–25% of all detected malignancies are DCIS.

If DCIS is treated with breast-ablative therapy, the prognosis is excellent. However, for many patients breast ablation may represent overtreatment, and therefore breast-conserving therapy is considered with increasing frequency. Several series of patients with DCIS who have been treated by breast-conserving therapy have been described in the literature (Lagios et al. 1989; Fisher et al. 1993; Solin et al. 1996). The largest series is the one described by Fisher et al. (1993). In this study of 818 patients with DCIS treated in a clinical trial, it was shown that lumpectomy alone resulted in 16% local recurrence; lumpectomy and breast irradiation resulted in 7% local recurrence. Approximately 50% of the local recurrences were invasive, the remainder were DCIS.

As histological classification is an important cornerstone for treatment decisions, this will be discussed in the next section. It is hoped that assessment of the genetic alterations in breast cancer, including DCIS, will greatly help in predicting tumour behaviour and thus guide treatment planning. The second section of this chapter will discuss present knowledge about genetic alterations in breast cancer, including DCIS.

Histological Classification of DCIS

It is clear that there are different histological types of DCIS. In most textbooks the following classification based on architectural growth pattern is used:
- Solid
- Comedo
- Cribriform
- (Micro)papillary.

In recent years it has become clear that the cytonuclear differentiation of tumour cells is more important than architectural growth pattern, and various new classifications of DCIS have been proposed. One proposal by our group (Holland et al. 1994) suggests a division into poorly differentiated, intermediately differentiated and well-differentiated DCIS (Table 1). This classification has not yet been correlated to follow-up after breast-conserving treatment. Silverstein et al. (1995) have proposed the so-called Van Nuys classification. This classification divides DCIS into three groups:
1. Non-high-grade DCIS without comedo-type necrosis
2. Non-high-grade DCIS with comedo-type necrosis
3. High-grade DCIS with or without comedo-type necrosis.

This classification has been tested in 238 patients after breast-conserving surgery followed by radiotherapy in 139 cases and no further treatment in 99 cases; local recurrence was seen in 3.8% of the patients in group 1, 11.1% in group 2, and 26.5% in group 3; median follow-up was 78 months. From this study it is very clear that for the well-differentiated type of DCIS (groups 1 and 2 in the Van Nuys classification) local control is very good with breast-conserving treatment. It is, however, possible that with longer follow-up, recurrences will be seen in the group of patients with well-differentiated DCIS. For well-differentiated DCIS, tumour excision without radiotherapy probably results in a low but continuing risk of local recurrence (Betsill et al. 1978; Page et al. 1995). An important factor in the usefulness of a classification of DCIS is its interobserver reproducibility (Schnitt et al. 1992). This will have to be evaluated in the future.

Table 1. Histological classification of DCIS by Holland et al. (1994)

Genetic Alterations in Breast Cancer

General

The pattern of genetic alterations present in a case of DCIS may also be associated with the clinical outcome. No attempts have been made to study the association between the profile of genetic alterations in DCIS and clinical outcome. In this section the genetic alterations identified in breast cancer, and particularly in DCIS, will be discussed.

The genetic alterations in breast cancer are amplification of a number of genes and inactivation of a number of tumour suppressor genes (Van de Vijver 1993). Translocations and point mutations are very rare and do not seem to play an important role in the development of breast cancer.

The techniques used to identify genetic alterations in breast cancer include Southern blot analysis; the polymerase chain reaction (PCR) to detect gene amplification and also to detect loss of heterozygosity (LOH); sequence analysis (which may be preceded by screening for altered gene sequences by, for instance, single-strand conformation polymorphism) to detect point mutations in tumour suppressor genes; and, in the past few years, comparative genomic hybridization (CGH) (Kallioniemi et al. 1994).

It is to be expected that more specific genes will be identified that are involved in breast cancer development. A number of amplified genes were already known; using CGH an increasing number of loci are being identified that also harbour amplified sequences (Kallioniemi et al. 1994; Isola et al. 1995). For most of these regions the gene, amplification of which has been selected for, has not yet been identified. Only a very limited number of tumour suppressor genes in breast cancer have been identified; given the very large number of loci for which loss of heterozygosity has been identified, the number of known tumour suppressor genes is expected to increase in the coming years.

Gene Amplification

The genes which have been found to be amplified in breast cancer are shown in Table 2. For each of these loci, some of the most important features are given below.

The neu/c-erbB-2 *gene (chromosome 17q12)*. This gene is amplified in 15%–25% of invasive carcinomas (Slamon et al. 1987, 1989; van de Vijver et al. 1987). The gene encodes a protein with the structure of a growth factor receptor located on the cell membrane. Amplification of this gene is associated with overexpression of c-erbB-2/neu mRNA (King et al. 1989) and of the protein, which can be detected using immunohistochemistry (Van de Vijver et al. 1988a). Tumours without gene amplification do not show detectable protein expression in paraffin sections. Overexpression of the protein is associated with the poorly differentiated type of DCIS (Van de Vijver et al.

Table 2. Genes known to be amplified in invasive breast cancer

Name of the gene	Chromosomal location	Wheater amplified in DCIS
c-myc	8q24	No
FGF-rec.I/flg	8p12	No
FGF-rec.II/bek	10q26	No
Cyclin D1	11q13	Yes
c-erbB-2/neu	17q12	Yes
CAS/AIB1	20q13	No

1988 b; Bartkova et al. 1990; Ramachandra et al. 1990; Liu et al. 1992). In invasive carcinomas, c-erbB-2/neu overexpression is associated with a large component of ductal carcinoma in situ.

The c-myc gene (chromosome 8q24). The c-myc gene encodes a nuclear protein involved in regulation of growth and apoptosis. c-myc gene amplification is found in approximately 20% of breast carcinomas and is associated with locally advanced disease and poor prognosis (Varley et al. 1987; Berns et al. 1992).

MDM-2 gene (chromosome 12q13/14). The MDM-2 gene encodes a nuclear protein which can form oligomeric complexes with the p53 tumour suppressor gene product. MDM-2 gene amplification has been reported in a very small percentage of breast carcinomas; clinicopathological correlations have not been reported (Marchetti et al. 1995; McCann et al. 1995). MDM-2 gene amplification results in overexpression, which can be detected as staining of nuclei of tumour cells in paraffin sections.

Cyclin D1 gene (chromosome 11q13). The cyclin D1 gene encodes a nuclear protein, a so-called cyclin, involved in cell cyclus regulation. The cyclin D1 gene is located in a large region of gene amplification, where amongst others the EMS gene is also located (Schuuring et al. 1995). It is assumed that the cyclin D1 gene is the important gene in this region; however, rare tumours exist where the 11q13 region is amplified without overexpression of the cyclin D1 gene. Cyclin D1 gene amplification is associated with estrogen receptor positivity. In estrogen-receptor-positive tumours, cyclin D1 gene amplification is associated with a relatively poor prognosis (Bartkova et al. 1994; Schuuring 1995). Overexpression of cyclin D1 messenger RNA has been reported in DCIS, but is absent in epithelial hyperplasia. This indicates that cyclin D1 overexpression may play a role in the transition to DCIS (Weinstat-Saslow et al. 1995).

CAS (cellular apoptosis susceptibility) gene and AIB1 gene (chromosome 20q13). The CAS gene encodes a protein which may have a function in apoptosis and cell proliferation. The gene is present in a region on chromosome 20 that is found to be amplified in approximately 15% of breast carcinomas (Brinkmann et al. 1996; Deng et al. 1996b). Another gene in this region is AIB1, which encodes a protein that binds to and co-activates the estrogen receptor.

EGF receptor gene (chromosome 7). This gene encodes a growth factor receptor located on the cell membrane. Amplification of this gene is found in less than 3% of breast carcinomas (Zeillinger et al. 1989). Elevated expression of the EGF receptor protein in the absence of gene amplification has been associated with estrogen receptor negativity (Sainsbury et al. 1987).

FGF-2 receptor (BEK) gene (chromosome 10q26). This gene encodes a cell-membrane-located receptor for fibroblast growth factor. This gene is amplified in approximately 12% of breast carcinomas (Adnane et al. 1992).

FGF-1R (FLG) gene (chromosome 8p12). This gene encodes another fibroblast growth factor receptor, which is also amplified in approximately 10% of breast carcinomas (Adnane et al. 1992). No clinical associations have yet been reported for the amplification of these two fibroblast growth factor receptors.

Using comparative genomic hybridization (CGH), other regions with amplification have been observed. For many of these regions, however, no gene probes have yet been isolated, and it is therefore impossible to say at this moment in what percentage of breast carcinomas these regions are amplified. One example of new candidate oncogenes identified using CGH are the CAS and AIB1 genes discussed above. For other regions, the oncogenes have not yet been identified.

Tumour Suppressor Genes

In breast cancer, as in other tumour types, inactivation of tumour suppressor genes plays an important role. The classical mechanism of inactivation is functional loss of both alleles of the tumour suppressor gene. In many cases, one allele is mutated by a relatively subtle mutation (point mutation, small insertion, small deletion) while the other allele is completely lost, resulting in loss of heterozygosity (LOH). The presence of these subtle mutations has made it possible to identify the tumour suppressor genes that are known today. In addition to the known tumour suppressor genes, a relatively large number of regions have been identified where frequent LOH is observed (Mackay et al. 1988; Chen et al. 1989; Sato et al. 1990; Devilee et al. 1991; Bieche et al. 1992; Cornelis et al. 1993; Cropp et al. 1990). Great efforts are being devoted to identify the tumour suppressor genes in these regions.

The tumour suppressor genes in breast cancer known to date are shown in Table 3. Some of the salient features of each of these genes are presented below:

The *p53 gene (chromosome 17p13.1)* encodes a nuclear protein that binds the DNA as a tetramer and is involved in regulation of transcription, DNA replication and apoptosis. Inactivating *p53* mutations are found in approximately 20% of breast carcinomas (Prosser et al. 1990; Varley et al. 1991; Cornelis et al. 1994). The presence of *p53* mutations has been associated with poor prognosis, resistance to chemotherapy and, in DCIS, the poorly differentiated histologic type (Chuaqui et al. 1997). In the majority of cases, *p53* mutations result in substitution of one amino acid; the resulting altered *p53* protein has an increased half-life. This increased half-life makes it possible to

Table 3. Tumour suppressor genes known to be inactivated in invasive breast cancer

Name of the gene	Chromosomal location	Whether inactivated in DCIS
IGF-II receptor	6q25–26	Yes
pTEN	10q23	?
E-cadherin	16q21	No; in LCIS, yes
Prohibitin	17q21	?
p53	17p13	Yes

detect the *p53* protein in the nucleus of tumour cells, whereas the wild-type *p53* protein cannot be detected. In this way it has become possible to identify tumours with *p53* mutations on the basis of the presence of *p53* protein overexpression. In the absence of *p53* mutations, *p53* overexpression is also observed in approximately 10%–20% of breast carcinomas.

The *E-cadherin gene (chromosome 16q22.1)* encodes a cell adhesion protein, involved in adhesion between epithelial cells. Complete loss of plasma-membrane-associated expression of E-cadherin is observed in the majority of invasive lobular carcinomas (Berx et al. 1995). In the majority of cases where E-cadherin expression is lacking, mutations in the E-cadherin gene are identified. In ductal carcinomas normal or somewhat reduced membrane-located expression of E-cadherin is always observed. These findings indicate that E-cadherin inactivation is a specific event in the development of lobular carcinoma but not in that of DCIS.

The *pTEN gene (chromosome 10q23)* is found to be mutated in human brain, breast and prostate cancer (Li et al. 1997). pTEN shares homology with the family of protein tyrosine phosphatases as well as with the cytoskeletal protein tensin. Germline mutations in pTEN are found in three related inheritable disorders characterized by an increased incidence of various forms of cancer: Cowden disease, Lhermitte-Duclos disease and Bannayana-Zonana syndrome (Liaw et al. 1997; Marsh et al. 1997; Nelen et al. 1997).

The *IGF-II-receptor gene (chromosome 6q26-27)* encodes a cell-membrane-located receptor for IGF-II; in addition this receptor functions as the mannose-6 phosphate receptor. Mutations in this gene have been identified in breast carcinomas (Hankins et al. 1996).

The *prohibitin gene (chromosome 17q21)*. There is frequent LOH in this chromosomal region; it was shown that the prohibitin gene, located in the region of frequent LOH, contained somatic mutation in some breast carcinomas (Sato et al. 1992).

Genetic Alterations in DCIS

As can be seen from Tables 2 and 3, almost every genetic alteration described in the previous section has been identified in DCIS. This indicates that most of the gene alterations identified to date are early events in breast tumorigenesis.

The only alterations that could be a relatively late event in breast tumorigenesis are amplifications of the c-*myc*, *flg* and *bek* genes. Of these, c-*myc* gene amplification has been found associated with locally advanced breast cancer. LOH on the short arm of chromosome 8 also seems to be associated with invasive behaviour (Yaremko et al. 1996).

A number of reports on LOH in DCIS have been published; in all cases, DNA was isolated from the DCIS tumour cells after microdissection. As for invasive carcinoma, regions with frequent LOH are found on chromosomes 16 and 17, indicating that these are early events in breast cancer development that precede the tumour cells' becoming invasive (Radford et al. 1993, 1995; Noguchi et al. 1994; Tsuda et al. 1994; Lakhani et al. 1995; Munn et al. 1995; Stratton et al. 1995; Zhuang et al. 1995; Fujii et al. 1996 a, b). Of interest is the finding that normal epithelial cells adjacent to invasive carcinoma show LOH for chromosome 3p (Deng et al. 1996 a).

Using fluorescent in situ hybridization (FISH), it has also been possible to demonstrate numerical chromosomal aberrations in DCIS (Harrison et al. 1995; Murphy et al. 1995). Another technical advance for the detection of genetic alterations in DCIS is FISH for the detection of amplified regions of DNA, which has for instance been used to show c-*erb*B-2/*neu* gene amplification (Pauletti et al. 1996).

Recently, we have analysed lobular carcinoma in situ (LCIS) and DCIS for expression of E-cadherin; all nine cases of LCIS were negative for staining, whereas all 150 cases of DCIS were positive. Using microdissection, we isolated tumour cells from an LCIS component adjacent to an invasive lobular carcinoma as two tumours with a known E-cadherin gene mutation. In the LCIS component we found the same truncating mutation as in the invasive lobular carcinoma, indicating that E-cadherin mutation is an early event in the development of invasive lobular carcinoma (Vos et al. 1998).

We and others (Simpson et al. 1997; Vos et al. submitted) have found cyclin D1 gene amplification in DCIS in a low percentage of cases; cyclin D1 overexpression was associated with the presence of cyclin D1 gene amplification, but was also found in the absence of cyclin D1 gene amplification. Overexpression of cyclin D1 in DCIS is associated with intermediately and poorly differentiated DCIS.

A multistep model of breast carcinoma development, similar to that developed for colon carcinoma, has not yet been developed. It is clear that there are a number of different types of breast cancer, each of which may have its own multistep genetic development scheme. The genetic alterations present in DCIS undoubtedly greatly influence the clinical behaviour of these lesions; in the future, this knowledge will help in planning therapy for this disease.

Summary

Ductal carcinoma in situ (DCIS) of the breast represents a proliferation of malignant epithelial cells within the ducts and lobules of the breast, without invasion through the basement membrane. It is believed that all invasive carcinomas are preceded by DCIS; however, it is not known what proportion of patients with DCIS will develop invasive carcinoma and after what interval. DCIS is heterogeneous with respect to its clinical presentation, mammographic abnormalities, histology and biology. The risk of progression to invasive carcinoma depends on the histologic type of DCIS and the size of the lesion; in the future, the analysis of the genetic alterations may also help in predicting the risk of progression to invasive breast cancer. As the risk of progression to invasive breast cancer (and the development of metastases) greatly influences the choice of treatment for DCIS, it is of importance to be able to make a reliable estimate of this risk of progression. In this chapter, the histologic classification of DCIS and the genetic alterations that have been found to date are discussed.

Acknowledgement. I would like to thank Carla Vos for critically reading the manuscript and giving helpful suggestions.

References

Adnane J, Gaudray P, Dionne CA, Crumley G, Jaye M, Schlessinger J, Jeanteur P, Birnbaum D, Theillet C (1992) BEK and FLG, two receptors to members of the FGF family, are amplified in subsets of human breast cancers. Oncogene 6:659–663

Anzick SL, Kononen J, Walker RL, Azorsa DO, Tanner MM, Guan XY, Sauter G, Kallioniemi OP, Trent JM, Meltzer PS (1997) AIB1, a steroid receptor coactivator amplified in breast and ovarian cancer. Science 15:965–968

Bartkova J, Barnes DM, Millis RR, Gullick WJ (1990) Immunohistochemical demonstration of c-erbB-2 protein in mammary ductal carcinoma in situ. Hum Pathol 21:1164–1167

Bartkova J, Lukas J, Muller H, Lutzhoft D, Strauss M, Bartek J (1994) Cyclin D1 protein expression and function in human breast cancer. Int J Cancer 57:353–361

Berns EMJJ, Klijn JGM, van Putten WLJ, van Staveren IL, Portengen H, Foekens JA (1992) c-myc amplification is a better prognostic factor than HER-2/neu amplification in primary breast cancer. Cancer Res 52:1107–1113

Berx G, Cleton-Jansen AM, Nollet F, De Leeuw WJF, Van de Vijver MJ, Cornelisse C, Van Roy F (1995) E-cadherin is a tumour/invasion suppressor gene mutated in human lobular breast cancers. EMBO J 14:6107–6115

Betsill WL, Rosen PP, Lieberman PH, Robbins GF (1978) Intraductal carcinoma: long-term follow-up after treatment by biopsy alone. JAMA 239:1863–1867

Bieche I, Champeme MH, Matifas F, Hacene K, Callahan R, Lidereau R (1992) Loss of heterozygosity on chromosome 7q and aggressive primary breast cancer. Lancet 1:139–143

Brinkmann U, Gallo M, Polymeropoulos MH, Pastan I (1996) The human CAS (cellular apoptosis susceptibility) gene mapping on chromosome 20q13 is amplified in BT474 breast cancer cells and part of aberrant chromosomes in breast and colon cancer cell lines. Genome Res 6:187–194

Chen L-C, Dollbaum C, Smith HS (1989) Loss of heterozygosity on chromosome 1q in human breast cancer. Proc Natl Acad Sci USA 86:7204–7207

Chitemerere M, Andersen TI, Holm R, Karlsen F, Børresen A-L, Nesland JM (1996) TP53 alterations in atypical ductal hyperplasia and ductal carcinoma in situ of the breast. Breast Cancer Res Treat 41:103–109

Chuaqui RF, Zhuang ZP, Emmertbuck MR, Liotta LA, Merino MH (1997) Analysis of loss of heterozygosity on chromosome 11q13 in atypical ductal hyperplasia and in situ carcinoma of the breast. Am J Pathol 150:297–303

Cornelis RS, Devilee P, van Vliet M, Kuipers-Dijkshoorn N, Kersenmaeker A, Bardoel A et al (1993) Allele loss patterns on chromosome 17q in 109 breast carcinomas indicate at least two distinct target regions. Oncogene 8:781–785

Cornelis RS, van Vliet M, Vos CBJ, Cleton-Jansen A, Van de Vijver MJ, Peterse JL et al (1994) Evidence for a gene on 17p13.3, distal to TP53, as a target for allele loss in breast tumours without p53 mutations. Cancer Res 54:1–7

Cropp CS, Lidereau R, Campbell G, Champene MH, Callahan R (1990) Loss of heterozygosity on chromosomes 17 and 18 in breast carcinoma: two additional regions identified. Proc Natl Acad Sci USA 87:7737–7741

Deng, G, Lu Y, Zlotnikov G, Thor AD, Smith HS (1996a) Loss of heterozygosity in normal tissue adjacent to breast carcinomas. Science 274:2057–2059

Deng G, Yu M, Chen LC, Moore D, Kurisu W, Kallioniemi A, Waldman FM, Collins C, Smith HS (1996b) Amplifications of oncogene erbB-2 and chromosome 20q in breast cancer determined by differentially competitive polymerase chain reaction. Breast Cancer Res Treat 40:271–281

Devilee P, van Vliet M, Kuipers Dijkshoorn N, Pearson PL, Cornelisse CJ (1991) Somatic genetic changes on chromosome 18 in breast carcinomas: is the DCC gene involved? Oncogene 6:311–315

Fisher B, Costantino J, Redmond C, Fisher E, Margolese R, Dimitrov N, Wolmark N, Wickerham DL, Deutsch M, Ore L, Mamounas E, Poller W, Kavanah M (1993) Lumpectomy compared with lumpectomy and radiation therapy for the treatment of intraductal breast cancer. N Engl J Med 328:1581–1586

Fujii H, March C, Cairns P, Sidransky D, et al (1996a) Genetic divergence in the clonal evolution of breast cancer. Cancer Res 56:1493–1497

Fujii H, Szumel R, Marsh C, Zhuo W, Gabrielson E (1996b) Genetic progression, histological grade, and allelic loss in ductal carcinoma in situ of the breast. Cancer Res 56:5260–5265

Hankins GR, De Souza AT, Bentley RC, Patel MR, Marks JR, Iglehart JD, Jirtle RL (1996) M6P/IGf2 receptor: a candidate breast tumor suppressor gene. Oncogene 12:2003–2009

Harrison M, Magee HM, O'Loughlin J, Gorey TF, Dervan PA (1995) Chromosome 1 aneusomy, identified by interphase cytogenetics, in mammographically detected ductal carcinoma in situ of the breast. J Pathol 175:303–309

Holland R, Peterse JL, Millis RR, Eusebi V, Faverly D, Van de Vijver MJ, Zafrani B (1994) Ductal carcinoma in situ: a proposal for a new classification. Sem in Diagn Pathol 11:167–180

Kallioniemi A, Kallioniemi OP, Piper J, Tanner M, Stokke T, Chen L, Smith HS, Pinkel D, Gray JW, Waldman FM (1994) Detection and mapping of amplified DNA sequences in breast cancer by comparative genomic hybridization. Proc Natl Acad Sci USA 91:2156–2160

King CR, Swain SM, Porter L, Steinberg SM, Lippman ME, Gelmann EP (1989) Heterogeneous expression of erbB-2 messenger RNA in human breast cancer. Cancer Res 49:4185–4191

Lagios MD, Margolin F, Westdahl PR, Rose MR (1989) Mammographically detected duct carcinoma in situ: frequency of local recurrence following tylectomy and prognostic effect of nuclear grade on local recurrence. Cancer 63:618–624

Lakhani SL, Collins N, Stratton MR, Sloane JP (1995) Atypical ductal hyperplasia of the breast: clonal proliferation with loss of heterozygosity on chromosomes 16q and 17p. J Clin Pathol 48:611–615

Li J, Yen C, Liaw D, Podsypanina K, Bose S, Wang S, Puc J et al (1997) pTEN, a putative protein tyrosine phosphatase gene mutated in human brain, breast and prostate cancer. Science 275:1943–1946

Liaw D, Marsh DJ, Li J, Dahia PL, Wang SI, Zheng Z, Bose S, Call KM, Tsou HC, Peacocke M, Eng C, Parsons R (1997) Germline mutations of the PTEN gene in Cowden disease, an inherited breast and thyroid cancer syndrome. Nat Genet 16:64-67

Liu E, Thor AHM, Barcos M, Ljung B-M, Benz C (1992) The HER2 (c-erbB-2) oncogene is frequently amplified in in situ carcinomas of the breast. Oncogene 7:1027-1032

Mackay J, Elder PA, Porteous DJ, Steel CM, Hawkins RA, Going JJ et al (1988) Partial deletion of chromosome 11p in breast cancer correlates with size of primary tumour and oestrogen receptor level. Breast 58:710-714

Marchetti A, Buttitta F, Girlando S, Palma PD, Pellegrini S, Fina P, Doglioni C, Bevilacqua G, Barbareschi M (1995) mdm2 gene alterations and mdm2 protein expression in breast carcinomas. J Pathol 175:31-38

Marsh DJ, Dahia PL, Zheng Z, Liaw D, Parsons R, Gorlin RJ, Eng C (1997) Germline mutations in PTEN are present in Bannayan-Zonana syndrome. Nat Genet 16:333-334

McCann AH, Kirley A, Carney DN, Corbally N, Magee HM, Keating G, Dervan PA (1995) Amplification of the MDM2 gene in human breast cancer and its association with MDM2 and p53 protein status. Oncogene 981-985

Munn KE, Walker RA, Varley JM (1995) Frequent alterations of chromosome 1 in ductal carcinoma in situ of the breast. Oncogene 10:1653-1657

Murphy DS, Hoare SF, Going JJ, Mallon EEA, George WD, Kaye SB, Brown R, Black DM, Keith WN (1995) Characterization of extensive genetic alterations in ductal carcinoma in situ by fluorescence in situ hybridization and molecular analysis. J Natl Cancer Inst. 87:1694-1704

Nelen MR, Staveren WC van, Peeters EA, Hassel MB, Gorlin RJ, Hamm H, Lindboe CF, Fryns JP, Sijmons RH, Woods DG, Marinan EC, Padberg GW, Kremer H (1997) Germline mutations in the PTEN/MMAC1 gene in patients with Cowden disease. Hum Nat Genet 6:1383-1387

Noguchi S, Motomua K, Inan J, Imaoka S et al (1994) Clonal analysis of predominantly intraductal carcinoma and precancerous lesions of the breast by means of polymerase chain reaction. Cancer Res 54:1849-1853

Page DL, Dupont WD, Rogers LW, Jensen RA, Schuyler PA (1995) Continued local recurrence of carcinoma 15-25 years after a diagnosis of low grade ductal carcinoma in situ of the breast treated only by biopsy. Cancer 76:1197-1200

Pauletti G, Godolphin W, Press MF, Slamon DJ (1996) Detection and quantitation of HER-2/neu gene amplification in human breast cancer archival material using fluorescence in situ hybridization. Oncogene 13:63-72

Prosser J, Thompson AM, Cranston G, Evans HJ (1990) Evidence that p53 behaves as a tumor suppressor gene in sporadic breast tumours. Oncogene 5:1573-1579

Radford DM, Fair KL, Thompson AM, Ritter JH, Holt M, Steinbrueck T, Wallace M, Wells, SA, Donis-Keller HR (1993) Allelic loss on chromosome 17 in DCIS of the breast. Cancer Res 53:2947-2950

Radford DM, Fair KL, Phillips NJ, Ritter JH, Steinbrueck T, Holt MS, Donis-Keller H (1995) Allelotyping in DCIS of the breast: deletion of loci on 8p, 13p, 16q, 17p and 17q. Cancer Res 55:3399-3405

Ramachandra S, Machin L, Ashley S, Monaghan P, Gusterson BA (1990) Immunohistochemical distribution of c-erbB-2 in in situ breast carcinoma - a detailed morphological analysis. J Pathol 161:7-14

Sainsbury JR, Farndon JR, Needham GK, Malcolm AJ, Harris AL (1987) Epidermal-growth-factor receptor status as predictor of early recurrence of and death from breast cancer. Lancet 1:1398-1402

Sato T, Tanigami A, Yamakawa K, Akiyama F, Kasumi F, Sakamoto G et al (1990) Allelotype of breast cancer: cumulative allele losses promote tumor progression in primary breast cancer. Cancer Res 50:7184-7189

Sato T, Saito H, Swensen J, Olifant A, Wood C, Danner D, Sakamoto T, Takita K, Kasumi F, Miki Y et al (1992) The human prohibitin gene located on chromosome 17q21 is mutated in sporadic breast cancer. Cancer Res 52:1643-1646

Schnitt SJ, Connolly JL, Tavassoli FA et al (1992) Interobserver reproducibility in the diagnosis of ductal proliferative breast lesions using standardized criteria. Am J Surg Pathol 16:1133–1143

Schuuring E (1995) The involvement of the chromosome 11q13 region in human malignancies: cyclin D1 and EMS1 are two new candidate oncogenes – a review. Gene 159:83–96

Sheikh MS, Shao ZM, Hussain A, Fontana JF (1993) The p53-binding protein MDM2 is differentially expressed in human breast carcinoma. Cancer Res 53:3226–3228

Silverstein MJ, Poller DN, Waisman JR et al (1995) Prognostic classification of breast ductal carcinoma-in-situ. Lancet 345:1154–1157

Silverstein MJ, Lagios MD, Craig PH, Waisman JR, Lewinsky BS, Colburn WJ, Poller DN (1996) A prognostic index for ductal carcinoma in situ of the breast. Cancer 77:2267–2274

Simpson JF, Quan DE, O'Malley F, Odom-Haryon T, Clarke PE (1997) Amplification of CCND1 and expression of its protein product cyclin D1 in ductal carcinoma in situ of the breast. Am J Pathol 151:161–168

Slamon DJ, Clark GM, Wong SG, Levin WJ, Ullrich A, McGuire WL (1987) Human breast cancer: correlation of relapse and survival with amplification of the HER-2/neu oncogene: Science 235:177–182

Slamon DJ, Godolphin W, Jones LA, Holt JA, Wong SG, Keith DE, Levin WJ, Stuart SG, Udove J, Ullrich A, Press MF (1989) Studies of the HER-2/neu proto-oncogene in human breast and ovarian cancer. Science 244:707–712

Solin LJ, Kurtz J, Fourquet A, Amalric R et al (1996) Fifteen-year results of breast-conserving surgery and definitive breast irradiation for the treatment of ductal carcinoma in situ of the breast. J Clin Oncol 14:754–763

Steeg PS, Clare SE, Lawrence JA, Zhou Q (1996) Molecular analysis of premalignant and carcinoma in situ lesions of the human breast. Am J Pathol 149:733–738

Stratton MR, Collins N, Lakhani SR, Sloane JP (1995) Loss of heterozygosity in ductal carcinoma in situ of the breast. J Pathol 175:195–201

Tavassoli FA, Norris HJ (1990) A comparison of the results of long-term follow-up for atypical intraductal hyperplasia and intraductal hyperplasia of the breast. Cancer 65:518–529

Tsuda H, Uei Y, Fukutomi T, Hirohashi S (1994) Different incidence of loss of heterozygosity on chromosome 16q between intraductal papilloma and intracystic papillary carcinoma of the breast. Jpn J Cancer Res 85:992–997

Van de Vijver MJ (1993) Molecular Genetics in Breast Cancer. Adv Cancer Res 61:25–56

Van de Vijver M, van de Bersselaar R, Devilee P, Cornelisse C, Peterse J, Nusse R (1987) Amplification of the neu (c-erbB-2) oncogene in human mammary tumors is relatively frequent and is often accompanied by amplification of the linked c-erbA oncogene. Mol Cell Biol 7:2019–2023

Van de Vijver MJ, Mooi WJ, Wisman P, Peterse, JL, Nusse, R (1988a) Immunohistochemical detection of the neu protein in tissue sections of human breast tumors with amplified neu DNA. Oncogene 2:175–178

Van de Vijver MJ, Peterse JL, Mooi WJ, Wisman P, Lomans J, Dalesio O, Nusse R (1988b) Neu-protein overexpression in breast cancer. Association with comedo-type ductal carcinoma in situ and limited prognostic value in stage II breast cancer. N Engl J Med 319:1239–1245

Varley JM, Swallow JE, Brammar WJ, Whittaker JL, Walker RA (1987) Alterations to either c-erbB-2(neu) or c-myc proto-oncogenes in breast carcinomas correlate with poor short-term prognosis. Oncogene 1:423–430

Varley JM, Brammar WJ, Lane DP, Swallow JE, Dolan C, Walker RA (1991) Loss of chromosome 17p13 sequences and mutation of p53 in human breast carcinomas. Oncogene 6:413–421

Vos CBJ, Cleton-Jansen AM, Berx G, de Leeuw WJF, ter Haar N, van Roy F, Cornelis CJ, Peterse JL, van de Vijver MJ (1998) E-cadherin inactivation in lobular carcinoma in situ: an early event in tumorigenesis. Br J Cancer 76:1131–1133

Weinstat-Saslow D, Merino MJ, Manrow RE, Lawrence JA, Bluth RF, Wittenbel KD, Simpson JF, Page DL, Steeg PS (1995) Overexpression of cyclin D mRNA distinguishes invasive and in situ breast carcinomas from non-malignant lesions. Nat Med 1:1257–1260

Yaremko ML, Kutza C, Lyzak J, Mick R, Recant WM, Westbrook CA (1996) Loss of hetero-
    zygosity from the short arm of chromosome 8 is associated with invasive behavior in
    breast cancer. Genes Chromosomes Cancer 16:189–195
Zeillinger R, Kury F, Czerwenka K, Kubista E, Sliutz G, Knogler W, Huber J, Zielinsk C, Rei-
    ner G, Jakesz R, Staffen A, Reiner A, Wrba F, Spona J (1989) HER-2 amplification, ste-
    roid receptors and epidermal growth factor receptor in primary breast cancer. Oncogene
    4:109–114
Zhuang Z, Merino MJ, Chuaqui R, Liotta LA, Emmert-Buck MR (1995) Identical allelic loss
    on chromosome 11q13 in microdissected in situ and invasive human breast cancer. Can-
    cer Res 55:467–471

Trials of Treatment for Non-invasive Breast Cancer

I. S. Fentiman

Guy's Hospital, London, SE1 9RT, UK

Background

Twenty years ago, ductal carcinoma in situ (DCIS) and lobular carcinoma in situ (LCIS) were rarely diagnosed conditions, poorly understood and usually treated by mastectomy like all other breast cancers. During the intervening years important changes have occurred with regard to both invasive and non-invasive breast cancer. In particular, several trials have demonstrated the safety of breast conservation therapy for selected patients with unifocal invasive breast cancers measuring up to 4 cm diameter (Veronesi et al. 1995; Fisher et al. 1989; Van Dongen et al. 1992; Jacobson et al. 1995; Blichert-Toft et al. 1988). The paradox then became apparent that women with invasive cancers were being treated by breast conservation therapy yet those with the non-life-threatening DCIS were still being subjected to mastectomy.

Additionally, the value of mammographic screening was demonstrated in women aged 50 years or over (Nystrom et al. 1993; De Koning et al. 1995). Because of the presence of X-ray microcalcifications, 15%–20% of cancers diagnosed are DCIS (Anderson et al. 1991). The incidence of LCIS is almost unchanged since there are no radiodiagnostic signs of LCIS on mammograms. With increasing specialisation in histopathology, however, subtle changes at the borderline of atypical lobular hyperplasia and LCIS are being recognised so that a few more cases are diagnosed. It is now more generally understood that LCIS or lobular neoplasia is a marker of risk rather than an obligate precursor of invasive cancer (Page et al. 1991). For this reason, LCIS has been selected as one of the entry criteria in the International Breast Intervention Study (Fentiman 1989). In this trial, women at a two- to four-fold increased risk of breast cancer are randomised to receive either tamoxifen 20 mg or placebo for 5 years. The end-point is the number of breast cancer cases in the two arms of the trial.

Considerations in Designing the Trials

Against this background the EORTC Breast Cancer Co-operative Group set about designing a trial of treatment for DCIS in the early 1980s (Fentiman 1997). It was recognised that wide excision of DCIS would be a pre-requisite because limited excision had been shown to be associated with a 25% risk of development of invasive cancer (Betsill et al. 1978; Rosen et al. 1980; Page et al. 1982). Additionally, unless a wide excision was performed there was a danger that DCIS found in a biopsy was a near miss representing the non-invasive element of an invasive carcinoma. This might explain the high proportion of invasive cancers diagnosed early on in a series of DCIS treated by local excision and radiotherapy (Morgan et al. 1984). In order to standardise histopathological handling of specimens a protocol of marking and sampling was drawn up by Dr. J. A. Peterse. The aim was to ensure that the specimen margins were systematically checked to minimise the risk of involved margins being missed.

All successful trials of breast conservation therapy had included axillary clearance so this procedure had to be considered as part of the surgical treatment. It was quickly dismissed. DCIS is by definition contained within the basement membrane of the ducts and has not attained the capability to break out of the normal domain of mammary epithelium. Hence neither vascular invasion nor axillary nodal involvement are accompaniments of pure DCIS. Although rare cases of axillary nodal involvement have been reported when the tumour was apparently pure DCIS, it is likely that foci of micro-invasion were missed, usually in more extensive lesions (Lagios et al. 1982). Since DCIS is not associated with axillary nodal involvement, not only could axillary surgery be omitted but so too could axillary irradiation. This would have an important consequence of reducing the morbidity of treatment within the trial.

With regard to the treatment of the breast itself, the randomised trials of treatment for invasive breast cancer had shown that a radiation dose of 46–50 Gy was adequate (Veronesi et al. 1995; Fisher et al. 1989; van Dongen et al. 1992; Jacobson et al. 1995; Blichert-Toft et al. 1988). With no available data on the radiosensitivity of DCIS, the dose was chosen arbitrarily as 50 Gy. Because the impact of radiotherapy on DCIS was unknown, the logical trial design was to compare breast irradiation with no radiotherapy in women who had had complete local excision of DCIS without evidence of micro-invasion. The basic trial design was thus:

Complete local excision – Randomise $\nearrow$ Breast irradiation (50 Gy)

$\searrow$ Observation

Unbeknown to the EORTC Breast Cancer Co-operative Group, at almost the same time the NSABP had started recruitment to B-17, a trial with similar inclusion criteria and treatment arms. Since then, various national groups have started trials but of these only four have been completed or are close to completion of accrual. The four randomised trials of treatment for DCIS and the numbers of cases entered and time of accrual are summarised in Table 1. Both NSABP B-17 and EORTC are now closed to entry and preliminary results of the former have been published (Fisher et al. 1993).

NSABP B-17 Trial

At the Fourth DCIS Consensus Meeting at Chateau Marquette, Amsterdam, on 23–24 January 1998, updated results from NSABP B-17 were presented. Qualitatively the data had not changed from those in the preliminary publication. As Table 2 shows, breast relapse occurred in 27% of the non-irradiated group; half of the recurrences were DCIS and half invasive. Radiotherapy reduced ipsilateral breast relapse from 27% to 12%. The major impact of radiotherapy was on invasive relapse (13% versus 4%), whereas DCIS relapse was reduced from 13% to 8%. The survival of both groups was similar, suggesting that the omission of radiotherapy has no deleterious effect on prognosis. Nevertheless, it must be remembered that this trial, like all the others, was not comparing breast conservation with mastectomy and so these results cannot be taken as showing that breast conservation for DCIS is the equivalent of total mastectomy.

Table 1. Accrual time and size of randomised trials of DCIS treatment

Trial	Accrual time	Number of cases
NSABP B17	1985–1990	818
EORTC 10853	1986–1996	1010
UK DCIS trial	1990–	1519
Swedish trial	1986–	>900

Table 2. Results of the NSABP B-17 trial presented at the Fourth DCIS Consensus Meeting, 23-24 January 1998, in Amsterdam (mean follow-up 90 months; *WLE* wide local excision)

	WLE ($n=405$) (%)	WLE + radiotherapy ($n=413$) (%)	p value
Event-free survival	62	75	<0.001
Overall survival	94	95	0.84
Ipsilateral relapse	27	12	<0.001
DCIS	13	8	<0.007
Invasive	13	4	<0.001

Table 3. Cumulative incidence of invasive breast cancer in NSABP B-17 by histological subgroup and treatment

Margins	Comedo	WLE ($n = 274$) (%)	WLE + radiotherapy ($n = 299$) (%)
Free	Absent/slight	15	11
Free	Moderate/Marked	34	9
Unknown/involved	Absent/slight	27	14
Unknown/involved	Moderate/Marked	41	12

Of the 818 cases in the trial, central pathological review has been conducted in 573 (70%). The histological features examined included nuclear grade, facility, comedo necrosis, cancerisation, stromal cellularity, lymphoid infiltrate, tumour size, margin status and tumour type. These were entered into a multivariate analysis of pathological factors and risk of relapse and the significant variables predicting for relapse were comedo/necrosis (relative risk 1.62, $p = 0.02$) and margin status (relative risk 1.57, $p = 0.055$). When these factors were analysed in relation to treatment (radiotherapy versus no radiotherapy) there appeared to be a benefit from breast irradiation in all sub-groups, as shown in Table 3.

Swedish DCIS Trial

This study is still underway; it has so far accrued more than 900 cases and will be closing within the next few months. No data are available at present.

UK DCIS Trial

Nation-wide breast cancer screening began in Britain in 1988 and as a consequence a boom in DCIS diagnoses was anticipated. To maximise the benefits of an expensive screening exercise a working party was set up under the chairmanship of Professor Charles Joslin. The final decision was to run a 2×2 factorial design trial, the outline of which is shown in Table 4. Participants had the option of a four-way randomisation or a two-way of radiotherapy versus no radiotherapy or tamoxifen versus no tamoxifen.

Eighty-five percent of cases were derived from the National Screening Programme in which triennial mammograms were taken of women between ages 50 and 64. Additionally, cases have been entered from Australia and New Zealand (co-ordinated by Professor John Forbes). A total of 1519 cases have been entered, of which 1357 came from the UK and 162 from Australia and New Zealand. There were 448 randomised to breast irradiation and 452 randomised to observation. The more popular choice was tamoxifen versus no tamoxifen, to which 723 and 705 were respectively randomised. Although

Table 4. Randomisation options in the UK DCIS trial

Complete local excision (CLE)	CLE + tamoxifen
CLE + radiotherapy	CLE + radiotherapy + Tamoxifen

it was originally planned to enter 1000 cases, because of the relative lack of cases in the radiotherapy versus no radiotherapy arms the trial will continue until 1000 have been randomised between these two options.

EORTC 10853 Trial

When this trial had been underway for 4 years the accrual rate was disappointingly low and so an analysis was conducted of all DCIS cases diagnosed between 1985 and 1989 in six of the participating centres: Centre Henri Becquerel, Rouen, Antoni van Leeuwenhoekhuis, Amsterdam, Daniel den Hoed Hospital Rotterdam, Longmore Hospital, Edinburgh, Guy's Hospital London and Centre Jules Bordet, Brussels (Fentiman et al. 1991). At that time these hospitals had entered into the trial 30, 14, 13, 7, 7 and 6 cases respectively. These 77 cases comprised, however, only 36% of the total of 216 patients diagnosed with DCIS.

Reasons for non-entry are outlined in Table 5. Of all the cases 46% were excluded because they did not fulfil non-pathological criteria, such as having had a prior invasive or non-invasive breast cancer (27, 19%), being too old or frail (4, 3%), or because of their refusal or the doctor's omission (8, 6%). The majority of patients who were not entered, however, had DCIS which was too extensive – 75, (54%), most of whom were treated by total mastectomy.

These results indicated that with stringent selection criteria, the majority of patients with DCIS would be unsuitable for breast conservation when diagnosed in units dealing mostly with symptomatic disease. At the time of that analysis the entry criteria excluded those with palpable lumps or microcalcification >3 cm (21, 15%). In order to try and improve accrual this was relaxed and patients with lumps or microcalcification up to 5 cm were eligible, provided that the DCIS was completely excised.

In total, 1010 cases have been entered of which 848 (84%) have been reviewed pathologically by Dr. Hans Peterse and site visits have been carried out by Dr. Nina Bijker. No data by treatment arm are available at present. The 5-year event-free survival is 78% and the local-relapse-free survival is 82%. The largest contributor to the trial was the National Cancer Institute, Milan, from which 151 cases were entered. Preliminary results have been presented after a median follow-up of 32 months and with a mean time to recurrence of 42 months (Salvadori et al. 1997). Table 6 gives the results and these indicate similar relapse rates with or without breast irradiation. No conclusions can be drawn from these early data other than the need for longer follow-up of the histologically well-characterised series of patients entered into EORTC 10853.

Table 5. Reasons for non-entry of cases to the EORTC 10853 trial

Protocol exclusions		Extent of DCIS	
Prior breast cancer	25	Margins involved	48
Patient refusal	6	Microcalcification >3 cm	16
Delay in histological diagnosis	9	Lump >3 cm	6
Borderline lesion	5	Multifocal DCIS	3
Protocol violation	4	Uncertain margins	2
Suspected invasive cancer	4		
Prior other malignancy	3		
Age over 70 years	2		
Contralateral DCIS	2		
Doctor's omission	2		
Unfit	2		

Table 6. Breast relapse rates after wide local excision and wide local excision plus radiotherapy in the Milan component of the EORTC 10853 trial

	WLE (n = 74)	WLE + radiotherapy (n = 77)
Ipsilateral relapse	10	9
DCIS	4	5
Invasive	6	4

Conclusions

It is still too early to draw definitive conclusions from the prospective randomised trials of DCIS treatment. The NSABP B-17 trial has furnished some evidence that radiotherapy does reduce the risk of progression to invasive cancer from DCIS, but this should not be taken as a blanket endorsement of the use of radiotherapy in patients with this condition. Some as yet unidentified patients do not need radiation, and this should emerge from the other trials when they become mature. Margins of excision are important but the necessary width is not yet defined. Probably the least welcome finding is the high rate of ineligibility for these trials, which indicates that many patients still need a mastectomy because of extensive DCIS. This may yet prove to be the optimal treatment for high-grade DCIS, but there may be a role for endocrine interventions in women with extensive well-differentiated DCIS.

Summary

Non-invasive breast cancer can be of either the ductal or the lobular type. While the former is often associated with progression to invasive cancer at the same site, lobular carcinoma in situ (LCIS) is a risk factor for invasive cancer rather than a precursor. As a result, LCIS has been used as one entry criterion for the International Breast Intervention Study in which women at increased risk because of histological findings or family history are randomised to receive either tamoxifen 20 mg daily or placebo for 5 years.

Four randomised trials have examined treatment options for ductal carcinoma in situ (DCIS) and all have demanded complete local excision as a necessary qualification for entry. Because of this, up to half the cases of DCIS were ineligible for entry since the disease was too extensive and was therefore usually treated by total mastectomy. In most studies – NSABP B-17, EORTC 10853 and Swedish trial – the randomisation was between breast irradiation and observation. Only one trial, NSABP B-17, has published results, and these suggest that progression to invasive cancer is reduced by irradiation. Withholding radiotherapy did not affect mortality. The UK DCIS trial is comparing the effects of both radiotherapy and tamoxifen, but as yet no results are available.

At present, radiotherapy should not be used as standard treatment of completely excised DCIS. Appropriate indications for irradiation will be determined when results of histologically characterised cases participating in mature trials become available. Total mastectomy remains the standard treatment for extensive DCIS, but the next generation of trials may examine the role of endocrine manipulation in cases with estrogen-receptor-positive tumours.

References

Anderson TJ, Lamb J, Donnan P et al (1991) Comparative pathology of breast cancer in a randomised trial of screening. Br J Cancer 64:108–113

Betsill WL, Rosen PP, Lieberman PH et al (1978) Intraductal carcinoma. Long-term follow-up after treatment by biopsy alone. JAMA 239:1863–1866

Blichert-Toft M, Brincker H, Andersen JA et al (1988) A Danish randomized trial comparing breast-preserving therapy with mastectomy in mammary carcinoma. Acta Oncol 27:671–677

De Koning HJ, Fracheboud J, Boer R et al (1995) Nation-wide breast cancer screening in the Netherlands: support for breast cancer mortality reduction. Int J Cancer 60:777–780

Fentiman IS (1989) The endocrine prevention of breast cancer. Br J Cancer 60:12–14

Fentiman IS (1997) EORTC trial 10853: Treatment options for DCIS of the breast. In: Silverstein MJ (ed) Ductal carcinoma in situ of the breast. Williams and Wilkins, Baltimore

Fentiman IS, Julien J-P, van Dongen JA et al (1991) Reasons for non-entry of patients with DCIS of the breast into a randomised trial (EORTC 10853). Eur J Cancer 27:450–452

Fisher B, Redmond C, Poisson R et al (1989) Eight-year results of a randomized clinical trial comparing total mastectomy and lumpectomy with or without irradiation in the treatment of breast cancer. N Engl J Med 320:822–828

Fisher B, Constantino J, Redmond C et al (1993) Lumpectomy compared with lumpectomy and radiation therapy for the treatment of intraductal breast cancer. N Engl J Med 328:1581–1586

Jacobson JA, Danforth DN, Cowan KH et al (1995) Ten-year results of a comparison of conservation with mastectomy in the treatment of stage I and II breast cancer. N Engl J Med 332:907–911

Lagios MD, Westdahl PR, Margolin FR et al (1982) Duct carcinoma in situ. Relationship of extent of non-invasive disease to the frequency of occult invasion, multicentricity, lymph node metastasis and short-term treatment failures. Cancer 50:1309–1314

Morgan DAL, Hinton CP, Blamey RW (1984) Management of intraduct carcinoma. Lancet 1:1082

Nystrom L, Rutqvist LE, Wall S et al (1993) Breast cancer screening with mammography: overview of Swedish randomised trials. Lancet 341:973–978

Page DL, Dupont AD, Roger LW et al (1982) Intraductal carcinoma of the breast: follow-up after biopsy alone. Cancer 49:751–758

Page DL, Kidd TE, Dupont WD et al (1991) Lobular neoplasia of the breast: higher risk for subsequent invasive cancer predicted by more extensive disease. Hum Pathol 22:1232–1239

Rosen PP, Braun DW, Kinne DF (1980) The clinical significance of pre-invasive breast carcinoma. Cancer 46:919-925

Salvadori B, Delledonne V, Rovini D (1997) National Cancer Institute Milan Experience. In Silverstein MJ (ed) Ductal carcinoma in situ of the breast. Williams and Wilkins, Baltimore

Van Dongen JA, Bartelink H, Fentiman IS et al (1992) Factors influencing local relapse and survival and results of salvage treatment after breast-conserving therapy in operable breast cancer: EORTC trial 10801, breast conservation compared with mastectomy in TNM stage I and II breast cancer. Eur J Cancer 28A:801-805

Veronesi U, Salvadori B, Luini A et al (1995) Breast conservation is a safe method in patients with small cancer of the breast. Long-term results of three randomised trials on 1,973 patients. Eur J Cancer 31A:1574-1579

Summary

J. M. Kurtz

Radiation Oncology Division, University Hospital, 1211 Geneva 14, Switzerland

Over the past 10 years carcinoma in situ has become a topic of intense interest. There are both scientific and practical reasons for this. From the standpoint of research, it is now believed that invasive breast carcinomas are preceded by an in situ phase. The study of non-invasive breast cancer may thus provide the key to understanding the multi-step genetic alterations leading to the development of invasive disease. From a clinical point of view, the interest is stimulated by the marked increase in the incidence of in situ breast cancer, particularly of the intraductal type (DCIS), essentially due to the increasing use of mammographic screening. Furthermore, the predominant role played by breast-conserving approaches makes it imperative to better define the optimal management of various types of in situ breast cancer with differing potentials for progression to invasive and possibly metastatic disease.

Although some attention was paid to molecular biological changes in breast cancer, this session was devoted largely to issues relating to the problem of breast conservation, particularly the question of histopathological classification, risk assessment in regard to local recurrence after conservation surgery, and information about randomised trials of adjuvant therapy. Epidemiological and diagnostic aspects, e.g. those relating to imaging and biopsy techniques, were not discussed at length. It was pointed out, however, that the current incidence of DCIS varies markedly between the United States and Europe, even European countries where mammographic screening is widely practised. This may reflect a greater tendency in the United States to biopsy mammographic lesions that are unlikely to be malignant. The possibility that American series may contain larger numbers of very small low-grade intraductal lesions must be borne in mind when attempting to extrapolate results from one side of the Atlantic to the other.

The first session speaker, Melvin J. Silverstein, discussed the clinical aspects of breast conservation in DCIS, based on a large series of 733 patients treated at the Breast Center in Van Nuys, California. Emphasising the heterogeneity of DCIS, Dr. Silverstein pointed out that no single treatment approach is likely to be appropriate for all patients. Compelling data were presented to show that the quantification of recurrence risk after breast-conserving therapy requires an assessment of three factors: (1) the extent of the lesion within the breast, (2) a parameter relating to the completeness of excision and, (3) a parameter expressing the biological aggressiveness of the particular lesion (e.g. the Van Nuys histological classification, see below under Prof. van de Vijver).

The Van Nuys Prognostic Index (VNPI) is essentially a numerical scoring system intended to integrate lesion size, resection margin width and histological classification into quantitative risk categories (Silverstein et al. 1996). Application of the VNPI to patients treated conservatively at the Breast Center suggests that the index can indeed potentially separate patients into subgroups of widely differing local recurrence risk. The practical usefulness of such a prognostic index might be to define patients who require no further treatment after local excision, those who might benefit additionally from breast irradiation, and perhaps a higher-risk group whose recurrence risk is unacceptably high despite breast irradiation and who might therefore benefit from mastectomy. Dr. Silverstein presented data suggesting that the margin width, i.e., the shortest distance from the microscopic lesion to the inked resection margin, might be the single most important factor predicging recurrence risk after excision. Data from the Van Nuys Breast Center suggest a very low recurrence risk of margins are greater than 10 mm, even in the presence of unfavourable histological features. Such low-risk patients would theoretically derive little benefit from breast irradiation. At the other end of the spectrum a high-risk subgroup was defined, consisting essentially of patients with large, rather high-grade lesions with positive margins. Here the recurrence risk approached 50% even in patients receiving radiotherapy, but only 27 patients fell into the latter category in the Van Nuys data set.

The influence of the VNPI in daily practice may be limited by difficulties in assessing lesion size and margin width for any but very small lesions. Larger lesions are often removed piecemeal, and meticulous pathological evaluation of excision specimens can be problematical even under the best of conditions. The Breast Center's experience suggests that the VNPI is a useful tool in a highly specialised multi-disciplinary setting, but it remains to be validated in other settings. Moreover, retrospective uncontrolled data such as those from the Breast Center cannot be used to draw reliable conclusions regarding the benefits of adjuvant treatments.

Dr. Silverstein also presented new data on outcome after local recurrence after breast conservation. About half of the local recurrences were invasive cancers, which tended to be diagnosed later (58 months median time) than non-invasive recurrences (22 months median). Although all the patients with non-invasive recurrences subsequently did well, patients with invasive recurrences sometimes presented with locally advanced disease, emphasising the importance of continued long-term clinical and mammographic follow-up. The 8-year breast-cancer-specific mortality for among patients with invasive recurrences was 14%.

The second speaker was Marc J. van de Vijver from the Pathology Department of the Netherlands Cancer Institute. In the first part of his talk he addressed the problem of pathological classifications. Because of the importance attached to breast preservation, classification systems can no longer be purely descriptive as in the past, but should reflect biological behaviour, particularly regarding the risk of progression to invasive carcinoma. Of several proposed classification systems, Prof. van de Vijver presented two in some detail: the one developed by an ad hoc EORTC pathology working party (Holland et al. 1994), and a second system called the Van Nuys classification (Silverstein et al. 1995). Although both systems attempt to define three distinct grades of differentiation, the European classification takes into account quite a large number of features, including cellular orientation. The Van Nuys classification, based only on the presence or absence of high cytonuclear grade and comedo necrosis, is much simpler to use. Future work will allow evaluation of the various classification systems, whose usefulness will be at least partially determined by interobserver reproducibility and ease of applicability. Whatever classification is currently favoured in any given centre, all important parameters should be noted and described in pathology reports so that cases can be classified according to various systems. A consensus conference on the pathology of in situ breast cancer was held in 1997 (Anonymous 1997).

The second half of Prof. van de Vijver's talk was devoted to genetic alterations, with particular emphasis on possible differences between the findings in invasive versus in situ lesions. Amplification of the c-erbB-2 and cyclin D1 genes has been well described in both invasive and in situ carcinomas, where the former gene is preferentially associated with poorly differentiated intraductal lesions. While these gene amplifications may reflect relatively early events in breast carcinogenesis, the amplification of certain other oncogenes has not yet been described in in situ carcinomas and thus may reflect later events in the evolution of invasive cancers. The inactivation of tumour suppressor genes is under intensive investigation. Mutation of the p53 gene has been demonstrated in both in situ and invasive carcinomas, particularly in the poorly differentiated subtypes. A large number of potential tumour suppressor genes have been postulated by demonstrating loss of heterozygosity (LOH) in specific regions of various chromosomes. Of particular interest in the E-cadherin gene, which is inactivated in invasive lobular but not in invasive ductal carcinomas, and which has been demonstrated in LCIS as well. E-cadherin inactivation may serve as a marker to distinguish between LCIS and low-grade DCIS, and its demonstration in LCIS militates against the widely held notion that LCIS is a "marker" rather than a true precursor lesion. Besides the apparent scientific interest associated with this domain of research, it is hoped that molecular markers will in future prove to be useful as prognostic factors for predicting the risk of progression after conservative treatment.

The last speaker of the session was Ian S. Fentiman from Guy's Hospital, who presented information regarding ongoing and completed prospective randomised trials concerning in situ breast cancer. The only trial open to patients with LCIS is the International Breast Intervention Study, in which patients are randomised to receive tamoxifen or placebo for 5 years. Of the DCIS trials, two have been completed and two are nearing completion of accrual. All four trials attempt to assess the benefits of breast irradiation following apparent complete excision, and the UK trial has an additional randomisation to tamoxifen or placebo. The only study with published results is the NSABP B-17 trial, in which 818 patients with DCIS were randomised after apparent complete excision to receive or not to receive 50 Gy breast irradiation. In the analysis at 8 years, breast irradiation was associated with a two-fold reduction in intraductal recurrence and an approximately four-fold reduction in invasive recurrence (Fischer et al. 1998). When analysed according to risk factors for recurrence (comedo-necrosis and margin status), radiotherapy appeared to benefit patients in all risk categories, although absolute benefits were very small in some subgroups. This study allowed for the first time a quantitative assessment of the relative risk reductions associated with radiotherapy in DCIS. However, the question still remains of defining subgroups whose absolute risks are so low that te security afforded by radiotherapy in unnecessary.

Professor Fentiman presented a progress report from the completed EORTC trial 10853. The reference pathologist has almost finished slide review. The overall number of observed events is similar in magnitude to that reported in the NSABP B-17 Trial, with a local relapse-free rate of 82% at 5 years. However, the EORTC has yet to authorise release of results according to randomisation arm; thus no conclusions can as yet be drawn regarding the effect of radiotherapy. Finally, Prof. Fentiman also stressed that a substantial proportion of patients have DCIS lesions that are too extensive to allow breast preservation, at least if the goal of treatment is to eliminate all "malignant" cells.

References

1. Anonymous (1977) Consensus conference on the classification of ductal carcinoma in situ. Cancer 80:1798–1802
2. Fisher B, Dignam J, Wolmark N et al (1998) Lumpectomy and radiation therapy for the treatment of intraductal breast cancer: findings from National Surgical Adjuvant Breast and Bowel Project B-17. J Clin Oncol 16:441–452
3. Holland R, Peterse JL, Millis RR et al (1994) Ductal carcinoma in situ: a proposal for a new classification. Semin Diagn Pathol 11:167–180
4. Silverstein MJ, Poller DN, Waisman JR et al (1995) Prognostic classification of breast ductal carcinoma-in-situ. Lancet 345:1154–1157
5. Silverstein MJ, Lagios MD, Craig PH et al (1996) A prognostic index for ductal carcinoma in situ of the breast. Cancer 77:2267–2274

V. Controversies About the Axilla

The Axilla: To Clear or Not to Clear?
That Is the Question!

M. Blichert-Toft

Rigshospitalet and DBCG Secretariat, 2100 Copenhagen, Denmark

> For few diseases does there exist
> a greater diversity of opinion
> regarding proper management
> than for mammary carcinoma.
>
> (William L. Donegan, 1967)

Introduction

Management of the axilla in patients with operable breast cancer is still hedged in by firm convictions. The most appropriate way of handling the axilla is a constant matter of great controversy. Views differ widely and opinions are strongly held (Fentiman et al. 1996). When the smoke had faded away, two main purposes remain, viz. (1) staging the axilla and (2) treating the axilla.

Predominantly, the debate is between believers in the Halsted concept and supporters of Fisher's theory. The Halstedians assume that breast cancer remains a localised disease for a long time, eventually spreading in an orderly fashion to the lymph nodes and blood stream, while the Fisher votaries assert that there is every probability that in the vast majority of patients the disease has already propagated and disseminated at an early stage before therapeutic intervention. Consequently, the Halsted spokesmen advocate extensive surgery including axillary dissection with the intention to cure, whereas the Fisher philosophy asserts the view that axillary surgery has no impact on the final outcome. According to Fisher's theory, the logical reason for axillary intervention, if any, is to implement a staging method, and not primarily to treat for cure.

There is every good reason, however, for emphasizing that a nihilistic attitude to the axilla should be avoided. It is generally that agreed accurate assessment of axillary node status is the single most reliable predictor of the final outcome of breast cancer and the primary determinant of the use of systemic therapy. It is also agreed that removal of axillary lymph nodes is the most reliable method of achieving accurate axillary staging (Fisher et al. 1981; Sacks et al. 1992; Rainsbury 1997). Finally, there is a growing approval of the role of locoregional tumour control is an important factor in survival (Overgaard et al. 1997; Ragaz et al. 1997). Thus, the views of both the Halstedians and the Fisher votaries should be taken into account in considering the proper approach to the axilla according to the "spectrum theory," which says that breast cancer is a heterogeneous disease – a spectrum ranging from a disease that remains local throughout its course to a disease which is systemic when first detected (Hellman 1994).

In the guidelines for surgeons in charge of the management of symptomatic breast cancer it is emphasized that histologic node status should be ascertained for all invasive tumors either by clearance or sampling of the axilla (British Association of Surgical Oncology 1995; Blichert-Toft et al. 1997). Admittedly, no surgeon favors surgical intervention in node-negative axillas. Therefore, the main question today is more like "How do we identify node-negative patients without complete axillary dissection?"

Frequency and Extent of Metastases Involving the Axilla

It has been argued that mammographic screening will minimize the dilemma about appropriate axillary management. More patients will be identified with small asymptomatic tumors with no axillary spread and a good prognosis (Dowlatshahi et al. 1995; Cady et al. 1996). This claim, however, has not been unanimously accepted (Fentiman et al. 1996; DBCG 1997).

Over the years, the Milan group has made a number of significant contributions to our knowledge about the extent of metastatic axillary involvement (Veronesi et al. 1990). The principal paper (Veronesi et al. 1990) reports on 1446 operable breast cancer patients treated by radical mastectomy, modified radical mastectomy, or breast-conserving surgery with additional axillary dissection irrespective of the breast surgical procedure. The average number of lymph nodes removed and examined was 20.3. In 839 patients (58%) axillary nodes were involved. The largest single group was the group of patients with one lymph node involved (26%). Groups became smaller with increasing number of metastatic lymph nodes, i.e., two positive nodes 16%, three nodes 10%, four nodes 6% etc. Remarkably, the proportion of patients harboring four positive nodes or more amounted to 48%. There was a direct correlation between tumor size and the number of metastatic nodes.

From the surgical angle the level of spread is of great significance. Level I was the only level involved in 54% of patients with a node-positive axilla, while level II and/or III was included as well in a further 45%. In 1%–2% of cases skip metastases were found, excluding level I. There was a close correlation between the number of metastatic lymph nodes involved at level I and the probability of lymph node involvement at a higher level. Further, with increasing tumor size there was an increasing risk of metastatic spread beyond level I. Risk of metastases at level III amounted to 35% for tumors 2 cm or less in size with involvement at levels I and II. Level III was the site of spread in 22% of all positive axillas.

The Milan study revealed that the incidence of metastatic spread to the axilla was quite considerable. Furthermore, level I was the level most often involved in metastatic spread, and removal of level I was reliable as a staging measure. If level I was the only level dissected there seemed to be a high risk of leaving behind residual disease at a higher level. If level I appeared without metastases there was a small risk of skip metastases at a higher level. Based on these findings, the authors concluded that the spread to the axilla followed a regular pattern invading level I first. Moreover, most problems regarding adequate surgery could be solved by complete axillary dissection.

In Denmark, breast cancer patients are treated according to nationwide protocols and approximately 95% of patients are registered in the Danish Breast Cancer Cooperative Group (DBCG) Data Center (DBCG 1997). The national figure of axillary node involvement amounted to 44%. The percentage of node positivity increased from 21% in tumors 1–10 mm in diameter to 72% in tumors more than 30 mm in diameter as measured by the pathologist (Fig. 1). The percentage of patients with four or more positive nodes increased from 23% for node-positive tumors of 1–10 mm up to 59% for node-positive tumors of more than 30 mm (Fig. 2). These data are based on a total of 16 600 DBCG patients below 75 years of age operated upon in the period 1990–1997 and with at least four axillary nodes retrieved. The results demonstrate that the frequency of metastatic spread to the axilla even in cases of small, impalpable tumors is considerable.

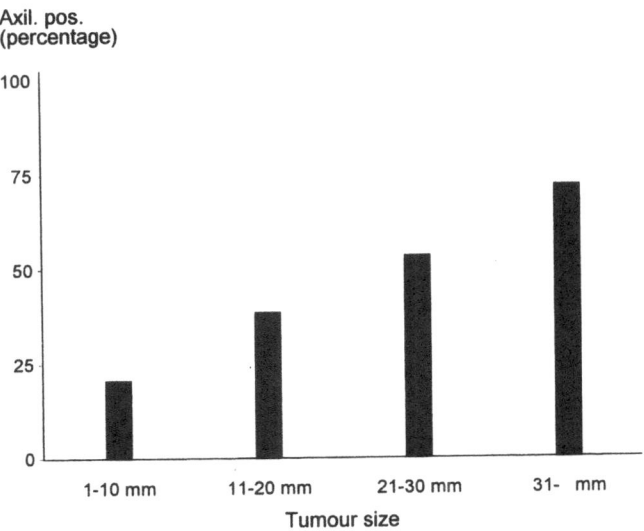

Fig. 1. Distribution of node positivity by axillary dissection in operable breast cancer patients, related to tumor size (16 660 patients under 75 years of age, median age 56 years, at least four nodes retrieved)

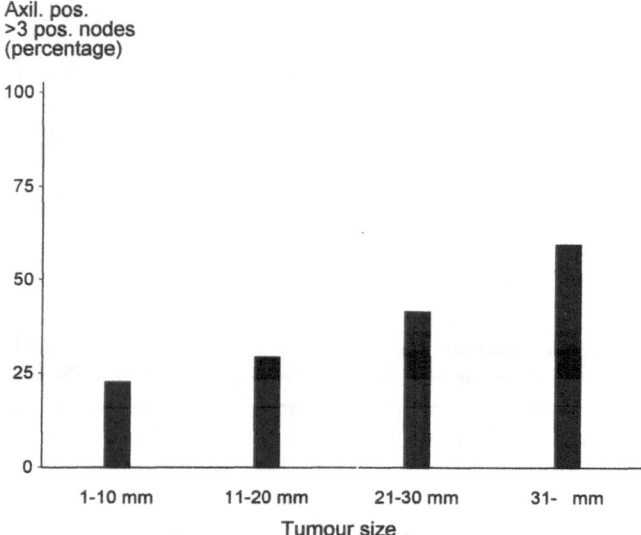

Fig. 2. Percentage of patients with four or more positive axillary nodes related to tumor size in node-positive-patients with operable breast cancer (7631 node-positive patients under 75 years of age, median age 56 years, at least four nodes retrieved)

Impact of Inaccurate Axillary Staging on Outcome

It is well established that accurate axillary staging can be performed by doing a less than complete axillary clearance (Fisher et al. 1981; Steele et al. 1985; Graversen et al. 1988; Veronesi et al. 1990; Axelsson et al. 1992). There is, however, a lower critical number of lymph nodes examined below which the likelihood of determining true nodal status turns out to be unreliable (Fisher et al. 1981). In treatment programs in which axillary nodal status decides patient allocation into risk groups, misclassification due to an unacceptably high rate of false negative nodal staging may be devastating (Graversen et al. 1988, 1992).

The calculated probability of false negative nodal staging has been analyzed in 3128 consecutive patients with operable invasive breast cancer initially characterized as node-negative and followed for up to 8 years (Graversen et al. 1988). The calculated 5-year probability for developing axillary relapse as first site was 19% in patients with no lymph nodes removed, 10% with one or two nodes removed and negative, 5% with three or four, 3% with five to ten, and 3% with more than ten nodes removed and negative at initial examination. Moreover, the study disclosed a significantly decreased overall survival in groups of patients with fewer than five nodes removed and negative at the initial examination compared with groups of patients who had five or more nodes excised. The decreased survival is explained as

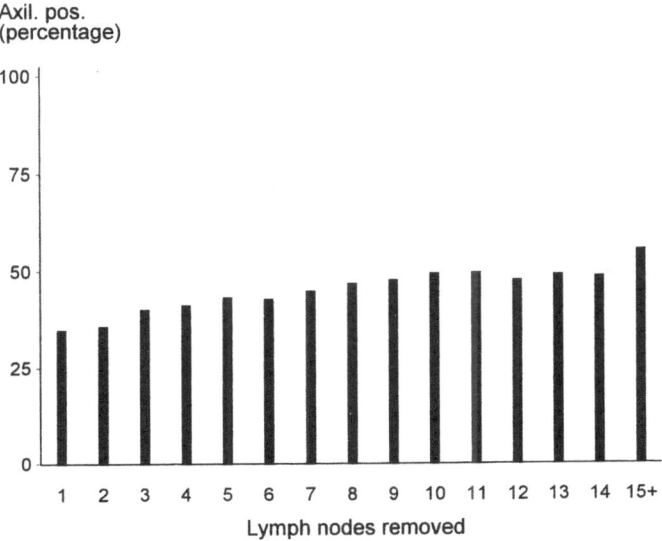

Fig. 3. Percentage of node positivity related to the number of axillary nodes removed in patients with operable breast cancer (42240 DBCG patients 1978–1997, median age 59 years, age range 14–96 years, at least one node retrieved)

a result of undertreatment, having deprived node-positive patients falsely staged as node-negative of optimal adjuvant therapy.

The study was enlarged and updated in 1990 (Graversen et al. 1992) and by now 6774 consecutive patients initially declared to be node-negative have been entered. A significant trend appeared showing a reciprocal relationship between the number of lymph nodes examined and axillary recurrence as first site. Survival differed highly significantly in a comparison between groups of patients with fewer than ten nodes removed and the group with ten or more nodes taken out.

The conclusion was that in DBCG programs at least ten nodes should preferably be recovered and examined by the pathologist in order to improve axillary staging. The minimum DBCG surgical requirement is a yield of four nodes. The DBCG quality measures are also based on the positive correlation between the total number of nodes removed and the proportion of node positivity as demonstrated in Fig. 3: at ten nodes excised the percentage of positivity seems to level out.

Patients Who Will Benefit from Meticulous Axillary Surgery

The advantage of axillary dissection in breast cancer management is often overlooked and over the years prevailing views have been colored by arguments valid in their era. Thus, in his Hunterian lecture presented in 1948

Victor Riddell said, "The views is taken that if the disease has spread to the axilla then surgery will only serve to disseminate it still further and if the disease is confined to the breast then dissection of the axilla is unnecessary". No wonder that many surgeons declined to dissect the axilla.

Further, the NSABP project (Fisher et al. 1985) presented its B-04 study which provided strong evidence against an advantage from axillary surgery. Eligible patients without clinically suspicious axillary lymph nodes were randomly assigned to one of three treatment arms: (1) radical mastectomy, (2) total mastectomy with postoperative radiation to the chest wall and the adjacent draining lymph node areas, and (3) total mastectomy alone. Respectively, 362, 352, and 365 patients were enrolled in the treatment arms. No significant difference in 10-year overall survival appeared among the three treatment groups. However, in the mastectomy-alone group the incidence of axillary failure was higher than in the two other arms. Subsequently, 17.8% of patients belonging to the mastectomy-alone group had histologically confirmed, positive ipsilateral axillary nodes, against 1%–3% in the other subgroups. There was no significant difference in distant disease rates among the three subsets. The conclusions of the B-04 study were that (1) axillary dissection had no bearing on survival and (2) subsequent removal of metastatic axillary nodes could be carried out as delayed surgery at the time of clinical presentation.

However, the B-04 study has been criticized (Harris and Osteen 1985). The main objection was that 35% of patients enrolled into the mastectomy-alone arm in fact had a lower axillary dissection at the initial operation. Taken this into account, the requirement for subsequent axillary dissection arose in 21% of the patients who had no nodes removed initially compared to 12% for the patients with one to five nodes recovered, and 0% for those who had at least six nodes taken out. This indicates that the requirement for delayed axillary surgery has been clearly underestimated in the Fisher trial. Besides, the criticism put forward by Harris and Osteen (1985) seriously affects the whole basis of the statistical analysis due to the reduced number of eligible probands in the mastectomy-alone group after correction for axillary intervention.

Although weight arguments have been raised against scepticism about axillary dissection, we still need to identify subsets of patients who will truly benefit from the procedure, i.e., in the form of increased survival. The value of axillary dissection as a staging procedure, prognosticator, and a safeguard against regional failure is highly acknowledged. What seems important to know is whether axillary metastases progress into distant disease. According to the Fisher spokesmen, axillary spread is an indicator rather than an instigator of distant disease. This statement, however, has become the object of serious doubt.

There are several studies in favor of the theory that axillary deposits might instigate distant spread and thereby influence survival in a negative way. This hypothesis is substantiated by the observation that a certain proportion of patients harboring axillary metastases have a similar survival to patients with local disease only – provided the axillary nodes are removed (Gardner and Feldman 1993). The excess mortality in the regional group disappeared by 7 years of observation after surgery. This segment of patients is estimated to amount 30% of patients with regional spread.

Similar results seem to appear from the DBCG 77 B and 77 C protocols (Dombernowsky et al. 1988; Mouridsen et al. 1988). Between 1977 and 1982 the two trials accrued a total of 1034 premenopausal and 1716 postmenopausal patients, respectively. All patients underwent mastectomy with partial axillary dissection. The main criterion for inclusion was axillary node positivity. Postsurgically, patients were allocated at random to receive radiotherapy alone or radiotherapy combined with systemic therapy, i.e., chemotherapy (CMF or C) in the premenopausal group and tamoxifen in the postmenopausal group. At 10 years of follow-up the probability of recurrence-free survival was about 30%–40% in the group of patients treated by locoregional therapy alone (DBCG 1997). This indicates that a substantial proportion of node-positive patients had not contracted distant disease at the time of surgery and were in fact true candidates to receive adequate axillary therapy.

The Milan group presented similar observations to the DBCG results in node-positive breast cancer patients treated with surgery alone (Cascinelli et al. 1987). Survival correlated with the number of nodes involved. Consequently, the study gave evidence of a subset of node-positive patients potentially curable by extensive surgery.

Recently, the DBCG presented substantial evidence in favor of locoregional tumor control as an influential factor on survival in node-positive premenopausal patients with operable breast carcinoma (Overgaard et al. 1997). After mastectomy and axillary dissection the patients were randomized to receive radiotherapy combined with chemotherapy (CMF) versus chemotherapy (CMF) alone. The study recruited 1708 eligible patients. Patients belonging to the CMF-alone arm experienced locoregional recurrence significantly more frequently than the group treated by radiotherapy as well. Remarkably, the 10-year survival differed highly significantly in favor of the radiotherapy arm. The conclusion was that the addition of radiotherapy to adjuvant therapy reduces locoregional relapse and improves survival. Quite similar observations were presented by Ragaz et al. (1997).

These studies seem to prompt a reevaluation of the need for axillary surgery. Thus, evidence is given in support of a true benefit on survival from axillary intervention in a certain subgroup of node-positive patients.

Extent of Axillary Dissection

The purpose of axillary dissection is accurate staging, reliable prognostic information, and to safeguard against regional failure. In order to achieve these goals complete axillary dissection is required (Mattheiem et al. 1989; O'Higgins 1994). Nonetheless, axillary dissection is undertaken in different ways, varying from complete clearance to partial dissection including one or more levels, sampling, and, finally, limited biopsies. Performing less than complete clearance entails a considerable risk of leaving behind residual disease. On the other hand, the benefits of extensive surgery have to be balanced against surgical sequelae. Today, most surgeons advocate modified axillary clearance involving level I or II or perhaps a sampling procedure (British Association of Surgical Oncology 1995; Blichert-Toft et al. 1997). Modified axillary clearance removing at least ten nodes including any grossly suspicious disease if present seems to be a reasonable and adequate compromise compared to complete clearance (Axelsson et al. 1992).

The sampling procedure may lead to improper treatment, local morbidity due to axillary failure not amenable to surgical excision, and false staging (Greenall 1995). Missing nodes has been described in up to 30% of cases due to poorly performed surgery. False negative axillary staging has been encountered in 3%–20% of cases and underdiagnosis of positivity in 5%–43%, depending on the number of nodes retrieved. Properly performed, the sampling procedure can allow qualitatively accurate staging (Steele et al. 1985). Nevertheless, a major disadvantage of the sampling procedure is inaccurate quantitative staging and a high probability of leaving residual disease in the axillary cavity that will require additional surgery or radiotherapy.

Only the DBCG studies (Graversen et al. 1988, 1992) and a study from the Institut Curie (Cabanes et al. 1992) have so far demonstrated a significant improvement in survival related to the yield of axillary dissection, while other trials have failed to reveal survival differences. Axillary failures and morbidity, however, relate clearly to the specific surgical procedure and the number of nodes recovered (Greenall 1995). Moreover, meticulous performance of axillary surgery is emphasized, due to records showing increased survival related to improved locoregional disease control (Overgaard et al. 1997; Ragaz et al. 1997).

Need for Radiotherapy After Axillary Clearance?

Arm morbidity, in particular lymphedema, is a serious and troublesome sequela after axillary surgery, often leading to deformity and disability of the ipsilateral arm. The combination of extensive axillary dissection and radiotherapy increases the risk of lymphedema by a factor 4–5, i.e., from 5%–10% without radiotherapy up to approximately 40% with irradiation.

In node-positive patients the axillary recurrence rate is unacceptably high unless an adequate number of nodes has been retrieved or radiotherapy is given as an adjunct to inadequate surgery. In the DBCG 82 B and 82 C adjuvant protocols (DBCG 1997) recruiting node-positive premenopausal (82 B) and postmenopausal (82 C) patients, the correlation between the number of lymph nodes recovered and the rate of axillary recurrence as first sile has been analyzed. In these two trials the patients underwent mastectomy and axillary dissection. After surgery, they were allocated at random to receive systemic therapy plus radiotherapy or systemic therapy alone. Comparison between the two regimes revealed that a yield of at least ten nodes ensured the smallest gap between axillary relapse rates at 5-year follow-up (Figs. 4, 5).

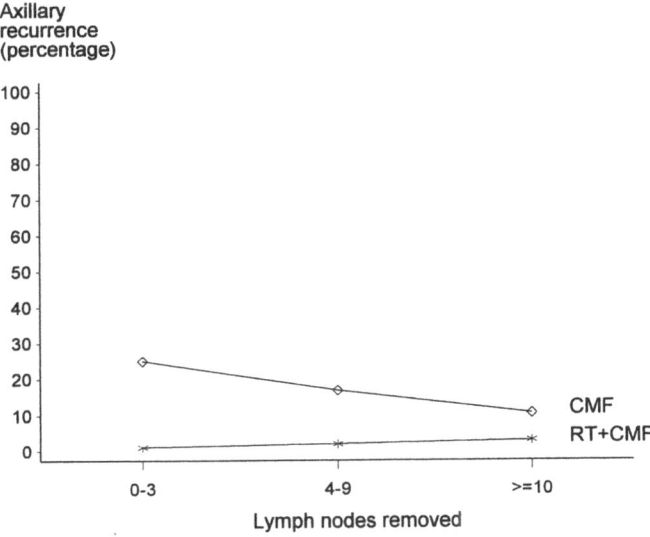

Fig. 4. Comparison of the frequency of axillary recurrence as first site at 5 years related to the number of axillary nodes removed: chemotherapy with or without radiation. The series comprised 1708 premenopausal node-positive patients (protocol DBCG-82 B) undergoing mastectomy with additional axillary dissection. Post-surgically, the patients were allocated at random to receive adjuvant chemotherapy (CMF) with or without radiotherapy

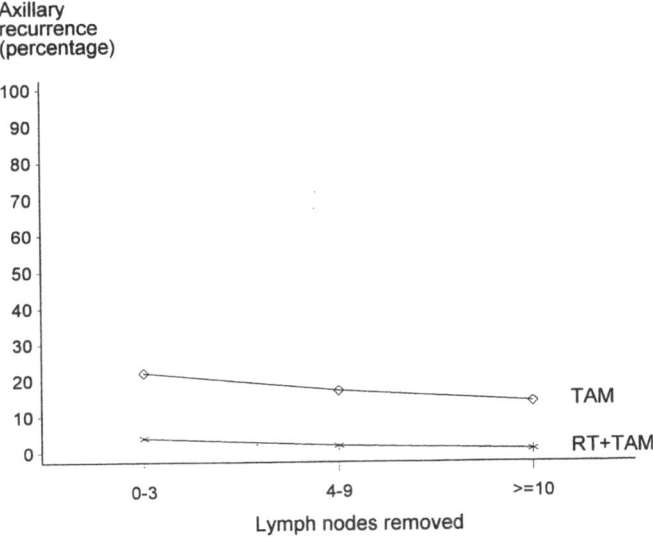

Fig. 5. Comparison of the frequency of axillary recurrence as first site at 5 years related to the number of axillary nodes removed: tamoxifen with or without radiation. The series comprised 1375 postmenopausal node-positive patients undergoing mastectomy with additional axillary dissection. Postsurgically, the patients were allocated at random to receive adjuvant tamoxifen with or without radiotherapy

In the future DBCG protocols, the axilla will no longer be irradiated in node-positive patients provided a yield of at least ten nodes and no grossly suspicious disease is left behind in the axillary cavity.

Conclusion

The main purposes of axillary dissection are (1) staging the axilla and (2) treatment of the axilla.

Most clinicians agree that axillary nodal status should remain the cornerstone of decision making in potentially curable invasive breast cancer. Nodal status is considered (1) the single best predictor of outcome and (2) the primary determinant of the use of systemic therapy. Most principal investigators also agree that no imaging technique can replace axillary dissection for accurate staging and no tumor marker can accurately predict axillary nodal status. At present, there are no nonsurgical staging alternatives for obtaining full axillary nodal status.

As to treatment to cure, there is increasing evidence indicating that control of locoregional disease plays an important role in survival for node-positive patients. Taking into account the extent of axillary spread, total or near-total dissection of the axilla is preferable to a sampling procedure in order to minimize the risk of leaving behind residual disease.

In future trials the main issue to be addressed should be how to avoid surgery of node-negative axillas and how to treat the node-positive axilla. The first must await results from ongoing trials addressing the reliability of the sentinel node technique. The second is obviously most properly dealt with by performing adequate axillary clearance. Reappraisal of the role of axillary lymph node dissection should be postponed until sentinel node biopsy has been widely adopted and the scientific results carefully examined (Morrow 1996). In the meanwhile the recommendation is to perform adequate axillary surgery rather than inadequate surgery with radiotherapy as an adjunct. As is wisely said by W. Mattheiem: "No woman afflicted with breast cancer can be cured if she is not cured locally."

Summary

The prime objectives for axillary dissection are staging and treatment to cure. No physical examination, no imaging techniques, and no tumor markers can replace axillary dissection for staging. Further, axillary node status in potentially curable breast carcinomas is still considered the single best predictor of outcome and the primary determinant of the use of systemic therapy. Finally, locoregional tumor control seems to improve survival, emphasizing meticulous axillary dissection. Today, the question to be asked is not whether or not to clear the axilla; rather, the question should go: How do we distinguish node-negative patients from those who are node-positive without clearing the axilla unnecessarily? No surgeon would advocate dissecting the axilla in node-negative patients if nodal status could be ascertained by a different technique. Ongoing trials addressing the reliability of the sentinel node technique seem promising, and this technique may perhaps in the near future solve the problem of distinguishing node-negative patients from those with axillary spread. For the time being, the necessity of determining axillary status and to treat for cure can hardly be questioned. Therefore, once axillary spread has been demonstrated in one way or another, an adequate and meticulous axillary dissection should be performed.

References

Axelsson CK, Mouridsen T, Zedeler K (1992) Axillary dissection of level I and II lymph nodes is important in breast cancer classification. Eur J Cancer 28 A:1415–1418

Blichert-Toft M, Smola G, Cataliotti L, O'Higgins N (1997) Principles and guidelines for surgeons – management of symptomatic breast cancer. Eur J Surg Oncol 23:101–109

British Association of Surgical Oncology (1995) Guidelines for surgeons in the management of symptomatic breast disease in the United Kingdom. Eur J Surg Oncol 21 Suppl A:1–13

Cabanes PA, Salmon RJ, Vilcoq JR, Durand JC, Fourquet A et al (1992) Value of axillary dissection in addition to lumpectomy and radiotherapy in early breast cancer. Lancet 339:1245–1248

Cady B, Stone MD, Schuler JG, Thakur R, Wanner MA et al (1996) The new era in breast cancer: invasion, size, and nodal involvement dramatically decreasing as a result of mammographic screening. Arch Surg 131:301–308

Cascinelli N, Greco M, Bufalino R, Clemente C, Galluzo D et al (1987) Prognosis of breast cancer with axillary node metastasis after surgical treatment only. Eur J Cancer Clin Oncol 23:795–799

DBCG (1997) Danish Breast Cancer Cooperative Group: Data collection, Secretariat. Righshospitalet, Copenhagen

Dombernowski P, Brincker H, Hansen M, Mouridsen HT, Overgaard M et al (1988) Adjuvant therapy of premenopausal and menopausal high-risk breast cancer patients. Acta Oncol 27:691–697

Dowlatshahi K, Snider HC, Kim R (1995) Axillary node status in nonpalpable breast cancer. Ann Surg Oncol 2:424–428

Fentiman IS, Epstein R, Barr L (1996) Is routine axillary nodal dissection necessary in the treatment of breast cancer? Eur J Cancer 32 A:1460–1461

Fisher B, Wolmark N, Bauer M, Redmond C, Gebhardt M (1981) The accuracy of clinical nodal staging and of limited axillary dissection as a determinant of histologic nodal status in carcinoma of the breast. Surg Gynecol Obstet 152:765–772

Fisher B, Redmond C, Fisher ER, Bauer M, Wolmark N et al (1985) Ten-year results of a randomized clinical trial comparing radical mastectomy and total mastectomy with or without radiation. N Engl J Med 312:674–681

Gardner B, Feldman J (1993) Are positive axillary nodes in breast cancer markers for incurable disease? Ann Surg 218:270–278

Graversen HP, Blichert-Toft M, Andersen JA, Zedeler K (1988) Breast cancer: risk of axillary recurrence in node-negative patients following partial dissection of the axilla. Eur J Surg Oncol 14:407–412

Graversen HP, Zedeler K, Andersen JA, Axelsson CK, Blichert-Toft M (1992) Axillary dissection at primary surgical treatment for cancer of the breast. The risk of false-negative axillary status. Ugeskr Laeger 154:3392–3395

Greenall MJ (1995) Why I favour axillary node sampling in the management of breast cancer. Eur J Surg Oncol 21:2–7

Harris JR, Osteen RT (1985) Patients with early breast cancer benefit from effective axillary treatment. Breast Cancer Res Treat 5:17–21

Hellman S (1994) Natural history of small breast cancers. J Clin Oncol 12:2229–2234

Mattheiem W, Bourgeois P, Delcorde A, Stegen M, Frühling J (1989) Axillary dissection in breast cancer revisited. Eur J Surg Oncol 15:490–495

Morrow M (1996) Role of axillary dissection in breast cancer management. Ann Surg Oncol 3:233–234

Mouridsen HT, Rose C, Overgaard M, Dombernowski P, Panduro J et al (1988) Adjuvant treatment of postmenopausal patients with high-risk primary breast cancer. Acta Oncol 27:699–705

O'Higgins N (1994) How I minimize morbidity in axillary dissection. Eur J Surg Oncol 20:80–81

Overgaard M, Hansen PS, Overgaard J, Rose C, Andersson M et al (1997) Postoperative radiotherapy in high-risk premenopausal women with breast cancer who receive adjuvant chemotherapy. N Engl J Med 337:949–955

Ragaz J, Jackson SM, Le N, Plenderleith IH, Spinelli JJ et al (1997) Adjuvant radiotherapy and chemotherapy in node-positive premenopausal women with breast cancer. N Engl J Med 337:956–962

Rainsbury RM (1997) New advances in the surgical treatment of breast cancer. Breast 6:349–353

Riddell V (1948) Hunterian lecture: carcinoma of the breast. Royal cCollege of Surgeons of England, London

Sacks NPM, Barr LC, Allan SM, Baum M (1992) The role of axillary dissection in operable breast cancer. Breast 1:41–49

Steele RJC, Forrest APM, Gibson T, Stewart HJ, Chetty U (1985) The efficacy of lower axillary sampling in obtaining lymph node status in breast cancer: a controlled randomized trial. Br J Surg 72:368–369

Veronesi U, Luini A, Galimberti V, Marchini S, Sacchini V et al (1990) Extent of metastatic axillary involvement in 1446 cases of breast cancer. Eur J Surg Oncol 16:127–133

Axillary Clearance in Operable Breast Cancer: Still a Necessity?

D. W. Kinne

Columbia Presbyterian Hospital, 622 West 168th Street, New York, NY 10032, USA

For many years, axillary lymph node dissection has been a routine part of the surgical treatment of breast cancer. This has been most often accompanied in the past by a total mastectomy (radical mastectomy or modified radical mastectomy); more recently, it has often been carried out at the time of or subsequent to segmental (breast conserving) mastectomy.

The attitudes and opinions of surgeons regarding the choice of therapy for breast cancer have gradually changed as we achieve earlier diagnoses and learn more of the biology of this disease. Questions regarding the role of axillary lymph node dissection in patients with primary operable breast cancer are a logical result.

The basic tenets of surgical oncology include that the surgical approach to primary operable cancer should afford maximal local control with an attempt to maximize preservation of function, have an impact on the natural history of the disease with a curative intent, and provide biologic information regarding the tumor as it relates to prognosis and efficacy of adjuvant therapy. The role and efficacy of axillary dissection for invasive breast cancer should be evaluated according to these parameters and compared to any other viable alternatives (Lindet et al. 1993; Moffat et al. 1992; Robinson et al. 1992; Fentimen and Mansel 1991).

Long-term survival exceeds 90% in patients with the earliest-detected lesions (Rosen et al. 1989a,b,1991). Survival is directly related to the size of the lesion and the involvement and number of involved axillary lymph nodes (Wilking et al. 1992; Haagensen 1986). There is a well-described linear relationship between tumor size and nodal involvement (Haagensen 1986). Even the smallest of lesions, such as a T1A lesion, are associated with a 10%–15% risk of axillary nodal disease (Stierer et al. 1992; Chada et al. 1994; Silverstein et al. 1994). The progression from primary tumor to nodal involvement and subsequent distant metastatic disease is often very orderly (Veronesi et al. 1987; Msuya and Hartveit 1991; Piggot et al. 1984; Boova et al. 1982; Reynolds et al. 1994). Tumor size is directly related to nodal involvement (Haagensen 1986). Ductal carcinoma in situ (DCIS) is rarely associated with nodal disease (Silverstein et al. 1991; Rosser et al. 1987) and DCIS with micro-invasion has been reported to have nodal disease about 10% of the time (Kinne et al. 1989). Small invasive cancers such as the T1A are reported to have a 10%–15% incidence of nodal disease (Rosen et al. 1989a; Boova et al. 1982). Similar information was reported by Winchester et al. (1996), who compiled more than 300 000 cases in the American College of Surgeons data bank and found a 15% frequency of axillary disease in the T1A lesion. Evaluation of all invasive breast cancers demonstrates 40% of the total to have involved axillary nodes, and subset analysis demonstrates 29% involvement with T1 lesions and 58% with T2 lesions (Danforth et al. 1986).

Quantitative progression of nodal involvement is also correlated with increasing involvement of nodal levels. In those patients with involved lymph nodes, approximately 60% have involvement of level I, 22% with levels I and II, and 17% with all three levels (Veronesi et al. 1987). A patient with a single involved lymph node at level I has an 8% chance of disease at levels II and III, a 25% risk with two level I nodes, and 66% with four or more involved level I nodes. A T1 tumor with involved lymph nodes in level I is associated with a 28.4% risk of involvement of the upper levels and T2 lesions with a 40% risk of upper level involvement. It is for this reason that a clinically suspicious axilla is fully dissected.

The intent of axillary dissection should be to remove all potentially involved lymph nodes. If clinically positive nodes are encountered, the dissection should be complete. Axillary dissection of the clinically and intraoperatively negative axilla should remove enough lymph nodes so as to be predictive that the remaining lymph nodes are also negative. A mathematical model of complete axillary dissection defines the minimum number of nodes removed per primary tumor size so as to predict with a high degree of confidence that the remaining nodes are negative. A minimum of ten nodes need to be removed to have a 93% predictive value (not a number the average cancer patient would find acceptable) that the remaining nodes are clear (Kiricuta and Tausch 1992). Axillary sampling achieves neither of the stated goals (Fentimen and Mansel 1991; Christensen and Jansson 1993).

Surgical removal of involved axillary nodes may be associated with long-term survival. The 30-year follow-up study of Adair et al. (1952) demonstrated 70% of T1N0 patients free of disease at 30 years and 45%–50% of all patients with nodal involvement surviving 30 years. These survival data come from an era when primary operable breast cancer was treated with radical mastectomy with complete axillary dissection and was without the benefit of adjuvant therapy. Similar survival data were reported in a more recent series with 83% of stage I breast cancer patients free of disease at the end of one decade and 79% at the end of the second decade (Rosen et al. 1989a).

Involvement of one lymph node decreased the survival to 71% at 10 years and 66% at 20 years, and involvement of two nodes diminished survival an additional 10% at each reference point. Further support comes from the occult axillary lymph node studies where survival in the 17% of cases with axillary metastasis noted only upon serial sectioning of the nodes was similar to the node-negative population (Wilkinson et al. 1992). It would seem that there was benefit from removal of this microscopic disease in that survival was equal to the node-negative without the benefit of adjuvant therapy.

It is important to recognize that although nodal involvement diminishes survival, many of the node-positive patients achieved long-term disease-free survival with surgery alone. Survival is directly related to nodal involvement; most of the attrition is early and there is little additional fall-off as time goes on. It would be difficult to understand the concept of breast cancer as a systemic disease from its inception in light of the long-term local control and disease-free survival seen with surgery alone. Similar information was reported by Haagensen (1986) directly relating survival to quantitative nodal involvement and reporting long-term survival with surgery alone.

The majority of breast cancer patients do not have an involved axilla and therefore do not derive survival benefit from the procedure. There is at present no accurate preoperative assessment of the axilla to select for those patients with a high probability of a disease-negative axilla. In addition, axillary recurrence is a negative prognostic event with high morbidity and mortality (Dekkers 1991). At present, axillary dissection is justified in all cases so as not to undertreat the involved axilla. It would be beneficial to have a preoperative assessment of the axilla so as to identify that group of patients with a very high probability of a negative axilla so as to potentially avoid axillary dissection in selected patients in the future.

Assessment of the Axilla

Several modalities have attempted to evaluate axillary lymph nodes prior to axillary dissection (Silverstein et al. 1994; Alex and Krag 1993; Noguchi et al. 1993; de Freitas et al. 1991; Ball et al. 1992; Fisher et al. 1981). Physical examination is remarkable for the impressive inaccuracy of the clinical examination, with a false negative rate of at least 25%. Danforth et al. reported on 136 patients with axillary dissections, and in those patients with a clinically negative axilla, 38% had a histologically proven disease in the nodes (Danforth et al. 1986). This is in line with other series reporting a false negative rate of physical examination at 29%–38% (de Freitas et al. 1991).

Attempts preoperatively to evaluate the axilla have ranged from mammography to computed axial tomography and positron emission tomography (Isaacs et al. 1993; Nieweg et al. 1993; Wahl et al. 1991). Mammography is of limited value in the assessment of axillary nodes and is accurate in only the analysis of the most clinically obvious nodes. CT scanning has been reported in a small number of patients with a positive predictive value of 89%, sensitivity of 50%, and specificity of 75%, and a negative predictive value of 20% (Isaacs et al. 1983). It was concluded that although the CT scan was superior to the physical examination, it was not an accurate predictor of lymph node involvement primarily because of the low negative predictive value. Other modalities include positron emission tomography utilizing 6-fluorodeoxyglucose metabolism (Nieweg et al. 1993; Wahl et al. 1991). A report of ten patients demonstrated the primary lesion in all patients and unsuspected nodal and bony disease in 40% (Nieweg et al. 1993).

Intraoperative assessment of axillary nodes includes sentinel node mapping and radioimmune-guided surgery (de Freitas et al. 1991; Giuliano et al. 1994; Krag et al. 1993). Both techniques require limited surgery of the nodal basin, and early results with sentinel node mapping suggest a correlation between the sentinel node and axillary nodal status. If the positive predictive value is high, such techniques would allow selective dissection of the positive axilla.

Axillary Recurrence

The issues with expectant observation of lymph nodes include the difficulty encountered in clinical examination of the axilla and those problems associated with local and distant control of the cancer. Clinical examination of the axilla is unreliable with up to one-third of involved axillary nodes not detected by standard means, which may lead to a significant delay in diagnosis. Local recurrences often lead to compressive symptoms in the axilla with impingement of vascular, lymphatic, or neural structures. Although the majority of symptoms are secondary to compressions rather than direct invasion, relief of the compression is not always associated with resolution of symptoms. In addition, there is the occasional patient with inoperable isolated axillary recurrence.

Local failure after complete axillary dissection is unusual and in the range of 0–2% (Fisher et al. 1981; Graversen et al. 1988). Axillary recurrence in the clinicallly node-negative in whom the axilla is not dissected occurs in the 16%–37% range. Graversen et al. (1988) quantified axillary recurrences according to the number of lymph nodes removed with a 19% 5-year recurrence rate in those in whom no nodes were removed, 10% in those with a limited dissection, and 3% in those with more than ten nodes removed. Similar information was reported from the NSABP B-04 with a 21.2% axillary recurrence in those with no axillary dissection, 12% if six or fewer nodes were removed, and 0.3% if more than ten nodes were removed (Fisher et al. 1981).

Axillary recurrence in breast cancer often has been compared to a similar event in melanoma with little or no reason to support such comparison. Isolated axillary recurrence in breast cancer is a poor prognostic event (Dekkers 1991). Axillary nodal recurrence as the sole site of disease was reported in 21% of the group randomized to no axillary therapy in the NSABP B-04 and 85% of this group eventually manifested systemic disease (Deckers 1991). The time to axillary recurrence ranged from 3 months to 134 months with a median of 14.8 months, and the time to subsequent systemic failure was a median of 17.2 months. Similar experience is noted by the authors with a 79% distant failure rate at 2 years in 42 patients who underwent complete axillary dissection after isolated axillary recurrence. All patients were free of distant disease at the time of axillary recurrence, and the initial axillary treatment was not the responsibility of the authors.

Analysis of NSABP Study B-04

Proponents of expectant observation of the axilla often quote NSABP B-04 as the basis of their position. The study involved 1665 patients randomized to one of three treatments: radical mastectomy, total mastectomy with radiation, and total mastectomy followed by axillary dissection only if axillary lymph nodes were later clinically positive. Isolated axillary recurrences – excluding preexisting or synchronous distant failure – were reported at 18%.

An analysis of the outcome in B-04 was reported by Harris and Osteen (1985). The original B-04 report acknowledged that 35% of the patients randomized to no axillary therapy had a limited axillary dissection, including some patients with >20 nodes removed (Fisher et al. 1981). A subsequent report related local regional failure to the extent of the axillary dissection in the group randomized to no axillary therapy. Of those who were randomized to no axillary therapy and actually had no nodes removed, 21% subsequently developed an isolated axillary recurrence. Excluded from the group of axillary recurrences were patients with either preexisting or synchronous distant failure. The analysis of Harris and Osteen (1985) suggests that B-04 does not have the statistical power to prove or disprove the efficacy of axillary dissection. In order to have a 90% chance of detecting a 7% difference between the two treatment groups, 2000 patients would have been required rather than the 550 patients assigned to each arm. In addition, the difficulty of axillary assessment is not addressed, meaning that many patients may harbor positive nodes not detected upon routine clinical follow-up. False negative clinical examination is reported to be about 30%, so a significant proportion of the total would have undetected axillary nodal disease.

Survival Benefit

There are several studies that support a survival benefit of axillary treatment. The second Guy's Hospital series randomized 253 clinical stage I patients to radical mastectomy with axillary dissection or wide local excision with postoperative radiation to the breast and axilla (Hayward 1983). At 8 years, there was a statistically significant difference in both distant recurrence and survival in the group with axillary dissection. A prospective randomized trial of axillary dissection in addition to lumpectomy and radiation was completed on 658 patients with a clinically negative axilla (Cabanes et al. 1992). With a median follow-up of 54 months, there was a significant advantage in survival in the axillary dissection group with less frequent visceral, supraclavicular, and axillary recurrences also noted. Adjuvant chemotherapy was given to 11 patients in the axillary dissection group and to none in the observation group. This study concluded that a survival benefit could be demonstrated with axillary dissection.

Biological Significance

Axillary lymph node status remains the most accurate predictor of outcome in breast cancer. Adjuvant hormonal or chemotherapy is most often predicted upon quantitative nodal status, and chemotherapeutic protocols differ according to quantitative axillary status. Adjuvant therapy in invasive breast cancer mandates therapy of all of the patients even though the majority of patients are cured with surgery alone and the incremental change in the node-negative is quite small. Axillary dissection provides information on those patients who are at highest risk for relapse and therefore stand to gain the most from adjuvant therapy.

Future Directions

It is clear that with increased mammographic screening, smaller breast cancers are being detected (Feig 1993). Tabar et al. (1992) have shown that these cancers carry a low risk of axillary metastases and present a rational case for omitting axillary treatment in selected cases. This approach has been championed by Cady et al. (1996). They present a statistical analysis showing the health care monies saved, avoiding complications of axillary dissection such as lymphedema, balanced against the advantage of systemic therapy in the few positive-node patients identified by axillary dissection.

However, the few patients with involved axillary nodes treated by this approach will have been done a disservice. A more rational management strategy would be to perfect sentinel node techniques. Surgeons who have perfected this technique, such as Giuliano et al. (1994) and Krag et al. (1993), report that only 1% or less will have an involved axillary node missed if careful serial sectioning of a sentinel node proves it to be negative. This will undoubtedly be the future approach to avoid surgical removal (or irradiation) for histologically negative nodes in breast cancer patients.

Conclusions

Axillary dissection for primary operable cancer follows the basic tenets of surgical oncology and achieves the stated goals. Local control is excellent with failure rates in the 0%–2% range. Long-term and disease-free survival is improved with axillary dissection. It is often stated that axillary dissection is not required for the smallest of lesions, but the 15% risk of axillary disease with the T1A lesion would suggest otherwise. Axillary sampling would not achieve the stated goals because of the high probability of retained, potentially resectable disease in the node-positive group. Axillary recurrence is associated with an unacceptably high morbidity and mortality. Although survival is similar in the three treatment groups of NSABP B-04, the inordinately high systemic failure rate with axillary recurrence would suggest that more aggressive local control could prevent many of these failures. After all, long-term survival free of disease is reported in many series even in patients with multiple involved nodes.

Axillary dissection also generates the most accurate prognostic variable upon which further therapeutic interventions are predicated. At present there is no other diagnostic or therapeutic approach that achieves all of these goals.

In summary, the value of axillary dissection is to provide accurate prognostic information as well as excellent local control and to improve the survival rate in the node-positive group. It is hoped that in the future a diagnostic test such as PET scanning or sentinel node mapping may identify those patients with a clear axilla who therefore do not require axillary dissection.

There has yet to be a primary operable carcinoma that benefits from preservation of potentially fully resectable disease. However, as discussed above, sentinel node lymphadenectomy for patients with small breast cancers and clinically uninvolved axillae will in all likelihood be the future approach. At present, axillary dissection should be done for those with clinically involved nodes or, in my opinion, for those with a positive node identified in a sentinel node biopsy. Even the latter is being subjected to trial, and it is possible that patients with positive sentinel nodes will undergo no further surgery.

Summary

Complete axillary dissection, as part of radical mastectomy, was the standard of care for the first three-quarters of this century. Long-term follow-up of these patients showed substantial cure rates for positive-node patients before systemic therapy was available, indicating a therapeutic value to nodal dissection. There was also good control of the axilla; axillary recurrence after removal of positive nodes was quite low. Even today, in patients with positive nodes, complete axillary clearance as part of a modified radical mastectomy or a breast conservation approach with lumpectomy leads to control of the axilla and complete axillary staging, allowing medical oncologists to tailor their systemic treatment to the total number of nodes involved. Today, due to a combination of factors including patient awareness and the ability of mammography to detect smaller lesions, many women present with small cancers that carry a much lower risk of axillary involvement. Whereas a complete dissection is indicated for patients with clinically involved nodes, a level I–II dissection is the standard in most centers for patients with clinically negative nodes. In those patients with very small (T1a, T1b) cancers, the role of sentinel lymphadenectomy is being explored; it may spare these patients the morbidity of complete axillary dissection.

References

Adair F, Berg J, Joubert L et al (1952) Long term follow up of breast cancer patients: the 30 year report. Cancer 5:992-997

Alex J, Krag D (1993) Gamma probe guided localization of lymph nodes. Surg Oncol 2:137-143

Ball ABS, Waters R, Fish S et al (1992) Radical axillary dissection in the staging and treatment of breast cancer. Ann R Coll Surg Engl 74:126-129

Boova R, Bonanni R, Rosato M (1982) Patterns of axillary nodal involvement in breast cancer: predictability of level one dissection. Ann Surg 196:642

Cabanes P, Salmon R, Vilcoq J et al (1992) Value of axillary dissection in addition to lumpectomy and radiotherapy in early breast cancer: the Breast Carcinoma Collaborative Group of the Institut Curie. Lancet 340:245-246

Cady B, Stone MD, Schuler JG et al (1996) The new era in breast cancer – invasion, size and nodal involvement dramatically decreasing as the result of mammographic screening. Arch Surg 131:301-308

Chada M, Chabon A, Friedman P et al (1994) Predictors of axillary lymph node metastases in patients with T1 breast cancer: a multivariate analysis. Cancer 73:350-353

Christensen S, Jansson C (1993) Axillary biopsy compared with dissection in the staging of lymph nodes in operable breast cancer. Eur J Surg Oncol 159:159-162

Danforth D, Findlay P, McDonald H et al (1986) Complete axillary lymph node dissection for stage I-II carcinoma of the breast. J Clin Oncol 4:655-662

De Freitas R Jr, Costa MV, Schneider SV et al (1991) Accuracy of ultrasound and clinical examination in the diagnosis of axillary lymph node metastases in breast cancer. Eur J Surg Oncol 17:240-244

Deckers PJ (1991) Axillary dissection in breast cancer: when, why, how much, and for how long? Another operation soon to be exstinct? J Surg Oncol 48:217-219

Feig S (1993) Mammographic screening: an historical perspective. Semin Roentgenol 28:193-203

Fentimen I, Mansel R (1991) The axilla: not a no-go zone. Lancet 337:221-223

Fisher B, Wolmark N, Bauer M et al (1981) The accuracy of clinical nodal staging and of limited axillary dissection as a determinant of histologic nodal status in carcinoma of the breast. Surg Gynecol Obstet 152:765-772

Forrest A, Stewart H, Roberts SR et al (1982) Simple mastectomy and axillary node sampling in the management of primary breast cancer. Ann Surg 196:371-378

Giuliano AE, Kirgan D, Guenther JM (1994) Lymphatic mapping and sentinel lymphadenectomy for breast cancer. Ann Surg 220:391-401

Graversen HP, Toft MB, Andersen JA et al (1988) Breast cancer: risk of axillary recurrence in node-negative patients following partial dissection of the axilla. Eur J Surg Oncol 14:407-412

Haagensen C (1986) Diseases of the breast. Saunders, Philadelphia, p 656

Harris J, Osteen R (1985) Patients with early breast cancer benefit from effective axillary treatment. Breast Cancer Res Treat 5:17-21

Hayward JL (1983) The Guy's Hospital trials on breast conservation. In: Harris JR, Hellman S, Silen W (eds) Conservative management of breast cancer. Lippincott, Philadelphia, pp 7-90

Isaacs RJ, Ford JM, Allan SG et al (1993) Role of computed tomography in the staging of primary breast cancer. Br J Surg 80:1137

Kinne D, Petrek J, Osborne M et al (1989) Breast carcinoma in-situ. Arch Surg 124:33-36

Kiricuta CI, Tausch J (1992) A mathematical model of axillary lymph node involvement based on 1446 complete axillary dissections in patients with breast carcinoma. Cancer 69:2496-2501

Krag DN, Weaver D, Alex JC et al (1993) Surgical resection and radiolocalization of the sentinel lymph node in breast cancer using a gamma probe. Surg Oncol 2:335-339

Lin PP, Allison DC, Wainstock J et al (1993) Impact of axillary lymph node dissection on the therapy of breast cancer patients. J Clin Oncol 11:1536-1544

Moffat F, Senofsky G, Davis K et al (1992) Axillary node dissection for early breast cancer: some is good but all is better. J Surg Oncol 51:8–13

Msuya CAD, Hartveit F (1991) Skip lesions in the axilla in breast cancer and their association with micrometastases. Breast Cancer Res Treat 19:277–281

Nieweg OE, Kim EE, Wong WH et al (1993) Positron emission tomography with fluorine-18-deoxyglucose in the detection and staging of breast cancer. Cancer 71:3920–3925

Noguchi M, Ohta N, Thomas M et al (1993) Clinical and biological prediction of axillary and internal mammary lymph node metastases in breast cancer. Surg Oncol 2:51–58

Piggot J, Nichols R, Maddox W et al (1984) Metastases to the upper levels of axillary nodes in carcinoma of the breast and its implications for nodal sampling procedures. Surg Gynecol Obstet 158:255–259

Reynolds J, Mercer P, McDermott E et al (1994) Audit of complete axillary dissection in early breast cancer. Eur J Cancer 30A:148–149

Robinson DS, Senofsky GM, Ketcham AS (1992) Role and extent of lymphadenectomy for early breast cancer. Semin Surg Oncol 8:78–82

Rosen PP, Groshen S, Saigo PE et al (1989a) A long-term follow-up study of survival in stage I (T1 N1 M0) breast carcinoma. J Clin Oncol 7:355–366

Rosen PP, Groshen S, Saigo PE et al (1989b) Pathological prognostic factors in stage I (T1 N0 M0) and stage II (T1 N1 M0) breast carcinoma: a study of 644 patients with median follow-up of 18 years. J Clin Oncol 7:1239–1251

Rosen PP, Groshen S, Kinne DW (1991) Prognosis in T2N0M0 stage I breast carcinoma: a 20-year follow-up study. J Clin Oncol 9:1650–1661

Rosser R, Gierson E, Waisman J et al (1987) Axillary lymph node dissection for intraductal cancer – is it indicated? Cancer 59:1819–1824

Silverstein M, Gierson ED, Colburn W et al (1991) Axillary lymphadenectomy for intraductal carcinoma of the breast. Surg Gynecol Obstet 172:211–214

Silverstein MJ, Gierson ED, Waisman JR et al (1994) Axillary lymph node dissection for T1a breast carcinoma. Cancer 73:664–667

Stierer M, Rosen HR, Weber R et al (1992) Long-term analysis of factors influencing the outcome in carcinoma of the breast smaller than one centimeter. Surg Gynecol Obstet 175:151–160

Tabar L, Fagerberg G, Duffy SW et al (1992) Update of the Swedish two-county program of mammographic screening for breast cancer. Radiol Clin North Am 30:187–210

Veronesi U, Rilke F, Luini A et al (1987) Distribution of axillary node metastases by level of invasion. Cancer 59:682–687

Wahl RL, Cody RL, Hutchins GD et al (1991) Primary and metastatic breast carcinoma: initial clinical evaluation with PET with the radiolabeled glucose analogue 2-[F-18]-fluoro-2-deoxy-D-glucose. Radiology 179:765–770

Wilking N, Rutqvist LE, Carstensen J et al (1992) Prognostic significance of axillary nodal status in primary breast cancer in relation to the number of resected nodes. Acta Oncol 31:29–35

Wilkinson EJ, Hause L, Hoffman RG et al (1982) Occult axillary lymph node metastases in invasive breast carcinoma: characteristics of the primary tumor and significance of the metastases. Pathol Annu 17:67–91

Winchester DP, Osteen RT, Mench HR (1996) The national cancer data base report on breast carcinoma characteristics and outcome in relation to age. Cancer 78:1837–1844

Sentinel Lymphadenectomy:
A Safe Answer to Less Axillary Surgery?*

C. E. Cox[1], S. S. Bass[1], N. N. Ku[2], C. Berman[3], A. R. Shons[1],
T. J. Yeatman[1], and D. S. Reintgen[1]

[1] Department of Surgery, University of South Florida, College of Medicine, and
the H. Lee Moffitt Cancer Center and Research Institute, 12902 Magnolia Drive,
Suite 2190, Tampa, Florida, USA
[2] Department of Pathology, University of South Florida, College of Medicine, and
the H. Lee Moffitt Cancer Center and Research Institute, 12902 Magnolia Drive,
Suite 2190, Tampa, Florida, USA
[3] Department of Radiology, University of South Florida, College of Medicine, and
the H. Lee Moffitt Cancer Center and Research Institute, 12902 Magnolia Drive,
Suite 2190, Tampa, Florida, USA

Introduction

The surgical evolution of breast cancer treatment over the past century from
Halsted through Haagensen and Urban has demonstrated the utility of radical and ultra-radical surgery. Patey, Meyer, and subsequently Fisher's studies
have initiated the movement toward surgical breast conservation. The continued progress toward lesser surgery has brought the value of axillary lymph
node dissection (ALND) under close scrutiny (Frazier et al. 1977; Silverstein
et al. 1987; Balch et al. 1993).

Controversy now rages regarding the role of axillary node dissection. The
need for axillary dissection in patients with ductal carcinoma in situ (DCIS)
or small invasive cancers has been rejected or questioned by several authors
(Silverstein et al. 1994; Fisher et al. 1981; Cady 1994). Data suggest that
ALND provides better local control of the disease, yet critics maintain that
the overall survival depends on the development of distant metastases (Fisher et al. 1981). It appears that removal of the axillary contents does not con-
vey a survival advantage. Regardless of that controversy, the status of the regional nodal basin remains the most important independent prognostic factor of survival (Moffatt et al. 1992). While other prognostic factors such as
tumor size, tumor grade, S-phase fraction, DNA index, tumor ploidy, and estrogen and progesterone receptor status are valuable in guiding the choice of
adjuvant therapy, none of these factors reliably identifies metastatic potential
of the individual tumor cells (Ravdin et al. 1994). Hence it remains impor-

* This study was supported by grant 30079 from the H. Lee Moffitt Cancer Center and Re-
search Institute, Tampa, Florida, by grant R21 CA66553-01 from the National Institutes of
Health, Bethesda, Maryland, by the McDonald Douglas Research Fund, and by the Joy
McCann Culverhouse Surgical Oncology Professorship of The University of South Florida
Foundation.

tant to identify those patients with nodal involvement in order to define their prognosis.

Clinical assessment of the axillary lymph node basin may vastly underestimate the existing pathology (Davies et al. 1980). The NSABP B-04 investigators demonstrated a false negative assessment rate of 38.6%. A more recent study has shown that 27% of clinically node-negative patients had pathologically positive nodes. Of particular interest, 8% of T1a and 10% of T1b tumors had positive axillary lymph nodes (Dees et al. 1997). These data demonstrate that very small invasive tumors can have a 12%–21% incidence of pathologically positive axillary nodes (Danforth et al. 1986; National Institutes of Health 1992). Limited axillary sampling has demonstrated staging error rates as high as 40% and therefore is not a useful technique. These data clearly support ALND for patients with small invasive primary breast cancer. However, ALND is a morbid procedure, especially if the total spectrum of its complications are considered, i.e., nerve ablation, paresthesia, wound infection, seroma, drain discomfort, acute and chronic lymphedema, and potential long delays in adjuvant treatment (Ivens et al. 1992; Recht and Houlihan 1995).

Morton et al. (1992) described the sentinel node as the first lymph node on a direct drainage pathway from the primary tumor in melanoma patients. Several authors have demonstrated that this sentinel node mapping technique applies equally well in breast cancer patients (Giuliano et al. 1994; Krag et al. 1993; Albertini et al. 1996), and the technique is gaining momentum in its application to the treatment of breast cancer. The sentinel lymph node (SLN) is defined as the first node or nodes in the lymphatic basin that receives primary lymphatic flow from the tumor site.

An important feature of sentinel node lymphadenectomy is that it makes it feasible to perform a more focused pathological examination, given the more limited number of sentinel node(s), using serial sections and special immunohistochemical stains. The significance of micro-metastatic disease in the lymph nodes has been questioned. However, studies conducted in Europe such as the Ludwig trial (International Breast Cancer Study Group 1990) have clearly demonstrated the recurrence potential of micro-metastatic disease. Indeed, the additional use of PCR analysis for the evaluation of SLN should further increase the sensitivity of the mapping technique to provide even more accurate staging.

The purpose of this paper is to describe the current methods employed by the present authors to identify the sentinel node(s) and to quantitatively assess the reliability, efficacy, and safety of the procedure as reported in this series of patients and those of other patients reported in the world's literature.

Patients and Methods

Patient Population

From June 1994 to April 1997, all patients presenting to the H. Lee Moffitt Cancer Center with breast cancer were evaluated for possible lymphatic mapping and SLN biopsy. Patients who were considered for this technique either had an invasive breast cancer clinically less than 5 cm in size or a high-grade DCIS-comedo type. Excluded were pregnant patients, patients with multicentric tumors, patients with axillary nodes clinically positive for metastatic disease, patients with a primary breast lesion clinically greater than 5 cm, patients with previous breast surgery that might interfere with the lymphatic drainage, and patients who were allergic to isosulfan blue dye. One hundred and sixty-seven (167) eligible patients (mean age 58.5±14.2 years) were enrolled in an IRB-approved study. All of the patients in this study were included in a phase I protocol which included the training phase of lymphatic mapping; these patients had an ALND performed after the SLN biopsy was completed.

Methods

Lymphatic Mapping

Lymphatic mapping was performed using a combination of approximately 5 nl vital blue dye (isosulfan dye, Lymphazurin blue dye, USSC, Connecticut, USA) and approximately 450 µCi filtered technetium-labeled sulfur colloid (Syncor International, Tampa, Florida). This technique has been previously outlined by Albertini et al. (1996). The peritumor site was injected with the radioactive agent 1–6 h prior to the operation. It is important to note that the injection of the radioactive agent is intraparenchymal; this differs from the intradermal injection technique used by Veronesi et al. (1997). The injection was accomplished either by palpation of the tumor or under mammographic or ultra-sonographic guidance. The isosulfan blue dye is injected in a similar fashion 15–60 min prior to the operation. The breast was scrubbed and prepared by the standard pre-operative method. This provides a moderate amount of massage which may improve the lymphatic flow, increasing the ability to identify the SLN in the axilla. A handheld gamma-detector probe (Neoprobe 1000/1500, Neoprobe Corp., Dublin, Ohio, USA; C-Trak System, Care Wise Medical, Massachusetts, USA; Navigator System, USSC, Connecticut, USA) is used to guide and locate the SLN intraoperatively. Meticulous dissection was performed to avoid staining of the surgical field with blood or premature disruption of the afferent lymphatic and staining of the surgical field with blue dye.

The SLN is defined as any blue node and/or "hot" node with a 10:1 ex-vivo radioactive count ratio of the SLN to non-sentinel lymph node (NSLN) and/or in-situ radioactive count at least three times that of the background count. After the removal of the SLN, the central bed was examined for activity. If the counts were greater than 150% than that of the background, the dissection is continued in search for additional SLN(s).

Histological Analysis

Excised lumpectomy margins were evaluated by touch preparation cytology, and on very rare occasions frozen sections were performed for the evaluation of intraoperative margins or tumor masses. All nodal tissue excised was submitted to the pathology department. Every SLN was identified by number (SLN 1, SLN 2, etc.). Non-sentinel nodes were also identified and remaining tissues were identified simply as axillary contents. All lymph nodes were identified and dissected from the surrounding fat and connective tissue. Intraoperative evaluation of bisected SLNs was accomplished utilizing imprint cytology. Following this, the bisected sentinel nodes were placed in paraffin blocks for embedding. Sections were obtained from the central cross-section of each block and stained with hematoxylin and eosin (H&E). Additional sections of each of the sentinel nodes were likewise stained for low molecular weight cytokeratin (CAM 5.2) with immunohistochemical techniques (Becton Dickinson Immunocytometry Systems, San Jose, California). A cytokeratin immunohistochemical stain was considered positive if there were cohesive clusters of malignant-appearing immunoreactive cells within the lymph node or if there were cytologically atypical individual cells in sinuses that could easily be correlated with H&E stains. The pathology of each histologically negative sentinel node was evaluated by cytokeratin immunohistochemical staining (CAM 5.2) of serial sections of these nodes. The remaining non-sentinel nodes were placed in blocks and evaluated by routine histological methods with H&E stains. A false negative SLN biopsy was defined as negative SLN(s) in the presence of other nodes in the basin positive for metastatic disease.

In addition to our data, we offer a review of the literature on lymphatic mapping, with a special emphasis on safety and efficacy data. One of the problems encountered in comparing data from multiple studies is the variance in the analytical methods employed by the investigators to define their results. We review the data and present them in a uniform manner using the analytical measures defined below:

Sensitivity = The proportion of patients with disease who tested positive
(TP/TP+FN)

Diagnostic Accuracy = The proportion of all true results to all test results
(TP+TN/TP+FP+TN+FN)

False Negative = The proportion of patients with disease who tested negative
(FN/TN)

Results

Present Series

From June 1994 to April 1997, 167 patients were successfully mapped. All of these patients were enrolled in the phase I protocol, in which they had sentinel node mapping followed by a complete axillary dissection. Fifty-nine (37.8%) patients were diagnosed by fine-needle aspiration, 89, (53.3%) patients by excisional biopsy and 19 (11.4%) patients by core biopsy. The biopsy method was thought to have an impact on the success of lymphatic mapping and thus was measured.

In 167 patients, a total of 337 sentinel nodes (SLN) were harvested, for an average of 2.01 SLN per patient. Fifty-two patients (31.1%) had metastasis in the SLN. In the 115 patients with negative SLN findings, one was found to have tumor in higher axillary nodes. These data demonstrated a false negative rate of 0.88%.

The tumor histology of the patients demonstrated 17 (10.2%) of the patients with DCIS. Infiltrating ductal lesions were documented in 115 (68.9%) patients. Infiltrating lobular histology was noted in 19 (11.4%) patients, while patterns of mixed cellularity were documented in 16 (9.6%) of the patients (Table 1).

Evaluation of the tumors by size was also done to identify the specific risk of tumor metastasis as it relates to T stage. T0 lesions were identified in 17 (10.2%) patients. T1a–T1b tumors were noted in 55 (32.9%) of the patients. T1c tumors were encountered in 58 (34.7%) patients. T2 tumors were seen in 30 (18.0%) patients, with T3 tumors in the remaining 7 (4.2%) patients (Table 2).

Of the 17 patients with DCIS, 1 (5.9%) had a positive SLN, and of the 115 patients with infiltrating ductal tumors, 33 (28.7%) had positive SLN. Of the 19 patients with infiltrating lobular tumors, 11 (57.9%) had positive SLN, and 7 (43.7%) of the 16 patients with mixed cellularity tumors had positive SLN (Table 1).

Of the 55 patients with T1a–T1b tumors, 7 (12.7%) had positive SLN, while 21 (36.2%) of the 58 patients with T1c tumors had positive SLN. Of the 30 patients with T2 tumors, 17 (56.7%) patients had positive SLN, and 6 (85.7%) of the 7 patients with T3 tumors had positive SLN (Table 2).

Table 1. Distribution of patients ($n=167$) by tumor histology and the proportion of each subgroup with metastasis in the sentinel lymph node (SLN)

Histological type	n	%	SLN+	
			n	%
Ductal in situ (DCIS)	17	10.2	1	5.9
Infiltrating ductal	115	68.9	33	28.7
Infiltrating lobular	19	11.4	11	57.9
Mixed cellularity	16	9.6	7	43.7

Table 2. Distribution of patients ($n = 167$) by tumor size and the proportion of each subgroup with metastasis in the SLN

Tumor stage	n	%	SLN+	
			n	%
T0	17	10.2	1	5.9
T1a–T1b	55	32.9	7	12.7
T1c	58	34.7	21	36.2
T2	30	18.0	17	56.7
T3	7	4.2	6	85.7

Table 3. Summary of the results of published series of lymphatic mapping and SLN biopsy, subjected to a uniform analytical method

Study	No. of patients mapped	Mapping technique	Sensitivity (%)	Diagnostic accuracy (%)	False negatives	
					Number	%
Giuliano et al. (1994)	114	B	88	95.6	5	6.5
Krag et al. (1993)	18	T	100	100	0	0
Veronesi et al. (1997)	160	T	95.3	97.5	4	5.1
Pijpers et al. (1997)	34	T	100	100	0	0
Neiweg et al. (1996)	22	B	100	100	0	0
Schneebaum et al. (1996)	13	B/T	75	92.3	1	10
Guenther et al. (1997)	103	B	90.3	97.1	3	4.2
Giuliano et al. (1997)	100	B	100	100	0	0
Cox et al. (present study)	167	B/T	98.1	99.4	1	0.9

Table 4. Summary of world experience (including the present study) with SLN biopsy

No. of patients mapped	Sensitivity (%)	Diagnostic accuracy (%)	False negative results	
			Number	%
731	95	98	14	3.1

Literature Review

Lymphatic mapping and SLN biopsy is being extensively investigated in several medical centers across the world. Table 3 represents a summary of the results of published series utilizing a uniform analytical method. The uniform format means that this data compilation may differ from the published results by the individual authors, due to the analytical methods used.

Several salient observations can be drawn from the data. The diagnostic accuracy (98%) and the sensitivity (95%) of lymphatic mapping are extremely high and improve with the operative experience of the surgeons. Furthermore, the false negative rate is low (3.1%) and, likewise, improves with the operative experience of the surgeons (Table 4). Most of these reported results represent the learning experience of the operative surgeons and should be viewed in that light, especially the series with less than 100 cases. Parenthetically, it is of importance to note that Veronesi's work represents a deviation from the methodology used for breast lymphatic mapping by the other authors in that the radiocolloid used is microcolloidal albumen and it is injected as in melanoma within the dermis overlying the breast tumor. Indeed this may be detecting sentinel nodes other than those being seen by intraparenchymal peritumoral injections as performed by the remaining authors and may explain the high rate of false negatives in that study.

Discussion

Although the controversy regarding the need for axillary dissection remains, axillary nodal status remains the most important prognostic factor in patients with carcinoma of the breast. Dees et al. (1997) have shown that accurate axillary staging impacts significantly on the treatment plans of patients with breast cancer. The early experience with SLN mapping has shown the technique to be safe and efficacious in the staging of the axilla. When looking at the review of the worldwide literature it is important to remember the learning curve associated with lymphatic mapping. Our review includes the initial experience with lymphatic mapping of several investigators. The more recent data seem to suggest that the false negative rate for intraparenchymal injection lies somewhere below 1%.

Upon review of our data, it became evident that approximately 29.2% of patients with a T1 or T2 lesion will be detected as having metastatic disease to the lymph nodes for which axillary dissection is required. With the application of lymphatic mapping and SLN biopsy to the treatment of early breast cancer, more than 70% of these patients would be spared an ALND with its associated morbidity. Furthermore, the intensity and cost of care can be greatly reduced to an outpatient setting for 70% of patients. A recent review at our institution has demonstrated that upstaging of breast cancer occurs in 9.4% of patients with the use of immunohistochemical staining (Schreiber et al. 1998). Ongoing investigations utilizing more rapid techniques for immunohistochemical staining of the SLN in the intraoperative setting should further decrease the rate of reoperation for ALND when immunohistochemical-positive nodes are detected by final pathology.

Perhaps the greatest benefit of SLN biopsy is that it allows a more focused examination of the nodes using serial sections and more sophisticated staining techniques to detect smaller foci of tumor. By more accurately staging patients with very small invasive tumors, we can better select patients for appropriate adjuvant therapy. Ultrastaging with PCR analysis may allow us to avoid adjuvant therapy in those patients who are PCR-negative and be more aggressive in patients with micro-metastatic disease.

Conclusion

The H. Lee Moffitt Breast Cancer Center experience combined with the worldwide experience of lymphatic mapping demonstrates that SLN biopsy has an extremely high sensitivity and diagnostic accuracy in predicting the axillary nodal status. It is a reproducible technique that is easily learned when combined dye techniques (radio-colloid and blue dye) are utilized. This technique affords a high rate of success and a low morbidity. The projected rate of false negative SLN biopsy is probably 1% or less when immunohistochemical techniques are employed and sufficient operative experience is gained. The mapping technique when performed in an outpatient environment will reduce costs with at the same time the improved diagnostic accuracy of being able to detect nearly 10% more nodal metastases than by the conventional means of complete axillary dissection. Finally, the future addition of more cost-effective and more sensitive methods such as PCR evaluation of nodal involvement may reduce the need for such widespread use of adjuvant chemotherapy with its high cost and attendant morbidity and mortality. We believe that this technique will eventually become the standard of care in the treatment of breast cancer, particularly for T1 and T2 lesions, and perhaps high-grade DCIS tumors.

Summary

Lymphatic mapping techniques have the potential of changing the standard of surgical care of breast cancer patients. This paper reports a prospective study documenting the safety and efficacy of sentinel lymph node biopsy in 167 breast cancer patients and reviews the world literature on the procedure. *Methods:* One hundred sixty-seven patients with newly diagnosed breast cancers underwent a prospective trial of intra-operative lymphatic mapping using a combination of vital blue dye and filtered technetium-labeled sulfur colloid. A sentinel lymph node (SLN) was defined as a blue node and/or "hot" node with a 10/1 ex-vivo gamma-probe ratio of SLN to non-SLN. All SLN were bi-valved, step-sectioned, and examined with routine H&E stains and immunohistochemical stains for cytokeratin. Cytokeratin-positive SLN were defined as any SLN with a defined cluster of positive staining cells which could be confirmed histologically on H&E sections. Finally, a review of the worldwide data was undertaken using a uniform analytical method to compare the rates of sensitivity, diagnostic accuracy, and false negatives of SLN mapping. *Results:* In 167 patients, 337 SLN were harvested, for an average of 2.01 SLN/patient. Fifty-two (31.1%) of the patients had metastasis in the SLN. In the 115 patients with negative SLN, 1 was found to have tumor in higher axillary nodes, for a false negative rate of 0.88%. Fifty-nine (37.8%) of the patients were diagnosed by fine-needle aspiration, 89 (53.3%) by excisional biopsy, and 19 (11.4%) by core biopsy. Positive SLN were identified in 1/17 (5.9%) patients with DCIS. Metastasis was found in 33/115 (28.7%) of the patients with infiltrating ductal tumors and in 11/19 (57.9%) of the patients with infiltrating lobular tumors. Positive SLN were identified in 7/16 (43.7%) of the patients with mixed cellularity tumors. Metastasis in the SLN was detected in 7/55 (12.7%) of the 59 patients with T1a–T1b tumors and in 21/58 (36.2%) of the patients with T1c tumors. Positive SLN were found in 17/30 (56.7%) of the patients with T2 tumors and in 6/7 (85.7%) of the patients with T3 tumors. A literature review of 731 patients (including this study) demonstrates a sensitivity rate of 95% and a diagnostic accuracy rate of 98%. The overall false negative rate is 3.1%. *Conclusions*: This study demonstrates that SLN biopsy is a highly sensitive and accurate method of predicting axillary nodal status. It is a reproducible technique that is easily learned. The future addition of more sensitive methods such as PCR evaluation of nodal involvement may reduce the need for widespread use of adjuvant chemotherapy with its high cost and attendant morbidity and mortality. We believe that this technique will eventually become the standard of care in the treatment of breast cancer, particularly for T1 and T2 lesions and perhaps also for high-grade DCIS tumors.

References

Albertini JJ, Lyman GH, Cox C et al (1996) Lymphatic mapping and sentinel node biopsy in the patient with breast cancer. JAMA 276:1818–1822

Balch CM, Singletary ES, Bland KI (1993) Clinical decision-making in early breast cancer. Ann Surg 217:207–225

Cady B (1994) The need to reexamine axillary lymph node dissection in invasive breast cancer. Cancer 73:505–508

Danforth DN Jr, Findlay PA, MacDonald HD et al (1986) Complete axillary lymph node dissection for stage I–II carcinoma of the breast. J Clin Oncol 4:655–662

Davies GC, Millis RR, Hayward JL (1980) Assessment of axillary lymph node status. Ann Surg 192:148–151

Dees EC, Shulman LN, Souba WW, Smith BL (1997) Does information from axillary dissection change treatment in clinically node-negative patients with breast cancer? Ann Surg 226:279–286

Fisher B, Wolmak N, Bauer M et al (1981) The accuracy of clinical nodal staging and of limited axillary dissection as a determinant of histologic nodal status in carcinoma of the breast. Surg Gynecol Obstet 152:765–772

Frazier TG, Copeland EM, Gallaher HS, Paulus DD Jr, White EC (1977) Prognosis and treatment in minimal breast cancer. Am J Surg 133:697–701

Giuliano AE, Kirgan DM, Guenther JM, Morton DL (1994) Lymphatic mapping and sentinel lymphadenectomy for breast cancer. Ann Surg 220:391–401

Giuliano AE, Jones RC, Brennan M et al (1997) Sentinel lymphadenectomy in breast cancer. J Clin Oncol 15:2345–2350

Guenther JM, Krishnamoorthy M, Tan LR (1997) Sentinel lymphadenectomy for breast cancer in a community managed care setting. Cancer J Sci Am 3:336–340

International (Ludwig) Breast Cancer Study Group (1990) Prognostic importance of occult axillary lymph node micrometastatses from breast cancers. Lancet 335:1565–1568

Ivens D, Hoe AL, Podd TJ, Hamilton CR, Taylor I, Royle GT (1992) Assessment of morbidity from complete axillary dissection. Br J Cancer 66:136–138

Krag DN, Weaver DL, Alex JC et al (1993) Surgical resection and radiolocalization of the sentinel lymph node in breast cancer using a gamma probe. Surg Oncol 2:335–339

Moffatt FL, Senofsky GM, Davis K et al (1992) Axillary node dissection for early breast cancer: some is good but all is better. J Surg Oncol 51:8–13

Morton DL, Wen DR, Wong JH et al (1992) Technical details of intraoperative lymphatic mapping for early stage melanoma. Arch Surg 127:392–399

National Institutes of Health (1992) Consumers Development Conference: National Institute of Health Consensus Statement 8:1–19

Neiweg DE, Kapteijn BA, Petuse JL et al (1996) Identification of the sentinel node in patients with breast carcinoma. Ned Tidschr Geneeskd 140:2235–2239

Pijpers R, Meijer S, Hoekstra OS et al (1997) Impact of lymphoscintigraphy on sentinel node identification with technetium-99m-colloidal albumin in breast cancer. J Nucl Med 38:366–368

Ravdin PM, DeLaurentiis M, Vendely T, Clark GM (1994) Production of axillary lymph node status in breast cancer patients by use of prognostic indicators. J Nat Cancer Inst 86:1771–1775

Recht A, Houlihan MJ (1995) Axillary lymph nodes and breast cancer: a review. Cancer 76:1491-1512

Schneebaum S, Stadler Y, Cohen M et al (1996) Sentinel lymph node localization in breast cancer: a feasibility study. Society of Surgical Oncology (SSO) Meeting, March 21–24, Atlanta, GA

Upstaging of breast cancer patients using cytokeratin staining of the sentinel lymph node. Ann Surg Oncol (in press)

Silverstein MJ, Rosser RJ, Gierson ED et al (1987) Axillary lymph node dissection for intraductal carcinoma: is it indicated? Cancer 59:1819–1824

Silverstein MJ, Gierson ED, Waisman JR, Senofsky GM, Colburn WJ, Gamagami P (1994) Axillary lymph node dissection for T1a breast carcinoma: is it indicated? Cancer 73:664–667

Veronesi U, Paganelli G, Galimberti V, Viale G et al (1997) Sentinel-node biopsy to avoid axillary dissection in breast cancer with clinically negative lymph nodes. Lancet 349:1864–1867

Endoscopic Surgery to the Axilla – A Substitute for Conventional Axillary Clearance?

F. Harder[1], M. Zuber[1], T. Kocher[1], and J. Torhorst[2]

[1] General Surgical Division, Department of Surgery, University of Basel, Basel, Switzerland
[2] Institute of Pathology, University of Basel, Basel, Switzerland

Introduction

Axillary clearance has for many decades been an integral part of breast cancer surgery. In fact, en bloc resection of the breast together with its lymph nodes draining into the axilla was probably the first example of good oncologic surgery.

Initially, axillary clearance aimed only at removing diseased nodes, thus significantly lowering the axillary recurrence rate to 2%. Additionally, axillary clearance permits selective identification of patients who will benefit from systemic therapy and have a survival advantage. Axillary dissection provides reliable prognostic information. It is a necessary basis for many prospective trials. To date, no imaging or molecular biological technique is able to consistently demonstrate diseased axillary nodes, which would allow it to replace conventional axillary clearance as a staging procedure. If, in operable breast cancer with clinically uninvolved nodes, axillary clearance is omitted altogether, axillary disease will develop in about 20% of the patients after 5 years (Graversen et al. 1988). For such late involvement of the axilla satisfactory treatment will not be possible in all cases, leading to considerable morbidity. However, even in 209 selected patients not undergoing axillary dissection with pT1 tumors (favorable prognostic factors: 56% smaller than 10 mm and 81% in postmenopausal women), after 4 years axillary recurrence was found in 13% (Agresti et al. 1995).

Following the increasing use of mammography and mammographic screening, smaller and impalpable tumors are being detected more frequently. In the 7 years from 1982 to 1989, the proportion of tumors detected with a diameter of less than 10 mm increased from 9 per 100 000 women per year to 63 per 100 000 women per year. Concomitantly, in-situ cancers went up from 12 to 45 cases per 100 000 women per year. In parallel with this, the proportion of tumors detected with a diameter of 30 mm or more has decreased accordingly (Miller et al. 1993).

pT1a cancers have a pN1 stage in the range of 3% (Silverstein et al. 1994). A large proportion of tumors less than 10 mm in diameter with uninvolved nodes are curable, and survival at 20 years is above 90%. Yet a very small proportion of these early cancers show aggressive behavior, with positive nodes, and patients with these cancers, if identified, could take advantage of systemic adjuvant treatment.

While there is general agreement that, for larger tumors and clinically involved nodes, conventional axillary clearance is to be recommended, in T1a and T1b lesions as well as in old patients without clinical disease in the axilla, at least the extent of surgery, if any, to the axilla is controversial. Earlier diagnosis of breast cancer is in fact leading to greater numbers of axillary dissections where nodes are disease-free and where the patient has no direct profit from this procedure. Where is the balance between risk and benefit for the patient, between long-term morbidity such as lymphedema, decreased sensation in the area of the intercostal brachial nerves, and painful or reduced range of shoulder motion caused by axillary surgery (Hoe et al. 1992; Larson et al. 1986; Paredes et al. 1990; Keramopulos et al. 1993). How often are therapeutic steps taken as a consequence of the information gained by lymph node analysis?

Axillary sampling, a procedure not precisely defined, neither protects as effectively against axillary recurrence as conventional axillary clearance does, nor is it an optimal staging procedure (Forrest et al. 1995). In 42% of patients who had undergone single node sampling, undetected cancer was later found (Davies et al. 1980).

Two new and completely different approaches to the axilla hold some promise in combining staging efficiency and prevention of recurrence. One technique is derived from experience in melanoma surgery, the other from minimally invasive surgery: the sentinel lymph node technique (Morton et al. 1992 a, b; Vanderven et al. 1994; Giuliano et al. 1994; Giuliano 1996; Turner et al. 1997; Veronesi et al. 1997) and liposuction with axilloscopic clearance (Suzanne et al. 1994). The sentinel lymph node (SLN) technique takes advantage of the known orderly progression of metastatic disease from the first to subsequent levels in the axilla. Skip metastases are found in less than 3% of cases (Büchels et al. 1997; Veronesi et al. 1986). The first draining node picks up dye or a radio-label after injection of material into the peritumoral area. The SLN histology will reflect the stage of the axilla. In experienced hands, accurate prediction of the axillary lymph node status is in a range well over 95% (Giuliano 1996; Veronesi et al. 1997). When the SLN is histologically negative, axillary clearance is not performed.

Endoscopic axillary clearance after liposuction of the axilla was first described by Suzanne et al. (1994) and Salvat et al. (1996) and transposes laparoscopic technique to the axilla. After axillary liposuction and under direct vision using a laparoscope, individual lymph nodes may be identified and removed. The vascular and neural structures of the axilla are clearly visualized during dissection of levels 1 and 2. Very early full arm mobilization, low morbidity, and excellent cosmesis are achieved thanks to there being only three 5- and 10-mm trocar incisions and an axillary wound of limited surface area. The number of lymph nodes removed is only slightly smaller than after conventional clearance of levels 1 and 2.

Materials and Method

Special Instrument Set

The special instrument set for axillary liposuction and endoscopy consists of:

- A 20-ml syringe and fine needle (as used for lumbar puncture)
- 500 ml liposuction solution (0.45% NaCl with 10 ml 4% lidocaine)
- Abortion canula no. 7 with a rounded tip and lateral opening (suction curette no. 7, 1602-R07 Wyss Pharma AG, 6330 Cham, Switzerland)
- Liposuction pump producing a vacuum between 800 and 1000 mbar
- Complete laparoscopy instrumentation with a 10-mm 25° angled laparoscope
- 5-mm (arthro-)scope
- One 10-mm and two 5-mm trocars
- Short (20 cm) 5-mm scissors that can be connected to electrocautery
- Short (20 cm) 5-mm grasper
- Electrocautery.

Technique

The patient is placed in a supine position and put under general anesthesia. One single dose of 2 g Zinacef (cefuroxime sodium) is given intravenously. The arm of the operated side is in 90° abduction, freely movable and draped.

The axillary fat pad is infiltrated with 200–300 ml of liposuction solution, depending on the volume of the axilla. Infiltration of the latissimus dorsi, pectoralis major, and puncture of the axillary vein must be avoided.

While the liposuction solution penetrates the tissues for about 20 min, the tumorectomy or medial part of the mastectomy is performed. Tumors situated at the lateral margin of the mammary gland are not suitable for liposuction and axilloscopy, since either liposuction would have to be done ahead of the tumorectomy, running the risk of cell seeding by the canula from injury to the primary tumor, or, if the tumorectomy is done before the liposuction (as is the rule), CO_2 gas leaks through the tumorectomy wound are difficult to control.

After tumorectomy the canula is introduced just 2–3 cm ventral to the middle axillary line, about 12 cm caudal of the axillary fold, through a 10 mm long incision. A subcutaneous tunnel penetrating the clavipectoral fascia and ending in the axillary fat pad is prepared with an appropriate clamp or with scissors to allow the introduction of the suction curette. Through this tunnel, careful liposuction will take about 10 min at a vacuum pressure of 800 mbar and will be continued until the axillary fat, initially yellow, stains pink.

The 25°-angled laparoscope is introduced through the liposuction incision and the incision tightened with a pursestring suture. Note that the CO_2 pressure used in the axilla is lower than that used in the abdomen – only 8 mmHg. Two additional accesses about 5 cm closer to the axillary fold in the anterior and posterior axillary line are created to accommodate the 5-mm trocars. Step by step, fibrous tracts and small blood and lymph vessels are coagulated and cut and individual or chains of lymph nodes carefully freed. These tissue fragments are deposited in front of the 10-mm trocar to be removed later on. As the axillary dissection progresses, the scapulothoracic nerve, the thoracodorsal neurovascular bundle, intercostobrachial nerves, the lateral pectoral nerve, and part of the axillary vein are visualized. Great care must be taken not to damage any of the motor nerve structures within this relatively small working space.

After completion of the dissection, small tissue fragments may be removed through the 10-mm trocar under visualization by a 5-mm arthroscope placed in one of the two 5-mm trocars. For larger fragments, the 10-mm trocar incision may be widened to accommodate a 20-mm trocar. Finally, the operative field is copiously rinsed with saline. The skin incisions are sutured. No drains are used in the axilla.

The liposuction material is filtered through fine gauze. The tissue fragments are carefully checked for lymph nodes aspirated during liposuction, and these are sent separately to the pathologist along with the nodes dissected by axilloscopy.

Results

In our series of 50 patients, all treated by one single surgeon in Basel (Table 1), we were able to confirm what Suzanne et al. (1994; personal communication) found in over 250 patients: decreased morbidity, almost unchanged range of motion without pain in the ipsilateral shoulder compared with the opposite side, absence of lymphedema, and an excellent cosmetic result. In three cases (3/53) the endoscopic procedure had to be converted to an open dissection, because of a very fatty axilla in two cases and because of bleeding from the thoracodorsal vein next to the accompanying nerve in one case, making axilloscopic hemostasis too hazardous.

In about 50% of the patients the carcinomas were staged as pT1 tumors (Table 2). There was one exceptionally large T2 cancer measuring 49 mm in

Table 1. Profile of 50 cases (out of 53 attempts) in which axilloscopic dissection was carried out

Mean patient age (years)	60
Ratio of pre- to postmenopausal patients	10:40
Mean duration of postop. hospital stay (days)	5.7 (range 1–16)
Mean duration of postop. hospital stay (days) in patients aged < 50 years	4.6 (range 1–8)
Averaged number of nodes removed	13.4 (range 5–25)
Number of pN+patients	17/50 (34%)

Table 2. pTpN Staging in 50 patients who underwent axilloscopic dissection

pT Stage	n	pN Stage	n
pTis	1		
pT1a	1	pN0	15
pT1b	4	pN1	9
pT1c	18		
pT2	26	pN0	18
		pN1	7
		pN2	1
Total	50		50

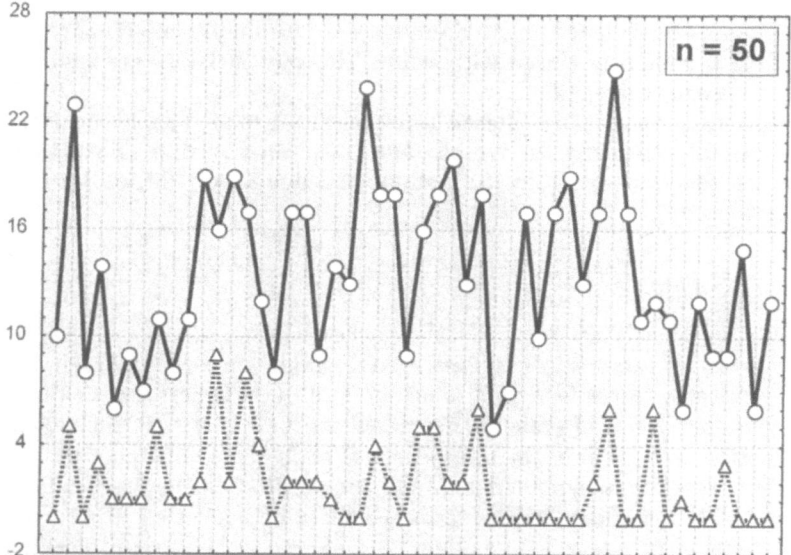

Fig. 1. *Upper curve:* Totalnumber of lymph nodes removed, by individual case in chronological order, in the 50 consecutive axilloscopic dissections carried out by one single surgeon. *Lower curve:* Number of lymph nodes counted in each case in the material aspirated by the liposuction canula

diameter. Nine (9/24) pT1 and 8 (8/26) pT2 tumors had involved axillary lymph nodes, giving an overall figure of 34% N1 tumors with a mean of 3.1 involved nodes (range 1–10; Fig. 1).

The average number of axillary lymph nodes removed was 13.4 (range 5–25; Table 1, Fig. 2). In the first 10 cases an average of 11 nodes were removed. This average increased slightly up to 14 nodes in cases 11–50. During liposuction an average of 2 lymph nodes (range 1–9) had already been aspirated. In only three cases were these lymph nodes histologically involved.

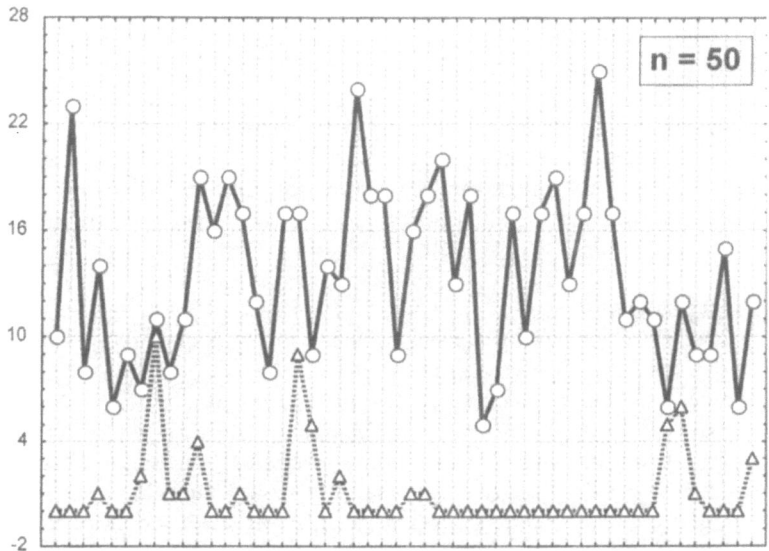

Fig. 2. *Upper curve:* Total number of lymph nodes removed, by individual case in chronological order, in the 50 consecutive axilloscopic dissections carried out by one single surgeon. *Lower curve:* Number of positive lymph nodes in each case (17 patients with involved nodes, out of 50 treated patients)

Table 3. Self-assessment of results by thefirst 40 of 50 patients who underwent axilloscopic dissection, after a median follow-up of 15 months (range 4–24 months)

	Subjective score[a]	
	Mean	Range
Pain in upper arm	9.4	5–10
Pain in lower arm	9.8	6–10
Pain in chest wall or breast	9.2	7–10
Shoulder mobility	9.3	4–10

[a] Scale of 1–10 with 1 = very bad and 10 = excellent.

One thoracodorsal nerve was injured by this procedure. Postoperative seroma necessitated aspiration in 8 of the 50 patients. No infections or hematomas were observed.

Patients were discharged on average 5.7 days postoperatively (range 1–16; Table 1), patients younger than 50 years after 4.6 days (range 1–8).

After an average follow-up period of 15 months (range 4–24 months) the first 40 patients were evaluated by means of a self-assessment questionnaire, an interview, and a physical examination (Table 3). Pain and shoulder mobility were rated between 9.2 and 9.8 on the self-assessment scale, 1 being very bad and 10 excellent. Two patients mentioned having a slightly swollen arm from time to time, but on physical examination no lymphedema could be detected. Objectively, nine patients had slight differences in upper arm circumference, in the range of 1–2 cm. In eight cases this correlated with the dominant arm and there were no signs of lymphedema. Patient no. 9 had a 2-cm very soft, flabby swelling on the upper arm on the nondominant side, not annoying the patient in any way and with normal arm motion and no pain.

No axillary recurrence and, especially, no trocar site implantation was found after this short median follow-up time of 15 months. Patients are being followed up in a hospital-based program every 4 months.

Discussion

While for larger tumors and for the clinically involved axilla, open axillary clearance is generally accepted for all risk and age groups with breast cancer, the dilemma about the need for axillary clearance exists for patients with small or nonpalpable lesions without clinical suspicion of axillary disease and where axillary lymph node staging in any individual patient is essential for adequate treatment planning. In this situation, is it justifiable today to proceed with formal level 1 and 2 (or even more) dissection which in over 80% of patients will yield only negative nodes? To the patient this offers no advantage and leaves her only with a certain risk of long-term morbidity.

Endoscopic exploration of the axilla has arrived at just the right time. It may perhaps not remain an important tool for very many years once dependable molecular biological markers allow us to correctly predict axillary nodal involvement or, in more general terms, define the aggressiveness of the disease. At that point treatment options based on validated nonsurgical data will rapidly be established. In the meantime, however, it is worth investigating any means that will allow more differentiated, subtle, and careful access to the axillary lymph nodes and combines very valuable information with low morbidity and excellent cosmesis.

Endoscopic lymphadenectomy is employed for pelvic and para-aortic nodes in different oncological settings. There liposuction is not necessary. However, the individual dissection of single nodes or small groups of lymph nodes is current practice and contrasts with the generally held view that such dissections should be made en bloc. Nevertheless, no observations such as of local tumor dissemination due to nonobservance of the rule of en-bloc lymphadenectomy have been published. For axilloscopy, the question remains whether the need for liposuction, the CO_2 gas insufflation, and the nonobservance of en-bloc dissection does not promote tumor cell implantation within the axilla or at the trocar sites. It is probably incorrect to compare axilloscopy in a lymph node area draining a primary tumor with laparoscopy performed for the treatment of a primary cancer, e.g., colorectal cancer within the abdominal cavity, where totally different conditions are found.

Dealing with lymph nodes draining a malignant primary tumor using techniques developed for abdominal minimally invasive surgery may very well be completely different to the laparoscopic handling of the primary tumor itself for which the techniques were developed, so far as the risk of tumor cell spillage is concerned. Certain precautions have to be taken: axilloscopy should be reserved for a clinically nonsuspect axilla, for small, preferably T1 lesions, and for tumors not reaching the axillary area exposed to liposuction and axilloscopy. Injury by the liposuction canula to the surface of the primary tumor might induce local tumor cell spillage. Following these precautions, it might be expected that axillary recurrences would not be seen in a range notably higher than that observed after conventional clearance for comparable tumor stages. Follow-up is too short in any series to make a final statement in this regard today, but Suzanne has compared histologically a large number of lymph nodes dissected by conventional open axillary clearance with lymph nodes removed by liposuction and axilloscopy; the lymph nodes showed comparable lesions in both groups with no significant difference in number (Suzanne 1998, personal communication).

The advantages of the liposuction and axilloscopy technique that are now evident are the clearly reduced invasiveness, the lower short- and long-term morbidity in comparison to open axillary clearance, the excellent cosmesis, and the high degree of patient satisfaction. At the same time, the desired prognostic information is obtained, with more than 13 nodes per treated axilla on average (personal series of one single surgeon).

It may very well turn out that in the future the sentinel lymph node technique and axilloscopy will become complementary. In a clinically uninvolved axilla in the case of a lesion up to 2 or 3 cm not in direct contact with the axilla, a negative sentinel lymph node precludes any further axillary treatment. If, by contrast, the sentinel lymph node removed at the time of tumorectomy is involved, axilloscopy a few days later in a second step may remove some additional involved nodes. Four or more involved nodes will rarely be found unless the work-up of the primary tumor has revealed signs of increased aggressiveness. In that case, open axillary clearance will be preferable to axilloscopy.

In such a one- to two-step procedure, depending on the findings of the sentinel lymph node and the characteristics of the primary tumor, the invasiveness of the axillary procedure may be adapted to the probability and extent of axillary nodal involvement of any individual patient. It must be clear, from what has been said above, that for the time being liposuction and axilloscopy to the axilla must be considered as a technique under investigation, not yet ready for general introduction. The technique requires wide experience in laparoscopic surgery and a good knowledge of the anatomy of the axilla. The working space within the axilla is quite small and there are a number of "noble" or important structures that must by all means be respected.

In any case, in the surgical field of breast cancer treatment alone, the years ahead will bring about significant changes for various types of invasive breast cancer, palpable and impalpable, in different age and risk categories. Breast conservation is certainly here to stay. The amount or extent of surgery will be further reduced for early breast cancer. The same is probably also true for the other form of local treatment, radiotherapy. In addition to all this, however, we continue to see locally very advanced forms of breast cancer that need extensive surgery, sometimes including parts of the chest wall and, accordingly, require plastic surgical reconstruction.

Summary

Nonpalpable, mammographically detected breast cancers are on the increase. The percentage of patients with histologically involved nodes is therefore decreasing. Axillary clearance aims at reducing the probability of later clinical involvement of the axilla and at establishing a sound basis for adjuvant treatment planning. Minimally invasive techniques have been applied to a growing number of surgical procedures now including exploration of the axilla. The technique used and results achieved in a series of 50 consecutive patients treated by liposuction and axilloscopy by one single surgeon, including all the patients from the very first attempt, are presented here. Patients were excluded with palpable lymph nodes or a primary tumor in the direct vicinity of the axilla that could be injured by the liposuction canula. The average number of lymph nodes removed was 13.4. Thirty-four percent of patients had involved nodes. The mean number of involved nodes in these patients was 3.1. After a median follow-up time of only 15 months no axillary recurrences or trocar site metastases have been found in the first 40 patients. Using a self-assessment questionnaire, the patients rate this technique as excellent. There was no lymphedema. The cosmetic result is certainly better than after conventional axillary clearance. Great experience of laparoscopic surgery and an excellent knowledge of the axillary anatomy are prerequisites for the practice of axilloscopic treatment of the axilla. The working space within the axilla is small and a number of structures need absolutely to be preserved. A longer follow-up period than the one so far achieved in this series or any other in the literature to date is necessary before this technique can be generally recommended.

References

Agresti R, Greco M, Raselli R et al (1995) Axillary surgery can be avoided in selected breast cancer patients: analysis of 401 patients. Eur J Cancer 31A Suppl 5:S214–S215

Büchels HK, Wagner T, Vogt H (1997) Mammakarzinom-Staging mittels Sentinel-Lymphadenektomie. Chirurg 68:1258–1261

Davies GC, Millis RR, Hayward JL (1980) Assessment of axillary node status. Ann Surg 192:148–152

Forrest APM, Everington D, McDonald CC et al (1995) The Edinburgh randomized trial of axillary sampling or clearance after mastectomy. Br J Surg 82:1504–1508

Giuliano AE (1996) Sentinel lymph adenectomy in primary breast carcinoma: an alternative to routine axillary dissection. J Surg Oncol 62:75–77

Giuliano AE, Kirgan DM, Günter JM et al (1994) Lymphatic mapping and sentinel lymph adenectomy for breast cancer. Ann Surg 220:391–401

Graversen HP, Blichert-Toft M, Andersen JA et al (1988) Breast cancer: risk of axillary recurrence in node-negative patients following partial dissection of the axilla. Eur J Surg Oncol 14:407-412

Hoe A, Iven D, Royle G, Taylor I (1992) Incidence of arm swelling following axillary clearance for breast cancer. Br J Surg 79:261-262

Keramopulos A, Tsionon C, Minaretzis D et al (1993) Arm morbidity following treatment of breast cancer with total axillary dissection. Oncology 50:445-449

Larson D, Weinstein M, Goldberg I et al (1986) Edema of the arm as a function of the extent of axillary surgery. Int J Radiat Oncol Biol Phys 12:1575-1582

Miller BA, Feuer EJ, Hankey BF (1993) Recent incidence trends for breast cancer in women and the relevance of early detection: an update. Cancer 43:27-41

Morton D, Wen D, Cochran A (1992a) Management of early-stage melanoma by intraoperative lymphatic mapping and selective lymph adenectomy: an alternative to routine elective lymph adenectomy or "watch and wait". Surg Oncol Clin North Am 1:247-259

Morton D, Wen D, Wong J et al (1992b) Technical details of intraoperative lymphatic mapping for early stage melanoma. Arch Surg 127:392-399

Paredes J, Puente J, Potel J (1990) Variation in sensitivity following sectioning the intercostal brachial nerve. Am J Surg 160:525-528

Salvat J, Knopf JF, Ayoubi JM et al (1996) Endoscopic exploration and lymph node sampling of the axilla. Eur J Obstet Gynecol Reprod Biol 70:165-173

Silverstein MJ, Gierson ED, Waisman JR et al (1994) Axillary lymph node dissection for T1a breast carcinoma. Is it indicated? Cancer 73:664

Suzanne F, Anton MC, Ducroz F et al (1994) Le curage axillaire dans le cancer du sein par aspiration graisseuse et ganglionnaire: à propos de 57 cas. Rev Fr Gynecol Obstet 3 (2):255-266

Turner RR, Ollila DW, Krasne DL et al (1997) Histopathologic validation of the sentinel lymph node hypothesis for breast carcinoma. Ann Surg 226:271-278

Vanderven H, Hoekstra OS, Paul MA et al (1994) Gamma-probe-guided sentinel node biopsy to select patients with melanoma for lymph adenectomy. Br J Surg 81:1769-1770

Veronesi U, Rilke F, Luini A et al (1986) Distribution of axillary node metastases by level of invasion: an analysis of 539 cases. Cancer 59:682-687

Veronesi U, Luini A, Galimberti V et al (1990) Extent of metastatic axillary involvement in 1446 cases of breast cancer. Eur J Surg Oncol 16:127-133

Veronesi U, Baganelli G, Galimberti V et al (1997) Sentinel-node biopsy to avoid axillary dissection in breast cancer with clinically negative lymph nodes. Lancet 349:1846-1867

VI. Integrated Therapy: Changing Surgical Procedures for Breast Cancer

Surgical Considerations in Preoperative Chemotherapy of Breast Cancer

R. G. Margolese

Jewish General Hospital, McGill University, 3755 Ch. Côte-Sainte-Catherine, Montreal, Canada H3T 1E2

Surgical considerations after primary systemic therapy will depend on which of the two main reasons for choosing primary chemotherapy prevails. Most European studies seek to decrease the size of some larger tumors so as to make them acceptable candidates for breast-conserving surgery (BCS). In the National Adjuvant Surgical Breast and Bowel Project (NSABP) study, the aim is to improve disease-free survival and overall survival by testing the hypothesis that existing micrometastases would be more sensitive to primary chemotherapy than they would be following surgical removal of the original tumor. Tumor reduction to permit BCS is a worthwhile but secondary goal.

In the European experience larger tumors have generally not been considered suitable for BCS, and those that are, are often treated by much wider local excisions such as quadrantectomy. In many cases, when tumors exceed certain preconceived size limits or appear to be "too close" to the nipple, mastectomy is performed. BCS has been evaluated by the NSABP (protocol B-06) (Fisher et al. 1985) on patients with tumors 4 cm or less in diameter, and in subsequent trials tumors measuring up to 5 cm have been included. On the other hand, European surgeons have obviously been concerned about tumor size and have usually concentrated on patients with 2- or 2.5 cm tumors as the upper limit for BCS (Table 1). Several clinical studies involving preoperative chemotherapy have been launched with the aim of reducing tumor size and increasing BCS (Jacquillat et al. 1990; Scholl et al. 1991; Mauriac et al. 1991). The impetus for these originated with treatment of patients with locally advanced disease in whom surgery was not considered initially appropriate. The patients received aggressive chemotherapy and showed some remarkable responses in tumor shrinkage and ultimate local control (Sorace et al. 1985). Subsequently, the technique was applied to less advanced breast cancers, those still considered too large for primary lumpectomy but without any of the grave signs indicating locally advanced disease. Two somewhat similar themes mark this approach. Several French studies sought to use chemotherapy and radiotherapy with the hope of avoiding or minimizing the use of surgery (Jacquillat et al. 1990; Scholl et al. 1991; Mauriac et al. 1991), while the Italian studies aimed at decreasing the size of the tumor so as to enable breast conserving surgery to be carried out. In one example, the

Table 1. Upper tumor size limits for aligibility in trials of breast-conserving surgery

NSABP B-06	4 cm
Milan QART	2 cm
Milan preop.	3 cm
NSABP subseq.	5 cm
NSABP B-18	No upper size limit

QART, Quadrantectomy and radiation therapy (see Veronesi et al. 1990).

Milan study (Bonadonna et al. 1990), an upper limit of 3 cm was chosen for primary BCS. Tumors larger than this would be treated with BCS only if the chemotherapy reduced them to below this size. In North America, the NSABP launched a clinical trial comparing standard postoperative adjuvant therapy with four cycles of adriamycin and cyclophosphamide to preoperative chemotherapy using the same chemotherapy regimen (protocol B-18). Decreasing tumor size to make lumpectomy more feasible was a secondary aim of this trial; the primary aim was to improve disease-free survival and overall survival and thus there was no upper size limit for this trial. Many NSABP surgeons are comfortable with lumpectomy for tumors up to 5 cm and would not necessarily have required preoperative chemotherapy to render most of these patients acceptable, but the issue of tumor-free margins and long-term local control might be factors that could be influenced by the use of preoperative chemotherapy.

Complete clinical response was obtained in 36% of patients (Fisher et al. 1997). Such tumor disappearance can create a problem in the placement of the lumpectomy incision because there is no palpable tumor. Simple techniques such as mapping the tumor with an overlying grid (Fig. 1) or simply making a small skin tattoo, as radiation therapists frequently do, will usually solve the problem.

Several surgeons noticed in their first few cases that even with good clinical response the pathologic extent of tumor did not always correlate favorably with the postchemotherapy clinical size. Tumors appeared to shrink not as a melting ice cube contracts but rather in a diffuse and irregular pattern, leaving islands of apparently viable tumor cells amid bands of fibrous tissue representing the chemotherapy effects on portions of the tumor mass. For this reason the NSABP conducted several workshops for its members in order to establish techniques of locating and excising the entire tumor mass.

Figure 2 is a photomicrograph of a whole-mount histology preparation showing how islands of tumor persist several millimeters apart. A lumpectomy which is tailored to the new clinical size, where the tumor was downsized by chemotherapy, might not attain clear margins as reliably as in a similar patient who had a traditional lumpectomy in which the resection was guided by the palpable tumor size. Thus, in patients treated by primary chemotherapy, risks of ipsilateral breast tumor recurrence (IBTR) may require

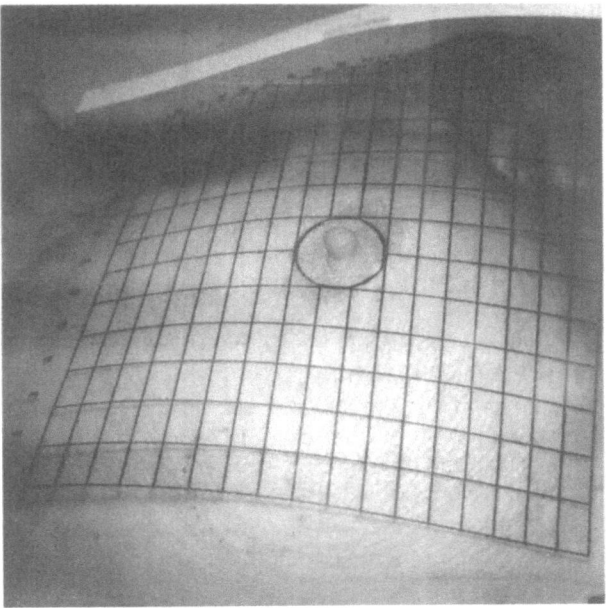

Fig. 1. Mapping the tumor with an overlying grid to allow accurate lumpectomy after tumor shrinkage due to preoperative chemotherapy

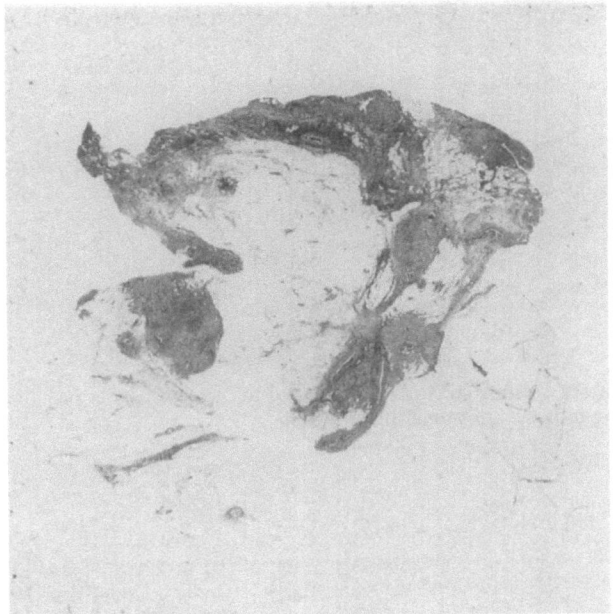

Fig. 2. Photomicrograph of a whole-mount histology preparation of a breast tumor showing typically irregular shrinkage in response to chemotherapy

different considerations. Several reports (Vicini et al. 1991; Veronesi et al. 1995a) support the view that risk of IBTR following traditional lumpectomy is related to original tumor size. However, a recent analysis of IBTR in B-18 shows that IBTR is uncommon in both pre- and postoperatively treated patients (Veronesi et al. 1995a). Although lumpectomy was performed more frequently in the preoperative than in the postoperative group, annual IBTR was only $\sim$8% and $\sim$6% in these two groups respectively (Table 2). It is worth noting, however, that smaller initial tumors were more likely to show clinical and even pathological complete response and these were more likely to remain free of IBTR (Tables 3, 4). Tumors larger than 3 cm were less likely to show complete clinical response and those that were downstaged to permit lumpectomy were more likely to recur locally, but this seemed to be more a function of age than tumor size (Table 5). It must be remembered that women younger than 50 years did not receive tamoxifen, and tamoxifen is known to decrease IBTR (Fisher et al. 1989).

In assuming that tumors smaller than 3 cm were unsuitable for BCS, the Milan group addressed the issue of tumor shrinkage and focused on aggressive wide local surgery exemplified by quadrantectomy. Patients received preoperative chemotherapy with the aim of reducing tumor size to 3 cm so that

Table 2. NSABP protocol B-18: local recurrence rates following lumpectomy in pre- and postoperatively treated patients according to age category and tumor size (*IBTR* ipsilateral breast tumor recurrence)

Group	Postoperative chemotherapy		Preoperative chemotherapy	
	No. of patiens	% with IBTR	No. of patients	% with IBTR
All patients	450	6	504	8
Age (years)				
≤49	235	8	256	13
≥50	215	3	248	3
Clinical tumor size (cm)				
<3	220	4	225	8
≥3	230	8	279	8

Table 3. NSABP protocol B-18: response to chemotherapy according to tumor size at initial presentation

Response	Tumor size prior to chemotherapy		
	≤2.0 cm (%)	2.1–4.0 cm (%)	≥4.1 cm (%)
Complete response	49	37	19
Partial response	29	46	56
Stable disease	17	13	23
Progressive disease	6	4	2

Table 4. NSABP protocol B-18: lumpectomy patiens who had a complete clinical response compared to those who had a lesser response

Group	Complete clinical response		Less than complete clinical response	
	No. of patients	% IBTR	No. of patients	% IBTR
Patients with follow-up	206	5	298	10
Age (years)				
≤49	115	10	141	16
≥50	91	0	157	5
Clinical tumor size (cm)				
<3	107	6	118	9
≥3	99	5	180	10

Table 5. NSABP protocol B-18: local recurrence rates by age and tumor size for patients who underwent lumpectomy only after chemotherapy reduced the size of (downstaged) their tumor, compared to patients considered suitable candidates for lumpectomy at the time of presentation

Group	Downstaged to lumpectomy		Lumpectomy proposed initially	
	No. of patients	% with IBTR	No. of patients	% with IBTR
All patients	69	15	435	7
Age (years)				
≤49	42	17	214	12
≥50	27	11	221	2
Clinical tumor size (cm)				
<3	13	15	212	7
≥3	56	14	223	7

lumpectomy would be acceptable according to their criteria. Nearly 80% of these patients had a tumor of 3–5 cm. However, tumors of this size were randomized in NSABP B-18 to primary surgery or primary chemotherapy. These differences in approach cause significant confusion in interpreting results, since the very definitions of BCS acceptability are so different. The NSABP, basing this treatment approach on a potential effect on micrometastases, used a traditional lumpectomy technique with routine margin sampling and routine radiation therapy postoperatively. There was a gain in successful attainment of lumpectomy for the preoperative chemotherapy group which, although statistically significant, did not represent a major clinical difference.

These differences in approach reflect other underlying differences in philosophy. Does successful local management depend on an aggressive rather than a moderate surgical approach? Does the lumpectomy have to be tightly controlled with postoperative X-ray of the specimen for calcifications and attainment of wide margins as in quadrantectomy, or does a simpler approach involving routine margin assessment suffice? In some reports, the risk of local recurrence does decrease as the volume of tissue removed increases (Vicini et al. 1991; Veronesi et al. 1995a), indicating a possible interaction between tumor size, extent of removal, and risk of IBTR, but this is usually a feature of cases where traditional margin control is not practised. In the NSABP lumpectomy trial (B-06) the risk of IBTR in the lumpectomy patients who did not receive radiation therapy also correlates with larger tumor size (Table 6). At first glance, this seems to confirm the need for wider excision, but this finding is not present in irradiated patients, where IBTR rates are low for all tumor sizes. Thus it appears that routine margin control and radiation therapy can produce good long-term local control with low rates of IBTR.

One consistent theme running through two decades of research on this subject is the lack of correlation between local treatment and long-term outcome. While IBTR is a predictor of increased likelihood of metastatic disease, the metastases do not appear to be a consequence of the initial surgical treatment selected. In protocol B-06 mastectomy patients and lumpectomy patients with or without radiation therapy had very different rates of local control but identical rates of long-term disease-free survival and overall survival (Fisher et al. 1995). In the Milan (Veronesi et al. 1995a) series comparisons of Halsted mastectomy, quadrantectomy with radiation therapy, tumorectomy with radiation therapy, and quadrantectomy without radiation therapy, had very different rates of local control but very similar long-term outcomes (all patients underwent axillary dissection). Therefore, the issue, even in preoperative chemotherapy programs, is one of local control and cosmesis, suggesting that aggressive local surgery with an increased likelihood of poor cosmesis may not be a worthwhile tradeoff, especially since local recurrence rates are generally low.

Another important point concerns the effect of adjuvant chemotherapy on local recurrence rates. The original lumpectomy trials were started in an era when adjuvant therapy was not common and certainly not routine for all patients. In subsequent NSABP trials it has become clear that adjuvant therapies, chemo or endocrine, reduce local recurrence rates significantly (Margolese 1992). Node-patients negative treated with lumpectomy and radiation therapy in protocols B-13 and B-14 have IBTR rates similar to patients with

Table 6. NSABP protocol B-06: local recurrence rates in patients who underwent lumpectomy with and without radiation therapy, related to tumor size

Tumor size (cm)	Precentage of patients tumor-fress	
	Lumpectomy	Lumpectomy+radiotherapy
0–1.0	87	94
1.1–2.0	75	97
2.1–3.0	73	93
3.1–4.0	67	92

the same characteristics in B-06, but those patients who received adjuvant therapies have their local recurrence rates diminished by half. Since preoperative chemotherapy is adjuvant therapy, the same low rate of local recurrence is not surprising and makes aggressive techniques aimed at local control more questionable.

With these differences in mind, surgical considerations in primary chemotherapy will fall into two categories depending on which of the abovementioned basic approaches is accepted. For a careful disciplined approach requiring very wide removal it will be necessary to localize the tumor with several tattoo marks. If tattooing is not practical, a simple grid on a large transparency can be used to map the tumor so that the site can be located if there is clinical disappearance. Using the grid a circle can be drawn around the coordinates. This drawing is kept in the patient's file and can be used at the time of surgery to redraw the size of the tumor on the skin in order to direct the lumpectomy (Fig. 1). Mammograms should be obtained at the beginning of chemotherapy and again just prior to surgery in order to be sure that an adequate wide local excision is performed. X-ray of the specimen would help by comparing the extent of calcifications preoperatively with those seen on specimen radiography. With this approach it will obviously be necessary to resect a volume of tissue as if the tumor had not shrunk in order to be sure that no islands of residual neoplasm are left.

On the other hand, since NSABP protocol B-06 (Fisher et al. 1995) showed that radiation is effective in controlling microscopic residual disease it may be just as reasonable to perform a traditional lumpectomy, verify negative margins pathologically, and rely on radiation for added control as we have always done. Although preliminary localization is still required to enable accurate excision of the site of the tumor, a more cosmetic approach with a smaller resection volume is reasonable in this situation. All of the early lumpectomy trials showed that radiation therapy reduced the risk of IBTR compared to lumpectomy alone. The best explanation for this difference is that even with pathologically clear margins, microscopic foci of tumor persist, but these are controlled by radiotherapy.

It is clear in several studies that significant tumor shrinkage is more likely with small tumors than with large. In an updated report on the Milan series (Veronesi et al. 1995b), tumor shrinkage to less than 3 cm occurred in 98% of patients with tumors 3-4 cm in size, compared to 80% for patients with tumors of 4.1-6 cm in size, and only 27% for larger tumors. NSABP B-18 patients showed a clear correlation of response by tumor size (Table 3). Do these results relate to IBTR risk? Protocol B-18 patients who were treated by BCS after downsizing by chemotherapy had a significantly higher rate of IBTR than patients allotted by their surgeons to BCS originally. This is a function of age more than tumor size since this was equally true whether patients had initial tumor size of more or less than 3 cm. This difference in IBTR among downsized patients was more obvious in younger women than those over 50 (Table 5). Since both groups of patients had the pathologic examination of margins performed by the same methodology, and these were in all cases determined to be negative, it is very likely that in the downsized patients the microscopic volume of tumor left behind is is more extensive and less likely to be controlled by radiotherapy, possibly because of nonuniform tumor shrinkage. The difference in age groups may be a function of tumor behavior in different ages, or may be related to the use of tamoxifen routinely in those aged over 50. In protocol B-27 all patients will take tamoxifen.

Therefore, the need for reduction is least likely to be met in those cases where the need is greatest. Small tumors shrink dramatically; they have the highest rate of complete response, but they would have been easily treated by lumpectomy without preoperative treatment with low IBTR rates. Large tumors which need size reduction are less likely to respond completely, and those that become eligible for lumpectomy after downsizing are more likely to recur locally. Therefore the gain in successful lumpectomy may not be much, especially if it is necessary to resect the original volume of tumor in order to have an acceptable local recurrence rate. It might make more sense to excise large tumors initially, with the advantage that it is easier to define the gross margins during surgery. This makes particular sense for those surgeons who are used to performing lumpectomies with tumors up to 5 cm in diameter. Nevertheless, it should be noted that even with a higher rate of IBTR, ∼90% of women older than 50 years of age and 83% of younger women had successful breast-conserving surgery, despite having a larger tumor size at presentation.

Conclusions

Initial chemotherapy can be aimed at both improving disease-free survival and overall survival and at improving the long-term success of local control with lumpectomy. Both are worthwhile objectives. Carefully identifying the extent of tumor remaining in the breast and performing of an appropriate (not too large, not too small) lumpectomy with negative margins are complex elements in the long-term preservation and cosmesis of the breast. Downsizing large tumors, even with its higher rate of IBTR, remains an option for women who wish to preserve their breast despite larger initial tumor size.

Summary

Primary sytemic chemotherapy for breast cancer was initially directed at downsizing tumors to make them acceptable candidates for breast-conserving surgery. Later trials used this approach in the hope of improving disease-free survival and overall survival. Results from NSABP protocol B-18 indicate significant initial tumor response and downstaging of lymph nodes in 30% of patients. Patients with small tumors were more likely to experience complete clinical response and complete pathologic response. Patients with larger tumors whose surgeons would have chosen mastectomy often responded with tumor decrease to a size at which lumpectomy was considered feasible. The local recurrence rate in these patients was higher than in those patients selected for lumpectomy primarily. Nevertheless, even with a higher rate of ipsilateral breast tumor recurrence, approximately 90% of women older than 50 years and 83% of younger women had successful breast-conserving surgery. There was no difference in disease-free survival or overall survival between preoperative and postoperative chemotherapy groups. The response of patients to initial chemotherapy can be a useful tool in exploring the biology of breast cancer.

References

Bonadonna G, Veronesi U, Brambilla C (1990) Primary chemotherapy to avoid mastectomy in tumors with diameters of three centimeters or more. J Natl Cancer Inst 82:1539–1545

Fisher B, Bauer M, Margolese RG (1985) Five-year results of a randomized clinical trial comparing total mastectomy and segmental mastectomy with or without radiation in treatment of breast cancer. N Engl J Med 312:665–673

Fisher B, Constantino J, Redmond C et al (1989) A randomized clinical trial evaluating tamoxifen in the treatment of patients with node-negative breast cancer who have estrogen-receptor-positive tumors. N Engl J Med 320:479–484

Fisher B, Anderson S, Redmond CK, Wolmark N, Wickerham DL, Cronin DM (1995) Reanalysis and results after 12 years of follow-up in a randomized clinical trial comparing total mastectomy with lumpectomy with or without irradiation in the treatment of breast cancer. N Engl J Med 333:1456–1461

Fisher B, Brown A, Mamounas E (1997) Effect of preoperative chemotherapy on local-regional disease in women with operable breast cancer: findings from National Surgical Adjuvant Breast and Bowel Project B-18. J Clin Oncol 15:2483–2493

Jacquillat C, Weil M, Baillet F (1990) Results of neoadjuvant chemotherapy and radiation therapy in the breast-conserving treatment of 250 patient with all stages of infiltrative breast cancer. Cancer 66:119–129

Mauriac L, Durand M, Avril A, Dilhuydy JM (1991) Effects of primary chemotherapy in conservation treatment of breast cancer patients with operable tumors larger than 3 cm. Ann Oncol 2:347–354

Margolese RG (1992) Treatment for early-stage breast cancer. J Natll Cancer Inst Monogr 11:1–5

Scholl SM, Asselain B, Palangie T, Dorval T, Jouve M, Garcia Giralt E, Vilcoq J, Durand JC, Pouillart P (1991) Neoadjuvant chemotherapy in operable breast cancer. Eur J Cancer 27:12 1668–1671

Sorace RA, Bagley CS, Lichter A (1985) The management of nonmetastatic locally advanced breast cancer using primary induction chemotherapy with hormonal synchronization followed by radiation therapy with or without debulking surgery. World J Surg 9:775–785

Veronesi U, Volterrari A, Luini A (1990) Quadrantectomy versus lumpectomy for small size breast cancer. Eur J Cancer 26:671–673

Veronesi U, Salvadori B, Luini A et al (1995a) Breast conservation is a safe method in patients with small cancers of the breast. Long-term results of three randomized trials on 1,973 patients. Eur J Cancer 31A:1574–1579

Veronesi U, Bonadonna G, Zurrida S (1995b) Conservation therapy after primary chemotherapy in large carcinomas of the breast. Ann Surg 222:612–618

Vicini F, Eberlein T, Connolly J (1991) The optimal extent of resection for patients with stage I–II breast cancer treated with conservative surgery and radiotherapy. Ann Surg 214:200–204

Integration of Plastic Surgery in the Course of Breast-Conserving Surgery for Cancer to Improve Cosmetic Results and Radicality of Tumor Excision

J.-Y. Petit, M. Rietjens, C. Garusi, M. Greuze, and C. Perry

European Institute of Oncology, Milan, Italy

Introduction

Reducing the psychological distress, which may result from the treatment of breast cancer is an important plastic surgical goal. Such distress occurs with both conservative surgery (CS) and total breast reconstruction (BR), as in the case of mastectomy. Immediate or delayed breast reconstructions are becoming increasingly common as their absolute contraindications are becoming less and less. For example, absolute contraindications to immediate breast reconstruction might only be limited to cases of locally advanced disease or inflammatory cancers. Today's plastic surgeons are called upon to improve the cosmetic results of aggressive conservative treatment. Indications for breast-preserving surgery, restricted initially to very small tumors, unifocal tumors, are now being proposed for tumors up to 4 or 5 cm in diameter, bifocal tumors located in the same quadrant, and even for large tumors which have been reduced in size by several courses of neoadjuvant chemotherapy. In some cancer protocols, the size reestriction on tumors suitable for CS relates only to tumor size as it compares to total breast volume, the main criterion being the final expected cosmetic result. In all cases, the cosmetic outcome correlates to the size of the specimen removed – more precisely, to the size of the specimen compared to the size of the breast and the size of the tumor including the width of the free margins.

What Should Be the Free Margins Around the Tumor?

Several authors such as Fisher and the NSABP group (Fisher and Redmond 1989) advocate a rather small free margin, provided that the margins are clear in all directions at the final histological examination. The problem that arises, however, is the risk of missing noncontiguous tumor foci located at some distance from the primary tumor mass. Holland et al. (1985) have shown that there is a risk of finding malignant cells in 57% of cases when tumors are resected with a 1-cm margin and in 17% of cases when tumors are resected with a 3-cm margin. Veronesi and Salvadori (1990) have demonstrated, in one of the Milan trials which compared tumorectomy plus brachytherapy with quadrantectomy followed by external radiotherapy, that the local recurrence rate was significantly higher in the group treated with smaller free margins, that is, the group treated with simple tumorectomy plus brachytherapy. At the Gustave Roussy Institute in Paris, long-term analysis of 753 consecutive cases treated with CS showed that the risk of local recurrence is only related to the radicality of the tumor excision and the age of the patient. These results confirm the need for more, not less, radical tumor excision, even if radiotherapy, which has been shown to reduce the risk of local recurrence, is to be performed (Sarrazin and Fontaine 1983; Dewar et al. 1995).

To put things into surgical perspective, consider a 3-cm breast cancer. Radical tumorectomy of a 3-cm tumor with a 2-cm free margin will result in a specimen at least 6 cm in diameter. A specimen of this magnitude will represent at least one-quarter of the total volume of a medium-sized breast. The final cosmetic result in such case depends primarily on the immediate closure techniques used. Suboptimal cosmetic results will be obtained if no attempt to reconstruct the breast is undertaken at the initial operation.

Deformations Observed in Cases of Poor Cosmetic Outcome

In a series of CS performed at the Gustave Roussy Institute without cosmetic surgical intervention at the time of the primary treatment, we observed a 20% rate of poor cosmetic results at a mean follow-up of 5 years (Petit and Rietjens 1991). The more disfiguring deformities were observed when the tumor bed was in the central and inferior portions of the breast. Initially, the glandular defects caused by surgery are masked by postoperative edema, local secretions, and/or hematomas. After reabsorption of the fluids and resolution of the edema, however, the defects become evident. Some of the more commonly seen defects are as follows:

1. When performing lymphadenectomy through the same incision as used for upper outer quadrantectomy, retraction of the resulting long linear scar can cause severe distorsion of the nipple-areola complex.
2. Glandular defects in the lower pole of the breast can cause retraction of the nipple in a downward direction and can distort the global shape of the breast.
3. Finally, if the paucity of postoperative glandular tissue is not problem enough, the contraction of the glandular tissue resulting from the surgical scarring is increased by the sclerosis induced by the application of adjuvant radiotherapy, which is included in the CS protocols.

All these deformations of the conservatively treated breast have been well described by Berrino et al. (1987).

What Can We Expect from Delayed Plastic Surgical Breast Reconstruction to Help Improve Bad Results?

Delayed plastic surgical breast reconstruction can be offered to patients with severe deformities resulting from ablative surgeries for breast cancer. Scar contractions can be modified with the help of "Z plasties." Local glandular flaps, prosthetic devices, as well as regional and distant musculocutaneous flaps can all be used to help improve glandular defects. Transfer of the nipple-areola complex to a more appropriate central position, together with glandular remodeling, can be performed using different mammaplastic techniques in an attempt to rebalance the surgically disrupted breast. Symmetrical considerations often warrant mammaplasty of the contralateral breast to help improve the overall esthetic appearance of the chest wall. These techniques, as well as others, are available, but considerations beyond the surgical techniques are required. For example, all of these procedures are to be performed on a breast that has been modified by a previous operation and/or radiotherapy. Because of the previous treatments, the risks of complications and recurrent sclerosis with deformity become a potentially greater problem than in operations on previously undisturbed breast tissue.

In the Gustave Roussy experience, delayed plastic surgery to improve poor esthetic results after initial conservative breast treatments resulted in only a 50% improvement in cosmetic outcome. Our conclusion from this disappointing French experience, therefore, was to combine the disciplines in an "onco-plastic" surgical procedure at the time of the primary treatment. Our hope was to lessen the cosmetic impact of the initial ablative procedure.

Immediate Partial Breast Reconstruction

The indication for plastic surgery intervention at the time of the quadrantectomy should be evaluated and discussed before the initial operation. The preoperative conference should include the cancer surgeon, the plastic surgeon, and the patient. The cancer surgeon must consider how much tissue will have to be removed from the breast to adequately treat the patient's cancer and also consider what the breast deformity and the final cosmetic outcome will be resulting from this intervention. Consultations with the plastic surgeon can help to improve the postoperative appearance of the surgically treated breast. Tumors located in the central or the lower part of the breast are prone to bad cosmetic results as already mentioned. The lack of glandular tissue in smaller breasts makes creation of glandular flaps more difficult and leads to a higher incidence of glandular distorsion. Extensive microcalcifications surrounding the main tumor foci require more radical resection of the involved area. With more extensive resection, more extensive reconstruction is required to adequately remodel the glandular tissue. These circumstances, as well as many more, illustrate the need for a full preoperative multidisciplinary conference so that choices can be made by the patient. Discussions with the patient should include talking about the possible need for a contralateral mammaplasty to help improve the overall symmetry of the chest wall. This kind of contralateral mammaplasty has been criticized by oncologists and radiologists, who say that the postoperative scarring makes later radiographic follow-up of the patient more difficult. Others claim that distinctions between postsurgical changes due to scarring and images caused by precancerous and cancerous lesions should be distinguishable to qualified radiologists (Tristant et al. 1988). Moreover, contralateral mammaplasties provide an excellent opportunity for thorough bimanual palpation of the contralateral breast, as well as an opportunity for visual inspection, and even for biopsy of any suspect areas, if warranted. Out of 450 mammaplasties performed at the Gustave Roussy Institute for the purpose of providing symmetry of the contralateral breast, we found occult carcinomas in the mammaplasty specimen in 4.5% of cases. Fifty percent of the carcinomas were found to be infiltrating and 50% were DCIS (Rietjens et al. 1997).

Plastic surgical techniques used at the time of quadrantectomy are similar to those proposed for delayed partial breast reconstruction. Local flaps, glandular flaps, mammaplasty techniques derived from reduction mammaplasty techniques (Garusi et al. 1997; Pitanguy 1981; McKissock 1976; Lejour 1990), or even regional and distant musculocutaneous flaps (Slavin et al. 1992) can also be used for both delayed and immediate reconstruction. Several surgical principles are used to help improve the final cosmetic outcome. For example, prevention of scar contraction is aided by making separate incisions for the tumorectomy and the axillary lymphadenectomy. In addition, special attention to the blood supply of the glandular flaps is required in order to avoid secondary infections and necrosis, especially in the case of fatty breasts. Skin resection in front of the tumor can be performed within the limits of a de-epithelialization in the periareolar area, combining the "round-block" mammaplasty and the quadrantectomy. In the case of central tumors, resection of the nipple-areolar complex is recommended to remove the ducts at risk of tumor spread. The glandular reconstruction can be performed immediately with an inferior glandular flap (Galimberti et al. 1993). In a second operation, performed under local anesthesia, the nipple-areolar complex can be reconstructed when the whole cancer treatment is completed (Little 1984).

European Institute of Oncology Experience

In Milan, 85 patients have undergone "onco-plastic surgery." That is, the oncologist eradicated the tumor and the plastic surgeon reconstructed the breast at the time of the primary treatment. These 85 patients represent almost 15% of the cases of conservative surgery performed at the EIO for the same period. Mean patient age was 49 years (range 26–70 years). Among the 85 cases, the final histological diagnosis was benign tumor in 7 cases (8%), infiltrating ductal carcinoma in 72 cases (85%), and DCIS in 6 cases (7%).

The tumor was located in the superior quadrants in 48 cases (56%), in the inferior quadrants in 27 cases (32%), and in the central area in 10 cases (12%). No axillary dissection was performed in 19 cases (22%). The mean follow-up was 21 months (range 6–36 months).

Adjuvant therapies were delivered as follows: hormonal therapy was given in 49 cases (58%). Adjuvant chemotherapy was given in 43 patients out of 85 (50.5%). Radiotherapy was delivered at the usual doses (45–50 Gy and 10 Gy on the tumor bed for boost) in all cases, except those of benign lesions and one case of Paget's disease.

Surgical Techniques

Put simply, we performed four different kinds of techniques. Glandular flaps were performed in 22 patients (25%), mammaplasties in 47 (55%), prostheses in 13 (15%) and distant flaps in 4 (5%). A contralateral mammaplasty was performed in 65 cases (76%). One occult in situ carcinoma was found in a specimen from a contralateral mammaplasty. The mean weight of specimens removed was 157.2 g (range 30–680 g).

Cosmetic Results

Evaluation of cosmetic outcome is always difficult. In order to try to avoid bias and prejudices, cosmetic results in our study were judged by surgeons who were not in charge of the operation. The photographs of the patients were rated according as follows:
– *Good:* The treated breast is hardly distinguishable on a front view.
– *Fair:* The treated breast is distinguishable, but the deformities and scars do not justify a second operation to improve the result.
– *Poor:* The deformity is significant and a secondary reconstruction can be offered to the patient.

Overall cosmetic results were rated as follows: good 57 patients (68%); fair, 22 (26%); poor 5 (6%) (Figs. 1–3). For cosmetic results in relation to specimen size, tumor location, and symmetry procedure on the contralateral breast, see Tables 1–3.

A prosthesis was placed in 13 cases, with a good result in 8/13 (62%), fair in 2/13 (15%), and poor in 3/13 (23%). Among these 13 cases, 7 have required surgical revision due to complications: 1 prosthesis ruptured, 1 prosthesis became infected, and 5 had to be revised owing to capsular contracture.

Forty-eight patients recorded an opinion, which was good in 38/48 cases (79%), fair in 8/48 (17%), and poor in 2/48 (4%).

Complications arose in a total of 18 cases (21%): infection in 2, hematoma in 2, skin necrosis in 3, fat necrosis in 1, capsular contracture in 9, and prosthesis rupture in 1.

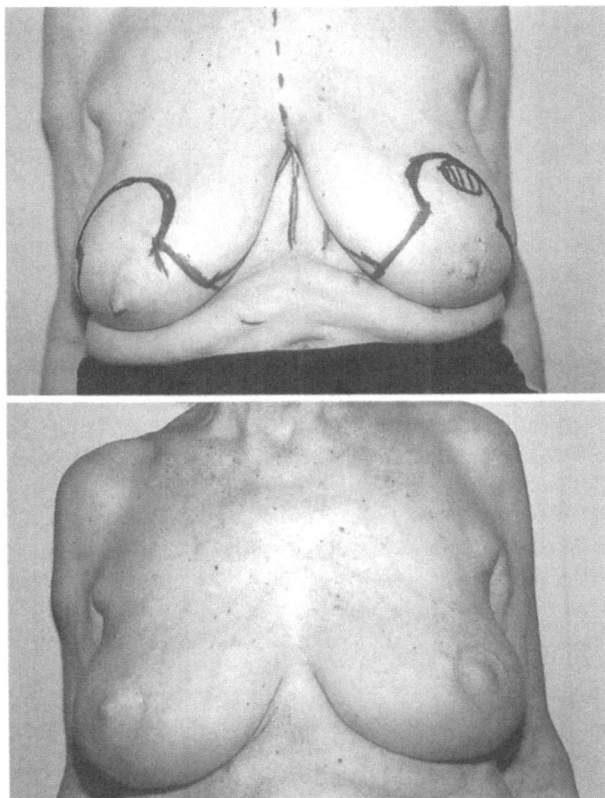

Fig. 1. a Preoperative drawings for a left breast quadrantectomy and bilateral reduction mammaplasty with inferior pedicle. **b** Three-month postoperative view. Example of good results

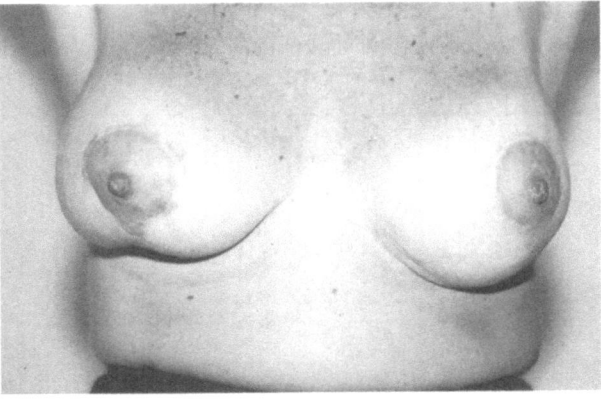

Fig. 2. Six-month postoperative view after left breast inferior quadrantectomy and bilateral reduction mammaplasty. Example of fair results, with scar retraction and deformity

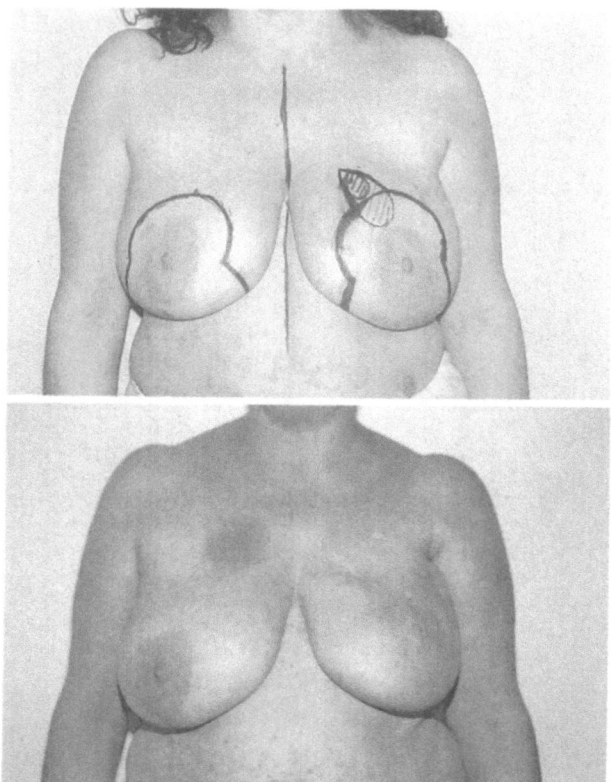

Fig. 3. a Preoperative drawings for a left breast quadrantectomy and bilateral reduction mammaplasty. The patient did not agree to the right breast correction. **b** One-year postoperative view. Example of poor results with asymetry of volume and shape

Table 1. Cosmetic results in relation to the size of the surgical specimen

	Good	Fair	Poor
< 100 g	27 (87%)	4 (13%)	0
>100 g	27 (56%)	17 (36%)	4 (8%)

Table 2. Cosmetic results in relation to tumor location

	Good	Fair	Poor
Superior quadrant	32/47 (68%)	12/47 (26%)	3/47 (6%)
Inferior quadrant	20/27 (74%)	6/27 (22%)	1/27 (4%)
Central quadrant	5/10 (50%)	4/10 (40%)	1/10 (10%)

Table 3. Cosmetic results in relation to symmetry procedure (if any) on the contralateral breast

	Good	Fair	Poor
Unilateral remodeling	8/19 (42%)	9/19 (47%)	2/19 (11%)
With symmetry procedure	49/66 (74%)	13/66 (20%)	3/66 (5%)

Discussion

The cosmetic results of the conservative treatment combining cancer surgery with an immediate plastic surgical procedure to reconstruct the breast in the series reported here should be considered as preliminary, because they require longer term follow-up. The mean follow-up of 21 months is insufficient, as demonstrated by other studies showing that the sequelae of the radiosurgical treatment require at least 5 years before they can be considered as final and stable (Avril et al. 1997). Despite the short follow-up period, however, it is already possible to draw several conclusions from these preliminary results.

First, the most important information in this series concerns the size of the specimen removed. The average weight is 157 g. This is at least four times the average weight of a tumorectomy specimen for a tumor of 2–3 cm with a free margin of 1 cm. This size discrepancy illustrates the radical means by which quadrantectomies are performed at the EIO. In our opinion, the combined "onco-plastic surgery" approach provides a better cosmetic result without compromising the oncologic surgical principle of radical excision of the tumor.

The second advantage of an onco-plastic surgical approach is complete bimanual exploration of the glandular tissue of the contralateral breast, if an operation is to be performed on it. The undermining required to remodel the contralateral breast allows excellent access to its glandular tissue for both visual and bimanual inspection. In our series, a symmetry procedure was performed in 76% of the cases. If indicated, an intraoperative biopsy could also be performed.

Radiologically suspect areas were underlined preoperatively and removed at the time of the reduction mammaplasty. Contralateral occult carcinoma was found in one case in this short series and six carcinomas (four DCIS and two infiltrating carcinomas) were found in the patients with a preoperative radiologically suspect area. These results are consistent with the published series of contralateral occult carcinomas (Rietjens et al. 1997).

Close collaboration between the oncologist and the plastic surgeon at all patients during the surgical treatment must be stressed, including in respect of the symmetry procedure on the contralateral breast.

Finally, the cosmetic evaluations warrant some remarks. As we have said, these results should be considered preliminary. They relate to a selected group of patients receiving conservative treatment and undergoing onco-plastic surgery. This group represents almost 15% of all the patients receiving conservative treatment in whom a poor cosmetic result was anticipated. The comparison between the results of the French series at Gustave Roussy and the Italian results at the EIO clearly show the role of onco-plastic surgery when poor cosmetic results are expected. Good results are less prevalent in the French series: 50% as compared to the 68% of the Milan series, while poor results are more prevalent in the French series, 20% as compared to 6% in the Milan study. However, such difference should be interpreted cautiously since the follow-up is too short in Milan. In addition, the Milan study shows clearly that cosmetic results correlate to the size of the specimen: 87% of patients had good results when the specimen size was less than 100 g, versus only 56% of patients who had good results when the specimen size was greater than 100 g.

In conclusion, looking at the overall cosmetic results and keeping in mind the preliminary nature of the Milan series, we see a positive role for oncoplastic surgery in the primary treatment of breast cancer, especially in cases where there is a high probability of a poor cosmetic result.

Summary

Integration of plastic surgery is currently widely practiced in cases of mastectomy. Immediate breast reconstruction with an implant or autologous tissue procedures is frequently proposed to the patient before the mastectomy. However, breast conserving surgery (BCS) is recognized as the treatment of choice in most cancers: breast conservation is proposed in more than 70% of the patients with primary cancer treated at the European Institute of Oncology in Milan. This high percentage of preservation has been made possible by the integration of plastic surgery at the time of primary surgery. The size of the tumorectomy remains a matter of discussion. Based on the Milan II trial and Holland's pathological studies, Veronesi recommended so-called "local radical surgery." For a tumor 1 cm in size, a free margin of 2 cm produces a final specimen at least 5–6 cm in diameter. In small or medium-sized breasts, such a resection results in a wide glandular defect and poor esthetic results if direct closure is carried out. Plastic surgery derived from reduction mammaplasty procedures allows much better final cosmetic results, which is the goal of conservative treatment. In 25% of our patients treated with BCS, the plastic surgeon is called upon by the general surgeon to close the glandular defect. However, such glandular remodeling changes the size and position of the breast. Therefore, in 15% of these cases a symmetry procedure is performed on the opposite breast. The reduction procedure in the opposite breast should be taken as a good opportunity to check the glandular tissue. Special attention should therefore be given to the contralateral mammogram in order to focus the glandular resection on the most dubious areas. Occult carcinomas, half of them infiltrating, were found in 4% of a series of 350 symmetry procedures performed during breast reconstruction at the Gustave

Roussy Cancer Institute. In conclusion, close collaboration between oncologists and plastic surgeons is required not only to obtain the best cosmetic results but also to allow improved radicality of the tumor resection and a histological check-up of the contralateral breast.

References

Avril M, Auperin A, Margulis A et al (1997) Basal cell carcinoma of the face: surgery or radiotherapy? Results of a randomized study. Bri J Cancer 76(1):100

Berrino P, Campora E, Santi PL (1987) Postquadrantectomy breast deformities. classification and techniques of surgical correction. Plast Reconstr Surg 79:567

Dewar J, Arriagada R, Benhamou S et al (1995) Local relapse and contralateral tumor rates in patients with breast cancer treated with conservative surgery and radiotherapy (Institut Gustave Roussy 1970–1982). Cancer 76:2260

Fisher B, Redmond C et al (1989) Eight year results of the NSABP randomized clinical trial comparing total mastectomy and lumpectomy with or without radiation in the treatment of breast cancer. N Engl J Med 320 (13):822

Galimberti V, Zurrida S et al (1993) Central small size breast cancer: how to overcome the problem of nipple and areola involvement. Eur J Cancer 29:1093

Garusi C, Petit J, Rietjens M, Lanfrey E (1997) La place de la chirurgie plastique dans le traitement conservateur du cancer du sein. Ann Chir Plast Esthet 42(2):168

Holland R, Veling SHJ et al (1985) Histologic multifocality of Tis T1-2 breast carcinoma. Implications for clinical trials of breast conserving surgery. Cancer 56:979

Lejour M (1990) Vertical mammaplasty without inframammary scar and with liposuction. Perspect Plast Surg 4(2):67

Little J (1984) Nipple-areola reconstruction. Plast Reconstr Surg 11(2):351

McKissock PK (1976) Reduction mammaplasty by the vertical bipedicle flap technique. Clin Plast Surg 3:309

Petit J, Rietjens M (1991) Deformities following tumorectomy and partial mastectomy. In: Noone B (ed) Plastic and reconstructive surgery of the breast. Decker, Philadelphia

Pitanguy I (1981) Reduction mammaplasty. In: Aesthetic plastic surgery of head and body. Springer, Berlin Heidelberg New York, p 3

Rietjens M, Petit JY, Contesso G, Bertin F, Gilles R (1997) The role of the reduction mammaplasty in oncology. Eur J Plast Surg 20:246

Sarrazin D, Fontaine MF (1983) Conservative treatment versus mastectomy in T1 or small T2 breast cancer: a randomized trial. In: Harris JR (ed) Conservative management of breast cancer. Lippincott, Philadelphia, p 101

Slavin S, Love S, Sadowsky N (1992) Reconstruction of the radiated partial mastectomy defect with autogenous tissues. Plast Reconstr Surg 90:854

Tristant H, Benmussa M, Bokobsa J (1988) Mammographie et echografie mammaire. Flammarion, Paris

Veronesi U, Salvadori B (1990) Conservative treatment of early breast cancer. Long-term results of 1232 cases treated with quadrantectomy, axillary dissection and radiotherapy. Ann Surg 211:250

Summary

W. C. Wood

Department of Surgery, Emory University School of Medicine, Emory University Hospital, 1364 Clifton Road, N.E., Atlanta, GA 30322, USA

The surgical management of the axilla in breast cancer is certainly among the most rapidly changing areas in this field of oncology. Dr. Blichert-Toft reviewed the importance of axillary lymph node staging as the dominant parameter in defining the prognosis of a breast cancer patient. Until we have better measures, planning for adjuvant therapy and stratification for clinical trial management will rely heavily on the results of axillary node dissection. He emphasized the role of local control in preventing recurrence of cancer and the ability of axillary dissection to control nodal metastases. The issue of whether such improved local control will issue in demonstrable survival advantage was discussed, but it seems clear that such a putative advantage will be of a size that a very large clinical trial would be required to address this question specifically.

The group from Milan agreed on the importance of axillary staging and control of axillary nodal metastases, so there was no advocate for avoidance of axillary nodal staging. They reported their experience with sentinel lymph node biopsy to determine whether or not axillary lymph node metastases were present and limiting dissection to the sentinel node-positive patient, as originally advocated by Drs. Morton and Giuliano. They have used the radionucleotide-labeled colloidal technique primarily. Those of us who have used the lymphazurin blue dye technique are similarly impressed with its utility and reliability when one has learned the technical tricks of the procedure and had sufficient personal experience to demonstrate the surgeon's ability to reliably identify and evaluate the sentinel node or nodes. I am convinced that the sentinel lymph node biopsy will replace axillary lymph node dissection as the initial axillary staging technique as rapidly as it can be learned and implemented. It will allow the benefits of axillary clearance to be confined to those with involved axillary lymph nodes. Clinical trials are in the planning stage to determine whether such dissection is of value even in women with positive sentinel lymph nodes but no clinical lymphadenopathy who will be having radiation to the breast as part of breast conservation, and that radiation will cover the level one and most of the level two nodes anyway. In addition, such node-positive patients will be receiving systemic adjuvant therapy.

The most frequent reason that mastectomy is performed for early breast cancer instead of breast conservation therapy is that the size of the tumor is judged to be too large relative to the size of the breast to allow conservation with good cosmesis. The NSABP trial of induction chemotherapy versus postoperative chemotherapy demonstrated identical survival and relapse-free survival in both groups. This has confirmed the phase II data of institutional trials and the smaller randomized trials suggesting the value of induction chemotherapy to allow breast conservation. Dr. Margolese made several cautionary comments. Among them was the reality that size is not an indication for mastectomy, per se. Tumors up to 5 cm in diameter can be managed with lumpectomy. Secondly, not all tumors regressing under the influence of chemotherapy will reduce totally from their periphery. Some may regress in an inhomogeneous fashion that will leave islands of viable tumor if only the residual mass is excised. This is a somewhat contentious point, although it seems reasonable enough. Further trial experience will allow a more confident statement about the ability of induction chemotherapy to downsize and permit smaller surgical excisions. Such have been done for some years without evidence of increased recurrence in several clinics, but larger numbers and additional publications are needed to resolve this issue.

The Milan group presented examples of immediate reconstruction with a variety of ablative surgical procedures. These demonstrated the good results to be obtained with careful planning to allow optimal radicality to assure local control and the preservation of good cosmesis. Our own experience is that skin-sparing mastectomy, removing only the nipple and areola, with autologous tissue reconstruction, allows a remarkably unchanged appearance of the breast for those women who require removal of the entire breast. Although these women represent a shrinking proportion of those with breast cancer, the ability to preserve excellent cosmesis without any evidence of diminished local control for this group is a major improvement.

Skin-sparing mastectomy, induction chemotherapy for larger tumors in smaller breasts to allow breast conservation, and the change to sentinel lymph node excision to replace axillary dissection for the majority of women with breast cancer are likely to modify the management of primary breast cancer as dramatically over the next decade as breast conservation therapy did in the last.

The other frontier being frequently discussed is the role of prophylactic mastectomy for women at increased risk of developing breast cancer. Two major drawbacks attend such a recommendation. The first is the morbidity of bilateral mastectomy. Even with skin-sparing techniques and the ability to achieve a commendable cosmetic result, the loss of all sensual sensation proves a more dramatic difference than many patients had anticipated. The second is the fact that some breast cells remain and there is no guarantee that cancer cannot still develop. Data from subcutaneous mastectomy series suggest that the reduction in risk is on the order of 90%. These data are derived from risk estimates based on family history, not on genetically defined risks of heritable breast cancer. Even such definition is in the process of study and uncertainty. The initial risk estimates were based on family linkage studies in families with an extremely high rate of penetrance of the BRCA 1 and 2 mutations. As population-based analyses are done, the rate of penetrance has been found to be lower (60% rather than over 80%). Many different mutations have been identified and some data suggest that these, too, may have differing rates of penetrance. All of this makes bilateral prophylactic mastectomy something not to be lightly recommended. The role of chemoprevention in lowering the risk of breast cancer in genetically defined individuals at increased risk is a further caution against too hasty recommendations for a surgical therapy that is not reversible. It is probably best to discuss the risk of genetic mutations in terms of risk over the next decade rather than lifetime risk, as new therapies may be available in the next few years.

It is ironic to note that mastectomy, devised for locally advanced breast cancer, migrated from that use to early stage breast cancer. As it was replaced there its use shifted in many places to in situ breast cancer, with invasive cancer treated with breast sparing techniques. Now as DCIS is usually treated with breast-conserving means, some are advocating mastectomy for women with no histologic abnormality at all, only genetically defined risk.

VII. Integrated Therapy: Primary Adjuvant Systemic Therapy

Is Primary Chemotherapy Useful for All Patients with Primary Invasive Breast Cancer?

S. M. Scholl[1], P. Beuzeboc[1], A. L. Harris[3], J. Y. Pierga[1], B. Asselain[2],
T. Palangié[1], T. Dorval[1], M. Jouve[1], V. Diéras[1], and P. Pouillart[1]

[1] Département de Médecine Oncologique, Institut Curie, 26 rue d'Ulm,
75231 Paris, Cedex 05, France
[2] Unité de Biostatistiques, Institut Curie, 26 rue d'Ulm, 75231 Paris, Cedex 05, France
[3] ICRF Clinical Oncology Unit, Radcliffe Hospital, Headington, Oxford OX3 7LJ, UK

Background

Following failed attempts to cure breast cancer by more surgery, the conservative management of early breast cancer, once controversial, has progressively been adopted as an alternative to mastectomy (Jacobson et al. 1995). The adjuvant treatment of breast cancer has a much shorter history and, while the radical Halstedian approach is obsolete, we have entered a radical adjuvant chemotherapy phase where 'earlier and more is better'. Given the still relatively small percentage of patients who do have a survival benefit from adjuvant manipulations (Early Breast Cancer Trialists' Collaborative Group 1992), this seems a reasonable point in time to question recent developments in our management of primary breast cancer.

Over recent years we have progressed in identifying patients who will most certainly be cured by local treatment or, on the contrary, are at very high risk for recurrence despite optimal systemic adjuvant therapy (Clark 1994; Scholl et al. 1996) (Table 1, Fig. 1). Due to the long interval from treatment to evaluation of adjuvant protocols, there has been little progress in matching patients with particular forms of therapy to which they are most likely to respond. The consensus goes that all patients 'at risk', that is with one or several parameters of poor prognosis, should receive some form of systemic treatment. Unfortunately the patients with the poorest prognosis are not the most likely to respond to systemic treatments.

Based on the concept of breast cancer as a systemic disease, the administration of primary chemotherapy was the logical next step, aiming at eradicating micrometastatic disease with the potential to increase cure rates. Yet, published clinical trials testing primary versus adjuvant chemotherapy have shown only minor (Scholl et al. 1994) or no statistical significant benefit. Did we go wrong? The latest update of the Curie trial (S6: 390 patients with an 8-year median follow-up) showed a minor survival advantage for the primary chemotherapy group (Wilcoxon 0.09; Breslow 0.05) (Fig. 2). A larger randomized trial comparing preoperative versus postoperative adjuvant chemotherapy (60/600) in patients who routinely received tamoxifen in the age group over 50 years (50%) did not show a difference in survival (Scholl et al.

Table 1. Risk profiles according to five parameters associated with poor outcome of breast cancer (from Scholl et al. 1996)

Profile no.	Node status (0.732)[a]	Int2 (1.092)	Membrane over expression of neu (0.750)	Vascular invasion (0.665)	T cells CD45RO+ (0.744)	N	No. of deaths	Relative risk
1	0[b]	0	0	0	0	34	4	1.00
2	1	0	0	0	0	41	16	2.08
3	0	0	0	0	1	4	2	2.11
4	0	0	1	0	0	6	2	2.13
5	0	1	0	0	0	8	2	2.98
6	1	0	0	1	0	17	6	4.05
7	0	0	0	1	1	2	0	4.10
8	0	0	1	1	0	2	2	4.14
9	1	0	0	0	1	6	3	4.38
10	1	0	1	0	0	12	4	4.42
11	0	0	1	0	1	1	1	4.48
12	1	1	0	0	0	8	5	6.21
13	0	1	1	0	0	3	2	6.34
14	1	0	0	1	1	3	3	8.53
15	1	0	1	1	0	10	7	8.61
16	1	0	1	0	1	2	1	9.31
17	1	1	0	1	0	2	2	12.08
18	1	1	1	0	0	3	2	13.19
19	1	1	1	1	0	1	1	25.67

[a] Parentheses contain the prognostic index for each variable.
[b] 0, normal or negative; 1, abnormal or positive

1995). Clinical response, our surrogate endpoint, was achieved in two-thirds of all patients (Scholl et al. 1994) and was highly predictive for breast conservative treatment, for lower local recurrence rates. Relapse-free survival figures have been shown to be significantly improved in an Italian series (Bonadonna et al. 1998) but were significant only in subgroups in the present series and not statistically different when complete and partial responders were compared to minor or non-responders (Fig. 3). Smaller tumour size (Scholl et al. 1994, 1995; Fisher et al. 1997), young age (Scholl et al. 1995; Fisher et al. 1997, and high mitotic rates (Scholl et al. 1995) were predictors of clinical response in both our and in the NSABP B18 series, and these criteria define a population who might benefit most from preoperative and intensified chemotherapy protocols.

Large international surveys of adjuvant chemotherapy estimate a gain of not more than 10% in survival (Early Breast Cancer Trialists' Collaborative Group 1992) at 10 years. According to these data, the vast majority will either not have needed this treatment or have a minimal therapeutic gain. The effects reported already with chemotherapy and hormone therapy may be due to a small effect for most patients or a large effect in a subset of patients. Based on the observations that in metastatic disease there is a subset of patients who achieve prolonged responses and the majority only have

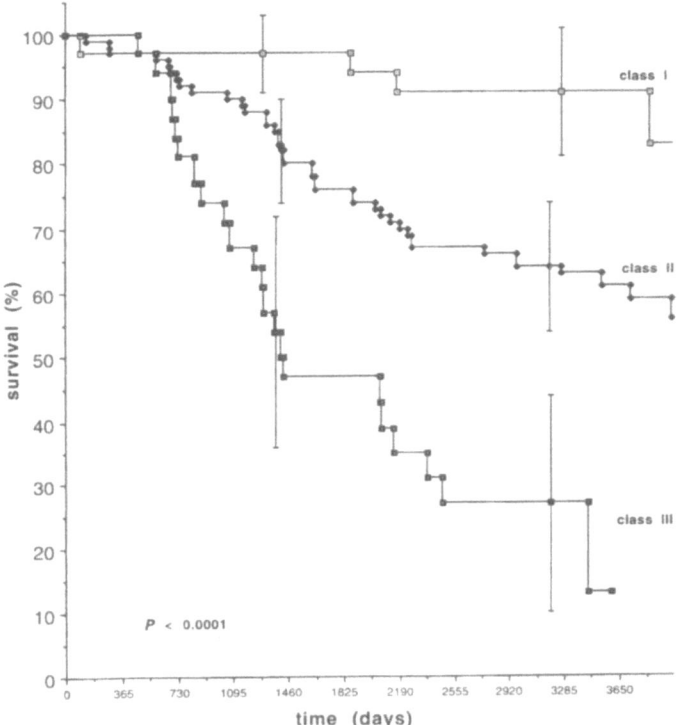

Fig. 1. Survival curves according to prognostic profiles (see Table 1). Patients with profile 1 (class I) were negative for all five of the dominant factors associated with a poor outcome. Profiles 2–11 group patients (class II) with one or two features of poer prognosis and with a PI>2. Profiles 12–19 group patients (class III) with a PI>2. $\chi^2=39.47$ (2 d.f.), p<0.0001; when comparing class I vs class II: $\chi^2 = 7.38$ (1 d.f.) p<0.005; comparing class II vs class III: $\chi^2=21.14$ (1 d.f.), p<10^{-5}; comparing class I vs class III: $\chi^2 = 35.49$ (1 d.f.), p<10^{-6}. (From Sholl et al. 1996)

short-lived responses, it is likely that beneficial effects are related to quite marked improvements for subsets. Thus, rather than giving all patients the same treatment, or all possible treatments to each patient (Fisher et al. 1997), therapeutic manoeuvres based on assessment of response following primary chemotherapy may greatly improve the efficacy/toxicity ratio.

Can We Predict Which Patients Will Benefit from Systemic Chemotherapy?

We addressed this question in a series of 195 stage II–III primary breast cancer patients who had been treated with chemotherapy at the Institut Curie, prior to local-regional treatments (Scholl et al. 1994). Not surprisingly, one of the major factors predictive for a response to chemotherapy was a high

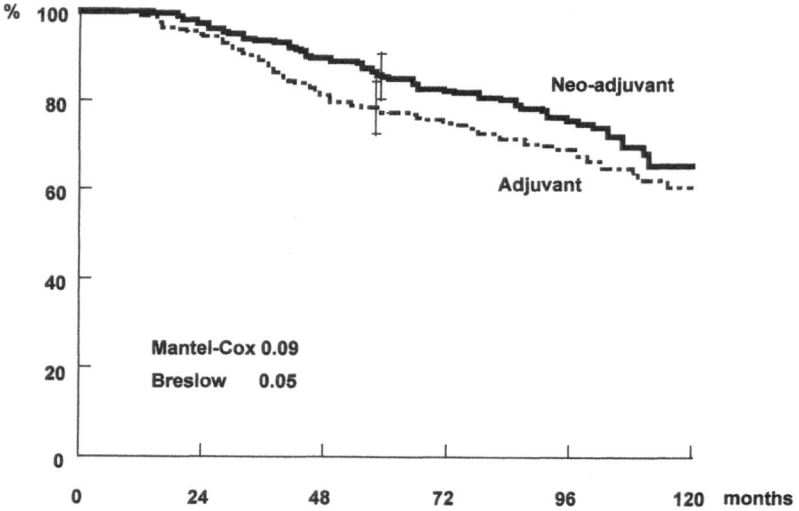

Fig. 2. Overall survival according to timing of chemotherapy at a median follow-up of 8 years. *n* = 200 (neoadjuvant), *n* = 190 (adjuvant)

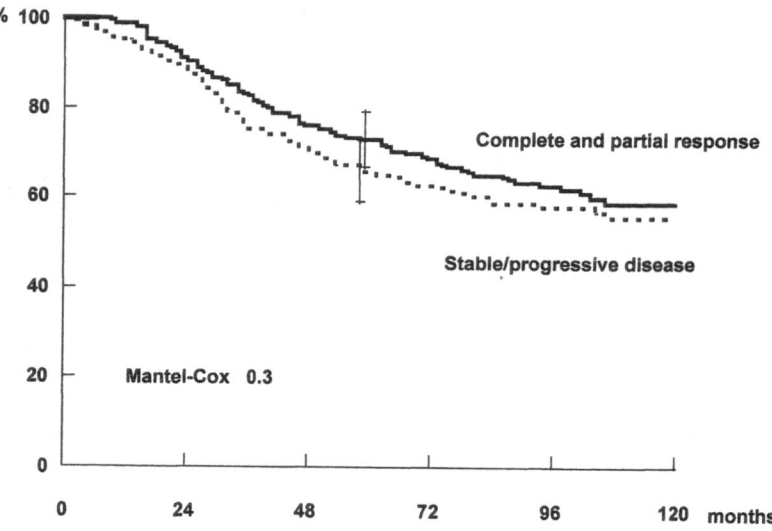

Fig. 3. Time to metastatic recurrence at a median interval of 8 years. One hundred and fifty-five patients were evaluable for response after four courses of neoadjuvant chemotherapy (Scholl et al. 1995), out of whom 124 patients had a complete or partial response while 31 patients had stable or progressive disease. Metastatic recurrence rates did not differ significantly

fraction of cells (>5%) in the S phase of the cell cycle. Patients aged below 35 years had a higher relative risk (RR = 2.46) for metastatic recurrences despite better response and higher mitotic rates, suggesting that the treatment may have been suboptimal for this subset (Scholl et al. 1995). Active cellular proliferation as measured by either S phase (Remvikos et al. 1989), BUdR (Wilson et al. 1988), or thymidine labelling (Silvestrini et al. 1985; Gamel et al. 1995; Frierson 1991) has been considered a prerequisite for the efficacy of cytotoxic regimes. Highly proliferative tumours have also been repeatedly associated with a poor prognosis (Kute et al. 1990). This finding was not confirmed in more recent studies in which all patients had received chemotherapy (Witzig et al. 1993; Allred et al. 1992), and several authors (Gamel et al. 1995; Frierson 1991; Witzig et al. 1993) have suggested that the correlation between high S phase and poor prognosis might be modified by the preferential efficacy of chemotherapy in tumours with a high proliferation rate. Chemotherapy dose intensification in solid tumours is being evaluated in many multicentre trials, its indication being based on a clinical response in high-risk patients, thus selecting for tumours with rapid proliferation and low resistance. However, results from randomized trials are still pending and data from open studies are misleading since they are heavily biased by patient selection. Patients with tumours overexpressing c-erbB2, a growth factor receptor of the EGF receptor family, earlier shown not to benefit from chemotherapy (Allred et al. 1992; Gusterson et al. 1992), were more recently shown to have a significant survival advantage in the higher dose regimen as compared to a less optimal treatment schedule (Muss et al. 1994).

Clinical response is a valuable surrogate endpoint following primary chemotherapy. It will allow one to distinguish between patients with a high S-phase fraction who still retain an apoptotic response to chemotherapy such that there is a high rate in cell kill and consequently an improvement in prognosis, and those patients (often with the most proliferative tumours) whose disease will progress rapidly due to resistance mechanisms or failure to show an apoptotic response. Thus the S-phase fraction can pick out a group that may be responsive, but additional markers will be needed to assess those that will be chemoresistant (Fig. 4). An example of the latter may be induction of MDR1 overexpression during the first course of chemotherapy (Chevillard et al. 1996). Interestingly, recent data indicate that, following acquisition of multi-drug resistance, tumour cells are refractory to fas-induced death because they express little or no fas (Cai et al. 1996).

For practical purposes, patients *at risk* (young age, rapidly progressing tumours, node-positive disease, vascular/lymphatic invasion, negative steroid receptor values, poor-grade and/or micrometastatic disease) and *capable of responding* (high mitotic rate, clinical response, no induction of multi-drug resistance, no downregulation of fas?) are the population of choice for primary systemic chemotherapy. Early clinical and biological monitoring of changes as the tumour regresses or grows and new clones are selected may help assess the likelihood of response and allow the adoption of different therapeutic strategies as well as provide novel biological information. Results

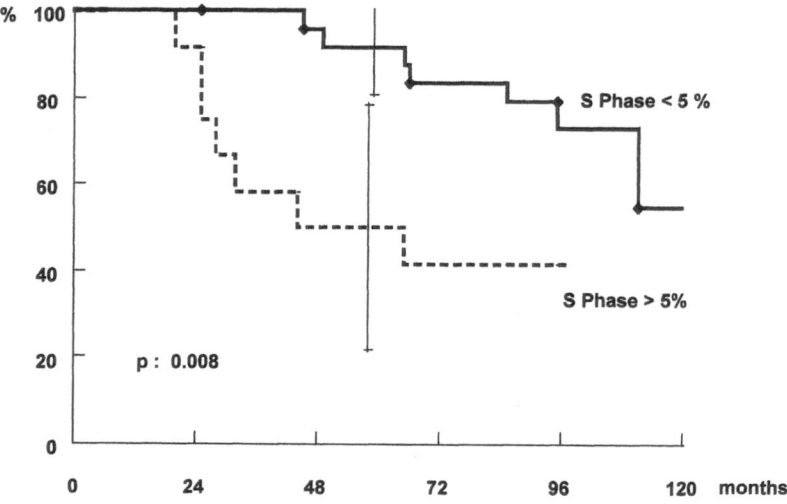

Fig. 4. S-phase fractions were evaluable in 35/70 patients who had shown no response following two courses of primary chemotherapy. Significantly better survival was seen in patients with tumours showing low proliferative rates (S phase <5%) as compared to patients with rapidly dividing tumours

of primary chemotherapy in breast cancer suggest high response rates compared to those reported in multi-treated metastatic cancer, again suggesting that genetic (and perhaps micro-environmental) changes may occur during treatment of metastases, producing drug resistance. The administration of chemotherapy, hormone therapy, or radiotherapy is likely to modify factors that are favourable for tumour survival. Examples of biological monitoring include measurement of apoptosis, which may give an indication of chemosensitivity, thus allowing cytotoxic therapy to be changed or omitted accordingly, provided that a good relationship between these early markers and outcome can be demonstrated. Another attractive strategy is monitoring for induction of resistance pathways, in particular during the early assessment of new agents. For instance, drugs that block a cell-cycle-dependent kinase such as CDK4 may be active only in a subset of patients with cyclin D1 overexpression. The therapeutic effect could be monitored ex vivo by flow cytometry. The techniques for these assessments are already available via fine needle aspirates and biopsy guns. Thus by investigating mechanisms of response and resistance in the first courses of treatment we may increase activity and decrease toxicity. The use of physiological modifications such as hypoxia and metabolism in the primary tumour (e.g. blood flow by PET scanning) before and after therapy may be worth assessing.

Are There Alternatives for Patients Who Fail to Respond to Primary Chemotherapy?

A number of immunotherapy and vaccination trials are being conducted in many different centres. There is a lot of anecdotal evidence that cancer vaccines could help patients, but little yet in the way of solid, reproducible clinical data. The patients in whom clinical phase I testing is carried out have advanced disease, have failed to respond to conventional treatments, and often cannot respond to immunological stimulation, for a number of reasons that increase with the extent of the tumour. Thus, tumours produce immunosuppressive cytokines that will hamper adequate antigen presentation and the development and maintenance of a cytotoxic response (Chonaib et al. 1997). MHC class I molecules are often downregulated (Cabrera et al. 1996), costimulatory molecules absent on tumour cells (Schwartz 1992), and some tumours are able to produce fas ligand (Walker et al. 1997), allowing counterattack of the immune system. Best responses to clinical testing would ideally be expected in early-stage disease because there is less tumour bulk and the patient's immune system is still able to respond.

The identification and cloning of several tumour antigens together with an improvement in the understanding of the mechanisms involved in antigen presentation and immune recognition has opened up the possibility of using active specific immunotherapy as a treatment for certain cancers. The polymorphic epithelial mucin (PEM), also called MUC1, is a potential target molecule since it is expressed, upregulated, and hypoglycosylated in a high proportion (>80%) of breast and ovarian cancers (Graham et al. 1996). This transmembrane protein is cleaved into the circulation where it is detectable in advanced disease as a tumour marker (CA 15.3) by a variety of antibodies. The objectives of a phase I clinical study at our centre were to examine the clinical and environmental safety and immunogenicity of a live recombinant vaccinia virus expressing the human MUC1 and IL-2 proteins (pTG1031). Vaccination resulted in no significant clinical side effects and there was no environmental contamination by live pTG1031. Peripheral blood lymphocytes of one patient at the intermediate dose level showed a proliferative response to repeat in vitro culture with MUC1 peptide molecules with a stimulation index of 7×, and to 14× after a boost injection. This patient had a concomitant drop in serum CEA levels, remained clinically stable for 10 weeks, and after progression had a major response to low-dose perfusion chemotherapy. MUC1-specific cytotoxic T lymphocytes, the effector mechanism most likely to be of therapeutic benefit, were detected in one other patient so far. Although antibody titers in the present study remained generally low, a spontaneous rise in antibody titers has been documented in a number of breast cancer patients and was thought to be protective against metastatic recurrence (Von Mensdorff-Pouilly et al. 1996). Patients with early breast cancer who are at high risk of recurrence and have failed primary chemotherapy might be given the option to participate in adjuvant vaccination trials following the completion of local therapy. A surrogate endpoint could be the development of a proliferative response in ex vivo testing of peripheral blood mononuclear cells, the primary endpoint being delay to recurrence.

Other major breast tumour targets currently under investigation are: HER2/neu overexpression (Baselga et al. 1994), *p53* mutated epitopes (Heise et al. 1997), neovasculature (Burrows and Thorpe 1993; Scott and Harris 1994), and metalloproteinases (Hodgson 1995). Humanized antibodies directed against HER2/neu have shown good tolerance in phase II and phase III clinical trial and results of these large multicentre trials should be available in the near future. The membrane overexpression of HER2/neu being associated with early recurrence and relative resistance to chemotherapy, the addition of antibodies to primary chemotherapy would appear to be useful and specific. Many different approaches, using either peptide vaccination or an E1b-defective adenovirus (Heise et al. 1997) capable of lytic reproduction in *p53* wild-type deficient (tumour) cells, are currently being tested in preclinical studies as well as in clinical studies of head and neck as well as in ovarian tumours. *p53* mutations are present on average in 20% of breast tumours, occasionally associated with signs of a spontaneous immune reaction (dendritic cells), and further clinical investigations in breast cancer patients are pending.

Conclusion

Intensified chemotherapy regimes may improve life expectancy in selected patients and the use of primary chemotherapy will permit optimization of drug combinations and schedules. However, it may be that our efforts should not be solely directed towards standardized high-tech, high-intensity treatments with the expectation of a small overall therapeutic gain but a certain high cost and morbidity. A more discerning attitude might be beneficial, and with new reagents becoming available, alternatives to cytotoxic chemotherapy can be tested. 'Primum non nocere' has always been a valuable guideline in difficult situations, but harm can be done not only by injudiciously over-treating patients, but also by failing to treat or, by extension, by lack of trying to find adequate treatments.

Summary

Chemotherapy dose intensification in breast tumours is being evaluated in many multicentre trials, its indication being based on a clinical response in high-risk patients, thus selecting for tumours with rapid proliferation and low resistance. However, results from randomized trials are still pending. Clinical and pathological responses to therapy are valuable surrogate endpoints following primary chemotherapy. They will make it possible to distinguish at an early stage between patients who still retain an apoptotic response to chemotherapy and those patients whose disease will progress rapidly due to resistance mechanisms. For practical purposes, patients *at risk* and *capable of responding* represent the population of choice for primary systemic chemotherapy. Thus, by investigating mechanisms of response and resistance during the first courses of treatment we may target chemotherapy at those patients likely to benefit most from this treatment. A number of immunotherapy and vaccination trials are being conducted in many different centres. There is a lot of anecdotal evidence that cancer vaccines could help patients, but little yet in the way of solid, reproducible clinical data. Best responses to clinical testing would ideally be expected in early-stage disease because there is less tumour bulk and the patient's immune system is still able to respond. Patients with early breast cancer who are at high risk of recurrence and who have failed to respond to primary chemotherapy might be given the option of participating in adjuvant vaccination trials following the completion of local therapy.

References

Allred CD, Clark GM, Tandon AK et al (1992) HET-2/neu in node-negative breast cancer. Prognostic significance of overexpression influenced by the presence of in-situ carcinoma. J Clin Oncol 10:599–605

Baselga J, Tripathy D, Mendelsohn J et al (1994) Ongoing phase II study of intravenous recombinant anti-p185 HER2 monoclonal antibody 4D5 (Mab 4D5) in patients with stage IV breast cancer overexpressing HER2. Breast Cancer Res Treat 32:8

Bonadonna G, Valagussa P, Brmabilla C et al (1998) primary chemotherapy in operable breast cancer: eight-year experience at the Milan Cancer Institute. J Clin Oncol 16:93–100

Burrows F, Thorpe PE (1993) Eradication of large solid tumors in mice with an immunotoxin directed against tumor vasculature. Proc Natl Acad Sci USA 90:8996–9000

Cabrera T, Fernandez MA, Sierra A, Garrido A, Garrido F (1996) High frequency of altered HLA class I phenotypes in invasive breast carcinomas. Hum Immunol 50:127–134

Cai Z, Stancou R, Korner M, Chouaib S (1996) Impairment of fas antigen expression in adriamycin resistant but not TNF resistant MCF7 tumor cells. Int J Cancer 68:535–546

Chevillard S, Pouillart P, Beldjord C et al (1996) Sequential assessment of multidrug resistance phenotype and measurement of S-phase fraction as predictive markers of breast cancer response to neoadjuvant chemotherapy. Cancer 77:292–300

Chouaib S, Asselin-Paturel C, Mami-Chouaib F, Caignard A, Blay JY (1997) The host-tumor immune conflict: from immunosuppression to resistance and destruction. Immunol Today 18:493–497

Clark GM (1994) Do we really need prognostic factors for breast cancer? Breast Cancer Res Treat 30:117–126

Early Breast Cancer Trialist's Collaborative Group (1992) Systemic treatment of early breast cancer by hormonal, cytotoxic or immune therapy. Lancet 339:1–15, 71–85

Fisher B, Brown A, Mamaounas E et al (1997) Effect of preoperative chemotherapy on local-regional disease in women with operable breast cancer: Findings from NSABP-18. J Clin Oncol 16:2483–2493

Frierson HJ (1991) Ploidy analysis and S-phase fraction determination by flow cytometry of invasive adenocarcinomas of the breast. Am J Surg Pathol 15:358–367

Gamel JW, Meyer JS, Province MA (1995) Proliferative rate by S-phase measurement may affect cure of breast carcinoma. Cancer 76:1009–1018

Graham R, Burchell JM, Taylor-Papadimitriou J (1996) The polymorphic epithelial mucin: potential as an immunogen for a cancer vaccine. Cancer Immunol Immunother 42:71–80

Gusterson BA, Gelber RD, Goldhirsh A et al (1992) Prognostic importance of c-erbB-2 expression in breast cancer. J Clin Oncol 10:1049–1056

Heise C, Sampson-Johannes A, Williams A, McCormick F, Von Hoff D, Kirn DH (1997) ONYX-015, an E1B gene-attenuated adenovirus, causes tumor-specific cytolysis and antitumoral efficacy that can be augmented by standard chemotherapeutic agents. Nat Med 3:639–645

Hodgson J (1995) Remodelling matrix metalloproteinase inhibitors. Biotechnology 13:654–657

Jacobson JA, Danforth DN, Cowan KH et al (1995) Ten-year results of a comparison of conservation with mastectomy in the treatment of stage I and breast cancer. N J Engl Med 233:907–911

Kute T, Muss H, Cooper M et al (1990) The use of flow cytometry for the prognosis of stage II adjuvant-treated breast cancer patients. Cancer 66:1810–1816

Muss HB, Thor AD, Berry D et al (1994) C-erbB2 expression and response to adjuvant therapy in women with node positive early breast cancer. N Engl J Med 330:1260–1266

Remvikos Y, Beuzeboc P, Zajdela A et al (1989) Correlation of pretreatment proliferative activity of breast cancer with the response to cytotoxic chemotherapy. J Natl Cancer Inst 81:1383–1387

Scholl SM, Forquet A, Asselain B et al (1994) Neoadjuvant versus adjuvant chemotherapy in premenopausal patients with tumours considered too large for breast conserving surgery: preliminary results of a randomized trial: S6. Eur J Cancer 30A:645–652

Scholl SM, Pierga JY, Asselain B et al (1995) Breast tumour response to primary chemotherapy predicts local and distant contral as well as survival. Eur J Cancer 31A:1969–1975

Scholl S, Bieche I, Pallud C et al (1996) Relevance of multiple biological parameters, in breast cancer prognosis. Breast 5:21–30

Schwartz D (1992) Costimulation of T lymphocytes: the role of CD28, CTLA-4 and B7/BB1 in interleukin-2 production and immunotherapy. Cell 71:1065–1068

Scott PAE, Harris AL (1994) Current approaches to targeting cancer using antigiogenesis therapies. Laboratory-clinic interface. Cancer Treat Rev 20:393–412

Silvestrini R, Daidone MG, Gasparini G (1985) Cell kinetics as a prognostic marker in node-negative breast cancer. Cancer 56:1982–1987

Von Mensdorff-Pouilly S, Gourevitch MM, Kenemans P et al (1996) Humoral immune response to polymorphic epithelial mucin (MUC1) in patients with benign and malignant breast tumours. Eur J Cancer 32A:1325–1331

Walker PR, Saas P, Dietrich PY (1997) Rôle of fas ligand (CD95L) in immune escape. The tumour strikes back. J Immunol 158:4521–4524

Wilson GD, McNally NJ, Dishe S et al (1988) Measurement of cell kinetics in human tumours in vivo using bromodeoxyuridine incorporation and flow cytometry. Br J Cancer 58:423–431

Witzig TE, Ingle JN, Schaid DJ et al (1993) DNA ploidy and percent of S-phase as prognostic factors in node-positive breast cancer: results from patients enrolled in two prospective randomized trials. J Clin Oncol 11:351–359

The Primary Use of Endocrine Therapies

A. Howell[1], E. Anderson[1], R. Blamey[2], R.B. Clarke[1], J.M. Dixon[3],
M. Dowsett[4], S.R.D. Johnston[4], W.R. Miller[3], R. Nicholson[5],
and J.F.R. Robertson[2]

[1] CRC Department of Medical Oncology and Department of Clinical Research,
Christie Hospital NHS Trust, Manchester M20 4BX, UK
[2] Department of Surgery, Nottingham City Hospital, Nottingham NG5 1PB, UK
[3] Edinburgh Breast Unit and ICRF Med Oncology Unit, Western General Hospital, Edinburgh EH4 2XU, UK
[4] Academic Department of Biochemistry, Royal Marsden Hospital,
London SW3 6JJ, UK
[5] Tenovus Institute of Cancer Research, Cardiff CF4 4XX, UK

Introduction

The major objective of nearly all studies of primary endocrine therapy has been to assess whether surgery can be deferred indefinitely without impairing survival, particularly in elderly infirm patients (Preece et al. 1982; Helleberg et al. 1982; Bradbeer and Kyngdon 1983; Allan et al. 1985; Richard 1989; Anderson et al. 1991; Foudraine et al. 1992; Bates et al. 1991; Robertson et al. 1992; Gaskell et al. 1992; Mustacchi et al. 1994; Gazet et al. 1994; van Dalsen and De Vries 1995; Bergman et al. 1995; Ciatto et al. 1996; Dixon et al. 1997). In contrast, the main objectives of primary chemotherapy have been to determine whether tumors can be downstaged in order to increase the possibility of breast conservation surgery, and to ask whether preoperative chemotherapy can improve survival compared with the same treatment given after primary surgery. Primary chemotherapy studies demonstrate high complete (CR) and partial response (PR) rates (CR+PR 60%–100%) and that response is associated with a good prognosis, but in randomised trials overall survival is not improved significantly by chemotherapy (Clemons et al. 1997).

Fisher and Mamounas (1995) pointed out the importance of establishing biologically plausible hypotheses which would underpin the clinical use of primary chemotherapy. They highlighted four hypotheses which might be tested. These may equally apply to primary endocrine therapy:

1. Tumor cells shed at the time of surgery are important for the development of metastases and patient survival.
2. Removal of the primary tumor causes release of factors which promote the growth of metastases (Fig. 1) (Gunduz et al. 1979; Fisher et al. 1989a,b).
3. Tumor resistance increases with time and the early introduction of effective chemotherapy, particularly alternating non-cross-resistant combinations of drugs, will lead to better survival (the Goldie-Coldman hypothesis) (Goldie and Coldman 1979).

4. The Skipper hypothesis (Skipper 1971) that primary and secondary tumors respond differently to chemotherapy; thus, even if there were no response in the primary tumor, secondary tumors would respond to the benefit of the host.

Primary chemotherapy might be expected to improve survival if any of these hypotheses were correct. Thus, if chemotherapy in women with breast cancer effectively inhibits tumor cell shedding and the effect of the primary tumors on metastases, and if primary chemotherapy supports the hypotheses of Goldie-Coldman and Skipper, survival may be improved. In the event, several randomised trials show that primary chemotherapy is not associated with a survival advantage. In terms of the first two hypotheses this may be because it is not normally administered during operations, which might be the optimal period to prevent cell shedding or the effect of the tumor on metastases. In terms of the Goldie-Coldman hypothesis, there is usually only a month or two's difference in time in the inception of chemotherapy, since postoperative chemotherapy is delayed only by the operative period. Finally, the observation that response to primary chemotherapy is related to survival appears to negate Skipper's hypothesis, since many data suggest that secondary tumors respond similarly to the primary.

Primary endocrine therapy has potential theoretical and practical advantages over chemotherapy, and its ease of administration during the operative

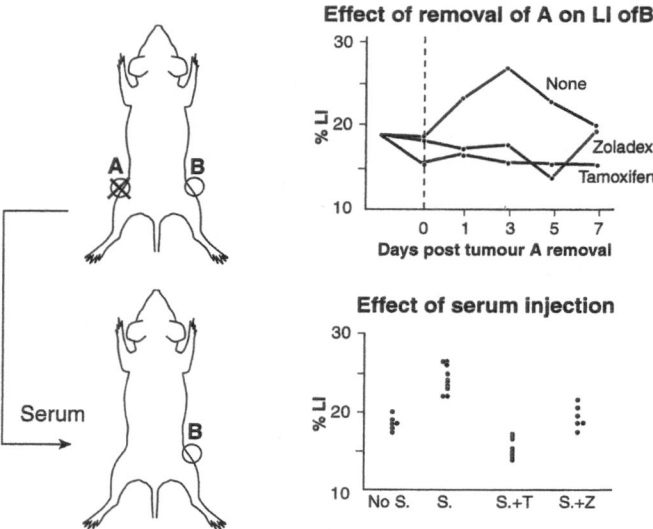

Fig. 1. *Upper part:* Effect of removal of tumor A on the proliferation of tumor B in untreated animals or in animals treated before, during, and after the operation with tamoxifen or zoladex. *Lower part:* Effect of serum taken after operation and infused into another mouse on growth of tumor B in untreated animals (no S.), in those infused with serum (S.) and in serum-infused animals treated with tamoxifen (S. + T.) or zoladex (S. + Z.). (Adapted from Fisher et al. 1989b)

period might allow testing of hypotheses 1 and 2. Inhibition of estrogen-stimulated enzyme relea (e.g. plasminogen activator, collagenases) may abrogate tumor-cell shedding. In addition, there is strong evidence that estrogen withdrawal reduces not only growth factor synthesis (e.g. TGFa) (Gregory et al. 1989; Noguchi et al. 1993) but also the function of a number of growth factor and hormone receptors and/or their second messenger signalling pathways (Fig. 2) (Vignon et al. 1987; Ignar-Trowbridge et al. 1992; Katzenellenbogen et al. 1997).

Adjuvant endocrine therapy for early breast cancer differs from chemotherapy in respect of duration of treatment. At present, 5 years appears to be the optimum treatment period for endocrine therapy, whereas chemotherapy is usually given for approximately 6 months. Differences in these treatment periods affect the design of trials of preoperative systemic therapy. For example 3–6 months of chemotherapy before operation is usually compared with the same treatment instituted some time after the operation. Since it is impractical, and probably unethical, not to give postoperative endocrine therapy, the optimal design for preoperative endocrine therapy trials should almost certainly compare a period (to be specified) of preoperative therapy in one arm versus nil in the other. Both arms should be given long-term adjuvant treatment. Such a design, although it would test all hypotheses outlined above, has not been formally implemented.

Preoperative chemotherapy has been tested in *appropriate* clinical trials much more frequently than endocrine therapy (Clemons et al. 1997). This is surprising, given the value of adjuvant endocrine therapy particularly in patients with receptor-positive tumors. Indirect comparisons in the World Overview indicate that survival using tamoxifen (or ovarian ablation) appears equivalent to chemotherapy in young women and superior to chemotherapy in older women with estrogen-receptor (ER) positive tumors (Table 1) (Early

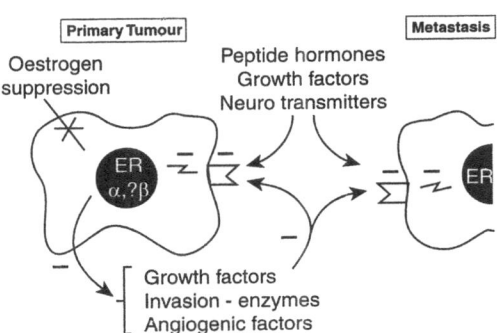

Fig. 2. Potential effects of estrogen withdrawal on tumor-metastasis interactions during the surgical period. Tumors are known to produce growth factors which may affect their own proliferation and, potentially, that of metastases. Peptide hormones (e.g. from the pituitary gland), neurotransmitters, and growth factors released in response to surgical injury may also affect tumor growth via cell surface receptors in endocrine-responsive tumor cells. Estrogen deprivation has been shown to inhibit tumor cell synthesis of growth factors and the activity of their cell surface receptors or second messengers

Table 1. Reduction in the odds of death by adjuvant tamoxifen and adjuvant chemotherapy in relationship to tumor estrogen receptor (ER) status and age of the patient. (Early Breast Cancer Trialists' Collaborative Group 1992, 1998)

	Patients <50 years		Patients ≥50 years	
	ER-pos.	ER-neg.	ER-pos.	ER-neg.
Tamoxifen (5 years)	26%	−3%	26%	−3%
Chemotherapy	~26%		~11%	

Breast Cancer Trialists' Collaborative Group 1992, 1998). Since the benefits of chemotherapy are unknown in women over 70 years of age, endocrine therapy is particularly important in this group, which represents about one-third of all breast cancers.

Although there are only four randomised trials of preoperative endocrine therapy, there are at least twelve small phase II trials. The purpose of this review is to indicate problems concerning their interpretation and to ask whether the trials answer the following questions:

1. Can preoperative endocrine therapy
   - Increase breast conservation?
   - Improve patient survival?
   - Give prognostic information?
2. Can we predict which patients are likely to benefit from preoperative endocrine therapy?
3. How does preoperative endocrine therapy compare with chemotherapy?

These are similar questions to those asked in the preoperative chemotherapy trials. In addition we will explore whether it is possible to predict which patients are likely to benefit from preoperative endocrine therapy and ask how well response rate to this treatment modality compares to that obtained with primary chemotherapy (Fisher and Mamounas 1995).

Problems with Interpretation of Data from Trials of Primary Endocrine Therapy

Table 2 gives an outline of the problems with interpreting the data from trials of primary endocrine therapy for breast cancer, which are discussed below.

Few Randomised Trials

There have been four randomised trials of primary endocrine therapy (Bates et al. 1991; Robertson et al. 1992; Mustacchi et al. 1994; Gazet et al. 1994). In all of them, the major question asked was whether use of preoperative endo-

Table 2. Trials of primary endocrine therapy: problems concerning interpretation of the available data

I	Few randomised trials – Tamoxifen vs surgery+tamoxifen (Bates et al. 1991) (Mustacchi et al. 1994) – Tamoxifen vs surgery (Robertson et al. 1992) (Gazet et al. 1994)
II	Trials (phase II and III) in elderly patients
III	Variable evaluation of response – Calipers – UICC criteria – Mammography – UICC criteria – 'Significant regression' – Best response at 2 years
IV	Variable duration of follow-up – Mean (11 studies) 39 months (range 1–132 months)
V	Number of patients studied – 1354 in 'phase II' studies

crine therapy could avoid the need for breast surgery in relatively infirm aged women and whether survival would be affected. In two trials, tamoxifen therapy and no immediate surgery was compared with immediate surgery and no tamoxifen (Bates et al. 1991; Robertson et al. 1992). In two other trials, tamoxifen alone was compared with tamoxifen and surgery (Mustacchi et al. 1994; Gazet et al. 1994). Not surprisingly, the time to local relapse was highly significantly shorter in the tamoxifen alone arm in all trials (Table 3). However, what *is* surprising is that the number of patients with distant relapse was slightly less in three out of the four trials in the no immediate surgery group. There were no significant differences in deaths from breast cancer or other causes (Table 3). In the immediate surgery arms, in all four trials either no tamoxifen was given ($n = 2$) or tamoxifen treatment was initiated after surgery, so that the period of surgery was not covered. In the tamoxifen alone arms there was no fixed period of treatment since the aim was to treat until local failure. Moreover, little or no information was given about other treatments that might have been used after surgery. Because these trials were designed to address the question whether delayed surgery is detrimental, it is not possible to use these studies to compare the value of a fixed period of primary endocrine therapy followed by surgery and adjuvant endocrine therapy for 5 years with surgery alone followed by adjuvant therapy. New randomised trials are required to answer this important question.

Table 3. Randomised trials of tamoxifen (T) versus surgery (S) or surgery and tamoxifen (S+T)

Treatments tested	Local relapse		Distant relapse		Study
	T (%)	S±T (%)	T (%)	S±T (%)	
Local and distant relapse rates					
TvS	40/68 (59)	20/67 (30)	16/68 (24)	22/67 (34)	Robertson et al. (1992)
TvS	56/100 (56)	44/100 (44)	8/100 (8)	14/100 (14)	Gazet et al. (1994)
TvS+T	60/236 (25)	15/237 (6)	19/236 (8)	33/237 (14)	Mustacchi et al. (1994)
TvS+T	51/183 (28)	22/177 (12)	6/183 (3)	6/171 (3)	Bates et al. (1991)
Deaths from breast cancer and other causes					
TvS	15/68 (22)	16/67 (24)	13/68 (19)	12/67 (18)	Robertson et al. (1992)
TvS	17/100 (17)	13/100 (13)	16/100 (16)	13/100 (13)	Gazet et al. (1994)
TvS+T	18/236 (7)	27/237 (11)	23/236 (10)	21/237 (9)	Mustacchi et al. (1994)

Trials Performed with Treatment Almost Exclusively in the Elderly

In addition to the four randomised trials outlined above, an additional twelve phase II trials have been reviewed (Preece et al. 1982; Helleberg et al. 1982; Bradbeer and Kyngdon 1983; Allan et al. 1985; Richard 1989; Anderson et al. 1991; Foudraine et al. 1992; Gaskell et al. 1992; van Dalsen and De Vries 1995; Bergman et al. 1995; Ciatto et al. 1996; Dixon et al. 1997). All studies except one treated patients over the age of 65 (Fig. 3). Data concerning the effects of preoperative therapy in younger patients are badly needed. However, as judged by the lack of effect of age on the value of tamoxifen in patients with ER-positive tumors in the World Overview (Fisher et al. 1989a; Early Breast Cancer Trialists' Collaborative Group 1998), it is likely that the effects of endocrine therapy will be similar in ER-positive tumors in patients above or below the age of 65.

Variation in Methods of Evaluating the Response to Tamoxifen

In general responses to tamoxifen treatment have been described using UICC criteria, but in some studies frequent measurements of multiple diameters have been made. In others, bidimensional measurements were made less frequently, and in others mammography or ultrasound were used instead. This multiplicity of method and timing of assessment may account for the wide range of responses reported (Fig. 4). For example, complete response rates varied from 8% to 58%, partial response rates from 15% to 75%, stable disease from 7% to 50%, and progressive disease from 0 to 23%.

The median duration of response to tamoxifen in studies where this was reported was 2 years. However, the durations in each category of response were highly variable (Table 4). In addition times to response were highly variable, often prolonged, and may reflect the assiduity with which response

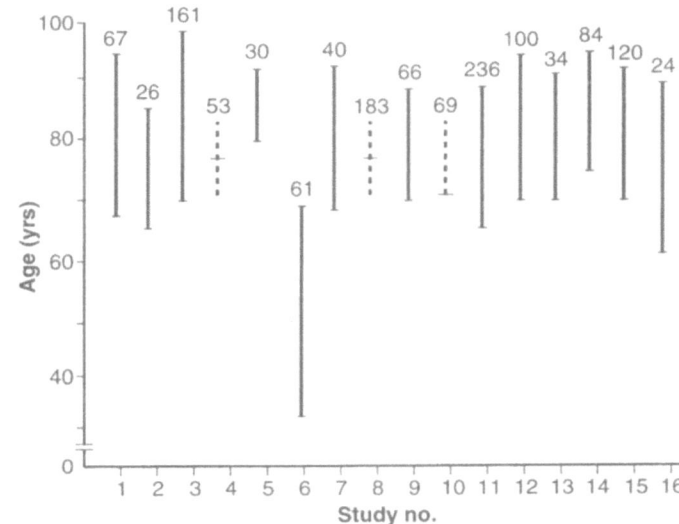

Fig. 3. Age range of patients studied in trials of primary endocrine therapy. Only median ages were cited in two trials (4, 8) and only lower age limit in one (10). The number of patients in each trial is shown; for the four randomised trials, number of patients in the primary tamoxifen therapy arm only are shown (8, 9, 11, 12). *Key: 1* Preece et al. 1982; *2* Helleberg et al. 1982; *3* Bradbeer and Kyngdon 1983; *4* Allan et al. 1985; *5* Richard 1989; *6* Anderson et al. 1991; *7* Foudraine et al. 1992; *8* Bates et al. 1991; *9* Robertson et al. 1992; *10* Gaskell et al. 1992; *11* Mustacchi et al. 1994; *12* Gazet et al. 1994; *13* Van Dalsen and De Vries 1995; *14* Bergman et al. 1995; *15* Ciatto et al. 1996; *16* Dixon et al. 1997

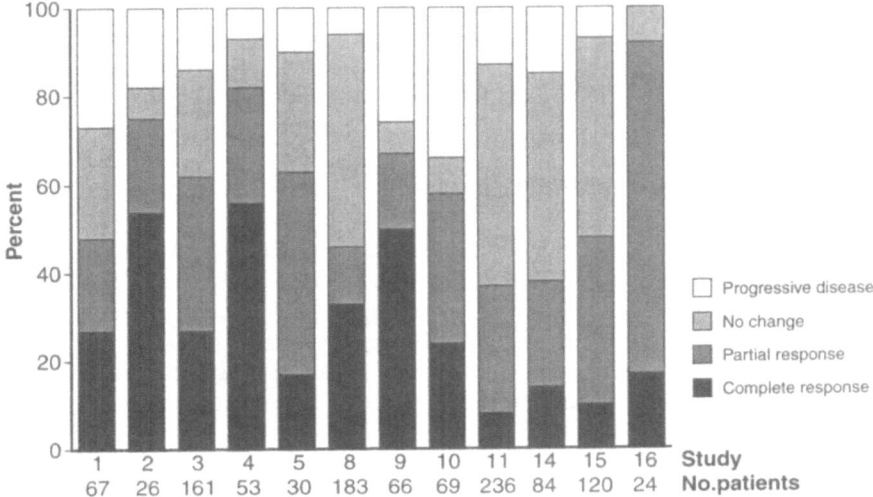

Fig. 4. Response categories after use of primary tamoxifen therapy in trials where these data were reported. *Key:* see Fig. 3 legend

Table 4. Variations in the response to primary endocrine therapy as reported in the literature

CR Months (range)	PR Months (range)	NC Months (range)	Study
Median duration of remission			
24 (6–36+)	12 (6–36+)	12 (6–36+)	Preece et al. 1982
25 (2–60)	14 (2–60)	–	Bradbeer & Kyngdon 1983
23 (5–48)	18 (6–55)	15	Allan et al. 1985
41	30		Ciatto et al. 1996
Time to response			
14 (3–25)	–	–	Helleberg et al. 1982
5 (2–24)	3 (2–7)	–	Bradbeer & Kyngdon 1983
	CR+PR 4 (1.51–34)		Allan et al. 1985
	CR+PR 9		Foudraine et al. 1982
6 (1–24)	7 (2–26)	14 (2–55)	Bergman et al. 1995
27	10	–	Ciatto et al. 1996

CR, Complete response; PR, partial response; NC, no change.

was assessed (Table 4). However, the new highly potent estrogen deprivation agents such as letrozole may act more rapidly than tamoxifen since 92% of patients were reported to respond within 3 months of the start of treatment (Dixon et al. 1997).

Number of Patients Studied

When tamoxifen only arms of randomised trials and phase II studies are considered, 1354 patients have been reported in the literature as being treated with preoperative endocrine therapy (Table 2). This number is considerably fewer than the numbers that have been entered into studies of primary chemotherapy (Clemons et al. 1997).

Use of Estrogen Receptor Measurements

In most studies, ER status has not been measured and thus an unknown proportion of patients with ER-negative tumors have been treated. Since the World Overview results show there is no significant benefit in terms of time to relapse or survival in patients with ER-negative tumors treated with tamoxifen, it is likely that such patients would not benefit from similar treatment given preoperatively. In patients with ER-positive tumors, complete and partial remission rates using tamoxifen range from 79% to 85% (Table 5). In the single study of preoperative treatment with letrozole, only patients with ER-positive tumors were entered. Of these patients, 17% had a complete remission and 75% a partial remission. These data emphasise the need to select patients with ER-positive tumors for entry into preoperative endocrine therapy trials.

Can Preoperative Endocrine Therapy Increase Breast Conservation?

The majority of the preoperative endocrine therapy trials outlined above were performed in the elderly and not designed to assess breast conservation. The prolonged time to response seen in some studies would suggest that primary endocrine therapy is not suitable for this approach although it is widely used to justify preoperative chemotherapy. However, in studies reported from Edinburgh, where response was monitored closely, 21 of 34 (62%) of patients responded to 6 months of treatment with a complete or partial remission, whereas 13/34 (38%) took longer than 6 months to respond (Gaskell et al. 1992). However, in the same unit 22/24 (92%) of post-menopausal patients with ER-positive tumors treated with letrozole had responses and were deemed suitable for conservation therapy after 3 months (Dixon et al. 1997). These impressive results, which indicate marked and rapid reductions in tumor size with a new endocrine therapy, need confirmation in further studies and pose the question whether similar rapid responses will be seen with the new anti-estrogens such as Faslodex (ICI 182780).

Can Primary Endocrine Therapy Improve Patient Survival?

The optimal test of primary endocrine therapy, which is initiated before and continued through and 4–5 years beyond surgery compared with therapy initiated after surgery, has not been performed. In the randomised trials of primary endocrine therapy reported to date, primary endocrine therapy continued until primary tumor progression and did not continue after surgery. Thus an appropriate randomised trial to test survival after primary endocrine therapy remains to be performed.

Can Preoperative Endocrine Therapy Give Prognostic Information?

Response to primary chemotherapy as a prognostic factor is well described. After primary tamoxifen therapy Bradbeer and Kyngdon (1983) demonstrated that the survival of responders to primary tamoxifen (CR+PR+no change) was greater than that of patients with progressive disease, although the statistical significance of this effect was not reported. Bergman et al. (1995) also showed a survival advantage for patients with an initial complete or partial response, but again the statistical significance of the effect was not reported. From these limited data we may tentatively conclude that response to primary endocrine therapy may be prognostic as it is in advanced disease, but once again more data from well-designed trials are required to be certain.

Can We Predict Which Patients are Likely to Benefit from Primary Endocrine Therapy?

Given that endocrine therapy is active in a large proportion of patients with ER-positive tumors and virtually inactive in those with ER-negative tumors, selection of the patients most likely to respond to primary endocrine therapy would enhance the power of clinical trials. The results of prediction of response on the basis of tumor ER status are shown in Table 5. In two of the four studies cited, only patients with ER-positive tumors were treated and thus we do not know the response rate in ER-negative tumors (Dixon et al. 1997; Low et al. 1992). In two other studies (Fisher and Mamounas 1995; Gaskell et al. 1989) the threshold values for ER positivity were respectively >25% and ≥20% of ER-positive cells by immunohistochemistry. In the first study 21 patients with ≤25% of cells staining were classified as ER-negative and one had a partial response whereas two had static disease (14%). In the second study, 13 patients had ER-negative tumors and two partial remissions and one static disease were seen (23%). The prediction of response (CR+PR+stable disease) in these studies was 100% and 91% respectively. Thus the positive predictive value of ER status for response is good but its negative predictive value is poor. In both studies there was not a single response in tumors with no ER-positive cells. This may be the most appropriate cut off point for clinical trial entry, as argued elsewhere by Elledge and Osborne (1997).

A series of other potential factors which predict response have been measured in tumors either before treatment or, in addition, after treatment to assess the biological effects of the endocrine agents (Table 6). Most studies were performed with tamoxifen as the primary endocrine therapy, but more recently studies using the 'pure' anti-estrogen Faslodex (ICI 182780) and the potent aromatase inhibitor letrozole have been reported. Since different responses were seen or different end points used with each endocrine agent, it is appropriate to summarise the data for each agent separately.

Table 5. Response to primary tamoxifen therapy in patients with ER-positive tumors

Study	Receptor value	n	CR+PR (%)	CR+PR+SD (%)
Low et al. (1992)	Score >100	47	85	98
Gaskell et al. (1989)	>25% cells positive	31	84	100
Gaskell et al. (1992)	≥20% cells positive	34	79	91
Dixon et al. (1997)	Score >80	24	92	100

SD, Stable disease.

Table 6. Potential markers for the prediction of response to primary endocrine therapy with tamoxifen, Faslodex, and letrozole

	Tamoxifen	Faslodex	Letrozole
Eestrogen receptor α $(?\beta)$	+	+	+
Progesterone receptor	+	+	+
PS2	+	+	+
Transforming growth factor α, β	+	+	+
EGFR, ERBB	+	+	+
Ki 67	+	+	+
Apoptosis	+	+	+
Tumor E_2	–	–	+
Aromatase	–	–	+

Other Predictors of Response to Tamoxifen

The predictive value of ER estimation is shown in Table 5. There appear to be no reports of the value of adding progesterone receptor (PR) estimations to those of ER. Several groups have shown that short-term treatment with tamoxifen stimulates expression of PR in primary tumors, which is presumed to be an agonist effect to tamoxifen on PR synthesis (Namer et al. 1980; Waseda et al. 1981; Montoya et al. 1992; Howell et al. 1987). In one study in advanced breast cancer, it was shown that an increase in PR expression during tamoxifen treatment was related of tumor response to treatment and subsequent survival (Fig. 5) (Howell et al. 1987). Transforming growth factor-a (TGF-a) expression is diminished by tamoxifen but has not been related to subsequent response to therapy (Gregory et al. 1989; Noguchi et al. 1993). Changes in the TGF-β isoforms do not appear to occur with sufficient regularity (Murray et al. 1994; MacCallum et al. 1996).

Rates of proliferation and cell death could potentially indicate responsiveness to tamoxifen. Expression of the proliferation marker Ki 67 is reduced during tamoxifen therapy and, surprisingly, the Bcl-2 proto-oncogene whose expression appears to block programmed cell death is increased in the short term (Clarke et al. 1993; Johnston et al. 1994; Keen et al. 1997). Tamoxifen also increases rates of apoptosis (Ellis et al. 1997). Potentially the short-term changes in rate of cell proliferation could be indicators of subsequent long-term endocrine responsiveness. However, the variable agonist activity of tamoxifen may be a confounding factor particularly in short-term studies, but to date the data do not suggest an induction of proliferation (Ki 67) in parallel with that of PR. The value of a number of other potential markers needs to be evaluated in this clinical situation (Le Roy et al. 1991; Soubeyran et al. 1996).

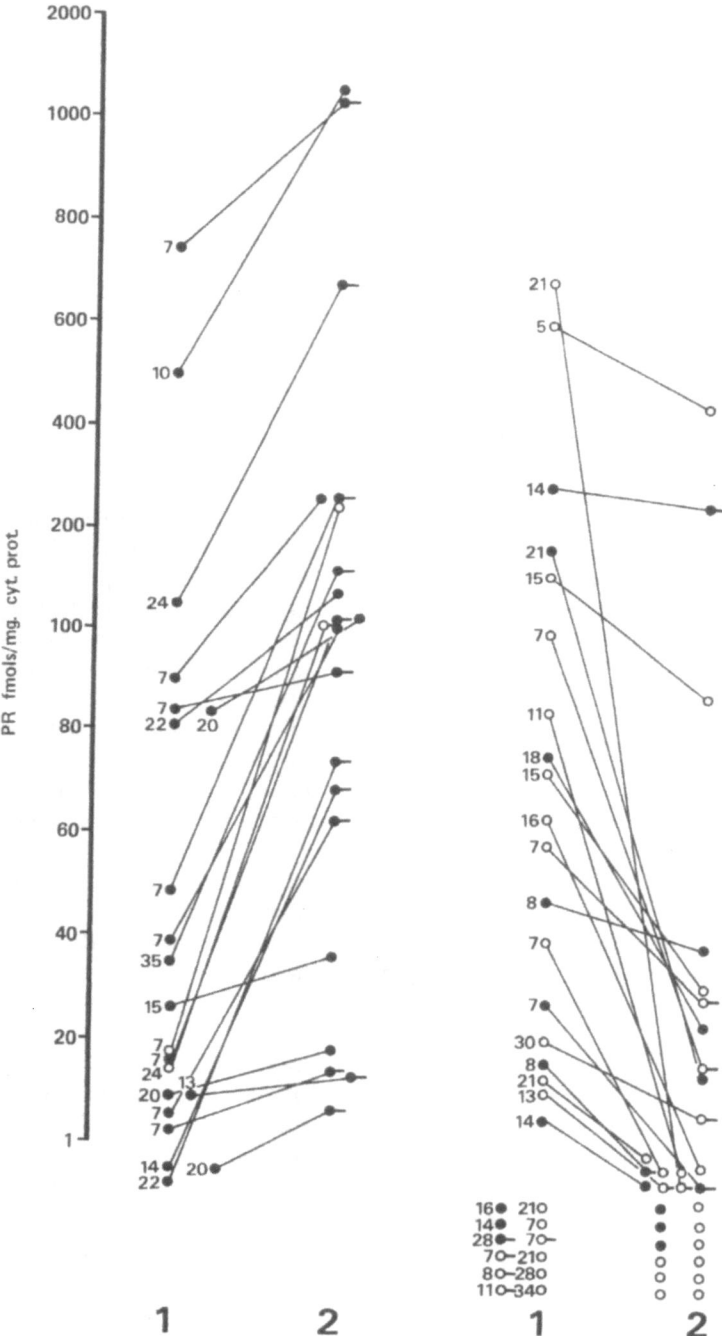

Fig. 5. Effect of tamoxifen on expression of progesterone receptor and its relation to subsequent response of the tumor to continued tamoxifen. *1* Increase in PR, *2* decrease in PR. ● Responders, ○ non-responders (from Howell et al. 1987)

Prediction of Response to Faslodex

The 'pure' steroidal anti-estrogen Faslodex (ICI 182780) has not been usede as primary endocrine therapy to induce responses. Its rapid and profound effect on reducing ER expression, a number of estrogen-induced proteins, and proliferation in preoperative studies in primary tumors appear to make Faslodex an ideal compound for preoperative treatment and prediction of tumor-responsiveness early in the course of therapy (Fig. 6) (Ellis et al. 1997; De Friend et al. 1994; Motta and Serio 1994; McClelland et al. 1996). It may be appropriate to compare short and long primary therapy (perhaps 1 and 6 months) with a no treatment arm.

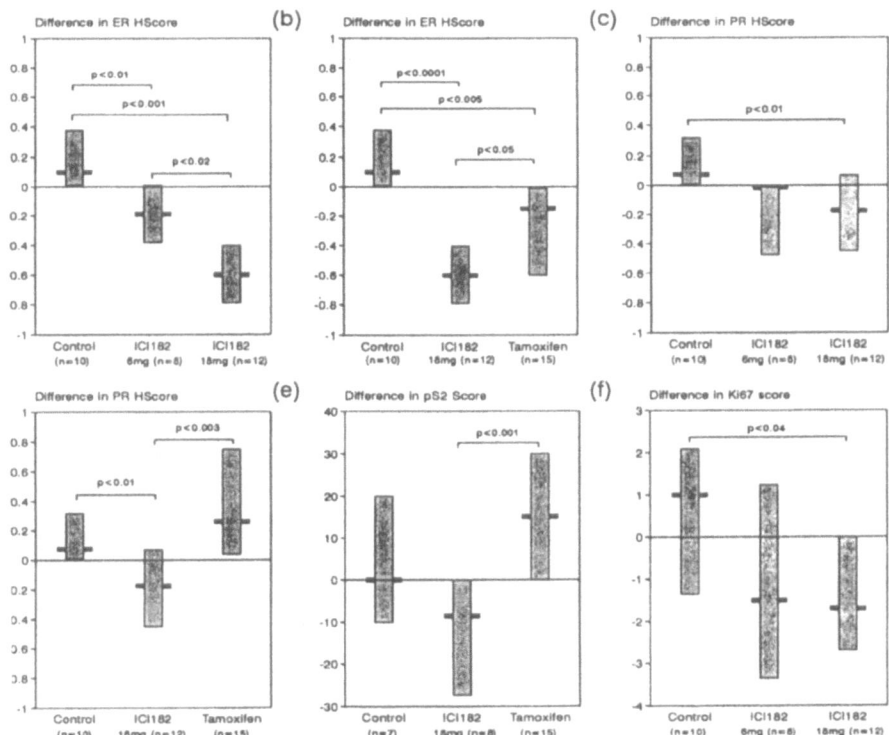

Fig. 6. Influence of the primary use of Faslodex (ICI 182780) on immunostaining for ER, PR, PS2 and Ki67. After obtaining a Trucut biopsy, Faslodex was given intramuscularly at doses of 6 mg ($n=12$) or 18 mg ($n=12$) per day. In a separate study, tamoxifen (20–40 mg/day) was given under similar circumstances. Assays were performed as described in Motta and Serio (1994). Faslodex inhibits expression of all antigens tested and was more potent than tamoxifen. The results are shown as median values with interquartile ranges

Prediction of Response to Letrozole

Although studies of primary endocrine therapy have almost exclusively involved tamoxifen, small numbers of patients have been treated with the aromatase inhibitors 4-OH androstenedione and letrozole. Prediction of response to aromatase inhibitors may require different assays compared to the anti-estrogens. For example, Miller et al. (1997) demonstrated that treatment with letrozole reduced tumor aromatase activity and estradiol levels when assessed after 3 months of treatment. It will be of great interest to see if these changes occur soon after the initiation of treatment and whether these have value in predicting response to primary treatment and survival in response to the aromatase inhibitors.

Comparison Between Primary Endocrine Therapy and Primary Chemotherapy

Primary chemotherapy is an attractive therapeutic option because of the often rapid responses, high response rates, and the prognostic value of response. However, when tumors which are expected to respond to therapy are selected (i.e., ER-positive ones) the complete plus partial remission rates for primary endocrine therapy range from 79% to 92% (Table 5). Because of the variability in evaluating responses, it is not clear exactly how quickly response occurs, but some responses to tamoxifen are obviously slow, which diminishes the chances of obtaining maximal downstaging within the usual 6-month duration of preoperative chemotherapy. In this regard it appears that newer endocrine therapies such as letrozole, and potentially Faslodex, may act more rapidly than tamoxifen and may make endocrine therapy equivalent to chemotherapy with respect to relatively rapid downstaging.

Summary and Conclusions

Primary endocrine therapy is potentially superior to primary chemotherapy in patients with ER-positive tumors. The ability to give endocrine therapy perioperatively may be a better test than chemotherapy of the hypothesis that the events accompanying surgery affect prognosis. However, a major problem in all studies of primary endocrine therapy is that there has been no clear experimental test of preoperative versus postoperative therapy. This is because the major thrust of treatment has been in the elderly with the purpose of determining whether surgery can be avoided altogether.

The fact that in ER-positive tumors primary endocrine therapy is associated with similar response rates to chemotherapy make it an attractive therapy for older women. This is the group where adjuvant chemotherapy has not been adequately tested ($\geq$70 years of age). In contradistinction, adju-

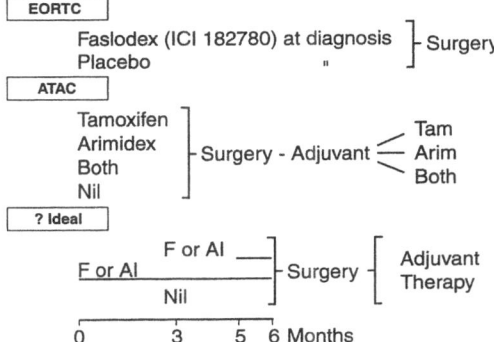

Fig. 7. Proposed and potential primary endocrine therapy trials. In the EORTC study it is projected that Faslodex be given as a single injection at the time of diagnosis. This will be effective throughout the operative period, and will be compared with a placebo injection. Subsequent postoperative therapy will be at the investigators choice. In the ATAC trial tamoxifen, Arimidex or both are to be compared with nothing immediately before surgery. An ideal trial would be a comparison of short lvs ong preoperative chemotherapy with perhaps Faslodex or an aromatase inhibitor

vant endocrine therapy shows marked survival benefits in patients with ER-positive tumors in these age groups (Table 1). It appears likely that primary endocrine therapy will allow breast conservation and prognostic information as is seen with chemotherapy. A major question which requires answering is whether primary endocrine therapy will improve survival more than adjuvant therapy alone.

Although ER status is a good marker of responsiveness, its specificity, in particular, is not optimal. The ability to assess the dynamic effects of primary endocrine therapy by sequential biopsy and measurement of biological responses to oestrogen deprivation may allow us to predict precisely the patients likely to benefit from treatment. This clinical scenario allows us to use other potentially useful assessments such as the non-invasive estimation of angiogenesis using quantitative imaging techniques of blood flow.

The newer anti-estrogens and aromatase inhibitors appear ideally suited to primary therapy since they have rapid and profound inhibitory activities, few or no agonist effects, and low side effect profiles. A preoperative trial of Faslodex is planned by the EORTC and another with Arimidex is under consideration by the ATAC (Arimidex, tamoxifen and combined) Trialist Group (Fig. 7). The precise design of these studies will require considerable thought.

References

Allan SG, Rodger A, Smyth JF et al (1985) Tamoxifen as primary treatment of breast cancer in elderly or frail patients: a practical management. Br Med J 290:358

Anderson EDC, Forrest AP, Hawkins RA et al (1991) Primary systemic therapy for operable breast cancer. Br J Cancer 63:561–566

Bates T, Riley DL, Houghton J et al (1991) Breast cancer in elderly women: a Cancer Research Campaign trial comparing treatment with tamoxifen and optimal surgery with tamoxifen alone. Br J Surg 78:591–594

Bergman L, Dongen L van, Ooijen B van et al (1995) Should tamoxifen be a primary treatment choice for elderly breast cancer patients with locoregional disease? Breast Cancer Res Treat 34:77–83

Bradbeer JW, Kyngdon J (1983) Primary treatment of breast cancer in elderly women with tamoxifen. Clin Oncol 9:31–34

Ciatto S, Cirillo A, Confortini M et al (1996) Tamoxifen as primary treatment of breast cancer in elderly patients. Neoplasma 43:43–45

Clarke RB, Laidlaw IJ, Jones LJ et al (1993) Effect of tamoxifen on Ki 67 labelling index in human breast tumors and its relationship to oestrogen and progesterone receptor status. Br J Cancer 67:606–611

Clemons M, Leahy M, Valle J et al (1997) Review of recent trials of chemotherapy for advanced breast cancer: studies excluding taxanes. Eur J Cancer 33:2171–2182

DeFriend DJ, Howell A, Nicholson RI et al (1994) Investigation of a new pure antiestrogen (ICI 182780) in women with primary breast cancer. Cancer Res 54:408–414

Dixon JM, Love CDB, Tucker S et al (1997) Letrozole as primary medical therapy for locally advanced and large operable breast cancer. Breast Cancer Res Treat 46(1):213

Early Breast Cancer Trialists' Collaborative Group (1992) Systemic treatment of early breast cancer by hormonal, cytotoxic, or immune therapy. Lancet 339:1–15

Early Breast Cancer Trialists' Collaborative Group (1998) Tamoxifen for early breast cancer: an overview of the randomised trials. Lancet (in press)

Elledge RM, Osborne CK (1997) Oestrogen receptors and breast cancer (Editorial). Br Med J 314:1843–1844

Ellis PA, Saccani-Jotti G, Clarke R et al (1997) Induction of apoptosis by tamoxifen and. ICI 182780 in primary breast cancer. Int J Cancer 72:608–613

Fisher B, Gunduz N, Coyle J et al (1989a) Presence of a growth-stimulating factor in serum following primary tumor removal in mice. Cancer Res 49:1996–2001

Fisher B, Saffer E, Rudosch C et al (1989b) Effect of local or systemic treatment prior to primary tumor removal on the production and response to a serum growth-stimulating factor in mice. Cancer Res 49:2002–2004

Fisher B, Mamounas EP (1995) Preoperative chemotherapy: a model for studying the biology and therapy of primary breast cancer. J Clin Oncol 13(3):537–540

Foudraine NA, Verhoef LCG, Burghouts JT (1992) Tamoxifen as sole therapy for primary breast cancer in the elderly patient. Eur J Cancer 28 A:900–903

Gaskell DJ, Hawkins RA, Sangsterl K et al (1989) Relation between immunocytochemical estimation of oestrogen receptor in elderly patients with primary breast cancer and response to tamoxifen. Lancet 1:1044–1046

Gaskell DJ, Hawkins RA, Carteret S de et al (1992) Indications for primary tamoxifen therapy in elderly women with breast cancer. Br J Surg 79:1317–1320

Gazet JC, Ford HT, Coombes RC et al (1994) Prospective randomized trial of tamoxifen vs surgery in elderly patients with breast cancer. Eur J Surg Oncol 20:207–214

Gee JMW, Robertson JF, Ellis IO et al (1994) Immunocytochemical localization of Bcl-2 protein in human breast cancers and its relationship to a series of prognostic markers and response to endocrine therapy. Int J Cancer 59:619–628

Goldie JH, Coldman AJ (1979) A mathematical model for relating the drug sensitivity of tumors to their spontaneous mutation rate. Cancer Treat Rep 63:1727–1733

Gregory H, Thomas CE, Willshire IR et al (1989) Epidermal and transforming growth factor α in patients with breast tumors. Br J Cancer 59:605–609

Gunduz N, Fisher B, Saffer EA (1979) Effect of surgical removal on the growth and kinetics of residual tumor. Cancer Res 39:3861–3865

Helleberg A, Lundgren B, Norin T et al (1982) Treatment of early localized breast cancer in elderly patients by tamoxifen. Br J Radiol 55:511–515

Howell A, Harland RNL, Barnes DM (1987) Endocrine therapy for advanced carcinoma of the breast: relationship between the effect of tamoxifen upon concentrations of progesterone receptor and subsequent response to treatment. Cancer Res 47:300–304

Ignar-Trowbridge DM, Nelson KG, Bidwell MC et al (1992) Coupling of dual signalling pathways: epidermal growth factor action involves the estrogen receptor. Proc Natl Acad Sci USA 89:4658–4662

Johnston SRD, MacLennan KA, Sacks NP et al (1994) Modulation of Bcl-2 and Ki-67 expression in oestrogen receptor-positive human breast cancer by tamoxifen. Eur J Cancer 30 A:1663–1669

Katzenellenbogen BS, Montano MM, Ekena K et al (1997) Antiestrogens: mechanism of action and resistance in breast cancer. Breast Cancer Res Treat 44:23–38

Keen JC, Dixon JM, Miller EP et al (1997) The expression of Ki-S 1 and Bcl-2 and the response to primary tamoxifen therapy in elderly patients with breast cancer. Breast Cancer Res Treat 44:123–133

Le Roy X, Escot C, Brouillet JP et al (1991) Decrease of c-erb-2 and c-myc RNA levels in tamoxifen-treated breast cancer. Oncogene 6:431–437

Low SC, Dixon AR, Bell J et al (1992) Tumor oestrogen receptor content allows selection of elderly patients with breast cancer for conservative tamoxifen treatment. Br J Surg 79:1314–1316

MacCallum J, Keen JC, Bartlett JM et al (1996) Changes in expression of transforming growth factor beta mRNA isoforms in patients undergoing tamoxifen therapy. Br J Cancer 74:474–478

McClelland RA, Manning DL, Gee JM et al (1996) Effects of short-term antiestrogen treatment of primary breast cancer on estrogen receptor mRNA and protein expression and on estrogen-regulated genes. Breast Cancer Res Treat 41:31–41

Miller WR, Telford J, Love CDB et al (1997) The effects of letrozole on in situ and in vitro oestrogen synthesis and endogenous oestrogen within the breast. Breast Cancer Res Treat 46(1):216

Montoya F, Barbazan MJ, Schneider J et al (1992) Variations in estrogen and progesterone receptor levels after short-term tamoxifen treatment in breast carcinoma. Oncology 49:422–425

Motta M, Serio M (eds) (1994) Sex hormones and antihormones in endocrine dependent pathology: basic and clinical aspects. Elsevier, Amsterdam

Murray PA, Gomm J, Ricketts D et al (1994) The effect of endocrine therapy on the levels of oestrogen and progesterone receptor and transforming growth factor-β1 in metastatic human breast cancer: an immunocytochemical study. Eur J Cancer 30 A(9):1218–1222

Mustacchi G, Milani S, Pluchinotta A et al (1994) Tamoxifen or surgery plus tamoxifen as primary treatment for elderly patients with operable breast cancer: the GRETA trial. Anticancer Res 14:2197–2200

Namer M, Lalanne C, Baulieu EE (1980) Increase of progesterone receptors by tamoxifen as a hormonal challenge test in breast cancer. Cancer Res 40:1750–1752

Noguchi S, Motomura K, Inaji H et al (1993) Down-regulation of transforming growth factor-α by tamoxifen in human breast cancer. Cancer 72:131–136

Preece PE, Wood RA, Mackie CR et al (1982) Tamoxifen as initial sole treatment of localised breast cancer in elderly women: a pilot study. Br Med J 284:869–870

Richard G (1989) Tamoxifen as an alternative to surgical resection for selected geriatric patients with primary breast cancer. Arch Surg 124:548–551

Robertson JFR, Ellis IO, Elston CW et al (1992) Mastectomy or tamoxifen as initial therapy for operable breast cancer in elderly patients: 5-year follow-up. Eur J Cancer 28 A:908–910

Skipper HE et al (1971) Kinetics of mammary tumor cell growth and implications for therapy. Cancer 28:1479–1499

Soubeyran I, Quenel N, Mauriac L et al (1996) Variation of hormonal receptor, pS 2, C-erbB-2 and GSTπ contents in breast carcinomas under tamoxifen: a study of 74 cases. Br J Cancer 73:735–743

Van Dalsen AD, De Vries J (1995) Treatment of breast cancer in elderly patients. J Surg Oncol 60:80–82

Vignon F, Bouton MM, Rochefort H (1987) Antiestrogens inhibit the mitogenic effect of growth factors on breast cancer cells in the total absence of estrogens. Biochem Biophys Res Commun 146:1502–1508

Waseda N, Kato Y, Imura H et al (1981) Effects of tamoxifen on estrogen and progesterone receptors in human breast cancer. Cancer Res 41:1984–1988

VIII. Integrated Therapy: Radiation Therapy/ Endocrine Treatment

Why and How to Combine Chemotherapy and Radiation Therapy in Breast Cancer Patients

A.K. Dubey[1], A. Recht[1,2], S. Come[2], L. Shulman[3], and J. Harris[1,3]

[1] Joint Center for Radiation Therapy and the Departments of Medical and Radiation Oncology, Harvard Medical School, Boston, MA 02115, USA
[2] Beth Israel Deaconess Medical Center, Harvard Medical School, Boston, MA 02115, USA
[3] Brigham and Women's Hospital and Dana-Farber Cancer Institute, Harvard Medical School, Boston, MA 02115, USA

Introduction

In this review, we discuss the reasons why it is important to consider combining adjuvant chemotherapy (CT) and radiotherapy (RT), the various considerations involved in designing the optimal combination, and the available evidence regarding the optimal combination. We stress here our past experience as well as information obtained from randomized controlled trials.

Many patients with early-stage breast cancer are currently being treated with both adjuvant CT and adjuvant RT. Meta-analyses performed of adjuvant CT trials have demonstrated a survival benefit for both premenopausal and postmenopausal females undergoing adjuvant CT (Early Breast Cancer Trialists' Group 1992). As a result, adjuvant CT is frequently prescribed for early-stage breast cancer patients. Radiation therapy is also frequently used in early-stage breast cancer patients, particularly in patients undergoing breast conservation surgery. Randomized trials have demonstrated that conservative surgery and RT are equivalent to mastectomy alone with regard to overall survival and are comparable with regard to local control (Fisher et al. 1989; Veronesi et al. 1990). There also is evidence that adjuvant RT is beneficial to patients undergoing mastectomy. Recent trials from British Columbia and Denmark (discussed below) have shown a survival benefit from postoperative RT in patients undergoing mastectomy and CT (Ragaz et al. 1997; Overgaard et al. 1997). Thus, there are many indications for the combined use of adjuvant CT and RT in early-stage breast cancer patients.

Influence of Local-Regional Control on Survival

A question raised by the use of adjuvant CT and RT is whether local-regional control affects survival. In the classic Halsted model, local control (achieved by radical mastectomy) was considered to be critical to survival. With the more recent Fisher hypothesis, micrometastases are considered to be present at the time of treatment and, therefore, local control is not predicted to affect systemic control and survival (Harris and Hellman 1996). The results of the recent Danish and British Columbia trials demonstrating an improved distant relapse-free and overall survival with postmastectomy RT suggest that local-regional control may affect both distant control and survival, particularly in the presence of effective systemic therapy. The Danish Trial 82b confirms the observation, established by previous studies, that moderate-dose (50 Gy) comprehensive local-regional RT, appropriately planned and delivered, reduces the risk of local-regional recurrence after total mastectomy and (partial) axillary dissection by a factor of about 4. In a premenopausal patient population with a cumulative risk of local-regional recurrence of about 30%, intensifying local-regional therapy (i.e., by administering RT) also reduced the proportional risk of total breast cancer recurrence by about 40% and resulted in a relative reduction in overall death by about 25% and an absolute improvement in 10-year overall survival by 9%. This effect is similar in magnitude to the effects of adjuvant systemic therapies demonstrated in the last published Overview (Early Breast Cancer Trialists' Collaborative Group 1992). This effect is not likely to be an artifact, given the size of the trial and as an identical effect is shown in the smaller British Columbia trial. Considerations in sequencing of CT and RT in patients treated with mastectomy may be different than with breast-conserving surgery. In such patients, the anticipated local tumor burden is small so that delays in RT would be less consequential. However, in both the British Columbia and Danish studies RT was delivered early, and it is not known whether this sequencing contributed to the favorable results observed by the addition of RT.

The results from the Danish and British Columbia trials suggest that the combined use of CT and effective local-regional treatment not only allows, in the absence of systemic involvement, the eradication of residual local-regional disease to prevent *seeding*, but also, in the presence of systemic involvement that is effectively treated by systemic therapy, the eradication of residual local-regional disease to prevent *reseeding*. RT in this setting may also eradicate drug, resistant tumor cells in the local tumor bed before they can metastasize. The new hypothesis is that, in the presence of adjuvant systemic therapy, local-regional treatment can have a substantial effect on survival. This hypothesis requires that current forms of effective systemic therapy are more effective systemically than locally, possibly because of the greater tumor burden locally and possibly because of a decreased blood supply to the tumor bed.

An important caveat in considering the effects of local control on survival is the toxicity of the local treatment; early reports demonstrated that postmastectomy RT was associated with an increased mortality (mainly cardiac toxicity from outdated RT techniques) (Cuzick et al. 1987). However, reanalysis of those trials suggested a cancer survival benefit that may have been masked by offsetting cardiac mortality (Cuzick et al. 1994). Thus, it is important in designing the optimal combination to consider not only efficacy, but also the toxicity. Reassuringly, in a recent review of our long-term experience with RT following breast conservation surgery using techniques that would still be considered current, we observed no increased cardiac or other non-breast-cancer mortality for patients with left-sided breast cancer compared to right-sided breast cancer through 12 years of follow-up (Nixon et al. 1998).

Effect of Delaying RT or CT:
The Potential Significance of the Surgery-Radiotherapy Interval

There are several issues involved in the optimal sequencing of CT and radiation therapy. A delay in systemic therapy may result in poorer systemic control. Likewise, a delay in RT may result in poorer local control. (Many authors have used the term "SRI" to denote "surgery-radiotherapy interval," or the length of time between the last surgery and the initiation of RT.) Additionally, there are the concerns that RT may affect the ability to deliver adequate CT dosages, as well as problems with excessive toxicity associated with CT and full-dose RT. Some of these issues are underscored by the recent Harvard "up-front/out-back" trial (Recht et al. 1996). In this trial, 244 women were randomized to receive a course of CT (12 weeks) either before or after RT. Median follow-up was 58 months. Patients in the RT-first arm had a higher rate of distant failure (37% vs 25%, $p = 0.05$), while patients in the CT-first arm had a higher rate of local failure (13% vs 5%, $p = 0.07$). This study suggests that a delay in CT adversely affects distant failure and survival, and that a delay in RT adversely affects local control.

The "up-front/out-back" trial is one of the few reported experiences describing the effect of delaying CT. In contrast, there have been many reports describing the effect of delaying RT. Our group was one of the first to retrospectively address the issue of sequencing of CT and RT in early-stage, node-positive breast cancer (Recht et al. 1991). We examined the results of 295 patients who had pathologically-positive axillary nodes and received at least three cycles of a CMF- or adriamycin-based regimen. Sequencing groupings (non-randomly assigned) were: (1) RT first, (2) "sandwich" therapy (RT given after one or more cycles of chemotherapy, followed by additional chemotherapy after RT), (3) concurrent CT and RT, and (4) CT-first (all CT given first). The actuarial local failure rates for the four groups were 4%, 8%, 6%, and 41% respectively. The actuarial local failure rate was 5% for patients who had a surgery-radiotherapy interval (SRI) of 16 weeks or less, and was 35% for patients with a SRI greater than 16 weeks. This report first suggested the hypothesis that a delay in the initiation of RT may result in an increased rate of local failure.

Another report demonstrating a negative treatment outcome with delayed RT was from Buchholz et al. (1993). They examined treatment outcome in 105 patients treated with surgery, RT and CT analyzed by whether patients began RT earlier or later than 6 months. The outcomes for local control, overall survival, and disease-free survival were superior in the early-RT group compared to the late-RT group. Eight-year local control was 98% in the early-RT group compared to only 76% in the delayed-RT group.

Other investigators, however, have failed to note an adverse effect with delaying RT. Wallgren et al. (1996) examined the issue of timing of RT (in the setting of sequential CT and RT) with regard to local control in patients with histologically confirmed negative margins. Peri-/premenopausal patients were randomized to receive CMF for either three or six cycles followed by RT (with median SRI of 4.0 and 6.6 months, respectively) and postmenopausal patients were randomized to receive either no CMF or CMF for three cycles (with median SRI of 2.3 and 3.9 months, respectively). No difference in local control rates between the "early" and "delayed" RT was observed in each group: the 4-year crude local failure rates were 8% and 9% respectively ($p = NS$) for peri-/premenopausal patients who had RT at 4 or 7 months after surgery, and 3% and 6% ($p = NS$) for postmenopausal patients who had RT at 2 or 4 months after surgery. No significant differences in failure patterns or disease-free survivals were noted between the "early" and "delayed" RT groups.

An important point regarding the effect of the SRI is the advancement of mammographic and pathologic evaluation. Surgeons may be better able to more fully excise lesions with such modern advancements. McCormick (1996) speculated that other factors, such as margin status and extent of resection, may take precedent over the sequencing of therapy. It has been hypothesized that the tumor burden following breast conservation surgery may be a major factor on the influence of the SRI on local-regional failure (Harris et al. 1993). Thus, if there is a significant amount of residual disease following surgery, then a delay of RT may be expected to produce a worse outcome. If the disease is more adequately resected and margins are negative, then it might be expected that a delay in the initiation of RT would not adversely affect outcome. A subset analysis of the up-front/out-back trial is consistent with this hypothesis: patients with close, positive, and unknown margins had a higher rate of local recurrence with delayed RT than to patients in the early RT group (23%, 26%, and 20% for the delayed RT group as compared to 0%, 14%, and 0% for the early RT group, respectively). However, such a post-hoc subset analysis with small number of patients cannot be considered as substantial evidence on this point and more definitive data is clearly needed.

Effect of CT on Local Control in Patients Treated With Breast Conservation Surgery and RT

There may also be a beneficial effect of CT combined with RT on local control. Rose et al. (1989) from the JCRT retrospectively studied a group of 74 premenopausal patients treated with conservative surgery, RT, and adjuvant CT. This was compared to a control group of 192 premenopausal patients treated with surgery and RT alone. Patients were less than age 50, had stage I or II disease, and underwent gross excision of the tumor. Of note, the patients in the CT arm had significantly larger and more node-positive cancers than did the surgery and RT alone group. The 5-year relapse rates for first site of failure were analyzed. For the CT/RT group, the 5-year initial local relapse rate was 4% compared to 15% for the RT group. The authors speculated that there may be a beneficial interaction between radiation and CT on local control. This hypothesis was corroborated by the NSABP B-13 trial (Fisher et al. 1996). The B-13 protocol randomized 760 patients to receive either surgery alone or surgery with adjuvant methotrexate and 5-FU. Among patients treated with breast-conserving surgery, local-regional failure was 13% in the surgery/RT arm, and 3% in the methotrexate and 5-FU arm ($p = 0.0003$). Possible mechanisms for this interaction include the radiosensitizing effects of some systemic agents (i.e., 5-FU), additive cytoreduction, and alteration of the hormonal milieu following systemic CT.

Effects of Sequencing CT/RT on the Cosmetic Result and Complications

Chemotherapy, however, may have effects on treatment outcomes other than on survival, local control, and distant control. Abner et al. (1991) at the JCRT examined the cosmetic outcome of 170 patients treated with breast conservation surgery, full-dose RT, and adjuvant CT. Patients received 45–50 Gy to the entire breast with 4–6 MV photons and a boost consisting of electrons, interstitial implant, and/or photons. Chemotherapy consisted of CMF in most patients. Using case-control methodology, a set of "control" patients treated with RT alone were identified, matching RT treatment factors found to be associated with poorer outcome (tumor size, boost technique, three-field vs tangents). At 36 months, 71% of patients treated with RT alone had excellent cosmetic results, 19% had good cosmetic results, and 9% had fair/poor cosmetic results, while 47% of patients treated with RT and CT had excellent cosmetic results, 36% had good cosmetic results, and 17% had fair/poor cosmetic results. The difference in percentage of patients rated with excellent cosmetic results was statistically significant ($p < 0.00001$) and it was concluded that the adjuvant CT shifted some patients from an excellent to a good cosmetic result. With regard to sequencing, patients undergoing concurrent therapy had worse cosmetic results than patients undergoing sequential therapy. In addition, concurrent CT and full-dose RT has been shown also to be associated with an increased rate of radiation pneumonitis and other toxicities compared with sequential treatment (Lingos et al. 1991; Pierce et al. 1992).

Concurrent CT and Reduced-Dose RT: A Pilot Study

The above studies suggest that tradeoffs in local or distant control may theoretically be minimized by concurrent CT and RT, but that the toxicity may be substantial. In order to improve upon the treatment outcome and minimize toxicity in patients treated with concurrent CT and RT, the JCRT conducted a prospective pilot study of a modified concurrent CT-RT regimen using reduced doses of RT designed to lessen treatment side effects by anticipating the known interaction of CT and RT (Dubey et al. 1997). One hundred twelve patients were entered into this prospective study. Eligible patients had clinical stage I or II unilateral invasive breast cancer, treated with complete gross excision of primary tumor, pathologic axillary staging with at least 6 nodes dissected, and 0–3 positive lymph nodes. Patients received 6 cycles every 28 days of CMF. On day 14 of cycle 1, patients started tangential field RT, consisting of 39.6 Gy in 22 fractions to the whole breast and a 16 Gy boost to the tumor bed using electrons. The most common acute toxicity observed during or shortly after RT was moist desquamation (seen in 50% of patients). Grade 4 neutropenia was noted in 16 patients during RT, but only 1 patient required hospitalization. Radiation pneumonitis was noted in only 1 patient (grade 2), who responded to steroid treatment. Fifty-one patients were evaluable for cosmetic scoring by JCRT physicians 2 years (±6 months) after the end of CT: 47% had excellent, 43% had good, and 10% had fair cosmetic scores. Seventy-nine percent of patients (89/112) were evaluable for CT dosages delivered; overall, 93% of patients received at least 85% of all drug doses. Based on these favorable early results, a randomized prospective trial comparing this concurrent approach (using 39.6+14 Gy) to CMF×6 followed by RT has just been activated.

Effects of RT on CT Administration

There is also concern whether prior RT has an adverse effect on the deliverable CT dosages. This did not appear to be the case in the JCRT concurrent pilot trial, where reductions were based on granulocyte counts and 93% of evaluable patients received at least 85% of prescribed drug dosages. However, other investigators have noted a deleterious effect of RT on deliverable CT dosages. Fentiman et al. (1989) prospectively randomized 399 patients to receive treatment with either modified radical mastectomy or by lumpectomy and RT. Patients with positive nodes were randomized to receive 12 cycles of CMF or no systemic adjuvant treatment. RT consisted of 46 Gy administered to the entire breast and 20 Gy administered by interstitial implant. They noted that patients in the mastectomy arm received a significantly higher percentage of planned CT dosages than did the patients in the RT group (85% vs 71% respectively, $p < 0.05$). The difference in dosage administered was not due to patient compliance, but rather due to drops in the total white cell count and subsequent reductions in CT dose. This was also true in the up-front/out-back study. These results indicate that it is important to use the granulocyte, and not the total white cell count in determining dose reductions, and that a brief delay in the next cycle is preferable to decreasing the CT dose.

Summary

The ideal sequencing of CT and radiation therapy in early-stage breast cancer treated with breast-conserving surgery and RT is not known. There is evidence that delaying CT might have an adverse impact on systemic control, while delaying RT might adversely affect local control. Concurrent CT and full-dose RT might minimize the above tradeoffs, but is associated with increased toxicity. Concurrent CT and reduced-dose RT is a novel approach to address these issues, but requires additional formal evaluation before clinical use. In the absence of definitive information, clinicians should balance each patient's risk for systemic recurrence and local-regional recurrence. For example, a patient with a large number of positive nodes but clearly negative margins would be an appropriate candidate for adjuvant therapy starting with CT and continuing with RT at the completion of CT. Alternatively, a patient with node-negative disease with close or focally positive margins might be an appropriate candidate for initiating RT sooner. Current treatment regimens which deliver CT in a "short" time period [i.e., Adriamycin (doxorubicin) and Cytoxan (cyclophosphamide) delivered in four 3-week cycles] may represent a reasonable tradeoff with regard to promptly starting systemic therapy while initiating RT within 3 months of surgery.

It is possible that optimizing the way RT and CT are combined is important in achieving the highest survival rate and in reducing long-term adverse effects. There is unfortunately very little solid information from randomized clinical trials addressing this question, and considerable controversy remains regarding the optimal approach to integrating these modalities. Additional randomized clinical trials addressing this important clinical question are needed.

References

Abner AL et al (1991) Cosmetic results after surgery, chemotherapy, and radiation therapy for early stage breast cancer. Int J Radiat Oncol Biol Phys: 21:331–338

Buchholz T et al (1993) Effect of delay in radiation in the combined modality treatment of breast cancer. Int J Radiat Oncol Biol Phys 26:23–35

Cuzick J et al (1987) Overview of randomized trials of postoperative adjuvant radiotherapy in breast cancer. Cancer Treat Rep 71:15–29

Cuzick J et al (1994) Cause-specific mortality in long-term survivors of breast cancer who participated in trials of radiotherapy. J Clin Oncol 12:447–453

Dubey AK et al (1997) Outcome following concurrent chemotherapy (CT) and reduced dose radiation therapy (RT) for patients with early stage breast cancer (Abstr). Int J Radiat Oncol Biol Phys

Early Breast Cancer Trialists' Collaborative Group (1992) Systemic treatment of early breast cancer by hormonal, cytotoxic, or immune therapy: 133 randomized trials involved 31,000 recurrences and 24,000 deaths among 75,000 women. Lancet 339:1–15, 71–85

Fentiman I et al (1989) Influence of radiotherapy on the dose of adjuvant chemotherapy in early breast cancer. Breast Cancer Res Treat 13:237–241

Fisher B et al (1989) Eight-year results of a randomized clinical trial comparing total mastectomy and lumpectomy with or without irradiation in the treatment of breast cancer. N Engl J Med 320:822–828

Fisher B et al (1996) Sequential methotrexate and fluorouracil for the treatment of node-negative breast cancer patients with estrogen receptor-negative tumors: eight-year results from National Surgical Adjuvant Breast and Bowel Project (NSABP) B-13 and first report of findings from NDABP B-19 comparing methotrexate and fluorouracil with conventional cyclophosphamide, methotrexate, and fluorouracil. J Clin Oncol 14:1982–1992

Harris JR, Hellman S (1996) Natural history of breast cancer. In: Harris JR, Hellman S, Lippman ME, Morrow M (eds) Diseases of the breast. Lippincott-Raven, Philadelphia

Harris JR et al (1993) Sequencing adjuvant chemotherapy and radiotherapy in breast cancer patients. Int J Radiat Oncol Biol Phys 26:183–185

Lingos TI et al (1991) Radiation pneumonitis in breast cancer patients treated with conservative surgery and radiation therapy. Int J Radiat Oncol Biol Phys 21:355–360

McCormick B (1996) Sequencing: one big tree in the forest of breast cancer management. Int J Radiat Oncol Biol Phys 35:843–844

Nixon A et al (1998) No long-term increase in cardiac-related mortality after breast-conserving surgery and radiation therapy using modern technique. J Clin Oncol (in press)

Overgaard M et al (1997) Postoperative radiotherapy in high-risk premenopausal women with breast cancer who received adjuvant chemotherapy. Danish Breast Cancer Cooperative Group 82b. N Engl J Med 337:949–955

Pierce SM et al (1992) Long-term radiation complications following conservative surgery (CS) and radiation therapy (RT) in patients with early stage breast cancer. Int J Radiat Oncol Biol Phys 23:915–923

Ragaz J et al (1997) Adjuvant radiotherapy and chemotherapy in node-positive premenopausal women with breast cancer. N Engl J Med. 337(14):956–962

Recht A et al (1991) Integration of conservative surgery, radiotherapy, and chemotherapy for the treatment of early-stage, node-positive breast cancer: sequencing, timing and outcome. J Clin Oncol 9:1662–1667

Recht A et al (1996) The sequencing of chemotherapy and radiation therapy after conservative surgery for early stage breast cancer. N Engl J Med 334:1356–1361

Rose MA et al (1989) Premenopausal breast cancer patients treated with conservative surgery, radiotherapy and adjuvant chemotherapy have a low risk of local failure. Int J 'Radiat Oncol Biol Phys 17:711–717

Veronesi U et al (1990) Breast conservation is the treatment of choice in small breast cancer: long-term results of a randomized clinical trial. Eur J Cancer 26:668–670

Wallgren A et al (1996) Timing of radiotherapy and chemotherapy following breast-conserving surgery for patients with node-positive breast cancer. Int J Radiat Oncol Biol Phys 35:649–659

Novel Approaches Using Radiation Therapies

L. E. Rutqvist

Oncologic Centre, Karolinska Hospital, Stockholm, Sweden

Introduction

New information has recently emerged concerning the role of adequate local control of breast cancer through the use of locoregional radiation therapy in conjunction with adjuvant cytotoxic chemotherapy. These data support the proposition that achieving initial local control is important to maximize breast cancer cure rates. At the same time it is important to minimize or avoid potential side effects of breast cancer radiation therapy, particularly cardiac side effects which may compromise overall survival. Novel approaches such as three-dimensional treatment planning can be of help clinically to quantitate such effects and to optimize therapy in individual patients. The increasing use of routine postoperative radiation therapy following conservative breast surgery highlights the need to identify those patient subsets that are likely to benefit from treatment. Studies that have aimed, using hitherto identified risk factors, to identify subgroups of patients at such low risk of breast recurrence that radiation therapy may not be warranted, have in general produced disappointing results. Searching for potential treatment-predictive assays may prove to be a more fruitful approach. Since the response to radiation therapy is probably related, at least in part, to the intrinsic radiosensitivity of the tumor cells, novel treatment-predictive assays based on molecular biology may perhaps turn out to be clinically useful. This paper will briefly review some recent information from the aforementioned fields of research.

The Danish and British Columbia Trials

Recent updates of these two trials have confirmed and extended previous studies in demonstrating statistically significant overall survival benefits from postoperative radiation therapy in conjunction with adjuvant cytotoxic chemotherapy among high-risk breast cancer patients.

The Danish DBCG 82b Trial

The Danish DBCG 82b trial included 1708 eligible premenopausal patients who had undergone a modified radical mastectomy between 1982 and 1989 (Overgaard et al. 1997). The inclusion criteria implied that all patients should have "high-risk" disease, defined as histopathologically positive axillary lymph nodes, or a primary tumor size exceeding 5 cm, or involvement of the skin or pectoral fascia. The axillary surgery included resection of level I and some level II nodes. The median number of nodes resected was seven. All patients were offered eight cycles of intravenous CMF (cyclophosphamide, methotrexate, fluorouracil) chemotherapy. Randomization was between radiation therapy plus cytotoxic chemotherapy versus chemotherapy alone. The radiation therapy, which was given to the chest wall and regional nodes including the internal mammary chain, was "sandwiched" in between the first and second chemotherapy cycle. The tumor dose was 50 Gy given in 25 fractions over a period of 5 weeks or 48 Gy given in 22 fractions over a period of 5.5 weeks. The recommended field arrangement involved the use of an anterior electron field against the internal mammary chain and the chest wall. At a median follow-up of 114 months there was a statistically significant benefit in terms of local control, disease-free survival, and overall survival. The life-table estimate of overall survival at 10 years was 54% among the patients allocated to radiation therapy versus 45% among those treated with chemotherapy alone ($p < 0.001$).

The British Columbia Trial

This Canadian trial included 318 premenopausal patients who had undergone a modified radical mastectomy between 1978 and 1986 (Ragaz et al. 1995). The inclusion criteria implied that all patients should have histopathologically positive axillary lymph nodes. All patients were offered intravenous CMF chemotherapy every 3 weeks. Initially the chemotherapy was given for 12 months, but among patients included after 1981 it was for 6 months. Randomization was between radiation therapy plus chemotherapy versus chemotherapy alone. The radiation therapy, which was given to the chest wall and regional nodes, was given between the fourth and fifth chemotherapy cycle. The tumor dose to the chest wall was 37.5 Gy given in 16 fractions over a period of 4–5 weeks. The mid-axilla and the internal mammary chain at a depth of 3 cm received a dose of 35 Gy. The recommended treatment technique involved the use of tangential fields to the chest wall, an anterior supraclavicular-axillary field with a posterior, axillary boost, and a direct, anterior field against the internal mammary chain. At a median follow-up of 150 months there was a statistically significant benefit in terms of disease-free ($p = 0.007$) as well as distant disease-free survival ($p = 0.006$). The differences in terms of breast-cancer-specific and overall survival in favor of the irradiated patients were of borderline significance ($p = 0.05$ and $p = 0.07$, respectively).

Translating Clinical Results into Clinical Practice

Given the results of the Danish and British Columbia trials, should all patients with node-positive disease be given postoperative radiation therapy including the peripheral lymphatics? Could the survival benefit be achieved with more limited radiation fields that might decrease the risk of potential long-term morbidity: arm edema, brachial plexopathy, pneumonitis, and cardiac problems? What is the absolute benefit with radiation therapy in more narrowly defined subgroups according to established prognostic factors such as tumor size and number of involved nodes? These questions and concerns are legitimate and show that the translation of trial results into clinical practice is not straightforward.

Risk of Postmastectomy Locoregional Recurrence

There is currently a wide consensus that all conservatively treated patients should receive postoperative radiation therapy to the breast parenchyma. However, as noted above, indications for postmastectomy radiation including the regional lymphatics remain controversial. To some extent this controversy is related to the relative lack of comprehensive information on the risk of postmastectomy locoregional recurrence in narrowly defined subgroups of patients.

In a study including about 7500 patients from the Stockholm Breast Cancer Database postmastectomy locoregional recurrences occurring as "first events" were analyzed according to tumor size, number of involved lymph nodes, and adjuvant systemic therapy given (Rutqvist and Liedberg, submitted). The median follow-up was 7.5 years. Among about 3200 patients treated with surgery alone the estimated cumulative 10-year recurrence rate among pathologically node-negative patients was consistently below 15% unless the tumor size exceeded 30 mm; in the latter subgroup the estimated cumulative risk at 10 years was 22%. In patients with 1–3 positive nodes the cumulative risk was consistently more than 15% unless the primary tumor size was below 10 mm. Among patients with 4 or more positive nodes the cumulative 10-year risk exceeded 25% in all subgroups studied. Among about 1900 estrogen-receptor-positive patients treated with adjuvant tamoxifen, all node-positive subgroups exhibited cumulative 10-year risks above 15%. Multivariate Cox analysis failed to demonstrate any statistically significant benefit in terms of a reduced risk of locoregional recurrence with the use of adjuvant CMF chemotherapy.

These results support the proposition that postmastectomy radiation therapy should be considered in node-negative patients with a large tumor size as well as in most node-positive patients irrespective of whether the patients also receive appropriate adjuvant systemic therapy.

Is Radiation Therapy After Breast Conservation Always Necessary?

Several controlled trials have convincingly demonstrated that the use of radiation therapy following breast-conserving surgery substantially reduces the risk of breast recurrence. However, the relatively low risk of such a recurrence among patients without specific risk factors, such as age under 50 years, multicentric disease, positive margins, extensive intraductal component, etc., has contributed to speculation about whether radiation therapy might safely be omitted in selected subgroups of patients.

The Boston Prospective Study

A recently published prospective study by Schnitt et al. (1996) included 87 patients with monocentric clinical stage I invasive breast cancers of ductal, mucinous, or tubular type without an extensive intraductal component, lymphatic vessel invasion, or histologically involved axillary lymph nodes. A wide excision was performed with a documented free margin of at least 1 cm. No postoperative radiation therapy or adjuvant systemic therapy was administered. The median tumor size was 0.9 cm and most tumors had been detected by mammography alone. Median patient age was 67 years. The trial had a sequential design and was originally intended to include 90 patients. However, the study was prematurely closed in 1992 when the predetermined stopping boundary was reached, that is, when the sixth breast recurrence was detected. At a median follow-up of 56 months the crude breast recurrence rate (first site of failure) was 14/87 (16%), giving an average annual local recurrence rate of 3.6%.

The Scottish Trial

The Scottish breast conservation trial included a total of 585 patients aged under 70 years with invasive breast cancer with a clinical tumor size less than 4 cm (Forrest et al. 1996). Surgical treatment consisted of a wide local excision with a 1-cm free margin (although histopathological confirmation of free margins was not obligatory) plus standard axillary surgery. Randomization was between postoperative radiation therapy to the breasts plus a boost to the original tumor site versus surgery alone. In addition, all patients received adjuvant systemic therapy according to their estrogen-receptor (ER) status: all ER-positive patients ($n = 331$) received adjuvant tamoxifen and all ER-negative patients ($n = 133$) adjuvant CMF chemotherapy. At a median follow-up of 5.7 years the breast recurrence rates among the nonirradiated patients were substantially higher than among those who had received radiation therapy, irrespective of which type of systemic therapy had been used. The respective crude percentages of breast recurrences among irradiated and nonirradiated patients in the tamoxifen group were 3 and 20; the corresponding percentages in the chemotherapy group were 10 and 39.

These two studies confirm and extend previous information from breast conservation radiation therapy trials in showing that even in highly selected subgroups of patients there is a substantial risk of early local recurrence for those treated with wide excision alone, irrespective of whether appropriate adjuvant systemic therapy is administered. These observations cast some doubt on the validity of the hypothesis that patient selection on the basis of hitherto known risk factors can effect a substantial decrease of the number of conservatively treated breast cancer patients who receive postoperative breast irradiation, without substantially compromising treatment outcome.

The time has probably come to focus on how to individualize radiation therapy, basing it more on potential predictors of the radiosensitivity of individual tumors rather than the widespread treatment of large groups of patients with or without selection on the basis of putative prognostic markers. However, this field of research is still in an early phase and so far results can only be regarded as tentative until supported by more large-scale studies.

Molecular Correlates of Radiation Responsiveness

The radiation responsiveness among breast cancer patients varies. Many patients are permanently cured locally by a conventionally fractionated "full-dose" regimen whereas others develop a breast recurrence despite the radiation. The outcome of treatment could probably be improved by increasing the dose of radiation, but acute and long-term side-effects limit the possible total dose. Accurate pretreatment prediction in individual patients of sensitivity or resistance of both tumor and healthy cells to radiation is not possible with today's prognostic and diagnostic methods. This implies that current methods to select patients for radiation therapy can only be based on prognostic factors, that is, the level of risk. Ideally, the selection should be based on both prognostic and treatment-predictive factors.

Genetic Factors Determining the Response to Radiation

To some extent clinical radioresponsiveness may be correlated with tumor growth rate and degree of oxygenation, but the intrinsic radiosensitivity of the tumor cells is probably also important. Currently relatively little information is available about the genetic factors, both in the healthy cell and in tumor cells, which determine the response to ionizing radiation. A number of candidate genes have been identified, however, which encode proteins with a central role in the cell's response to radiation damage. Sequence variation in these genes which results in a functional change in the encoded protein may have a profound effect on this response. If one could characterize the sequence of these genes in a significant number of individuals, and at the same time clinically validate the contribution of different variants to the response to radiation therapy, new opportunities for patient management could emerge.

The antineoplastic properties of ionizing radiation are thought to be primarily related to DNA damage. Three different intracellular pathways can be activated when DNA damage is detected: DNA repair, cell growth arrest, and programmed cell death (apoptosis) (Brown and McCarthy 1997; Kroemer 1997). Each pathway involves a distinct set of gene products and, when activated, proceeds independently of the other two pathways. The three different pathways must therefore be coordinated when DNA damage is recognized. DNA damage caused by ionizing radiation is detected by a dedicated DNA damage-sensing apparatus which triggers, via the *p53* protein, one of the possible pathways leading to DNA repair, growth arrest, or apoptosis. The damage-sensing apparatus is not fully described or understood, but some of the critical genes with central functions have been identified. Two of the most interesting are the ATM and ABL genes.

The ATM gene has been presented as the "most common cancer gene found so far". It is estimated that 1 in 100 people are carriers of a mutation in one copy of the ATM gene. Estimates are that there are two million carriers in the US, one million men and one million women – clearly more than the approximatley 600 families affected by ataxia telangiectasia. It has also been estimated that between 8% and 18% of breast cancer tumors carry a mutation in the ATM gene. Mutation of one of the germ-line ATM alleles confers increased susceptibility to cancer. Carriers have a three to four times increased risk of cancer in general; female carriers have a five-fold increased risk of breast cancer. The ATM protein is presumably, therefore, an important component of a multiprotein signal transduction system. As such it has a critical role in avoiding the loss of genome stability that has occurred in cancer cells and in establishing the level of radiosensitivity or radioresistance of tumor cells.

It has been reported that the ABL protein and the ATM protein are associated with one another in the normal cell. The *c-abl* gene encodes a nonreceptor protein tyrosine kinase whose targets include the RNA polymerase II. When the cell is treated with ionizing radiation, ABL is activated, but only in the presence of a functional ATM. One amino acid (ser 465) in the ABL protein is critical for its activation by ATM. The mechanism by which the existence of DNA is sensed by the ATM protein is not known. It is possible that another protein senses the damage and reports it to the ATM-ABL complex. DNA damage also triggers a direct association between ABL and *p53*. In addition, ABL also interacts with the Rb protein, which is a key regulator of the G1/S cell cycle transition.

The GADD45 (growth arrest and DNA damage inducible) gene is induced by DNA damage in human cells. The GADD45 protein binds to proliferating cell nuclear antigen (PCNA), which is a normal component of cyclin-dependent kinase complexes and is involved in DNA replication and repair. GADD45 also interacts with p21, the cell growth inhibitor which mediates *p53*-dependent cell growth inhibition. The effect of GADD45 is to stimulate DNA repair and to bring about cell growth arrest. It therefore forms an important link between DNA repair and *p53*-dependent cell growth inhibition. The *p53* gene product has a central role in coordinating the response to DNA damage, i.e., deciding between activation of DNA repair, growth arrest, or apoptosis. The retinoblastoma protein is responsible for transmitting the growth signal from the cyclin D proteins further into the transcription control machinery of the cell. *p53* acts to inhibit the process either at the level of the cyclin D-dependent kinases or the cyclin A-dependent kinases and it acts via the kinase inhibitors p21 or p27. Of these two, p27 may be of most direct importance in cell cycle arrest. The p15/16 proteins are highly related and act to specifically inhibit the cyclin D-dependent kinases. These gene products are critical for the negative regulation of the cell cycle and have been found to be frequently mutated in cancers. Growth inhibition (more specifically, G1 arrest) and apoptosis appear to be alternative *p53*-induced outcomes. Cooperation between *p53* and Rb pathways is thought to be the process by which it is determined whether *p53* will activate growth arrest or apoptosis.

Clinical Significance of Mutations in *p53*

At present relatively little clinical information is available on correlations between the outcome of radiation therapy and the afore-mentioned putative molecular markers of radioresponsiveness. Most studies have concerned *p53*. For instance, in a study by Jansson et al. (1995) the primary tumor was analyzed with regard to mutations in *p53* among 168 conservatively treated patients with node-negative breast cancer. A cDNA-based sequencing method was used which is probably more accurate in comparison with commercially available immunohistochemical methods to detect mutations. Relapse-free survival was significantly better among patients with detected *p53* mutations who had received radiation therapy than among those with mutations who had not received radiation therapy ($p = 0.0007$). Their overall survival was also significantly improved ($p = 0.02$). Among patients with wild-type *p53* no significant differences were observed between irradiated and nonirradiated patients. However, due to the small number of patients studied these results can only be regarded as tentative.

Novel Methods to Avoid Cardiac Risks with Radiation Therapy

Individual studies as well as the overviews of randomized radiation therapy trials have convincingly demonstrated that some types of postmastectomy radiation therapy used in the past were associated with cardiac effects resulting in increased mortality due to ischemic heart disease (Early Breast Cancer Trialists' Collaborative Group 1995). Such effects have been shown to be correlated with the cardiac dose-volume. In radiation therapy after breast conservation the target volume is typically restricted to the breast parenchyma alone, so cardiac problems should theoretically be much less common than with some types of postmastectomy treatment, particularly those that include the internal mammary chain. However, relatively little information on cause-specific mortality is available from randomized radiation therapy trials including conservatively treated patients.

The Stockholm Study

In a study of 684 patients treated with conservative surgery and breast irradiation (typically 50 Gy/5 weeks) in the Stockholm area during 1976–1987, their risk of acute myocardial infarction (AMI) was compared to that among 4996 concurrent mastectomized patients who had not received radiation therapy (Rutqvist et al. 1998). At a median follow-up of 9 years the relative hazard of AMI adjusted for differences in age among the irradiated patients versus the mastectomized women was 0.6 (95% confidence interval: 0.4–1.2). The corresponding relative hazard for patients with left-sided disease was also 0.6 (0.2–1.4). These results indicate that radiation-induced ischemic heart disease is in general not a significant problem in patients treated with breast irradiation after breast conservation using modern treatment techniques.

Cardiac Risks with Left-Sided Irradiation?

In a study by Gyenes et al. (1997) of the three-dimensional treatment plans for 100 consecutive patients with left-sided stage I disease it was found that the cardiac dose-volumes in a small subgroup of women were nearly as large as those estimated for women with left-sided breast cancer treated with deep tangential fields in the First Stockholm Radiation Therapy Trial. In a previous analysis that treatment technique was found to be associated with a significant excess of mortality due to ischemic heart disease during long-term follow-up. The study by Gyenes et al. illustrates that there is small subgroup of women that have an "unfavorable anatomy" with the heart located anteriorly in the mediastinum. If such a woman is treated for a left-sided breast cancer with conventional tangential photon fields, the resulting cardiac dose-volume may be so high that the risk of excess cardiac mortality during long-term follow-up may be in the order of 5% even if the target volume only includes the breast parenchyma (Gagliardi et al., submitted). In a study by Gagliardi et al. (submitted) it was demonstrated that the excess risk of cardiac mortality could be reduced to 0.4%–0.6% by blocking part of the beam hitting the heart through conventional or multileaf collimation. The most effective method to decrease the cardiac risk, however, was through an optimized general fluence modulation method based on multiple beams.

With that technique the excess long-term cardiac risk was more or less completely avoided. However, there are still many technical problems that need to be addressed before such sophisticated treatment techniques can be used routinely.

Conclusions

Recent clinical data have confirmed that locoregional radiation therapy as part of the primary mangement of early-stage breast cancer clearly has a role beyond simple local control of the disease. In-depth analyses of individual studies have indicated that the prevention of breast-cancer-related death by radiation therapy is mediated through eradication of subclinical foci of tumor cells in the breast or on the postmastectomy chest wall which, if left untreated, would give rise to distant dissemination (Arriagada et al. 1995). This observation indicates that those patients who are most likely to benefit from radiation therapy are those that are at high risk of local recurrence with surgery alone or even surgery followed by appropriate adjuvant systemic therapy. There is still some controversy as to the absolute risk of local failure in narrowly defined subgroups of patients and whether the survival benefit with radiation therapy could be achieved with more limited fields of irradiation that carry a lower risk of potential late side effects.

Selection of conservatively treated patients for breast irradiation on the basis of hitherto known risk factors has not been demonstrated to be a valid approach since even supposedly "low risk" groups seem to have a substantial risk of local recurrence despite stringent selection criteria or administration of appropriate systemic treatment. Long-term follow-up of patients treated with conservative surgery plus breast irradiation indicates that such treatment is not in general associated with such adverse cardiac side effects as have been demonstrated with some types of treatment used in the past in the postmastectomy setting. However, there is a small subgroup of women who have an "unfavorable anatomy" with the heart located anteriorly in the mediastinum. If irradiated for left-sided breast cancer such women may be at risk of significant excess, i.e., radiation-induced, cardiac mortality. Three-dimensional treatment planning can be used to identify such women and to modify the treatment technique so that cardiac problems are more or less completely avoided.

A number of candidate genes have be identified which encode proteins with a central role in the cell's response to radiation damage. At present little clinical information is available on correlations between the outcome of radiation therapy and putative molecular markers of radiosensitivity, although some preliminary studies have indicated that mutations in *p53* may be clinically significant. Further research concerning such markers will probably in provide new opportunities for patient management in the near future.

Summary

The updates of the Danish DBCG 82b trial and the British Columbia trial have confirmed a significant overall survival benefit with postoperative radiation therapy in patients with high-risk disease. These trials together with in-depth analyses of previous studies suggest that the mechanism of the survival benefit is eradication of subclinical locoregional deposits of tumor cells with a potential for further dissemination if left untreated. Despite these findings, several questions remain largely unanswered concerning the optimal way to integrate radiation therapy into routine clinical practice. For instance, which subgroups are likely to benefit from comprehensive treatment including the peripheral lymphatics as opposed to treatment of the breast/chest wall alone? The available randomized trials and overviews have convincingly demonstrated that it is essential to minimize long-term radiation side effects in the myocardium in order to achieve an overall survival benefit. An appropriate treatment technique is therefore essential. Individual treatment planning should be encouraged since some patients have an "unfavorable anatomy" with the heart located anteriorly in the mediastinum. Such patients may receive a high cardiac dose-volume even with conventional tangential field irradiation that does not include the internal mammary nodes.

References

Arriagada R et al (1995) Adequate locoregional treatment for early breast cancer may prevent secondary dissemination. J Clin Oncol 13:2869–2878

Brown L, McCarthy N (1997) DNA repair. A sens-abl response? Nature 387:450–451

Early Breast Cancer Trialists' Collaborative Group (1995) Effects of radiotherapy and surgery in early breast cancer. An overview of the randomized trials. N Engl J Med 333:1444–1455

Forrest P et al (1996) Randomised controlled trial of conservation therapy for breast cancer: 6-year analysis of the Scottish trial. Lancet 348:708–713

Gyenes G et al (1997) Evaluation of irradiated heart volumes in stage I breast cancer patients treated with postoperative adjuvant radiotherapy. J Clin Oncol 15:1348–1353

Jansson T et al (1995) p53 status predicts survival in breast cancer patients treated with or without postoperative radiotherapy: a novel hypothesis based on clinical findings. J Clin Oncol 13:2745–2751

Kroemer G (1997) The proto-oncogene Bcl-2 and its role in regulating apoptosis. Nat Med 3:614

Overgaard M et al (1997) Postoperative radiotherapy in high-risk premenopausal women with breast cancer who receive adjuvant chemotherapy. N Engl J Med 337:949–955

Ragaz J et al (1995) Adjuvant radiotherapy and chemotherapy in node-positive premenopausal women with breast cancer. N Engl J Med 337:956–962

Rutqvist LE et al (1998) Myocardial infarction among women with early stage breast cancer treated with conservative surgery and breast cancer. Int J Radiat Oncol Biol Phys (in press)

Schnitt S et al (1996) A prospective study of conservative surgery alone in the treatment of selected patients with stage I breast cancer. Cancer 77:1094–1100

Molecular Biology of the Estrogen Receptor Aids in the Understanding of Tamoxifen Resistance and Breast Cancer Prevention with Raloxifene*

V. C. Jordan

Robert H. Lurie Cancer Comprehensive Cancer Center, Northwestern University Medical School, Chicago, IL 60611, USA

Introduction

Tamoxifen (Nolvadex) (Fig. 1), a nonsteroidal antiestrogen, is the endocrine treatment of choice for all stages of breast cancer. The drug has ten million women-years of clinical experience and is described by the World Health Organization as an essential treatment for breast cancer. The clinical pharmacology of tamoxifen has been studied in great detail because it is currently being tested as a preventive for breast cancer in high-risk women (Jordan 1993). This strategy is based on three important facts. Firstly, tamoxifen prevents rat mammary carcinogenesis (Jordan 1974, 1976). Secondly, tamoxifen reduces the incidence of contralateral breast cancer (Cuzik and Baum 1985) and, thirdly, when the preliminary studies were started in 1986 (Powles et al. 1989), tamoxifen was believed to have a low incidence of side effects (Furr and Jordan 1984).

As a prelude to the testing of tamoxifen in healthy women, studies were conducted to evaluate the effect of antiestrogens on bone density. Remarkably, tamoxifen exhibits target site-specific effects in animals; bone density is maintained in ovariectomized rats but estrogen-stimulated uterine weight is blocked (Jordan et al. 1987). The action in bone translated to the clinic (Love et al. 1992), but regrettably the finding of the target site-specific effects of tamoxifen to stimulate endometrial cancer growth while preventing the estrogen-stimulated growth of breast cancer (Gottardis et al. 1988a) also translated to the clinic. There is a documented two-fold increase in the incidence of endometrial cancer in breast cancer patients who take tamoxifen (Assikis et al. 1996). Although no woman being treated for breast cancer with tamoxifen should have the drug stopped because of concerns about endometrial cancer, this troublesome side effect is unacceptable if tamoxifen is to be used

---

* This article is dedicated to Professor E. V. Jensen on the occasion of the 40th anniversary of the first report of the specific binding of estrogen in estrogen target tissues.
These studies were supported by the NIH grant CA-56143. The author is grateful for the continuing support of the Lynn Sage Breast Cancer Foundation of Northwestern Memorial Hospital.

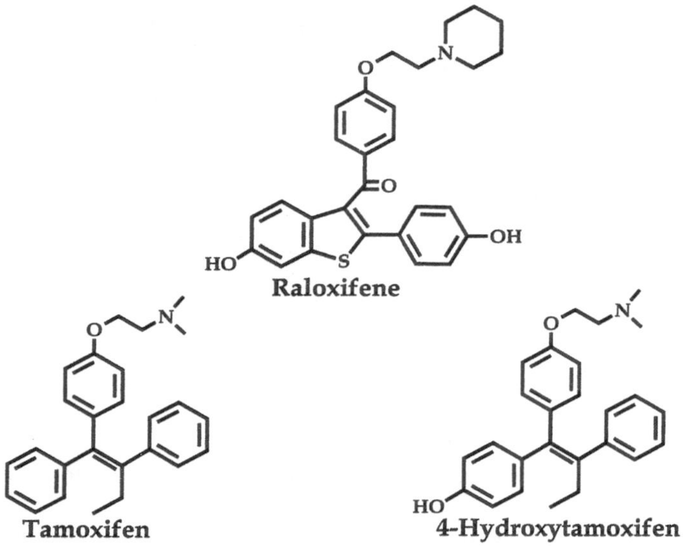

Fig. 1. Chemical structures of nonsteroidal antiestrogens: raloxifene, tamoxifen, and 4-hydroxytamoxifen

by the general population to prevent breast cancer. In the late 1980s there was a paradigm change for the prevention of breast cancer. If targeted drugs could be identified as preventives for osteoporosis then the beneficial side effect would be the prevention of breast and endometrial cancer (Lerner and Jordan 1990). The widespread use of the therapy in postmenopausal women would have a significant impact on the incidence of breast cancer.

Raloxifene (Evista) has recently been approved by the Food and Drug Administration in the USA for the prevention of osteoporosis in postmenopausal women. Raloxifene (originally named LY156,750 or keoxifene) (Fig. 1) is a nonsteroidal antiestrogen with a high affinity for the estrogen receptor (ER) (Black et al. 1983). Drug development was originally targeted towards breast cancer therapy but was discontinued in the late 1980s. However, the finding that raloxifene maintained bone density in rats (Jordan et al. 1987), prevented rat mammary carcinogenesis (Gottardis and Jordan 1987), and inhibited tamoxifen-stimulated endometrial carcinoma growth (Gottardis et al. 1990) laid the foundation for drug development as a preventive for osteoporosis in the mid 1990s.

The drugs, originally classified as antiestrogens, are having an enormous impact on therapeutics. Raloxifene and tamoxifen are now classified as selective ER modulators because of their diverse pharmacology. Remarkably, an examination of their molecular biology is providing insight not only into the mechanism of antiestrogen action, but also into a mechanism of drug resistance to tamoxifen.

Crystal Structure of the Raloxifene-Estrogen-Receptor Complex

The ER was first identified by Jensen and Jacobson in 1962 and isolated from the rat uterus by Gorski's group in the mid 1960s (Gorski et al. 1968). However, Jensen et al. (1971) subsequently suggested that ER determinations could be used as a marker for the hormone dependency of breast cancer, and for two decades the ER protein has played a central role in the management of breast cancer as the target for antiestrogen action (Jordan 1995)..

For the past 30 years there has been a quest to solve the crystal structure of the estradiol-ER complex and define the molecular events of estrogen action. In 1997, the ligand binding domain of the ER was crystallized with estradiol and raloxifene (Brzozowski et al. 1997). Estradiol forms a complex in the hydrophobic ligand binding pocket through hydrogen bonding at amino acids Glu 353 and Arg 394 with the 3-phenolic hydroxyl and amino acid His 524 with the 17β hydroxyl (Fig. 2A). As a result, there is a conformational change in the protein that re-orients helix 12 to snap shut on the ligand binding pocket and to seal the steroid inside the protein (Fig. 3). Helix 12 contains the important AF-2 region and three amino acids (Asp 538, Glu 542, Asp 545) (Danielian et al. 1992; Tzukerman et al. 1994) have been identified that are essential for the subsequent activation of the receptor complex as a transcription unit at an estrogen-sensitive gene. Site-directed mutagenesis in this region destroys AF-2 activity and nonsteroidal antiestrogens also silence AF-2 activity (Berry et al. 1990).

Raloxifene is anchored at the same two amino acids as estradiol (Fig. 2B); however, the aminoethoxy side chain extends away from the molecule. The alkylaminoethoxy side chain is known to be the essential structural feature of all antiestrogens (Jordan 1984). Changes in the distance between the oxygen and the nitrogen (Lednicer et al. 1996), restriction in the conformation of the side chain (Clark and Jordan 1976), or the basicity of the nitrogen (Robertson et al. 1982) all result in a decrease in antiestrogenic activity. Indeed, removal of the side chain results in either an increase in estrogenic properties or a complete loss of activity (Jordan and Gosden 1982).

An earlier model of estrogen and antiestrogen action, based on experimental evidence with polyclonal antibodies to the ER, described estradiol as being "locked" into the ligand binding site but that antiestrogens were wedged into the site because of multipoint attachment via the alkylaminoethoxy side chain (Tate et al. 1984). Similarly, a model of antiestrogen action based on the structure-function assays of antiestrogens in cell culture proposed that the aminoethoxy side chain would bind to an "antiestrogenic region" of the ligand binding domain to prevent the closure of the ligand binding pocket (Lieberman et al. 1983). That interaction was the key to antiestrogen action.

By reference to the crystal structure of the raloxifene-ER complex the alkylaminoethoxy side chain binds to amino acid 351 (aspartate) (Fig. 2B). The consequence of this interaction is a macromolecular perturbation in the complex that moves helix 12 to a new position, thereby masking the critical

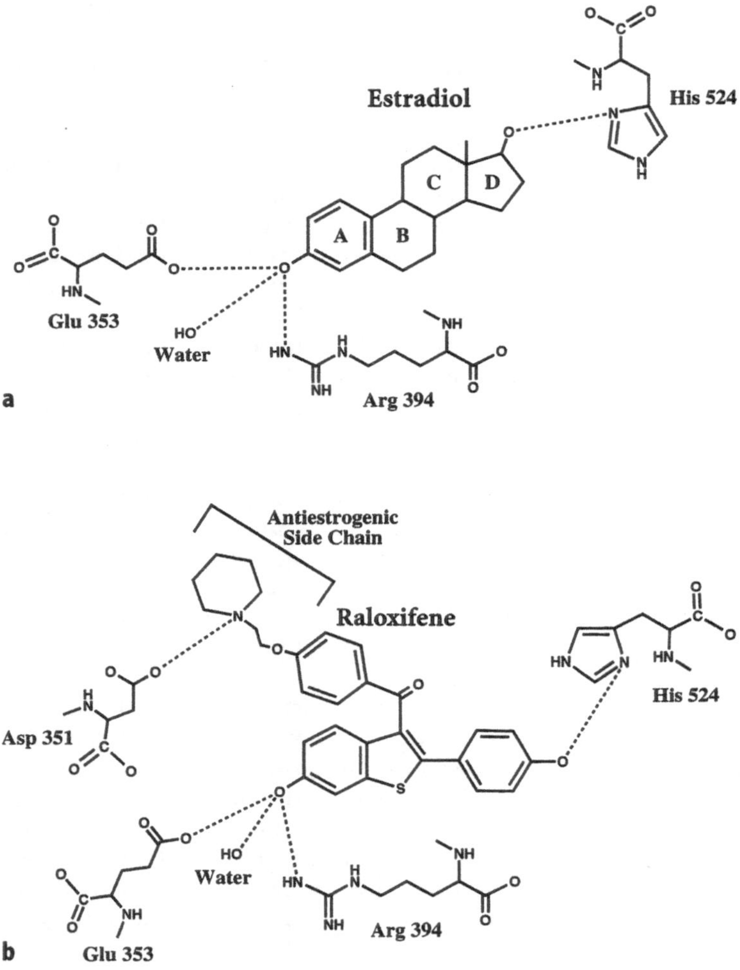

Fig. 2. The interaction of **a** estradiol and **b** raloxifene in the ligand binding domain of the ER. (Adapted from Brzozowski et al 1997)

three amino acids in the AF-2 region: Asp 538, Glu 542, Asp 545 (Tzukerman et al. 1994). Raloxifene has silenced AF-2 activity (Fig. 3). It is proposed that the coactivators that are needed to form a transcription complex can no longer bind to ER. However, the most compelling evidence to support the molecular model of antiestrogen action for raloxifene comes from the study of drug resistance to tamoxifen.

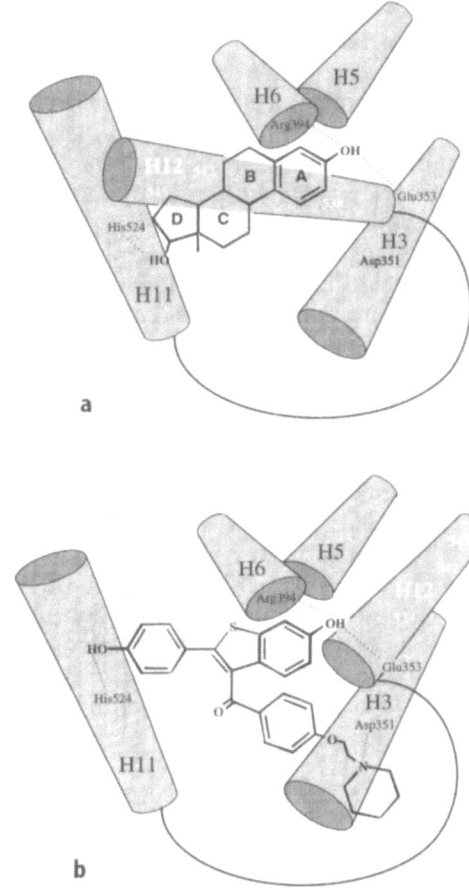

Fig. 3. A molecular mechanism of estrogen and antiestrogen action. **a** Helix 12 snaps shut on the ligand binding pocket and seals the steroid inside the protein. This allows coactivators to bind to the critical amino acids (538, 542, 545) to complete the formation of a transcriptional complex. **b** By contrast, raloxifene causes a shift in helix 12 because the piperazine ring binds to amino acid 351. This repositions the helix and masks the AF-2 site

Drug Resistance to Tamoxifen

Drug resistance to tamoxifen can take many forms (Morrow and Jordan 1993), but the type that has attracted most interest is tamoxifen-stimulated growth. This phenomenon is observed clinically because patients whose tumors begin to grow during tamoxifen treatment can exhibit a withdrawal response when tamoxifen is stopped (Howell et al. 1992; Canney et al. 1987).

During the early 1980s when the strategy of long-term adjuvant tamoxifen therapy was being translated from the laboratory to the clinic (Jordan 1983), it was clear that breast cancer would ultimately become resistant to tamoxifen, so laboratory models were necessary to understand the process and to be used to test new therapeutic agents. Osborne et al. (1987) in San Antonio first demonstrated that tamoxifen treatment would not control the eventual growth of MCF-7 (ER-positive) breast cancer cells inoculated into athymic animals. However, he demonstrated that the tumor cells retained the appropriate estrogen and antiestrogen sensitivities in vitro. Similarly, we found that implanted MCF-7 tumors would initially respond to tamoxifen as an antiestrogen, but when therapy was stopped estrogen could reactivate tumor growth (Gottardis et al. 1988b). However, tamoxifen-stimulated tumors eventually grow and can be retransplanted into young athymic mice (Gottardis and Jordan 1988). The tumors are ER-positive and require either estradiol or tamoxifen for growth (Gottardis and Jordan 1988). We discovered that it is the direct effect of the tamoxifen on the tumor that provokes growth, and that the host can be either an athymic mouse or rat (Gottardis et al. 1989a). Species-specific metabolism, known to be a fundamental difference between mice and rats (Robinson et al. 1991), or local tumor metabolism of tamoxifen (Wolf et al. 1993) was not relevant. The "estrogenicity" of an antiestrogen is the critical factor for growth; the pure antiestrogen ICI 164,384 (Gottardis et al. 1989b) or ICI 182,780 (Osborne et al. 1995) are able to control tamoxifen-resistant tumor growth. The question of major importance, though, is the mechanism of tamoxifen-stimulated growth. On the basis of the crystal structure of the raloxifene-ER complex, two pathways merit consideration: a mutant receptor or a selective increase in coactivator molecules (or both).

A Mutant Receptor in Tamoxifen-Stimulated Tumors

During the early 1990s, a popular theory to explain drug resistance to tamoxifen was the selection of breast cancer cells containing a mutant receptor that translates an antiestrogenic response into an estrogenic response. Mahfoudi et al. (1995) proposed a mutation hypothesis for the AF-2 region based on their work with the mouse ER. However, sequencing of the AF-2 region of tamoxifen-stimulated breast and endometrial tumors demonstrated that this was not the cause of tamoxifen-stimulated growth in reproducible laboratory models (Bilimoria et al. 1996). None of the appropriate mutations were found. By contrast, we addressed the hypothesis by developing different transplantable MCF-7 tumor lines in athymic mice, describing their biological characteristics (Wolf and Jordan 1994a), and sequencing the whole receptor in each tumor line (Wolf and Jordan 1994b).

One tumor line was found that contained a codon 351 Asp→Tyr mutation as the majority of receptor present (Wolf and Jordan 1994b). However, the problem was to test the efficacy of the receptor appropriately. The biology was not tested in animal or yeast cells because of a concern that the results would reflect the wrong cellular context, with either inappropriate or insufficient levels of supporting transcription factors. In contrast, stable transfectants were prepared with clone 10A of the ER-negative breast cancer cell line MDA-MB-231. The reasoning for this was that the receptors might function optimally in the correct context, i.e., a breast cancer cell, replete with coactivators.

In 1992, the first stable transfectants of MDA-MB-231 cells with cDNAs from wild-type and codon 400 Gly→Val mutant ERs were reported (Jiang and Jordan 1992). The goal at that time was to determine whether reintroduction of the ER into receptor-negative breast cancer would reassert control by estrogen. Interestingly, estrogen decreased growth rather than increased growth and the pure antiestrogen ICI 164,384 blocked estrogen action. Although the precise mechanism for the phenomenon could not be discovered, the end point of growth inhibition was used as an assay for the "estrogenicity" of any ligand receptor complex.

4-Hydroxytamoxifen (Fig. 1) and a steroidal antiestrogen RU 39,411 with a structural similarity to 4-hydroxytamoxifen (Jiang et al. 1993) were found to be more estrogenic in cells transfected with the codon 400 Gly→Val mutant ER cDNA. Raloxifene, by contrast, is an antiestrogen in transfectants with either wild-type or codon 400 Gly→Val mutant cDNAs (Jiang et al. 1993). 4-Hydroxytamoxifen, therefore, appears to be more promiscuous with estrogen-like activity in the codon 400 Gly→Val mutant transfectants (Jiang et al. 1992).. Although these data with the 400 mutant ER are of interest, the receptor is a cloning artifact rather than a natural mutant (Tora et al. 1989). By contrast, the codon 351 Asp→Tyr mutant is the first natural mutant to be identified that could possibly have a role in drug resistance. Stable transfectants with the cDNA for the mutant receptor in MDA-MB-231 cells were prepared (Catherino et al. 1995) and an analogue of 4-hydroxytamoxifen was found to be a potent estrogen and inhibited cell growth. A strategy of using single, double, and triple vitellogenin estrogen response elements (Catherino and Jordan 1995) with a luciferase reporter gene was used to show that the mutant receptor was more estrogenic than the wild-type receptor. However, it is extremely hard to retransfect the transfectants so a gene target was selected in situ.

The Key to the Antiestrogenic Activity of Raloxifene

Estradiol increases the transcription of transforming growth factor-α (TGFα) mRNA in MDA-MB-231 cells transfected with the cDNA for the ER (Jeng et al. 1994). This action of estradiol is blocked by the pure antiestrogen ICI 164,384 (Jordan et al. 1994). Since the regulation of TGFα is well recognized as an estrogen-dependent event, this gene was chosen to use as a precise assay, in human cells, to document the efficacy of ligand ER complexes. Raloxifene is a complete antiestrogen in the wild-type ER transfectant (Levenson et al. 1997) (Fig. 4). However, when raloxifene is liganded to the 351 mutant receptor, raloxifene induces TGFα mRNA. The pure antiestrogen ICI 182,780 blocks the induction of TGFα mRNA by both estradiol and raloxifene. It is

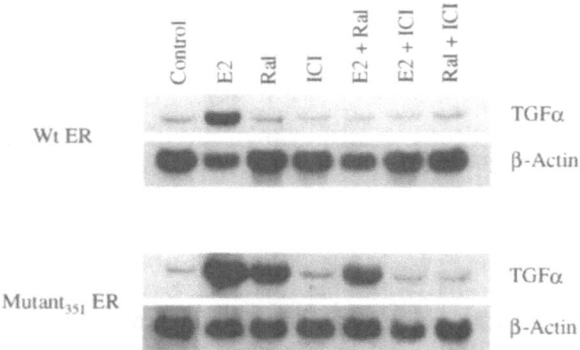

Fig. 4. Effects of estradiol and antiestrogens, or combinations of compounds, on TGFα mRNA expression in ER transfectants analyzed by Northern blot. The sources for RNAs were following: *Control*, cells treated with EtOH vehicle; *E2*, cells treated with 10^{-9} *M* estradiol [wild-type (wt) ER], and 10^{-8} *M* estradiol (mutant$_{351}$ER); *Ral*, cells treated with 10^{-6} *M* raloxifene; *ICI*, cells treated with 10^{-6} *M* ICI 182,780; *E2+Ral*, cells treated with 10^{-9} *M* or 10^{-8} *M* estradiol (depending on the cell line) and 10^{-6} *M* raloxifene; *E2+ICI*, cells treated with 10^{-9} *M* or 10^{-8} *M* estradiol (depending on the cell line) and 10^{-6} *M* ICI 182,780; *Ral+ICI*, cells treated with 10^{-6} *M* raloxifene and 10^{-6} *M* ICI 182,780. β-Actin was used as a loading control. (Adapted from Jordan et al 1994)

therefore clear that the specific mutation at amino acid 351 changes the pharmacology of raloxifene from an antiestrogen to an estrogen. The data derived from a natural mutant ER are extremely important as they confirm the key role of amino acid 351, aspartate, which is identified in the crystal structure as interacting with the alkylaminoethoxy side chain (Brzozowski et al. 1997). Additionally, these studies identify, for the first time, a specific mechanism for the development of drug resistance to tamoxifen. The mutation clearly provides a growth advantage for breast cancer cells by exploiting the increased estrogenicity of the receptor complex. Nevertheless, it is important to appreciate that the mutation does not compromise the effectiveness of the pure antiestrogen ICI 182,780 as an appropriate second-line breast cancer therapy following tamoxifen treatment failure.

Future Advances in Understanding Drug Resistance to Tamoxifen

Although a mechanism of drug resistance to tamoxifen has been identified and the molecular mechanism for the antiestrogen raloxifene has been confirmed, the molecular mechanisms of action of tamoxifen and 4-hydroxytamoxifen are subtly different. This in turn has implications for the eventual development of tamoxifen-stimulated tumor growth. The great majority of tamoxifen-stimulated tumors in the laboratory have a wild-type ER so a growth mechanism other than mutation must be amplified in these tumor cells.

The current hypothesis for tamoxifen resistance was developed based on evidence recently published using the stable transfectants with cDNAs from

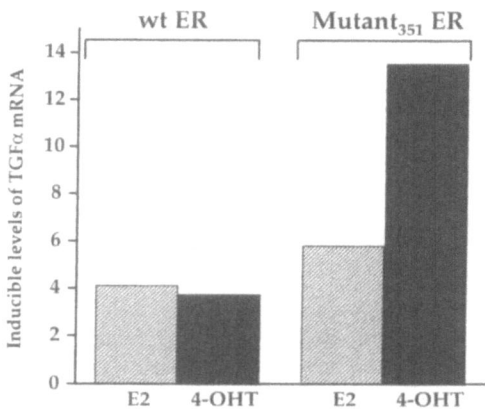

Fig. 5. Induction of TGFα mRNA expression by estradiol (E2) and 4-hydroxytamoxifen (4-OHT) in cells with wild-type (wt) ER and mutant$_{351}$ ER. Cells were treated with 10^{-7} M E2 or 4-OHT for 24 h and analyzed by Northern blot. The graph shows inducible levels of TGFα mRNA (ratio of normalized TGFα mRNA in cells treated with compounds to normalized levels in untreated cells) as determined by densitometric analyses. (Adapted from Levenson et al 1997)

either wild-type or 351 mutant ER. Unlike raloxifene, which exhibits estrogen-like activity only with the 351 mutant ER (Levenson et al. 1997), 4-hydroxytamoxifen exhibits estrogen-like properties to initiate TGFα mRNA synthesis with either wild-type or 351 mutant ER (Levenson et al. 1998) (Fig. 5). The 4-hydroxytamoxifen-ER complex is more promiscuous than the raloxifene ER complex. It is therefore reasonable to suggest that the 4-hydroxytamoxifen-ER complex is subtly different from the raloxifene-ER complex so that large concentration of coactivators in the MDA-MB-231 cells can bind to the complex. Indeed, the stable transfectant containing the 351 mutant is supersensitive to the action of 4-hydroxytamoxifen (Levenson et al. 1998). So the enhanced efficacy of the receptor complex would provide a clearcut growth advantage in the development of a tumor from the original MCF-7 cells. These data support the proposition (McDonnell et al. 1995) that antiestrogen receptor complexes are subtly different in shape and this conclusion should act as a stimulus for investigators to crystallize the 4-hydroxytamoxifen-ER complex. Additionally, it is clearly a priority to determine how the family of coactivator (or corepressor) proteins regulate gene activation.

Conclusion

The recent crystallization of the estradiol- and raloxifene-ER complex (Brzozowski et al. 1997) has provided fascinating clues to the mechanism of action of antiestrogens and confirmed, for the first time, a mechanism of drug resistance for tamoxifen. The new strategy to prevent breast cancer as a beneficial side effect of the prevention of osteoporosis (Jordan et al. 1987; Lerner and Jordan 1990) is poised to revolutionize health care for postmenopausal women. The convergence of molecular biology and medicine has the potential to open up new therapeutic opportunities for the discovery of novel targeted antiestrogens.

Acknowledgment. I wish to thank Henry Muenzner for excellent assistance in preparing the figures.

References

Assikis VJ, Neven P, Jordan VC et al (1996) A realistic clinical perspective of tamoxifen and endometrial carcinogenesis. Eur J Cancer 32A:1464–1476

Berry M, Metzger D, Chambon P (1990) Role of the two activating domains of the oestrogen receptor in the cell-type and promoter-context dependent agonistic activity of the anti-oestrogen 4-hydroxytamoxifen. EMBO J 9:2811–2818

Bilimoria MM, Assikis VJ, Muenzner HD et al (1996) An analysis of tamoxifen-stimulated human carcinomas for mutations in the AF-2 region of the estrogen receptor. J Steroid Biochem Mol Biol 58:479–488

Black LJ, Jones CD, Falcone JF (1983) Antagonism of estrogen action with a new benzothiophene-derived antiestrogen. Life Sci 32:1031–1036

Brzozowski AM, Pike ACW, Dauter Z et al (1997) Molecular basis of agonism and antagonism in the oestrogen receptor. Nature 389:753–758

Canney PA, Griffiths T, Latief TN et al (1987) Clinical significance of tamoxifen withdrawal response. Lancet 1:36

Catherino WH, Jordan VC (1995) Increasing the number of tandem estrogen response elements increases the estrogenic activity of a tamoxifen analogue. Cancer Lett 92:39–47

Catherino WH, Wolf DM, Jordan VC (1995) A naturally occurring estrogen receptor mutation results in increased estrogenicity of a tamoxifen analogue. Mol Endocrinol 9:1053–1063

Clark ER, Jordan VC (1976) Oestrogenic, antiestrogenic and antifertility properties of a series of compounds related to ethamoxytripheno (MER-25). Br J Pharmacol 57:487–493

Cuzik J, Baum M (1985) Tamoxifen and contralateral breast cancer. Lancet 2:282

Danielian PS, White R, Lees JA et al (1992) Identification of a conserved region required for hormone dependent transcriptional activation by steroid hormone receptors. EMBO J 11:1025–1033

Furr BJA, Jordan VC (1984) The pharmacology and clinical uses of tamoxifen. Pharmacol Ther 25:127–205

Gorski J, Toft D, Shyamala G et al (1968) Hormone receptors: studies on the interaction of estrogen with the uterus. Recent Prog Horm Res 24:45–80

Gottardis MM, Jordan VC (1987) The antitumor action of keoxifene (raloxifene) and tamoxifen in the N-nitrosomethylurea-induced rat mammary carcinoma model. Cancer Res 47:4020–4024

Gottardis MM, Jordan VC (1988) Development of tamoxifen-stimulated growth of MCF-7 tumors in athymic mice after long-term antiestrogen administration. Cancer Res 48:5183–5187

Gottardis MM, Robinson SP, Satyaswaroop PG et al (1988a) Contrasting actions of tamoxifen on endometrial and breast tumor growth in the athymic mouse. Cancer Res 48:812–815

Gottardis MM, Robinson SP, Jordan VC (1988b) Estradiol-stimulated growth of MCF-7 tumors implanted in athymic mice: a model to study the tumoristatic action of tamoxifen. J Steroid Biochem 20:311–314

Gottardis MM, Wager RJ, Borden EC et al (1989a) Differential ability of antiestrogens to stimulate breast cancer cell (MCF-7) growth in vivo and in vitro. Cances Res 49:4765–4769

Gottardis MM, Jiang SY, Jeng MH et al (1989b) Inhibition of tamoxifen stimulated growth of an MCF-7 tumor variant in athymic mice by novel steroidal antiestrogens. Cancer Res 49:4090–4093

Gottardis MM, Ricchio MD, Satyaswaroop PG et al (1990) Effect of steroidal and nonsteroidal antiestrogens on the growth of a tamoxifen-stimulated human endometrial carcinoma (EnCa101) in athymic mice. Cancer Res 50:3189–3192

Howell A, Dodwell DJ, Anderson H (1992) Response after withdrawal of tamoxifen and pro-gestogens in advanced breast cancer. Ann Oncol 3:611–617

Jeng M-H, Jiang S-Y, Jordan VC (1994) Paradoxical regulation of estrogen-dependent growth factor gene expression in estrogen receptor (ER)-negative human breast cancer cells stably expressing ER. Cancer Lett 82:123–128

Jensen EV, Jacobson HI (1962) Basic guides to the mechanism of estrogen action. Recent Prog Horm Res 18:378–414

Jensen EV, Block GE, Smith S et al (1971) Estrogen receptors and breast cancer response to adrenalectomy. In: Hall TC (ed) Prediction of response in cancer therapy. Monogr Natl Cancer Inst 34:55–70

Jiang SY, Jordan VC (1992) Growth regulation of estrogen receptor-negative breast cancer cells transfected with complementary DNAs for estrogen receptor. J Natl Cancer Inst 84:580–591

Jiang SY, Langan-Fahey SM, Stella A et al (1992) Point mutation of the estrogen receptor (ER) in the ligand binding domain changes the pharmacology of antiestrogens in ER-negative breast cancer cells stably expressing cDNAs for ER. Mol Endocrinol 6:2167–2174

Jiang SY, Parker CJ, Jordan VC (1993) A model to describe how a point mutation of the es-trogen receptor alters the structure function relationship of antiestrogens. Breast Cancer Res Treat 26:139–148

Jordan VC (1974) Antitumour activity of the antioestrogen ICI46,474 (tamoxifen) in the di-methylbenzanthracene (DMBA)-induced rat mammary carcinoma model. J Steroid Bio-chem 5:354

Jordan VC (1976) Effect of tamoxifen (ICI46,474) on initiation and growth of DMBA-in-duced rat mammary carcinoma. Eur J Cancer 12:419–424

Jordan VC (1983) Laboratory studies to develop general principles for the adjuvant treat-ment of breast cancer with antiestrogens: problems and potential for future clinical ap-plications. Breast Cancer Res Treat 3 Suppl:73–86

Jordan VC (1984) Biochemical pharmacology of antiestrogen action. Pharmacol Rev 36:245–276

Jordan VC (1993) Current view of the use of tamoxifen for the treatment and prevention of breast cancer. Gaddum Memorial Lecture. Br J Pharmacol 110:507–517

Jordan VC (1995) Studies on the estrogen receptor in breast cancer: 20 years as a target for the treatment and prevention of breast cancer. William L. Maguire Memorial Lecture. Breast Cancer Res Treat 36:267–285

Jordan VC, Gosden B (1982) Importance of the alkylaminoethoxy side chain for the estro-genic and antiestrogenic actions of tamoxifen and trioxifene in the immature rat uterus. Mol Cell Endocrinol 27:291–306

Jordan VC, Phelps E, Lindgren JU (1987) Effects of antiestrogens on bone in castrated and intact female rats. Breast Cancer Res Treat 10:31–35

Jordan VC, Jiang SY, Catherino WH et al (1994) Regulation of cell growth with the trans-fected estrogen-receptor gene. In: Motta M, Serio M (eds) Sex hormones and antihor-mones in endocrine dependent pathology: basic and clinical aspects. Elsevier, Amster-dam, pp 243–248

Lednicer D, Lyster SC, Aspergren BD et al (1996) Mammalian antifertility agents. III. 1-Anyl-2-phenyl-1,2,3,4-tetrahydro-1-naphthols, 1-anyl-2-phenyl-3,4-dihydronaphthalenes and their derivatives. J Med Chem 9:172–176

Lerner LJ, Jordan VC (1990) Development of antiestrogens and their use in breast cancer. English Cain Memorial Lecture. Cancer Res 50:4177–4189

Levenson AS, Catherino WH, Jordan VC (1997) Estrogenic activity is increased for an anti-estrogen by a natural mutation of the estrogen receptor. J Steroid Biochem Mol Biol 60:261–268

Levenson AS, Tonetti DA, Jordan VC (1998) The estrogen-like effect of 4-hydroxytamoxifen on transforming growth factor alpha mRNA in MDA-MB-231 breast cancer cells stably expressing the oestrogen receptor. Br J Cancer (in press)

Lieberman ME, Gorski J, Jordan VC (1983) An estrogen receptor model to describe the regulation of prolactin synthesis by antiestrogens in vitro. J Biol Chem 258:4741–4745

Love RR, Mazess RB, Barden HS et al (1992) Effects of tamoxifen on bone mineral density in postmenopausal women with breast cancer. N Engl J Med 326:852–856

Mahfoudi A, Poulet E, Dauvois S et al (1995) Specific mutations in the estrogen receptor change the properties of antiestrogens to full agonists. Proc Nat Acad Sci̇USA 92:4206–4210

McDonnell DP, Clemm DL, Hermann T et al (1995) Analysis of estrogen receptor function in vitro reveals three distinct classes of antiestrogens. Mol Endocrinol 9:659–669

Morrow M, Jordan VC (1993) Molecular mechanism of resistance to tamoxifen therapy in breast cancer. Arch Surg 128:1187–1191

Osborne CK, Coronado EB, Robinson JP (1987) Human breast cancer in athymic nude mice: cytostatic effects of long-term antiestrogenic activity. Eur J Cancer Clin Oncol 23:1189–1196

Osborne CK, Coronado-Heinsohn EB, Hilsenbeck SG et al (1995) Comparison of the effects of a pure steroidal antiestrogen with those of tamoxifen in a model of human cancer. J Natl Cancer Inst 87:746–750

Powles TJ, Hardy JR, Ashley SE et al (1989) A pilot trial to evaluate the acute toxicity and feasibility to tamoxifen for prevention for breast cancer. Br J Cancer 60:126–133

Robertson DW, Katzenellenbogen JA, Hayes JR et al (1982) Antiestrogen basicity-activity relationships: a comparison of the estrogen receptor binding and antituterotrophic potencies of several analogues of (Z)-1,2-diphenyl-1-[4-[2-(dimethylamino) ethoxy]phenyl]-1-butene (tamoxifen, Nolvadex) having altered basicity. J Med Chem 25:167–171

Robinson SP, Langan-Fahey SM, Johnson DA et al (1991) Metabolites, pharmacodynamics and pharmacokinetics of tamoxifen in rats and mice compared to the breast cancer patient. Drug Metab Dispos 19:36–43

Tate AC, Greene GL, DeSombre ER et al (1984) Differences between estrogen and antiestrogen-estrogen receptor complexes identified with an antibody raised against the estrogen receptor. Cancer Res 44:1012–1018

Tora L, Mullick A, Metzger D et al (1989) The cloned human oestrogen receptor contains a mutation which alters its hormone binding properties. EMBO J 8:1981–1986

Tzukerman MT, Esty A, Santiso-Mere D et al (1994) Human estrogen receptor transactivational capacity is determined by both cellular and promoter context and mediated by two functionaly distinct intramolecular regions. Mol Endocrinol 18:21–30

Wolf DM, Jordan VC (1994a) Characterization of tamoxifen stimulated MCF-7 tumor variants grown in athymic mice. Breast Cancer Res Treat 31:117–127

Wolf DM, Jordan VC (1994b) The estrogen receptor from a tamoxifen stimulated MCF-7 tumor variant contains a point mutation in the ligand binding domain. Breast Cancer Res Treat 31:129–138

Wolf DM, Langan-Fahey SM, Parker CP et al (1993) Investigation of the mechanism of tamoxifen-stimulated breast tumor growth using non-isomerizable analogs of tamoxifen and metabolites. J Natl Cancer Inst 85:806–812

Aromatase Inhibitors and Their Use in the Adjuvant Setting

R. C. Coombes

Department of Cancer Medicine, Division of Medicine, Imperial College School of Medicine, Charing Cross Hospital, Fulham Palace Road, London, W6 8RF, UK

Introduction

The aromatase enzyme is a cytochrome-P450-mediated enzyme complex responsible for the conversion of the androgens androstenedione and testosterone to estrone and oestradiol respectively. The idea of treating estrogen-dependent breast cancer with aromatase inhibitors has been recognised for several years. Indeed, aminoglutethimide was the first compound with which this approach was shown to be clinically effective (Santen et al. 1978). Trials using aminoglutethimide in advanced breast cancer showed that responses occurred in between 20% and 40% of women so treated and the remission duration ranged from 6 to 12 months (Harris et al. 1983; Santen et al. 1978). A major feature that emerged from these studies was the toxicity of aminoglutethimide. Side effects included skin rash, drowsiness and the inhibition of cortisol synthesis, which necessitated the use of corticosteroids with their concomitant side effects. These observations led to various studies in which lower doses of aminoglutethimide were used in the treatment of patients with breast cancer (Harris et al. 1983; Stuart-Harris et al. 1985). However, the responses seen with lower doses of aminoglutethimide were generally lower and the duration of response was reduced compared with higher dosages, although formal trials comparing different dose regimens and using sufficient numbers of patients to provide the necessary statistical power have not been adequately carried out and confirmed.

Second-Generation Aromatase Inhibitors

4-Hydroxyandrostenedione

4-Hydroxyandrostenedione is a compound that has been shown to possess irreversible binding to the enzyme substrate binding sites (Brodie et al. 1981). This effect would lead one to expect that the compound would cause permanent inactivation and a high degree of selectivity for aromatase. Prolonged inhibition of the enzyme would be likely to result, since recovery of activity is dependent on the rate of neosynthesis of the enzyme. Several studies have been carried out using 4-hydroxyandrostenedione over the past 13 years. Essentially these studies were initially conducted using a lyophilised microcrystalline material given at a dosage of 250 mg every 2 weeks. Peak levels were seen on the 1st and 2nd day after injection with a fall to less than 50% of peak levels by day 4. Thereafter the fall in serum 4-hydroxyandrostenedione was approximately log-linear with an apparent half-life of between 5 and 10 days.

4-Hydroxyandrostenedione is principally metabolised to the 4-hydroxyandrostenedione glucuronide, which is found in the patients' urine to between 14% and 35% of the administered dose. Major routes of metabolism are via dehydrogenation, reduction of the ketone functional groups, reduction of the C4/C5 double bond and hydroxylation at the C5 position (Poon et al. 1991).

Clinical studies began, as mentioned, at the dosage of 250 mg every 2 weeks (Coombes et al. 1984). This dosage selection was based on plasma estrogen measurements in which we compared the suppression obtained with a single injection of 4-hydroxyandrostenedione at dosages of 125 mg to 500 mg. Comparison of 250 mg and 500 mg showed equivalent degrees of initial suppression but there was an indication of minor recovery in the patients receiving the lower dose. The slightly lower pharmacological effectiveness was confirmed in studies using in vivo aromatisation in which the 250-mg dose reduced peripheral aromatisation to 15.2% of base-line in comparison to a reduction to 8.1% with the 500-mg dose ($p<0.05$) (Jones et al. 1992). Serum estrone levels measured by GCMS have been found to fall in parallel with estradiol levels during intramuscular treatment. Comparison of parenteral with oral administration of 4-hydroxyandrostenedione has shown that there is a trend in favour of the intramuscular route of administration, but this is not statistically significant.

Other endocrine effects of 4-hydroxyandrostenedione were generally not seen. There were no significant effects on luteinising hormone, follicle stimulating hormone, sex hormone binding globulin (SHBG) or dehydroxyepiandrostenedione sulphate (DHEAS), testosterone, 5a-dihydroxyhydrotestosterone or androstenedione when the drug is given intramuscularly. However, when the drug is given orally a small increase in DHEAS levels are seen. Oral administration of 4-hydroxyandrostenedione is also associated with a dose-related fall in SHBG (Dowsett et al. 1992), and this may be a reflection of the minor androgenic activity associated with the drug.

The drug is clinically extremely effective. In the studies which we carried out (Coombes et al. 1992) we treated 186 patients of whom 136 received therapy for at least 4 weeks. The overall complete and partial response rate was 26%. A major determinant of response was estrogen receptor status of the primary tumor, since 93% of objective responders whose estrogen receptor staturs was known had estrogen-receptor-positive tumors. Prior successful therapy with endocrine therapy was also a determinant, since only 2 of 35 patients responded amongst those who had failed to respond to other prior endocrine therapy. In these studies the drug was extremely well tolerated, with only a minority having any adverse effects; thus, 13% of patients on the dosage of 250 mg every 2 weeks complained of some local side effect, principally pain and inflammation at the site of the injection. Only one patient showed androgenic side effects, but anaphylactoid reactions occurred in five patients, presumed to be due to inadvertent intravenous administration.

4-Hydroxyandrostenedione has been given in combination with other endocrine agents. Encouraging results were obtained with a combination of 4-hydroxyandrostenedione and goserelin, the GNRH agonist which is currently used for medical ovariectomy. Goserelin is not able to affect peripheral aromatisation, but in patients who respond to goserelin and then relapse the subsequent addition of 4-hydroxyandrostenedione led to further reduction in estradiol and subsequent response in a high proportion of patients (Stein et al. 1990). Others (Lonning et al. 1992) have also studied the combination of aminoglutethimide and 4-hydroxyandrostenedione in post-menopausal breast cancer patients. Significant further falls in estradiol, estrone and estrone sulphate were achieved on the addition of aminoglutethimide, with the greatest fall effect being on estrone sulphate. Two patients achieved an objective tumor response on the further addition of aminoglutethimide.

4-Hydroxyandrostenedione has also been used in the neo-adjuvant setting (Gazet et al. 1996). In this study patients with invasive breast cancer were assigned to pre-treatment based on estrogen receptor status. Although patients with hormone-receptor-negative tumors received chemotherapy, patients with estrogen-receptor-positive tumors received 4-hydroxyandrostenedione if they were post-menopausal. Treatment was continued for 3 months and 34 patients received 4-hydroxyandrostenedione with an overall response rate of 35%.

This suggests that 4-hydroxyandrostenedione could be used as a neo-adjuvant therapy to reduce the size of large or unresectable primary breast carcinomas.

Fadrozole Hydrochloride

Fadrozole hydrochloride is a tetra-hydro-imidazole pyridine derivative and is an example of a non-steroidal aromatase inhibitor. Initial studies by Dowsett et al. (1994) in a double-blind randomised endocrine study of three dosages of oral fadrozole hydrochloride in 80 post-menopausal patients showed substantial falls in estradiol, estrone and estrone sulphate. However, complete suppression was not maintained throughout the 12-h dosing period, and there were significant increases in 17-hydroxyprogesterone and androstenedione thought to be due to a block of 11-β-hydroxylase. A statistically non-significant fall in aldosterone levels ($p = 0.06$) during treatment was seen but no electrolyte changes were observed. The clinical efficacy of fadrozole hydrochloride was studied by Bonnefoi et al. (1996) in this same group of women and an objective response rate of 17% was seen with no complete responders. Fifteen patients (21%) had stable disease and 45 patients (63%) had progressive disease. Median duration of objective response was 36 weeks and the time to treatment failure was 12.7 weeks. There was no difference between the three dosages (1 mg, 2 mg and 4 mg per day) used. The most common side effect was moderate nausea in 11 patients.

Fadrozole hydrochloride appeared to be an effective and relatively safe aromatase inhibitor which possessed the possible disadvantage of inhibition of aldosterone synthesis.

Third Generation Aromatase Inhibitors

New aromatase inhibitors include letrozole, anastrozole and vorozole, all of which are non-steroidal aromatase inhibitors, and exemestane, which is an example of a steroidal third-generation aromatase inhibitor.

Regarding the non-steroidal aromatase inhibitors, several clinical studies have now been done to assess their efficacy and tolerability. Johnston et al. (1994) studied vorozole at three separate doses (1, 2.5 and 5 mg) in 24 postmenopausal patients with breast cancer. Increasing doses of vorozole showed more potent suppression of estradiol, estrone and estrone sulphate. Eight out of 24 patients achieved an objective response: these were principally patients who had responded to tamoxifen. Aside from a slight reduction in serum cortisol, no other endocrine changes were seen.

Vorozole has also been compared to aminoglutethimide in tamoxifen-treated patients. In one study 277 patients received vorozole and 279 patients received aminoglutethimide; responses were seen in 23% and 18% respectively. Drug-related adverse events were seen in only 31% of patients receiving vorozole and in 53% of patients receiving aminoglutethimide (Bergh et al. 1997). Vorozole has also been compared with Megace (megestrol acetate) in tamoxifen-treated patients; complete and partial response rates were seen in 10.5% of vorozole and 7.6% of patients receiving Megace but weight gain occurred in 14% of patients receiving Megace compared with only 1% of patients receiving vorozole. These preliminary results were presented to the American Society of Clinical Oncology (Goss et al 1997).

Anastrozole was assessed in an early clinical study (Plourde et al. 1994) and this showed considerable suppression at doses between 1 and 20 mg. No other endocrine changes were observed. A study by Buzdar et al. (1997) compared Arimidex (anastrozole) 1 mg, Arimidex 10 mg and Megace 160 mg in 386 tamoxifen-treated patients. No differences in response rates were seen. However, side effects differed, with weight gain being more prevalent in Megace-treated patients and gastrointestinal side effects in anastrozole-treated patients.

In a further study letrozole was given at 0.5 and 2.5 mg with aminoglutethimide at 500 mg daily and more than 170 patients were accrued in each arm of the study. Complete and partial responses were seen in 16.7% of the patients receiving the lower dose of letrozole and 17.8% of those receiving the higher dose, whereas only 11.2% of aminoglutethimide patients responded. Treatment-related adverse events were seen in 28%, 32% and 45% respectively (Marty et al. 1997).

Exemestane (FCE 24304) was developed some 15 years ago. It is a compound which causes a time-dependent inactivation of human placental aromatase (TR 13.9 min) and to have a Ki of 26 nm, thus showing an affinity for the enzyme to be 2.6-fold higher than the substrate androstenedione. In preclinical studies exemestane induced a high rate of regression in DMBA-induced mammary tumors in rats (30% at 10 mg/kg and 73% at 50 mg/kg) and these dosages caused an 86% and a 93% decrease in total ovarian aromatase activity respectively (di Salle et al. 1989; Zaccheo et al. 1991). A phase I endocrine study of exemestane was carried out by Evans et al. (1992). In this study, exemestane was given at dosages between 0.5 and 800 mg to groups of three or four patients. The minimal dose which produced a maximum suppression of plasma estrogen was 25 mg. Although in this study there was evidence that some of the metabolites of exemestane interfered with some of the assays used, estrone, estradiol and estrone sulphate were reduced to 35%, 28% and 39% of basal values. No clinically adverse events were attributed to the drug during this study.

Subsequent to this, 27 post-menopausal, heavily pre-treated patients with metastatic breast cancer were selected for exemestane treatment. Exemestane was given again at between 5 and 600 mg daily to three or four subjects per dosage; treatment was given for at least 12 weeks and, if the disease had stabilised of response by the end of the 12-week period, continued until tumor progression. Minor side effects were seen including dizziness, headaches, hot flushes and nausea. Objective response was seen in 8 (2 CR and 6 PR) of the 24 evaluable patients (33%), (95% confidence intervals 18%–53%). Mean duration of response was 42 weeks (range 12–72 weeks plus). These studies indicated that exemestane was an effective and relatively well tolerated third-generation aromatase inhibitor, and other subsequent studies have confirmed that the drug is highly active.

Adjuvant Studies with Aromatase Inhibitors

The first study of aromatase inhibitors in the adjuvant setting was published by Coombes et al. (1987), in which aminoglutethimide at a dose of 1g daily with hydrocortisone supplementation was given to patients with breast cancer in a randomised trial. Although this study showed an improvement in disease-free survival, the side effects of the drug were significant and many patients had to reduce or stop treatment early. The second study in which aromatase inhibitors have been given in the adjuvant setting was published by Gazet et al. in 1996. In this study, 4-hydroxyandrostenedione was given to patients with primary breast cancer but was continued for a total of 18 months. This study, in which endocrine treatment was randomised to be given before or after surgery, is due to be published shortly (Gazet et al., in preparation).

These studies have spurred on the development of adjuvant studies using the newer aromatase inhibitors. Studies proposed include trials in which letrozole is being compared directly with tamoxifen and in which letrozole is being given in sequence after tamoxifen or vice versa. Further studies are comparing anastrozole with tamoxifen, both given for 5 years, and anastrozole and tamoxifen in combination given for 5 years compared with each drug given alone.

The exemestane study group has been set up to evaluate the use of exemestane when given after tamoxifen therapy. In this study we are intending to compare disease-free survival and survival of women who received tamoxifen for 5 years compared with women who received tamoxifen for 2–3 years and exemestane for 2–3 years (total treatment duration 5 years). The study is now underway in several countries around the world.

Summary

Over the past decade several novel aromatase inhibitors have been introduced into clinical practice. The discovery of these drugs followed on from the observation that the main mechanism of action of aminoglutethemide was via inhibition of the enzyme aromatase, thereby reducing peripheral levels of estradiol in post-menopausal patients. The second-generation drug 4-hydroxyandrostenedione was introduced in 1990, and although its use was limited by its need to be given parenterally, it was found to be a well-tolerated form of endocrine therapy. The third-generation inhibitors include vorozole, letrozole, anastrozole and exemestane, the former three being non-steroidal inhibitors, the latter being a steroidal inhibitor. All these compounds are capable of reducing estrogen levels to within 5%–10% of baseline levels compared with 20%–30% base line levels in the case of 4-hydroxyandrostenedione. Studies are currently in progress to determine the value of these third-generation aromatase inhibitors in the adjuvant setting. These studies include head-to-head comparison of aromatase inhibitor with tamoxifen, sequential aromatase inhibitor after tamoxifen and first-line aromatase inhibitor followed by adjuvant tamoxifen. Current issues revolve around the toxicity of these compounds in terms of effects on the cardiovascular system and bone.

References

Bergh J, Bonneterre J, Illiger HJ, Murray R, Nortier J, Paridaens R, Rubens RD, Samonigg H, Van Zyl J for the Vorozole Study Group (1997) Vorozole (Rivizor) versus aminoglutethimide (AG) in the treatment of postmenopausal breast cancer relapsing after tamoxifen. Meeting of the American Society of clinical Oncology (ASCO), Denver, CO, 17–20 May 1997, Abstract 543

Bonnefoi HR, Smith IE, Dowsett M, Trunet PF, Houston SJ, da Luz RJ, Rubens RD, Coombes RC, Powles TJ (1996) Therapeutic effects of the aromatase inhibitor fadrozole hydrochloride in advanced breast cancer. Br J Cancer 73:539–542

Brodie AMH, Garrett WM, Hendrickson JR, Tsai-Morris CH, Marcotte PA, Robinson CH (1981) Inactivation of aromatase in vitro by 4-hydroxy-4-androstene-3,17-dione and 4-acetoxy-4-androstene-3,17-dione and sustained effects in vivo. Steroids 38:693–702

Buzdar AU, Jones SE, Vogel CL, Wolter J, Plourde P, Webster A for the Arimidex Study Group (1997) A phase III trial comparing anastrozole (! and 10 milligrams), a potent and selective aromatase inhibitor, with megestrol acetate in postmenopausal women with advanced breast carcinoma. Cancer 79:730–739

Coombes RC, Goss P, Dowsett M, Gazet J-C, Brodie A (1984) 4-Hydroxyandrostenone in treatment of postmenopausal patients with advanced breast cancer. Lancet 2:1237–1239

Coombes RC, Powles TJ, Easton D, Chilvers C, Ford HT, Smith IE, McKinna A, White H, Bradbeer J, Yarnold J, Nash A, Bettelheim R, Dowsett M, Gazet J-C Investigators of the Collaborative Breast Cancer Project (1987) Adjuvant aminoglutethimide therapy for postmenopausal patients with primary breast cancer. Cancer Res 47:2496–2499

Coombes RC, Hughes SWM, Dowsett M (1992) 4-hydroxy-androstenedione: a new treatment for postmenopausal patients with breast cancer. Eur J Cancer 28A:1941–1945

Di Salle E, Briatico G, Giudici D, Ornati G, Zaccheo T (1989) Aromatase inhibition and experimental antitumor activity of FCE24304, MDL 18962 and SH489. J Steroid Biochem 34:431–434

Dowsett M, Mehta A, King N, Smith IE, Powles TJ, Stein RC, Coombes RC (1992) An endocrine and pharmacokinetic study of 4 oral doses of formestane in post-menopausal breast cancer patients. Eur J Cancer 28:415–420

Dowsett M, Smithers D, Moore J, Trunet PF, Coombes RC, Powles TJ, Rubens R, Smith IE (1994) Endocrine changes with the aromatase inhibitor fadrozole hydrochloride in breast cancer. Eur J Cancer 30A:1453–1458

Evans RTJ, Di Salle E, Ornati G, Lassus M, Benedetti MS, Pianezzola E, Coombes RC (1992) Phase I and endocrine study of exemestane (FCE24304), a new aromatase inhibitor, in postmenopausal women. Cancer Res 52:5933–5939

Gazet J-C, Coombes RC, Ford HT, Griffin M, Corbishley C, Makinde V, Lowndes S, Quilliam J, Sutcliffe R (1996) Assessment of the effect of pretreatment with neoadjuvant therapy on primary breast cancer. Br J Cancer 73:758–762

Goss P, Wine E, Tannock I, Schwartz IH, Kremer AB for the North American Vorozole Study Group (1997) Vorozole versus Megace in postmenopausal patients with metastatic breast carcinoma who had relapsed following tamoxifen. Meeting of the American Society of Clinical Oncology (ASCO), Denver, CO, 17–20 May 1997, Abstract S42

Harris AL, Dowsett M, Smith IE; Jeffcoate SL (1983) Endocrine effects of low dose aminoglutethimide alone in advanced postmenopausal breast cancer. Br J Cancer 47:621–627

Johnston SRD, Smith IE, Doody D, Jacobs S, Robertshaw H, Dowsett M (1994) Clinical and endocrine effects of the oral aromatase inhibitor vorozole in postmenopausal patients with advanced breast cancer. Cancer Res 54:5875–5881

Jones AL, MacNeil F, Jacobs S, Lonning PE, Dowsett M, Powles TJ (1992) The influence of intramuscular 4-hydroxyandrostenedione on peripheral aromatisation in breast cancer patients. Eur J Cancer 28:1712–1716

Lonning PE, Dowsett M, Jones A, Ekse D, Jacobs S, MacNeill F, Johannessen DC, Powles TJ (1992) Influence of aminoglutethimide on plasma estrogen levels in breast cancer patients on 4-hydroxyandrostennedione treatment. Breast Cancer Res Treat 23:57–62

Marty M, Gershanovich M, Campos B, Romieu G, Lurie H, Bonaventura T, Jeffrey M, Buzzi F, Ludwig H, Bodrogi I, Reichardt P, Higgins N, Chaudri HA, Friederich P, Biachoff MA for the Letrozole International Trial Group (AR/BC3) (1997) Letrozole, a new potent selective aromatase inhibitor (Al) superior to aminoglutethimide (AG), in postmenopausal women with advanced breast cancer (ABC) previously treated with anti-estrogens. Meeting of the American Society of Clinical Oncology (ASCO), Denver, CO, 17–20 May 1997, Abstract 544

Plourde OV, Dyroff M, Dukes M (1994) Arimidex, a potent an selective fourth-generation aromatase inhibitor. Breast Cancer Res Treat 30:103–111

Poon GK, Jarman M, Rowlands MG, Dowsett M, Firth J (1991) Determination of 4-hydroxy-andros-4-ene-3,17-dione metabolism in breast cancer patients using HPLC/MS. J Chromatogr 565:75–88

Santen RJm Santner S, Davis B, Veldhuis J, Samojlik E, Ruby E (1978) Aminoglutethimide inhibits extraglandular estrogen production in postmenopausal women with breast carcinoma. J Clin Endocrinol Metab 47:1257–1265

Stein RC, Dowsett M, Hedley A, Coombes RC (1990) The clinical and endocrine effects of 4-hydroxyandrostenedione alone and in combination with goserelin in premenopausal women with advanced breast cancer. Br J Cancer 62:679–683

Stuart-Harris R, Dowsett M, DeSouza A (1985) Endocrine effects of low dose aminoglutethimide as an aromatase inhibitor in the treatment of breast cancer. Clin Endocrinol 22:219–226

Zaccheo T, Giudici D, Ornati G, Panzeri A, Di Salle E (1991) Comparison of the effects of the irreversible aromatase inhibitor, exemestane, with atamestane and MDL 18962 in rats with DMBA-induced mammary tumors. Eur J Cancer 27:1145–1150

GnRH Analogues and Ovarian Ablation: Their Integration in the Adjuvant Strategy

K. I. Pritchard

Department of Medical Oncology, Sunnybrook Health Science Center, Bayview Regional Cancer Center, 2075 Bayview Avenue, Toronto M4N 3M5, Canada

Ovarian ablation has been used for the treatment of metastatic breast cancer since the 1890s. It may have been first used by Beatson, who found it useful in shrinking tumors in pre-menopausal women with widespread metastatic disease (Beatson 1896). It was probably Schinzinger, however, who first suggested the use of (surgical) ovarian removal before or at the time of mastectomy in order to "involute the breast" and thus "contain tumour cells" (Schinzinger 1889). The subsequent development of methods for irradiating the ovaries led to the suggestion that ovarian radiation ablation might prove useful as adjuvant therapy at or around the time of breast removal (Taylor 1934). A series of small studies of ovarian ablation were subsequently carried out, but they were difficult to interpret due to their small size and the lack of sophisticated methodologic approaches to analysis. Enthusiasm for adjuvant ovarian ablation dwindled following the promising early results of adjuvant chemotherapy in the mid-1970s (Bonadonna et al. 1976; Fisher et al. 1975).

In the early 1980s, however, a number of factors combined to reawaken interest in adjuvant hormonal therapy. First, it became apparent that chemotherapy was not the panacea for the prevention of recurrence in this situation. Several new and more easily administered hormonal agents became available for the treatment of metastatic disease (Santen et al. 1977; Legha et al. 1978; Legha and Carter 1976), and estrogen and progesterone receptors were becoming widely used to assess the potential responsiveness of tumors to endocrine approaches. The development, in 1984, of the Early Breast Cancer Trialists' Collaborative Group (EBCTCG) led to a broad and very useful meta-analysis approach to the available trials of both chemotherapy and ovarian ablation in the adjuvant setting. This approach clarified for the first time that ovarian ablation did have a substantial effect when given as adjuvant therapy in pre-menopausal women.

If one examines the EBCTCG meta-analysis of ovarian ablation as adjuvant therapy, one can look at three separate groups of trials which can then be combined for an overall impression. The first is a series of ten small randomized trials of ovarian ablation compared to no systemic therapy (Table 1). Most of these trials included both pre- and post-menopausal patients,

Table 1. Randomized trials of ovarian ablation versus no systemic therapy

Trial	Ovarian treatment	Accrual period	No of. randomized patients		Data available	Published
			< 50 years	> 50 years		
Paterson (Christie)	450 rad	1948–50	178	11	Yes	Yes (Paterson et al. 1959; Cole 1975)
Nissen-Meyer (Norwegian)	1000 rad	1957–63	151	195	Yes	Yes (Nissen-Meyer 1967, 1975, 1991)
Nevinny (Boston)	Surgery	1961–[a]		143	No	Yes (Nevinny et al. 1969)
Ravdin (NSABP)	Surgery	1961–67	184	0	Yes	Yes (Ravdin et al. 1970)
Bryant & Weir (Saskatchewan)	Surgery	1964–74	255	124	Yes	Yes (Bryant et al. 1981)
Meakin & Hayward (Princess Margaret Hospital Toronto)	2000 rad[b]	1965–72	349	430	Yes	Yes (Meakin et al. 1979, 1983, 1996)
Ontario Cancer Treatment and Research Foundation	1500 rad	1968–77	9	323	Yes	Yes (Clarke et al. 1990)
CRFB Cancer Agency	900/1400 rad	1971–76	1	51	Yes	Yes (Delozier et al. 1990)
Bradford Royal Infirmary	Surgery	1974–85	42	9	Yes	No
Subtotal (except Nevinny)		1948–85	1169	1143	Yes	

NSABP, National Surgical Adjuvant Breast Project; CRFB, Centre Régionale François Baclesse.
[a] 143 patients were randomized but there are no individual patient data available on accrual period, age distribution or outcome.
[b] Stratum 1: control vs 2000 rad.

but the small majority of women were under 50. These trials were carried out between 1948 and 1985 and include over 1200 pre-menopausal women. When one looks at each of these studies individually, none is large enough to show a statistically significant improvement in either event-free or overall survival, although all trend in that direction. When the meta-analysis technique is applied, however, it is clear that the annual odds of an event (recurrence or death) are significantly reduced by about 25% [standard deviation (SD)±7] ($p = 0.0005$) (Fig. 1). The annual odds of death are similarily reduced by 24% (SD±7) ($p = 0.0006$) (Fig. 2).

A second group of trials which accrued patients between 1974 and 1985 consisted of five small randomized studies of ovarian ablation plus chemotherapy versus the same chemotherapy used alone (Table 2). Most of the patients in these studies were pre-menopausal. Over 900 were studied in all. Here once again, most of the trials trend toward, showing a benefit in favor of ovarian ablation (4/5 in event-free survival; 3/5 in survival) but, when summed, the overall reduction in annual odds of event is only 10% (SD±9) ($p > 0.1$; not significant) (Fig. 1). Similarly, the annual odds of death are reduced by 8% (SD =±10) ($p > 0.1$; not significant) (Fig. 2b). Thus, perhaps because of the smaller number of patients studied and/or less prolonged follow-up, or perhaps because of a smaller effect in this setting, it seems less

Table 2. Randomized trials of ovarian ablation plus chemotherapy versus chemotherapy alone

Trial	Ovarian treatment	Common systemic therapy	Accrual period	No of. randomized patient < 50 years	> 50 years	Data available	Published
Bradford RI	Surgery	M+TT	1974–85	38	5	Yes	No
Toronto-Edmonton study group	1500 rad +P	CMF[a] (some±TT)	1978–88	241	56	Yes[b]	No
Ragaz BCCA Vancouver	1600 rad +P	CMF	1979–85	111	23	Yes[b]	Yes (Ragaz et al. 1988)
IBCSG/ Ludwig II	Surgery	CMF+P	1978–81	281	75	Yes[b]	Yes (LBCSG 1985)
SWOG 7827 B	Surgery	CMFVP	1979–89	262	52	Yes[b]	No
Subtotal			1974–89	933	211		

RI, Radiotherapy Institute; IBCSG, International Breast Cancer Study Group; BCCA, British Columbia Cancer Agency; SWOG, SouthWest Oncology Group; LBCSG, Ludwig Breast Cancer Study Group. Treatments: IT, immunotherapy; F, 5-fluorouracil; TT, thiotepa; C, cyclophosphamide; V, vincristine; M, methotrexate; P, prednisone.
[a] First patients were cross-randomized to receive or not to receive immunotherapy with oral BCG (bacillus Calmette-Guerin).
[b] Estrogen receptor status available only in these studies.

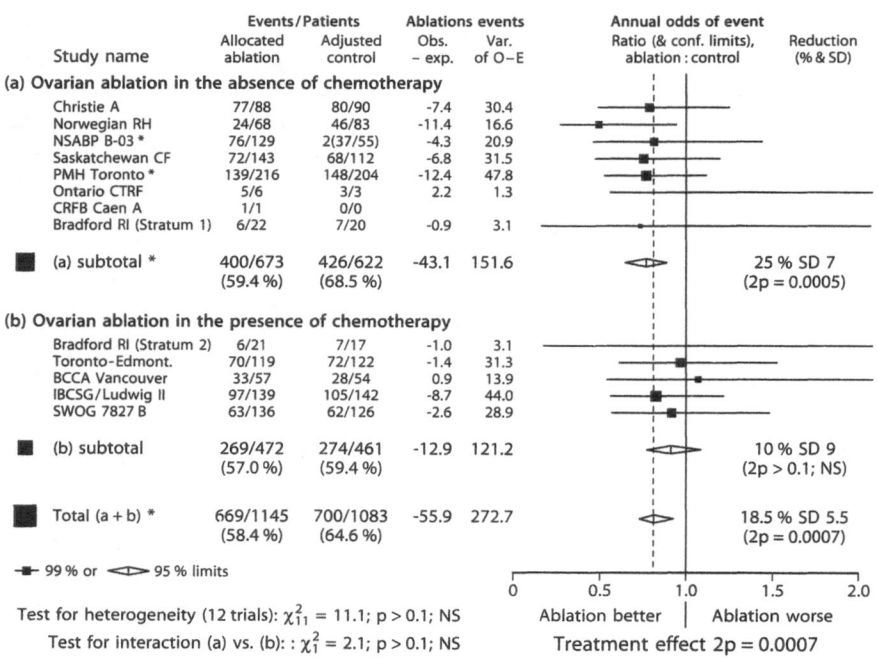

Study name	Events/Patients Allocated ablation	Adjusted control	Ablations events Obs. – exp. of O–E	Var.	Annual odds of event Ratio (& conf. limits), ablation : control	Reduction (% & SD)
(a) Ovarian ablation in the absence of chemotherapy						
Christie A	77/88	80/90	-7.4	30.4		
Norwegian RH	24/68	46/83	-11.4	16.6		
NSABP B-03 *	76/129	2(37/55)	-4.3	20.9		
Saskatchewan CF	72/143	68/112	-6.8	31.5		
PMH Toronto *	139/216	148/204	-12.4	47.8		
Ontario CTRF	5/6	3/3	2.2	1.3		
CRFB Caen A	1/1	0/0				
Bradford RI (Stratum 1)	6/22	7/20	-0.9	3.1		
■ (a) subtotal *	400/673 (59.4 %)	426/622 (68.5 %)	-43.1	151.6		25 % SD 7 (2p = 0.0005)
(b) Ovarian ablation in the presence of chemotherapy						
Bradford RI (Stratum 2)	6/21	7/17	-1.0	3.1		
Toronto-Edmont.	70/119	72/122	-1.4	31.3		
BCCA Vancouver	33/57	28/54	0.9	13.9		
IBCSG/Ludwig II	97/139	105/142	-8.7	44.0		
SWOG 7827 B	63/136	62/126	-2.6	28.9		
■ (b) subtotal	269/472 (57.0 %)	274/461 (59.4 %)	-12.9	121.2		10 % SD 9 (2p > 0.1; NS)
■ Total (a + b) *	669/1145 (58.4 %)	700/1083 (64.6 %)	-55.9	272.7		18.5 % SD 5.5 (2p = 0.0007)

━■━ 99 % or ◁▷ 95 % limits

Test for heterogeneity (12 trials): χ^2_{11} = 11.1; p > 0.1; NS
Test for interaction (a) vs. (b): : χ^2_1 = 2.1; p > 0.1; NS

Ablation better | Ablation worse
Treatment effect 2p = 0.0007

* Adjustment: for balance, control patients in 2:1 randomisations contribute twice.
PMH contributes Stratum 1: 49/68 vs. 50/62 plus Stratum 2: 90/148 vs. 2(49/71)

Figs. 1, 2. Proportional effects of ovarian ablation in each trial and overall, with subdivisions by absence or presence of chemotherapy, among women aged under 50 at entry. Recurrence-free survival (Fig. 1) and overall survival (Fig. 2) for women aged under 50 when randomized, with subtotals for strata in the absence and in the presence of routine cytotoxic chemotherapy. Each trial, or part of a trial, is described by a single line of information, showing the numbers of events and patients and summary logrank statistics. For each of these strata, the ratio of the annual event rate in the ovarian ablation group to that in the control group (the odds ratio) is plotted as a *solid square*, with the 99% confidence interval shown. For the subtotals and total, the 95% confidence interval is represented by a *diamond*. The *solid vertical line* indicates an odds ratio of 1.0 (i.e., no difference between ovarian ablation and control), whereas the *broken vertical line* indicates the "typical odds ratio" in the total of all these trial results. For balance, control patients in the 2:1 randomizations (i.e., NSABP and part of PMH) are counted twice in the adjusted control totals but not in the statistical calculations. *NSABP,* National Surgical Adjuvant Breast Project; *CTRF,* Cancer Treatment and Research Foundation; *CRFB,* Centre Régionale François Baclesse; *RI* Royal infirmary; *BCCA,* British Columbia Cancer Agency; *IBCSG,* International Breast Cancer Study Group; *SWOG,* South West Oncology Group, Princess Margaret Hospital

clear that ovarian ablation adds significantly to the role of chemotherapy in this setting.

A third group of trials have been carried out between 1987 and the present (Table 3). These include four randomized studies of medical ovarian ablation versus control. In two of these studies, all patients also received 5-fluorouracil, adriamycin and cyclophosphamide (FAC) or 5-fluorouracil, epirubicin and cyclophosphamide (FEC) chemotherapy, while in three of the trials there was also a second randomization for patients to receive or not receive adjuvant tamoxifen. These trials include only pre-menopausal women,

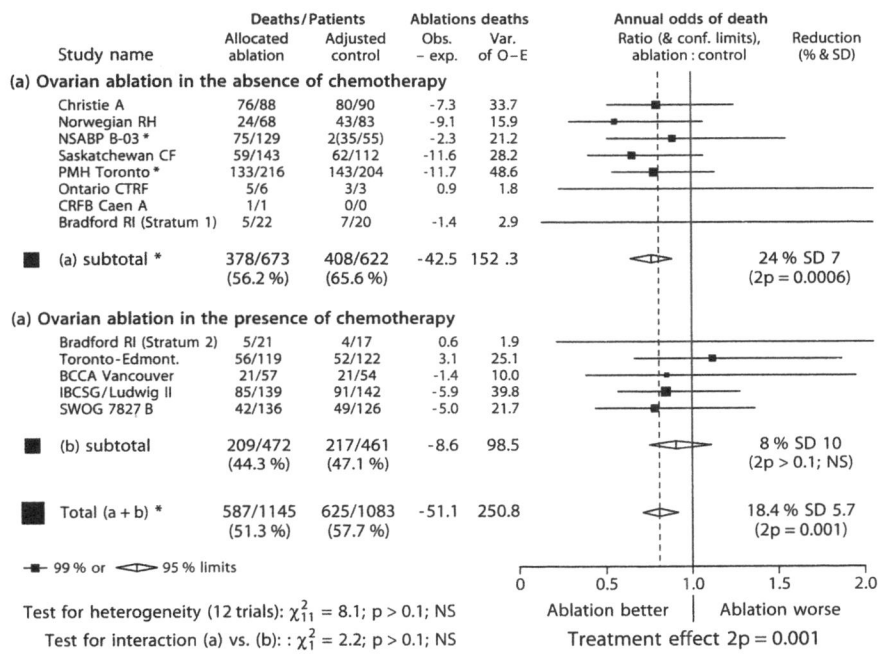

Fig. 2.

Table 3. Randomized trials of medical ovarian ablation

Trial	Ovarian treatment	Common systemic therapy	Accrual period	No. of randomized patients		Data available	Published
				<50 years	>50 years		
CRC under 50's	Goserelin (Zoladex)	± Tamoxifen	1987-SR	972	0	No	No
FNCLCC (France)	Triptorelin or goserelin (Zoladex)	FAC or FEC	1989-SR	746	120	No	No
Southeast Sweden	Goserelin (Zoladex)	± Tamoxifen	1989-SR	191	0	No	No
ECOG EST 5188	Goserelin (Zoladex)	FAC±tamoxifen	1989–94	1382	155	No	No
Subtotal			1987	3291	275		

CRC, Cancer Research Campaign; FNLCC, Fédération Nationale des Centres de Lutte contre le Cancer; ECOG, Eastern Cooperative Oncology Group.
F, 5-Fluorouracil; C, cyclophosphamide; V, vincristine; A, adriamycin (doxorubicin); E, epirubicin; SR, still randomizing patients; ±, randomization.

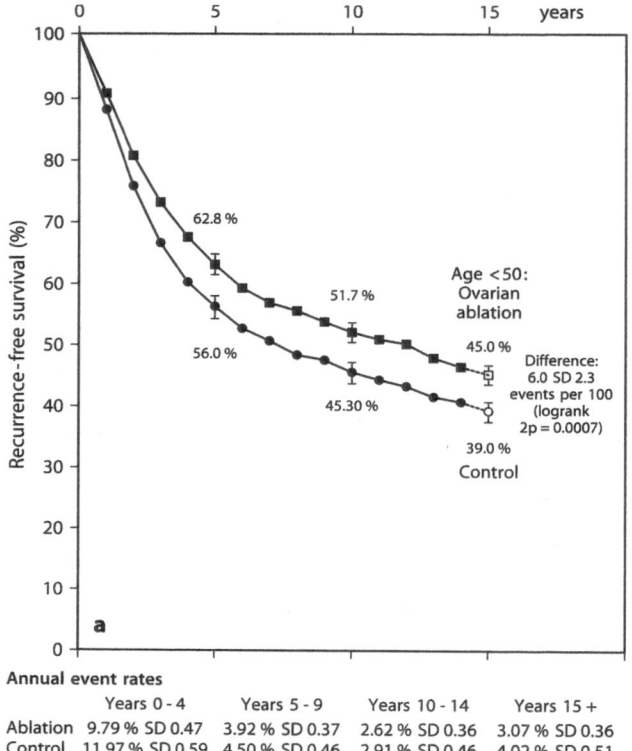

Fig. 3a, b. Absolute effects of ovarian ablation in all trials combined among women aged under 50 at entry. Recurrence-free survival (**a**) and overall survival (**b**) for 2102 women aged under 50 when randomized between ovarian ablation (*squares*) and control (*circles*). *Bars* indicate standard deviations (SD)

although a few are over the age of 50. There are 3291 pre-menopausal women under 50 included in these trials. As yet, however, no outcome data have been published or made available to the EBCTCG analysis group.

When one looks at all of these data on ovarian ablation combined, without regard to whether the control arms of the studies included chemotherapy or not, one sees a clear benefit for ovarian ablation overall. Event-free survival is reduced by 18.5% (SD±5.5) ($p=0.0007$), while annual odds of death are reduced by 18.4% overall (SD±5.7) ($p=0.001$) (Fig. 3). Perhaps most significant of all, the difference between the women receiving ovarian ablation and those in the control arms persists out to 15 or more years of follow-up. At 15 or more years of follow-up, recurrence-free survival for women receiving ovarian ablation is 45% in comparison to 49% in the control arm, while at 15 or more years of follow-up, overall survival is 52.4% for the women receiving ovarian ablation in comparison to 46.1% in the control arm (Fig. 3b). Similarly when one divides women as to whether or not they had tumour involvement of their nodes at the time of surgery, one sees a significant recurrence-free survival difference

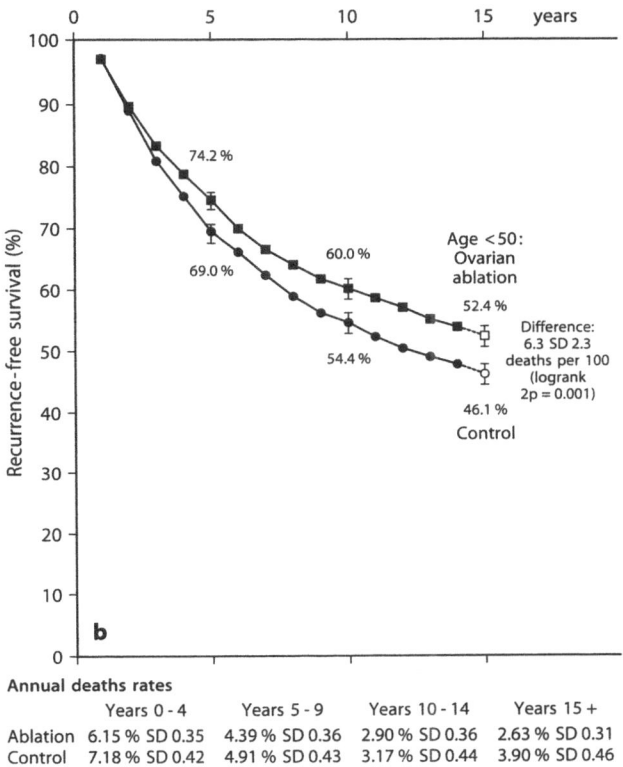

Annual deaths rates

	Years 0 - 4	Years 5 - 9	Years 10 - 14	Years 15 +
Ablation	6.15 % SD 0.35	4.39 % SD 0.36	2.90 % SD 0.36	2.63 % SD 0.31
Control	7.18 % SD 0.42	4.91 % SD 0.43	3.17 % SD 0.44	3.90 % SD 0.46

Fig. 3 b

at 15 or more years, of 75.4% versus 66.5% for node-negative women and of 37.4% versus 24% for node-positive women (Fig. 4a), and a significant differ-ence in survival of 76.6% versus 70.9% for node-negative women and of 41.7% versus 29.2% for node-positive women at 15 or more years of follow-up (Fig. 4b). Thus, it seems clear that, overall, ovarian ablation adds significantly to the prevention of recurrence and to improvement of survival, but that this effect is more clearly seen when ovarian ablation is compared to no other sys-temic treatment, than when ovarian ablation plus chemotherapy is compared to the same chemotherapy given alone. The numbers of women in these sub-groups are small, however, and the trends, even in the group receiving ovarian ablation added to chemotherapy, are in a positive direction. Thus, the addition of data from larger studies such as those of medical ablation added to chemo-therapy will provide additional data which will clarify this situation.

It is of interest to look at the limited data on other causes of death in the EBCTCG results. One would think that women undergoing ovarian ablation prematurely might suffer from additional heart disease and osteoporosis and/or that they might be spared some risk of second breast primaries. Overall, however, these results do not seem to be seen in the EBCTG Over-

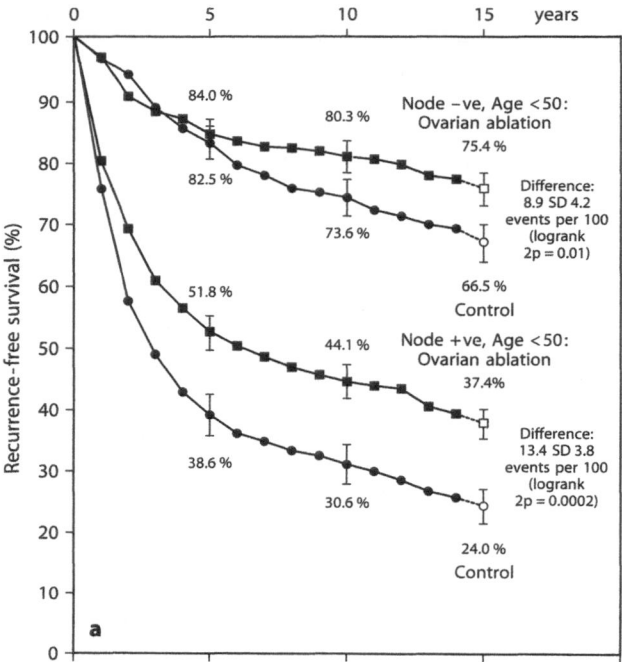

Fig. 4 a, b. Absolute effects of ovarian ablation in the absence of routine chemotherapy in all trials combined among women aged under 50 at entry. Recurrence-free survival (**a**) and overall survival (**b**) for 473 node-negative and 696 node-positive women who were aged under 50 when randomized between ovarian ablation (*squares*) and control (*circles*) in the trials, or parts of trials, where cytotoxic therapy was not routinely used. Among node-negative women, in years 0–4 there were 28 deaths out of 1170 person-years in the ablation group versus 25 of 1037 in the controls (annual death rates: 2.4% SD 0.5 versus 2.4% SD 0.5); in years 5–9, there were 15 of 1030 versus 21 of 884 (1.5% SD 0.4 versus 2.4% SD 0.5); in years 10–14, there were 12 of 931 versus 15 of 779 (1.3% SD 0.4 versus 1.9% SD 0.5); and in years 15+ there were 33 of 1580 versus 43 of 1309 (2.1% SD 0.4 versus 3.3% SD 0.5). Among node-positive women, the corresponding values are years 0–4, 166 of 1620 versus 134 of 997 (10.3% SD 0.8 versus 13.4% SD 1.2); years 5–9, 55 of 1077 versus 37 of 577 (5.1% SD 0.7 versus 6.4% SD 1.1); years 10–14, 29 of 870 versus 23 of 426 (3.3% SD 0.6 versus 5.4% SD 1.1); and years 15+, 40 of 1151 versus 28 of 491 (3.5% SD 0.6 versus 5.7% SD 1.1). Format as in Fig. 3

view. In fact, non-breast-cancer deaths are 22/922 in the ovarian ablation arm versus 20/824 in the control arm, while vascular deaths are 44/929 versus 30/824 respectively. Neither of these differences are significant. There are 30/712 and 32/679 second primaries. Once again, these differences are not significant. These rates of other causes of death and of second malignancies have been corrected for differences in event-free and overall survival in the two arms, related to the positive effects of ovarian ablation on breast cancer recurrence. It is worth stressing that few of these studies were designed to collect specific causes of death, or even occurrence of second primaries. Thus, these data in a meta-analysis situation must be regarded with some caution (Early Breast Cancer Trialists' Collaborative Group 1990, 1992, 1996).

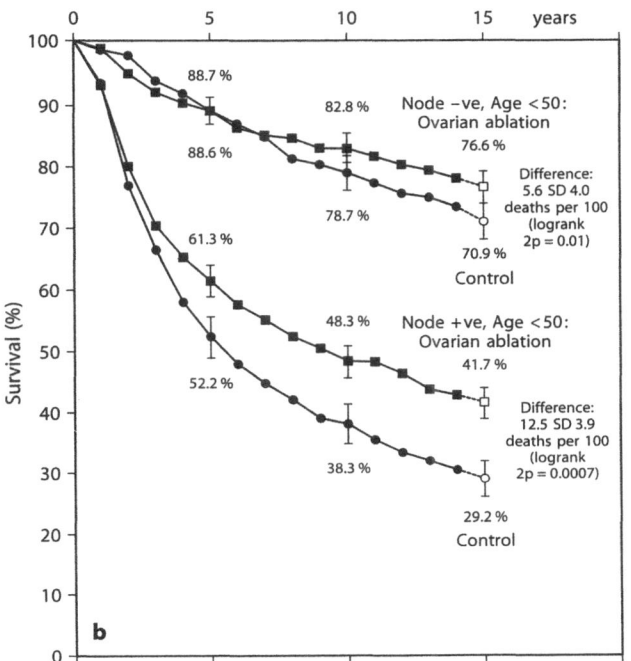

Fig. 4 b

If one looks at individual studies of ovarian ablation plus chemotherapy versus the same chemotherapy alone, of course one sees much the same results as those in the meta-analysis, since it is these results that make up the meta-analysis itself. One study worth discussing individually, however, is that of the International Breast Cancer Study Group (IBCSG, Ludwig Group), in which 356 women with four or more positive lymph nodes were randomized to receive cyclophosphamide, methotrexate, 5-FU and prednisone (CMFP) chemotherapy with or without ovarian surgical removal. Overall, there was no benefit for the addition of ovarian removal, but for estrogen-receptor-positive patients there was a trend approaching significance for improvement in disease-free and overall survival. Once again, there seems to be some effect of ovarian ablation added to this type of chemotherapy, but the effect is small. It is interesting that this effect has persisted in the IBCSG/Ludwig trial in spite of the fact that over 80% of patients in either arm of that study became amenorrhoeic as the result of CMFP therapy (Ludwig Breast Cancer Study Group 1985 a, b).

There are very few trials that directly compare chemotherapy to ovarian ablation. One notable exception is that of the Scottish Group, in which a number of pre-menopausal women with pathologic stage II breast cancer were randomized to receive cyclophosphamide, methotrexate, and 5-FU (CMF) chemotherapy versus adjuvant ovarian ablation (Scottish Cancer Trials Breast Group

1993). In this group, ovarian ablation was comparable in its effects to CMF in terms of recurrence and overall survival. When the women were divided by estrogen receptor status, however, it was clear that in those who were estrogen-receptor-positive, ovarian ablation tended to produce a better effect, while in those who were estrogen-receptor-negative, chemotherapy seemed somewhat better. It is worth noting that the chemotherapy given in this trial was somewhat less dose-intensive than standard Bonadonna CMF (Bonadonna et al. 1976). It is, of course, unclear whether any different chemotherapy dose or schedule would have produced different results.

In awaiting the results of the newer trials of medical ablation, one should consider whether the GnRH analogues are indeed equivalent to the more traditionally used surgical or radiation methods of ovarian ablation. First, it should be stated that radiation ablation was not always effective or complete. In a variety of studies, many women resume menstruation after ovarian irradiation. In that of Nissen-Meyer (1967, 1975, 1991) the failure rate was up to 13%, while in that of Meakin et al. (1979, 1983, 1996) the rate was 3.3%, but 7% in women under 45 years of age at the time of the ovarian ablation. Medical castration with GnRH analogues in most of the current group of trials is given for 2–5 years for medical ablation trials. It seems that the effect of GnRH analogues is reversible and that most women resume menstruation within a month or two after stopping administration of these drugs (West and Baird 1987). Thus, there is no reason to assume that 2–5 years of administration of these substances is necessarily equivalent to a permanent ovarian ablation. We do know, however, from at least one large trial in metastatic disease, that treatment with a GnRH analogue is equivalent to ovarian ablation (Taylor et al. 1998), so that at least in the short term these two manoeuvres should be relatively similar.

Last but not least, it is interesting to consider whether adjuvant chemotherapy in pre-menopausal women works in part through the mechanism of a medical castration. It has been long appreciated that similar chemotherapies appear to produce somewhat greater effects in pre- than in post-menopausal women, and long hypothesized that the reason for this differential effect may relate to chemical ovarian ablation. The incidence of amenorrhoea in several trials of adjuvant chemotherapy in pre-menopausal women ranges from 40%–90% (Rubens et al. 1983; Fisher et al. 1979; Bonadonna et al. 1981; Ludwig Breast Cancer Study Group 1985 a,b; Pourquier 1981; Howell et al. 1984). Several investigators have dissected the data from their studies in an attempt to see whether patients who become amenorrhoeic have a better result from adjuvant chemotherapy than those who do not. Three investigators have found a positive correlation (Ludwig Breast Cancer Study Group 1985 b; Pourquier 1981; Howell et al. 1984), but three others have not (Rubens et al. 1983; Fisher et al. 1979; Bonadonna et al. 1981). It seems likely that part of the effect of cytotoxic chemotherapy in pre-menopausal women is indeed endocrine. This would fit well with the data suggesting that similar chemotherapies produce greater results in pre-menopausal than in post-menopausal women, and also with the data just outlined suggesting that the addition of ovarian ablation to chemotherapy may be less effective than ovarian ablation given alone in the adjuvant setting.

In conclusion, it seems that ovarian ablation is effective therapy for pre-menopausal women, probably particularly for those who have high or positive estrogen and/or progesterone receptor levels. It also seems apparent that ovarian ablation may contribute a small additional benefit, particularly in es-trogen-receptor-positive and/or progesterone-receptor-positive women when given in addition to chemotherapy. Although at least one study shows that ovarian ablation may be equivalent to chemotherapy in estrogen-receptor- and progesterone-receptor-positive women in this setting, it is unclear that the chemotherapy that was compared is either a standard or the best available today. Newer chemotherapeutic agents may cause ovarian ablation in any case. Thus, the role of adding ovarian ablation in this situation is somewhat unclear, although in at least one trial (Ludwig) this still seemed to provide a small additional benefit. The role of medical ovarian ablation in comparison to the more standard surgical or radiation ablation is also somewhat unclear, particularly when the medical ablation is only given for 2–5 years. Furthermore, the role of ovarian ablation in comparison to tamoxifen in pre-menopausal women has not been well explored.

The upcoming data from our next EBCTCG meta-analysis (2000) should provide interesting results from four trials of medical ovarian ablation in pre-menopausal women. The total group of women studied is larger than that available for some of the earlier meta-analyses. Two studies will look at the question of medical ovarian ablation added to chemotherapy versus the same chemother-apy alone. These data should be of considerable additional benefit. In the meantime, further trials of the addition of ovarian ablation or of other endo-crine manoeuvres to standard current chemotherapy, or trials comparing endo-crine therapy directly to chemotherapy, would be of great interest.

Summary

Ovarian ablation, either by surgery or radiation, has been clearly shown to be an effective adjuvant therapy for pre-menopausal women following breast cancer surgery. The 1995 Oxford Overview confirmed this effect in trials of ovarian ablation compared to no other systemic adjuvant therapy. In trials of chemotherapy plus ovarian ablation compared to the same chemotherapy alone, however, the addition of ovarian ablation, although tending to add benefit, did not achieve a statistically significant positive effect. Data exist from a variety of randomized trials of adjuvant chemotherapy suggesting that pre-menopausal women who become amenorrhoeic after chemotherapy achieve a better outcome than those who continue to menstruate. These data are not consistent among all trials, however. There are few trials that com-pare ovarian ablation directly to chemotherapy, but those few that exist, as well as indirect comparisons, suggest that the effects of ovarian ablation, par-ticularly in estrogen-receptor-positive women, are similar in magnitude to those of chemotherapy. Several large trials comparing chemotherapy to the LH-RH analogue Zoladex (goserelin) and studying the addition of Zoladex to adjuvant chemotherapy will be available by 1999 or 2000 and will provide considerable additional information on this matter.

References

Beatson GT (1896) On the treatment of inoperable cases of carcinoma of the mamma: suggestions for a new method of treatment with illustrative cases. Lancet 2:104–107

Bonadonna G, Brusamolino E, Valagussa P, Rossi A, Brugnatelli L, Brambilla C, De Lena M, Tancini G, Bajetta E, Musumeci R, Veronesi U (1976) Combination chemotherapy as an adjuvant treatment in operable breast cancer. N Engl J Med 294:405–410

Bonadonna G, Valagussa P, DePalo G (1981) The results of adjuvant chemotherapy are predominantly caused by the hormonal changes such therapy induces. In: Van Scoy-Moscher MB (ed) Medical oncology. Controversies in cancer treatment. Hall, Boston, pp 100–109

Bryant AJS, Weir JA (1981) Prophylactic oophorectomy in operable instances of carcinoma of the breast. Surg Gynecol Obstet 153:660–664

Clarke EA, Fetterly JC, Ryan NC (1990) The Ontario Cancer Treatment and Research Foundation Clinical Trial on the comparative effect of ovarian irradiation in carcinoma of the breast in the postmenopausal patient. In: Early Breast Cancer Trialists' Collaborative Groud (ed) Treatment of early breast cancer. I. Worldwide evidence 1985–1990. A systematic overview of all available randomized trials of adjuvant endocrine and cytotoxic therapy. Oxford University Press, Oxford, p 106

Cole MP (1975) A clinical trial of an artificial menopause in carcinoma of the breast. In: Namer M, Lalanne CM (eds) Hormones and breast cancer. INSERM, Paris, pp 143–150

Delozier T, Juret P, Couette JE, Mace-Lesech J (1990) Ovarian irradiation in postmenopausal women with breast cancer and positive axillary nodes. In: Early Breast Cancer Trialists' Collaborative Group (ed) Treatment of early breast cancer. I. Worldwide evidence 1985–1990. A systematic overview of all available randomized trials of adjuvant endocrine and cytotoxic therapy. Oxford University Press, Oxford, p 114

Early Breast Cancer Trialists' Collaborative Group (1990) Treatment of early breast cancer. In: Early Breast Cancer Trialists' Collaborative Group (ed) Treatment of early breast cancer. I. Worldwide evidence 1985–1990. A systematic overview of all available randomized trials of adjuvant endocrine and cytotoxic therapy. Oxford University Press, Oxford

Early Breast Cancer Trialists' Collaborative Group (1992) Systemic treatment of early breast cancer by hormonal, cytotoxic, or immune therapy. Lancet 339:71–85B

Early Breast Cancer Trialists' Collaborative Group (1996) Ovarian ablation in early breast cancer: an overview of the randomized trials. Lancet 348:1189–1196

Fisher B, Carbone P, Economou SG, Frelick R, Glass A, Lerner H, Redmond C, Zelen M, Band P, Katrych DL, Wolmark N, Fisher ER (1975) L-phenylalanine mustard (L-PAM) in the management of primary breast cancer: a report of early findings. N Engl J Med 292:117–122

Fisher B, Sherman B, Rockette H, Redmond C, Margolese R, Fisher ER (1979) L-phenylalanine mustard (L-PAM) in the management of premenopausal patients with primary breast cancer: lack of association of disease-free survival with depression of ovarian function. Cancer 44:847–857

Howell A, George WD, Crowther D, Bush H, Howat JM, Sellwood RA, Rubens RD, Hayward JL, Bulbrook RD, Fentiman I.S (1984) Controlled trial of adjuvant chemotherapy with cyclophosphamide, methotrexate and fluorouracil for breast cancer. Lancet 2:307–311

Legha SS, Carter SK (1976) Antiestrogens in the treatment of breast cancer. Cancer Treat Rev 3:205–216

Legha SS, Davis HLJ, Muggia FM (1978) Hormonal therapy of breast cancer: new approaches and concepts. Ann Intern Med 88:69–77

Ludwig Breast Cancer Study Group (1985 a) Chemotherapy with or without oophorectomy in high risk premenopausal patients with operable breast cancer. J Clin Oncol 13:1059–1067

Ludwig Breast Cancer Study Group (1985 b) Adjuvant combination chemotherapy with or without prednisone in premenopausal breast cancer patients with metastases in 1 to 3 axillary lymph nodes: a randomized trial. Cancer Res 45:4454–4459

Meakin JW, Allt WEC, Beale FA, Brown TC, Bush RS, Clark RM, Fitzpatrick PJ, Hawkins NV, Jenkin RD, Pringle JF, Reid JG, Rider WD, Hayward JL, Bulbrook RD (1979) Ovarian irradiation and prednisone therapy following surgery and radiotherapy for carcinoma of the breast. Can Med Assoc J 19:1221–1238

Meakin JW, Allt WEC, Beale FA, Bush RS, Clark RM, Fitzpatrick PJ, Hawkins NV, Jenkin RDT, Pringle JF, Reid JG, Rider WD, Hayward JL, Bulbrook RD (1983) Ovarian irradiation and prednisone following surgery and radiotherapy for carcinoma of the breast. Breast Cancer Res Treat 3:45–48

Meakin JW, Hayward JL, Panzarella T, Allt WEC, Beale FA, Bulbrook RD, Bush RS, Clark RM, Fitzpatrick PJ, Hawkins NV, Jenkin RDT, Pringle JF, Rider WD (1996) Ovarian irradiation and prednisone therapy following surgery and radiotherapy for carcinoma of the breast. Breast Cancer Res Treat 37:11–19

Nevinny HB, Nevinny D, Roscoff CB, Hall TC, Muench H (1969) Prophylactic oophorectomy in breast cancer therapy. Am J Surg 117:531–536

Nissen-Meyer R (1967) The role of prophylactic castration in the therapy of human mammary cancer. Eur J Cancer 3:395–403

Nissen-Meyer R (1975) Ovarian suppression and its supplement by additive hormonal treatment. In: Namer M, Lalanne CM (eds) Hormones and breast cancer. INSERM, Paris, pp 151–158

Nissen-Meyer R (1991) Primary breast cancer: the effects of primary ovarian ablation. Ann Oncol 2:343–346

Paterson R, Russell MH (1959) Clinical trials in malignant disease. Part II – Breast cancer: value of irradiation of the ovaries. J Faculty Radiologists 10:130–133

Pourquier H (1981) The results of adjuvant chemotherapy are predominantly caused by the hormonal changes such therapy induces. In: Van Scoy-Moscher MB (ed) Medical oncology. Controversies in cancer treatment. Hall, Boston, pp 83–89

Ragaz J, Jackson S. Nilson K, Plenderleith IH, Knowling M. Basco V, Ng V (1988) Randomized study of locoregional radiotherpay and ovarian ablation in premenopausal patients with breast cancer treated with adjuvant chemotherapy (abstract. Proc Am Soc Clin Oncol 7:12

Ravdin RG, Lewison EF, Slack NH, Gardner B, State D, Fisher B (1970) Results of a clinical trial concerning the worth of prophylactic oophorectomy for breast carcinoma. Surg Gynecol Obstet 131:1055–1064

Rubens RD, Knight RK, Fentiman IS, Hayward JL, Bulbrook RD, Chaudary M, Howell A, Bush H, Crowther D, Sellwood RA, George WD, Howat JM (1983) Controlled trial of adjuvant chemotherapy with melphalan for breast cancer. Lancet 1:839-843

Santen RJ, Samojik E, Lipton A, Harvey H, Ruby EB, Wells SA, Kendall J (1977) Kinetic, hormonal and clinical studies with aminoglutethimide in breast cancer. Cancer 39:2948–2958

Schinzinger A (1889) Über Carcinoma Mammae. Verh Dtsch Ges Chir 18:28–29

Scottish Cancer Trials Breast Group (1993) Adjuvant ovarian ablation versus CMF chemotherapy in pre-menopausal women with pathological stage II breast carcinoma: the Scottish trial. Lancet 341:1293–1298

Taylor GW, Green S, Dalton WS, Martino S, Rector DJ, Ingle JN, Robert NJ, Budd GT, Paradelo JC, Natale RB, Bearden JD, Mailliard JA, Osborne CK (1998) Multicenter randomized clinical trial of goserelin versus surgical ovariectomy in premenopausal patients with receptor-positive metastatic breast cancer: an intergroup study. J Clin Oncol 16:994–999

Taylor GW (1934) Artificial menopause in carcinoma of the breast. N Engl J Med 211:1138–1140

West CP, Baird DT (1987) Suppression of ovarian activity by Zoladex depot (ICI 118,630), a long acting luteinizing hormone releasing hormone agonist analogue. Clin Endocrinol (Oxf) 26:213–220

Summary

A. Wallgren[1] and H. T. Mouridsen[2]

[1] Department of Oncology, University of Göteborg,
Sahlgrenska University Hospital, 41345 Gothenburg, Sweden
[2] Department of Oncology, Copenhagen University Hospital, Rigshospitalet,
Blegdamsvej 9, 2100 Copenhagen Ø, Denmark

Radiation Therapy

The treatment of breast cancer has changed over the last decades from a locally aggressive treatment to a systemic treatment in which the local treatment only had a locally curative aim, reflecting changing concepts about the
nature of the disease. Radiation therapy, in spite of its ability to reduce the
risk of local and regional recurrences, became mainly used when surgery was
considered unsuitable or in recurrent cases. The reasons for this were not
only the supposed lack of influence on survival, but also the increased complication rate after radiotherapy, including arm edema, inhibition of shoulder
mobility, plexus problems and increased risk of cardiac death.

Breast conservation treatment became the new indication for radiation
therapy. Several trials of breast-conserving surgery with or without radiotherapy, some of which also included adjuvant systemic treatment, indicated
that radiation therapy reduced the risk of breast relapse, and most prospective studies have failed to show sub-groups with such low rate of breast failure that radiation therapy was not needed.

Problems concerning the timing of radiotherapy and systemic treatment,
as well as technical aspects of delivering radiotherapy were the subjects of
the presentations by Drs Rutqvist and Harris at the symposium. In addition,
both authors claimed that results of individual studies and overviews of
radiotherapy trials have shown that the present hypothesis of breast cancer
as a systemic disease in all cases must be questioned.

The results of an overview of studies comparing surgery with the same
type of surgery plus radiotherapy have indicated that the addition of radiation therapy to the chest wall and the regional glands, besides reducing recurrences in these regions, may also improve survival from breast cancer, but
increase deaths from other causes. Excess cardiac mortality has been shown
to be a cause of this. Two of the studies included in the overview have been
updated recently. Both studies on the combination of adjuvant chemotherapy
versus adjuvant chemotherapy plus radiation therapy in pre-menopausal
women with a follow-up of 10–15 years have reported an overall survival

benefit in the group of patients given radiotherapy. As pointed out in the presentations on radiation therapy, this supports the idea that secondary dissemination from cancer cells remaining after surgery may cause distant failure and breast cancer deaths. These two studies also showed that it is possible to achieve eradication of local and regional deposits using radiation therapy without increasing the risk of cardiac death.

In the Danish study there was a high rate of local and regional recurrence, 32%, which was reduced to 9% by radiation therapy. This study has been criticised as the surgery has been considered to be sup-optimal, as indicated by the low median number of seven lymph nodes found in the axilla. Almost half of the recurrences indeed occurred in the axilla and more than half in the chest wall. Another source of criticism also acknowledged by the authors is that the adjuvant chemotherapy consisted of intravenous CMF given every 4 weeks, which gave a dose intensity of the drugs lower than in, for instance, the classical oral CMF regimen. It is therefore possible that more extensive surgery and/or more intensive chemotherapy might have reduced the residual tumor in local and axillary sites with less detrimental effect on survival than in the chemotherapy arm of the Danish study, even without radiation therapy.

Both Dr. Rutquist and Dr. Harris discussed questions concerning the integration of radiation therapy into a treatment programme which also included adjuvant systemic treatment. Several studies have indicated that delaying radiotherapy after breast-conserving surgery until after completion of the systemic treatment programme does not seem to increase the frequency of breast recurrence. On the other hand, a Boston prospective study of four cycles of CAMFP given before or after radiation therapy indicated a higher frequency of local and regional recurrence if radiation therapy was given after chemotherapy, but when chemotherapy was given after radiation therapy the frequency of distant metastases was increased. As Dr. Harris pointed out, there is a need for future studies on how best to combine the two treatment modalities.

When is there an indication for postoperative radiation therapy? The afore-mentioned studies show that a high risk of residual cancer in the local and regional area may be hazardous for the patient and cannot always be controlled by systemic adjuvant treatment. It is obvious that "high risk" can only be evaluated in the context of other treatments. The addition of radiation therapy to surgery and systemic treatments may increase the frequency and intensity of side effects such as plexus and shoulder/arm problems. Irradiation of the internal mammary nodes or the left breast or chest wall may include a volume of the heart, with the risk of increased cardiac morbidity. It is thus essential both to restrict treatment to the patients who need it and to develop treatment techniques which avoid side effects but retain efficacy against residual cancer.

Most studies on postoperative radiotherapy after breast-conserving surgery have failed to reveal sub-groups with a very low rate of breast recurrence without radiation therapy. Patient age, the radicality of the surgery and histological type and grade all seem to be factors prognostic of recurrence. Indeed, in a prospective trial the Milan group identified a sub-group of patients consisting of women over 55 years of age who were treated with a quadrantectomy alone for a tumor less than 2.5 cm in diameter and had a local recurrence rate of only 3.8% after a median of 39 months. As reported by Dr. Harris, a prospective series on selected patients who were treated without radiation therapy after locally radical breast conservative surgery had to be closed prematurely, since the breast recurrence rate was higher than anticipated. At a median follow-up of nearly 5 years, 14 of 87 patients have relapsed – a relapse rate similar to the 15% at 5 years in women over the age of 60, with tumors less than 2 cm and with other histology than comedo or lobular carcinoma, in a retrospective analysis of a Swedish study. Even though no clinical study so far has shown worse survival after breast conservation without radiation therapy, the finding of an increased incidence of distant metastases in women with stage I tumours treated without radiation therapy in NSABP B-04 is a warning that residual cancer in the breast may not be quite as innocent as has been believed.

Drs. Rutquist and Harris also showed that the available prognostic factors are not good enough to select patients for different treatment modalities. Not only is it essential to select patients who need a certain type of treatment because of a high rate of recurrent disease, but also to select those who would benefit from the treatment in question. Predictors for the effect of radiotherapy as well as for chemotherapy are lacking, but there is hope that in the future molecular biology will provide us with such tools. A small retrosprective analysis of a prospective study found mutated *p53* to be prognostic for the effect of radiation therapy. This as well as other candidate predictive factors will have to be tested prospectively before their place if any in the clinic can be established.

The two papers presented on radiation therapy indicate that radiation therapy may have a substantial role in the overall improvement of survival of breast cancer. It seems reasonable that radiation therapy should be included in future trials to define when it should be used, what regions should be treated and to what doses, as well as the timing of radiation therapy in relation to other treatment modalities. Future technical development of radiation therapy is possible, which might for instance include radiation triggered by the patient's breathing in order to avoid inclusion of the heart in the irradiated volume; this should make radiation therapy in the initial treatment more efficient.

Endocrine Therapy

Ovarian ablation was introduced in the treatment of advanced breast cancer nearly 100 years ago and in the adjuvant setting some 30 years ago. Several other endocrine treatment modalities have been introduced over the past 50 years in advanced disease. Until recently none of these modalities demonstrated significant superiority in terms of efficacy in advanced disease. However, as a consequence of the relative lack of toxicities associated with treatment with tamoxifen, this drug has since long been considered the first-line endocrine therapy of choice in advanced breast cancer in post-menopausal patients, and the benefit achieved with the drug in the adjuvant setting is now well established.

The response to endocrine therapy is related to receptor status. However, even among receptor-positive patients nearly 50% are primarily resistant to tamoxifen, and all responding patients will ultimately demonstrate clinical resistance in terms of progression of the disease. Similarly, in the adjuvant situation a substantial proportion of the patients offered tamoxifen will experience recurrence. There is therefore a need to gain more knowledge about the mechanisms involved in primary and acquired resistance to endocrine therapy, and to develop new agents less likely to be associated with resistance.

V. C. Jordan presented data demonstrating that amino acid 351 in the estrogen receptor is the key to the anti-estrogenic activity. Thus mutation prevents the necessary change in receptor conformation resulting in estrogenic stimulation of the tumor cell. This is the first example of a molecular mechanism for stimulation, rather than inhibition, of tumor cell growth by tamoxifen, and future studies within this fascinating area may perhaps lead to means to improve outcome with anti-estrogenic therapy.

New endocrine treatment modalities introduced recently were presented by R. C. Coombes and K. I. Pritchard. R. C. Coombes reviewed the third generation of aromatase inhibitors (AI) in present development. These include the non-steroidal AIs anastrozole and letrozole and the steroidal AI exemestane. Compared with the first-generation AI (aminoglutethimide) these drugs are more potent in their oestrogenic suppression and they are highly selective, i.e. substitution with corticosteroids can be avoided. As second-line therapy the non-steroidal AI have proven superiority in randomised trials over recently used alternatives (medroxyprogesterone acetate, aminoglutethimide) in terms of increased efficacy and/or decreased toxicity. The third-generation AI have therefore been introduced in clinical trials as first-line therapy in advanced disease and in the adjuvant setting. The latter studies compare tamoxifen as a reference with AIs or with tamoxifen and AIs given sequentially. An essential part of these studies would be careful registration of potential long-term toxicities with the two modalities, especially with regard to endometrial carcinoma and the effect on the cardiovascular system and bone.

As reported by K. I. Pritchard, ovarian ablation is effective as adjuvant therapy in pre-menopausal patients. However, this conclusion stems from patients unselected according to receptor status and the relative benefit of ablation compared with chemotherapy in receptor-positive patients has yet to be analysed in a randomised trial.

As emphasised by K. I. Pritchard, the role of combined chemotherapy and ablative therapy in pre-menopausal patients with receptor-positive tumors remains controversial. Thus no benefit was observed in trials adding ablation to chemotherapy, and results from ongoing trials adding GnRH analogues to chemotherapy are not yet available.

IX. Adjuvant Systemic Treatments: Cytotoxic Strategies

Putting the Taxanes to Work: Unanswered Questions

P. F. Conte and L. Del Mastro

Division of Medical Oncology, Department of Oncology, St. Chiara Hospital and University, 56100 Pisa, Italy

Introduction

Adjuvant polychemotherapy improves the outcome of early breast cancer: 10-year relapse-free and overall survival are 44% and 51% respectively in patients treated with chemotherapy and 36% and 45% in controls (Early Breast Cancer Trialists Group 1992) Although encouraging in terms of treatment success, these results, also mean that, despite adjuvant chemotherapy, more than 60% of the patients have suffered relapse and nearly 50% have died. Improved therapeutic options are therefore necessary, particularly in node-positive breast cancer patients. Taxanes have shown promising activity in advanced breast cancer patients; in particular, two phase III studies have demonstrated that single-agent paclitaxel as first-line therapy induces response rates ranging from 25% to 33%, i.e., similar or slightly lower than those observed with doxorubicin, which range from 41% to 34% (Awada et al. 1997; Sledge et al. 1997). Moreover, docetaxel has shown a higher activity than doxorubicin: the observed response rates were 47% and 32%, respectively, in a population of patients pretreated with alkylating-containing regimens (Chan et al. 1997). Beside their activity, taxanes are very interesting because of their incomplete cross-resistance with anthracyclines: a response rate ranging from 27% to 48% was observed with paclitaxel in patients resistant to prior anthracyclines (Seidman et al. 1993; Wilson et al. 1994; Gianni et al. 1995a). Similarly, data from a randomized study showed that docetaxel has a higher activity than a regimen with mitomycin-vinblastine (overall response: 28% vs 14%) in anthracycline-pretreated patients (Nabholtz et al. 1997).

Because of the high level of activity and the incomplete cross-resistance, the combination of anthracyclines and taxanes has been extensively studied. Several phase II studies have reported that the combination of doxorubicin and paclitaxel is extremely active, with an overall response rate around 90% and exciting complete remission rates ranging from 24% to 41% (Gianni et al. 1995b; Gehl et al. 1996; Amadori et al. 1996). Unfortunately the incidence of cardiotoxicity was also significantly high, and with this combination the cumulative doxorubicin dose should not exceed 360 mg/m^2. The substitution of epirubicin for doxorubicin in this combination resulted in reduced cardiotoxicity with an interesting level of activity (overall response rate 84% with 19% complete responses) (Conte et al. 1997). Preliminary data indicate similar high activity with the combination docetaxel-anthracyclines (Dieras 1997).

The high activity of taxane-containing regimens in metastatic breast cancer patients has prompted the investigators to explore their role in the adjuvant setting; however, methodological issues and as yet unsolved pharmacokinetic and pharmacodynamic problems might jeopardize these attractive regimens and should be taken into account in the design and interpretation of adjuvant trials.

Methodological Issues

In order to reduce methodological weaknesses, it may be of interest to run through the history of the introduction of anthracyclines in the adjuvant setting. Anthracyclines were first introduced for the treatment of metastatic breast cancer in the 1970s and are still considered the most active single agent for the treatment of this disease. Surprisingly, more than 20 years after their introduction, only a few high-power studies which correctly addressed the question of the role of these drugs in adjuvant setting are available. These studies showed no difference (Fisher et al. 1990; Carpenter et al. 1994) or superiority (Tormey et al. 1992; Levine et al. 1995; Coombes et al. 1996) of anthracycline-containing regimens in comparison to CMF-based regimens in terms of disease-free survival and/or overall survival. In the majority of the other studies results are actually misleading because the sample sizes were too small to detect a "realistic" difference. Comparing a standard chemotherapy regimen with a taxane combination it is realistic to expect a reduction in risk of death lower than that induced by CMF versus control. On the other hand, new, more toxic and/or more expensive regimens are justified only if a worthwhile improvement is achieved. A reduction in risk of death not higher than 20% can be considered both realistic and clinically worthwhile. In node-positive patients, this reduction in the risk of death would translate into an absolute survival increase of 5% at 5 years and 7% at 10 years. Only large trials enrolling more than one thousand patients will have the power to detect these differences. Besides the sample size, the endpoints of adjuvant trials also deserve some comment. It has been shown that adjuvant therapies can affect the activity and efficacy of treatments received at the time of recurrence, thus compromising the overall survival of relapsed patients (Venturini et al. 1996). Therefore, an improvement in recurrence-free survival induced by an adjuvant treatment might not necessarily lead to an improvement in overall survival. This might be even more true nowadays when aggressive drug combinations with or without hematopoietic progenitor cell support have the potential to prolong survival in a fraction of patients with advanced disease.

Taxane-Specific Issues

Schedule and Pharmacokinetic Interferences

The use of paclitaxel in combination with anthracyclines is complicated by pharmacokinetic interactions which are different according to the schedule of paclitaxel (24 vs 3 h) and the anthracycline employed. The early phase I/II studies used paclitaxel by prolonged infusion (24 or 72 h) with doxorubicin given concomitantly for 72 h (Fisherman et al. 1996), by 48-h infusion immediately before or after paclitaxel (Holmes et al. 1996), or as an i.v. bolus 4 h before or after paclitaxel (Sledge et al. 1994). With these regimens the dose-limiting toxicities appear at relatively low doses and are schedule-dependent, with doxorubicin followed by paclitaxel being less toxic. Moreover, the overall and complete response rates were lower than expected, suggesting that the cytotoxicity of this combination is subadditive. Preliminary results of a large phase III study (Sledge et al. 1997), indeed, indicate that the combination of doxorubicin with 24-h infusion paclitaxel produces a higher response rate than either agent alone, but this response rate (46%) is lower than that expected on the basis of previous phase II studies. The demonstration of the safety and activity of paclitaxel given as a short infusion (Eisenhauer et al. 1994; Hainsworth and Greco 1994) led to trials using bolus doxorubicin and paclitaxel over 3 h. The most relevant findings of these studies were the lack of sequence-dependent toxicity, the high incidence of symptomatic congestive heart failure, and the striking antitumor activity. The antitumor activity and the cardiac effects of this combination suggest the possibility of a therapeutic and toxic synergism between the two drugs. The cardiotoxicity occurred at median cumulative doses of 392–480 mg/m^2; therefore, the cumulative dose of doxorubicin when used in combination with paclitaxel should not exceed 360 mg/m^2. Interestingly, when doxorubicin was given 16 h before paclitaxel, no cardiotoxicity was observed (Amadori et al. 1996). Ongoing clinical trials in metastatic breast cancer patients will clarify whether a gap between the administration of doxorubicin and paclitaxel is necessary and, if so, how long it should be, in order to maintain the antitumor activity and reduce the cardiotoxicity. In the meanwhile, the risk of cardiotoxicity should be carefully considered in the adjuvant setting by limiting the doxorubicin dose and restricting eligibility criteria to patients without cardiac risk factors.

Another possible way to reduce the cardiotoxicity is to use epirubicin in place of doxorubicin. Several clinical studies have shown that epirubicin and doxorubicin have similar antitumor activity and hematologic toxicity, but the cardiotoxicity of epirubicin appears at cumulative doses which are double those of doxorubicin. The epirubicin-paclitaxel combination, indeed, showed a very low incidence of cardiotoxicity (Conte et al. 1997). Such reduced cardiotoxicity could be partly due to the pharmacokinetic interferences between epirubicin and paclitaxel: co-administration of epirubicin and paclitaxel induces increased glucuronidation of epirubicin and of epirubicinol, the metabolite involved in the pathogenesis of cardiac damage, and the increased glucuronidation leads to increased urinary elimination, which could account for the decreased cardiotoxicity of such combination (Gianni et al. 1997). On the other hand, it is unknown whether these pharmacokinetic interferences alter the antitumor activity of the combination. Data on potential pharmacokinetic interferences between docetaxel in combination with doxorubicin or epirubicin are not yet available. In evaluating the role of taxane-anthracycline combinations in early breast cancer patients, investigators should be aware of potential pharmacokinetic interactions which may be responsible for unexpected side effects and/or subadditive cytotoxicity.

The pharmacokinetic interferences between taxanes and anthracyclines are avoided in trials based on sequential administration of the two drugs. This treatment approach allows the administration of optimal doses and schedules of each drug, or established combination of drugs (e.g., CMF). Moreover, the sequential approach has been shown to be particularly effective with doxorubicin and CMF (Bonadonna et al. 1995). Sequential use of anthracyclines and taxanes compared to combination of the two drugs is under evaluation in ongoing randomized studies in advanced breast cancer patients.

Treatment Duration

Clinical trials have demonstrated that 12 cycles of adjuvant CMF are not better than six, and four courses of AC are as effective as six CMF. For this reason, in clinical practice, adjuvant chemotherapy is administered for no more than four to six courses. However, the optimal use of taxanes could mean a longer duration of treatment. Laboratory data indicate that paclitaxel could have additional mechanisms of cytotoxicity, i.e., induction of apoptosis (Saunders et al. 1997) and antiangiogenic activity (Klauber et al. 1997), which could require prolonged treatments and/or a different schedule, e.g., weekly administration. Clinical data in metastatic breast cancer seem to confirm the importance of treatment duration; in the study of Gianni et al. (1995b) the administration of doxorubicin was stopped after a maximum of eight cycles and patients were treated with additional cycles of paclitaxel alone. Interestingly, 15% of the patients achieved the best response while on paclitaxel alone. These observations have prompted studies aimed at evaluating the role of maintenance therapy or weekly prolonged paclitaxel in advanced breast cancer patients.

In the majority of ongoing adjuvant trials, planned cycles of taxanes alone or in combination are equal to or less than six; therefore, trials evaluating different schedules and treatment duration are warranted.

Interaction with Endocrine Therapy

The combination of tamoxifen with adjuvant CMF-based chemotherapy has produced similar or better results than has tamoxifen alone, while its combination with anthracycline-containing chemotherapy was always better, thus

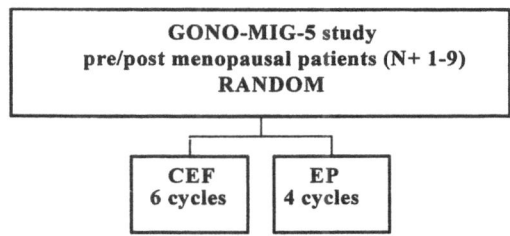

Fig. 1. Design of GONO (Gruppo Oncologico Nord Ovest) MIG-5 (Mammella Intergruppo) study. *CEF:* Cyclophosphamide (600 mg/m^2), epirubicin (60 mg/m^2), 5-fluorouracil (600 mg/m^2) given on day 1 every 21 days ; *EP* epirubicin (90 mg/m^2), paclitaxel (175 mg/m^2, 3-hour infusion) given on day 1 every 21 days; *N+1–9*, 1–9 involved lymph nodes

confirming laboratory findings of synergistic effects between tamoxifen and anthracyclines.

Possible interactions between taxanes and tamoxifen are still unclear. Early laboratory data indicate that tamoxifen might have a synergistic antiproliferative effect and no additive cytotoxicity when combined with docetaxel (Ferlini et al. 1997) and paclitaxel (Cheng et al. 1995), respectively. Clinical data are necessary to clarify these interactions in order to allow recommendations in the adjuvant clinical setting.

On the other hand, the high activity of the taxane-anthracycline combination and recent data, reporting the limited value of intermediate- and high-dose cyclophosphamide in the adjuvant setting (Fisher et al. 1997), led to the design of studies such as GONO-MIG5 (Fig. 1) in which the alkylating agent is not used in the experimental arm based on the combination of epirubicin and paclitaxel. A potential advantage of dropping the alkylating agent could be decreased incidence of amenorrhea in pre-menopausal patients. The high cytotoxic effect of the taxane-anthracycline regimen is expected to counterbalance the loss of the indirect endocrine effect related to drug-induced amenorrhea, and at the same time to avoid side effects of early menopause induced by chemotherapy (Del Mastro et al. 1997).

Interactions with Radiotherapy

The optimal sequencing of chemotherapy and radiotherapy after conservative surgery is still a matter of controversy. Recent data indicate that giving chemotherapy first gave better overall results but was associated with an increased risk of local recurrence (Recht et al. 1996). On the other hand, the simultaneous administration of chemotherapy and radiotherapy could induce increased toxicity. Some studies reported an increased incidence of skin reactions, radiation pneumonitis, and cardiotoxicity following simultaneous treatments, but these increased side effects were not observed in other studies. The radiosensitizing effects of taxanes might represent a major obstacle to the use of simultaneous radio- and chemotherapy because of the risk of radiodermitis and/or impaired cosmetic results. Moreover, two recent reports have described recall dermatitis induced by taxanes given after radiotherapy (Raghavan et al. 1993; Yeo et al. 1997); therefore, radiotherapy should be given at the end of adjuvant chemotherapy even in regimens in which the taxane is administered after drugs which allow the simultaneous use of radiotherapy. The necessity of careful evaluation of possible detrimental effects of delayed radiotherapy following adjuvant taxanes is strengthened by the recently reported benefit induced by radiotherapy after mastectomy (Overgaard et al. 1997; Ragaz et al. 1997).

Toxicity and Long-Term Sequelae

The majority of acute side effects of taxane-containing regimens, i.e., neutropenia and neuropathy, are short-lasting and reversible, but other potential toxicities, such as the cardiotoxicity associated with the combination of paclitaxel and doxorubicin, need careful monitoring not only during treatment but also in long-term follow-up.

Specific side effects of taxanes are prevented by the use of steroids. These drugs are used for hypersensitivity prophylaxis in paclitaxel-containing regimens and to reduce the fluid retention due to docetaxel. The premedication regimen is usually based on oral steroids starting the night before the administration of taxane. One disadvantage of this premedication, patient compliance, has been overcome in paclitaxel-containing regimens. It has been reported that the intravenous administration of steroids 30 min before paclitaxel is as safe as the oral premedication (Gennari et al. 1996; Bookman et al. 1997). However, prolonged use of steroids can have other disadvantages. The International Breast Cancer Study Group has reported that the use of low-dose continuous prednisone added to adjuvant CMF chemotherapy (CMFp) was associated with an increased risk of bone metastases (relative risk compared to CMF alone was 2.06; 95% confidence interval 1.23–3.46; $p = 0.004$) and a small, not statistically significant increased incidence of second malignancies (relative risk = 3.34; 95% confidence interval 0.91–12.31; $p = 0.09$) (Marini et al. 1996). The authors hypothesized that the impaired bone metabolism induced by steroids may play a major role in the process of seeding cancer cells in the bone. Moreover, the potential immunosuppressive effect of steroids could explain the slightly increased incidence of second primary tumors in patients treated with CMFp. Although these data need to be confirmed, they prompt an accurate evaluation of these potential side effects when high-dose steroids are being given as premedication for taxanes.

Conclusions

The potential role of taxanes in the adjuvant setting will be clarified by ongoing clinical trials large enough to demonstrate a realistic difference in treatment outcomes. Due to unresolved issues about pharmacokinetic interactions with other drugs, optimal schedule, and treatment duration, the use of these drugs outside clinical trials in early breast cancer patients should be discouraged.

The introduction of new drugs or new strategies in the treatment of curable cancer patients, such as early breast cancer patients, requires careful evaluation of potential side effects which may reduce the expected benefits. Acute and delayed cardiotoxicity, potential disadvantages due to the necessity to delay radiotherapy at the end of taxane-containing chemotherapy, and possible negative effects of high-dose steroids should be taken into account. Despite these words of caution, it may be hoped that ongoing clinical trials will allow measurement of the efficacy of adjuvant taxanes less than 10 years after their introduction into clinical practice. If we look back over the time needed to prove the effects of adjuvant anthracyclines, we can say that the speed and quality of clinical research in early breast cancer have substantially improved.

Summary

The promising activity of taxanes in advanced breast cancer patients has prompted the investigators to explore their role in the adjuvant setting. Methodological issues, still unsolved pharmacokinetic and pharmacodynamic problems, and potential severe toxicities could jeopardize these attractive regimens and should be taken into account in the design and interpretation of adjuvant trials. In order to minimize the methodological drawbacks, the potential role of taxanes in the adjuvant setting should be assessed in clinical trials powered to detect an absolute survival increase of near 7% at 10 years. The use of paclitaxel in combination with anthracyclines is complicated by pharmacokinetic interactions which may be responsible for unexpected side effects and/or subadditive cytotoxicity. Moreover, possible interactions between taxanes and tamoxifen are still unclear, and therefore more data are necessary before recommending the combined use of the two drugs in the adjuvant setting. Nowadays, the majority of breast cancer patients receive conservative surgery followed by radiotherapy; when adjuvant taxanes are used, radiotherapy should be delayed because of their radiosensitization effect, with potential detrimental effects. Finally, the majority of side effects of taxane-containing regimens are short-lasting and reversible, but other potential toxicities, such as the cardiotoxicity and long-term possible sequelae of the use of high-dose steroids, need long-term evaluation.

References

Amadori D, Frassineti GL, Zoli W et al (1996) A phase I/II study of sequential doxorubicin and paclitaxel in the treatment of advanced breast cancer. Ann Oncol 23 (Suppl 11):16–22

Awada A, Paridaens R, Bruning P et al (1997) Doxorubicin or taxol as first line chemotherapy for metastatic breast cancer: results of an EORTIC-IDBBC/ECSG randomized trial with crossover (EORTC 10923). Breast Cancer Res Treat 46:23

Bonadonna G, Zambetti M, Valagussa P (1995) Sequential or alternating doxorubicin and CMF regimens in breast cancer with more than three positive nodes. Ten-year results. JAMA 273:542–547

Bookman MA, Kloth DD, Korer PE et al (1997) Short-course intravenous prophylaxis for paclitaxel related hypersensitivity reactions. Ann Oncol 8:611–614

Carpenter JT, Velez-Garcia E, Aron BS et al (1994) Five-year results of a randomized comparison of cyclophosphamide, doxorubicin and fluorouracil (CAF) vs cyclophosphamide, methotrexate, and fluorouracil (CMF) for node positive breast cancer: a Southeastern Cancer Study Group trial. Proc Am Soc Clin Oncol 13:66

Chan S, Friedrichs K, Noel D et al (1997) A phase III study of taxotere vs doxorubicin in patients with metastatic breast cancer who have failed an alkylating containing regimen. Breast Cancer Res Treat 46:23

Cheng L, Zheng S, Norris JS et al (1995) Long-term treatment with tamoxifen in vitro inhibits taxol-induced apoptosis in human breast cancer cells. Proc Annu Am Assoc Cancer Res 36:A2492

Conte PF, Baldini E, Gennari A et al (1997) Dose-finding study and pharmacokinetics of epirubicin and paclitaxel over 3 hours: a regimen with high activity and low cardiotoxicity in advanced breast cancer. J Clin Oncol 15:2510–2517

Coombes RC, Bliss JM, Wils J et al (1996) Adjuvant cyclophosphamide, methotrexate, and fluorouracil versus fluorouracil, epirubicin, and cyclophosphamide chemotherapy in premenopausal women with axillary node-positive operable breast cancer: results of a randomized trial. J Clin Oncol 14:35–45

Del Mastro L, Venturini M, Sertoli MR et al (1997) Amenorrhea induced by adjuvant chemotherpy in early breast cancer patients: prognostic role and clinical implications. Breast Cancer Res Treat 43:183–190

Dieras V (1997) Review of docetaxel/doxorubicin in metastatic breast cancer. Oncology 11 Suppl 8:31–33

Early Breast Cancer Trialists' Collaborative Group (1992) Systemic treatment of early breast cancer by hormonal, cytotoxic, or immune therapy. Lancet 339:1–15, 71–85

Eisenhauer EH, ten Bokkel Huinink W, Swenerton KD et al (1994) European-Canadian randomized trial of taxol in relapsed ovarian cancer: high vs low dose and long vs short infusion. J Clin Oncol 12:2654–2666

Ferlini C, Scambia G, Di Stefano M et al (1997) Synergistic antiproliferative activity of tamoxifen and docetaxel on three oestrogen receptor-negative cancer cell lines is mediated by the induction of apoptosis. Br J Cancer 75:884–891

Fisher B, Brown AM, Dimitrov NV et al (1990) Two months doxorubicin-cyclophosphamide with or without interval reinduction therapy compared with 6 months of cyclophosphamide, methotrexate and fluorouracil in positive node breast cancer patients with tamoxifen non responsive tumor: results from National Surgical Adjuvant Breast and Bowel Project B-15. J Clin Oncol 8:1483–1496

Fisher B, Anderson S, Wickerham DL et al (1997) Increased intensification and total dose of cyclophosphamide in a doxorubicin-cyclophosphamide regimen for the treatment of primary breast cancer: findings from National Surgical Adjuvant Breast and Bowel Project. J Clin Oncol 15:1858–1869

Fisherman JS, Cowan KH, Noone K et al (1996) Phase I/II study of 72 hour infusional paclitaxel and doxorubicin with granulocyte-stimulating factor in patients with metastatic breast cancer. J Clin Oncol 14:774–782

Gehl J, Boesgard M, Paaske T et al (1996) Combined doxorubicin and paclitaxel in advanced breast cancer: effective and cardiotoxic. Ann Oncol 7:687–693

Gennari A, Salvadori B, Tognoni A, Conte PF (1996) Rapid intravenous premedication with dexamethasone prevents hypersensitivity reactions to paclitaxel. Ann Oncol 7:977–979

Gianni L, Munzone E, Capri G et al (1995a) Paclitaxel in metastatic breast cancer: a trial of two doses by a 3-hour infusion in patients with disease recurrence after prior therapy with anthracyclines. J Natl Cancer Inst 87:1169–1175

Gianni L, Munzone E, Capri G et al (1995b) Paclitaxel by 3-hour infusion in combination with bolus doxorubicin in women with untreated metastatic breast cancer: high antitumor efficacy and cardiac effects in a dose-finding and sequence-finding study. J Clin Oncol 13:2688–2699

Gianni L, Vigano' L, Locatelli A et al (1997) Different interference of paclitaxel on human pharmacokinetics of doxorubicin and epirubicin. Proc Am Soc Clin Oncol 16:786

Hainsworth JD, Greco FA (1994) Paclitaxel administered by 1 hour infusion: preliminary results of a phase I-II trial comparing two schedules. Cancer 74:1377–1382

Holmes FA, Madden T, Newman RA et al (1996) Sequence-dependent alteration of doxorubicin pharmacokinetics by paclitaxel in a phase I study of paclitaxel and doxorubicin in patients with metastatic breast cancer. J Clin Oncol 14:2713–2721

Klauber N, Parangi S, Flynn E et al (1997) Inhibition of angiogenesis and breast cancer in mice by the microtubule inhibitors 2-methoxyestradiol and taxol. Cancer Res 57:81–86

Marini G, Murray S, Goldhirsch A et al (1996) The effect of adjuvant prednisone combined with CMF on patterns of relapse and occurrence of second malignancies in patients with breast cancer. Ann Oncol 7:245–250

Levine M, Bramwell V, Bowman D et al (1995) A clinical trial of intensive CEF versus CMF in premenopausal women with node positive breast cancer. Proc Am Soc Clin Oncol 14:112

Nabholtz JM, Thuerlimann B, Bezwoda WR et al (1997) Taxotere vs mitomycin C-vinblastine in patients with metastatic breast cancer who have failed an anthracycline containing regimen. Breast Cancer Res Treat 46:93

Overgaard M, Hansen PS, Overgaard J et al (1997) Postoperative radiotherapy in high-risk premenopausal women with breast cancer who receive adjuvant chemotherapy. N Engl J Med 337:949–955

Ragaz J, Jackson SM, Le N et al (1997) Adjuvant radiotherapy and chemotherapy in node-positive premenopausal women with breast cancer. N Engl J Med 337:956–962

Raghavan VT, Bloomer WD, Merkel DE (1993) Taxol and radiation recall dermatitis. Lancet 341:1354

Recht A, Come SE, Henderson IC et al (1996) The sequencing of chemotherapy and radiation therapy after conservative surgery for early-stage breast cancer. N Engl J Med 334:1356–1361

Saunders DE, Lawrence WD, Christensen C et al (1997) Paclitaxel-induced apoptosis in MCF-7 breast cancer cells. Int J Cancer 70:214–220

Seidman AD, Nortol L, Reichman BS et al (1993) Preliminary experience with paclitaxel (Taxol) plus recombinant human granulocyte colony-stimulating factor in the treatment of breast cancer. Semin Oncol 20:40–45

Sledge GW Jr, Robert M, Sparana JA et al (1994) Paclitaxel (taxol)-doxorubicin combinations in advanced breast cancer: the Eastern Cooperative Oncology Group experience. Semin Oncol 21 Suppl 8:15–18

Sledge GW, Neuberg D, Ingle J, Martino S, Wood W (1997) Phase III trial of doxorubicin vs paclitaxel vs doxorubicin + paclitaxel as first line therapy for metastatic breast cancer: an intergroup trial. Proc Am Soc Clin Oncol 16:1a

Tormey DC, Gray R, Abeloff MD et al (1992) Adjuvant therapy with a doxorubicin regimen and long-term tamoxifen in premenopausal breast cancer patients: an Eastern Cooperative Oncology Group trial. J Clin Oncol 10:1848–1856

Venturini M, Bruzzi P, Del Mastro L et al (1996) Effect of adjuvant chemotherapy with or without anthracyclines on the activity and efficacy of first-line cyclophosphamide, epidoxorubicin, and fluorouracil in patients with metastatic breast cancer. J Clin Oncol 14:764–773

Wilson WH, Berg SL, Bryant G et al (1994) Paclitaxel doxorubicin-refractory or mitoxantrone-refractory breast cancer: a phase I/II trial of 96-hour infusion. J Clin Oncol 12:1621–1629

Yeo W, Leung SF, Johnson PJ (1997) Radiation recall dermatitis with docetaxel: establishment of a requisite radiation threshold. Eur J Cancer 33:698–699

Putting Taxanes to Work in Operable Breast Cancer: A Search for Selective Indications from Empirical Studies

L. Gianni, G. Capri, P. Valagussa, and G. Bonadonna

Divisione di Oncologia Medica, Istituto Nazionale Tumori, 20133 Milan, Italy

Introduction

Based on their unique and novel mechanism of action, the taxanes paclitaxel (PCT) and docetaxel (DCT) have been extensively studied in solid tumors. The two drugs found in the field of breast cancer an arena of most intensive investigation (Gianni and Capri 1997). The huge body of studies and reports in the literature has prompted enthusiasm, some concern and occasionally confusion on the actual role of the two drugs in breast cancer. The risk of the unprecedented investigational effort on taxanes in breast cancer is one of generating confusion, due to their already widespread use when key aspects of their pharmacology and their optimal application are still undefined. This risk is very much present in the case of adjuvant or neo-adjuvant use of PCT and DCT. Some remarks may help in putting the problems into perspective.

Evidence on the Use of Taxanes in Metastatic Breast Cancer

Data from a large number of trials have clearly defined the antitumor activity of PCT in metastatic breast cancer (Gianni et al. 1996b; Nabholtz et al. 1996; Seidman 1995; Seidman et al. 1995). In these studies, many investigators have also demonstrated efficacy of the drug in women who failed prior treatment with anthracyclines. In addition, comparative efficacy and safety trials showed that PCT has a therapeutic value similar to that of doxorubicin (Sledge et al. 1997) and superior to that of CMFP (cyclophosphamide, methotrexate, fluorouracil and prednisone) in terms of survival and quality of life (Bishop et al. 1997). Studies with docetaxel in metastatic breast cancer have rapidly closed the gap to those completed earlier with paclitaxel. The first and, to date, the only analog of paclitaxel has outstanding antitumor activity at the cost of frequent and severe hematological toxicity and unusual side effects, such as a total-dose dependent fluid-retention syndrome and skin/nail toxicity which may limit its administration for prolonged periods (Gianni and Capri 1997). For docetaxel, major responses, including a high complete response rate, were observed in 50%–70% of patients. In addition, response was uninfluenced by prior treatment with anthracyclines, and was equally high in non-visceral and visceral metastases (Ravdin 1995; Ravdin et al. 1995).

The above studies contributed to rank single-agent taxanes among the most active new drugs in women with breast cancer, and justified the conducting of studies of combination chemotherapy with anthracyclines due to the lack of complete clinical cross-resistance between the two classes of drugs. Combinations with paclitaxel were not a straightforward process due to possible drug–drug interactions in combination, and to the dependence of the pharmacological effects of paclitaxel on the duration of infusion and on the sequence of administration in respect to that of the combined drug (Gianni 1995). The very high antitumor effects of a 3-h infusion of paclitaxel with bolus doxorubicin have raised considerable interest, but also some concern because of the high rate of cardiac toxicity reported in two dose-finding studies (Gianni et al. 1995a; Dombernowsky et al. 1996). Cardiac risk is dependent on the total dose of doxorubicin, and it is now clear that limiting the anthracycline to a maximum of 360 mg/m^2 in combination with paclitaxel is not associated with enhanced cardiac effects (Gianni et al. 1997; Moliterni et al. 1997). Cardiac toxicity does not appear to be a problem with the combination of epirubicin and paclitaxel (Frassineti et al. 1996; Schwartsmann et al. 1996; Conte et al. 1997), nor in the only reported study of doxorubicin and docetaxel (Bourgeois et al. 1996).

Table 1 is a compilation of selected studies of paclitaxel and docetaxel given in combination with doxorubicin or epirubicin in metastatic breast cancer, and clearly shows the very high rate of overall and complete response observed in these trials. The overall assessment of the merits and limits of the two taxanes in metastatic breast cancer is largely in favor of expanding their role in treating the disease. Table 2 summarizes the main characteristics of the two taxanes as they have emerged from the intense effort of development in metastatic breast cancer (for a detailed discussion of the points listed see Gianni and Capri 1997). These features have prompted evaluation of the use of paclitaxel and docetaxel in operable breast cancer in an effort to exploit their high antitumor activity to increase overall and disease-free survival in adjuvant or neo-adjuvant treatment programs.

Table 1. Selected studies of paclitaxel or docetaxel in combination with anthracyclines in women with metastatic breast cancer

Reference	Anthracycline (dose, mg/m^2)	Taxane (dose, mg/m^2)	Response rate (%)	Complete response (%)
Gianni et al. (1995b)	DOX/60	PCT/125–200	94	38
Dombernowsky et al. (1996)	DOX/50–60	PCT/125–200	83	24
Schwartsmann et al. (1996)	DOX/60	PCT/250	80	28
Frassinetti et al. (1996)	DOX/50	PCT/130–250	79	32
Conte et al. (1997)	EPI/90	PCT/135–225	80	16
Bourgeois et al. (1996)	DOX/50–60	DCT/75–60	90	NA

DOX, Doxorubicin; EPI, Epirubicin; PCT, Paclitaxel; DCT, Docetaxel; NA, Not available.

Table 2. Main characteristics of paclitaxel and docetaxel as they emerged from studies in women with metastatic breast cancer (for references see Gianni and Capri 1997)

Paclitaxel	Docetaxel
Active at all doses and by all schedules (1 h, 3 h, 24 h and 96 h)	*Near maximum tolerated dose used (dose-response?)*
Dose-response?	Similar high activity in untreated and pretreated patients
More active in less heavily pretreated patients	Equally active on all sites of metastases
Active in anthracycline-resistant patients	Response to prior anthracycline not predictive of response to docetaxel
Similar activity to doxorubicin	Activity superior to that of doxorubicin
Prolonged therapy feasible (mostly limited by cumulative neurotoxicity)	*Unusual toxicity (fluid retention; skin limits prolonged therapy*
High overall response and complete response rate by short infusion when combined with doxorubicin/epirubicin	High overall response and complete response rate when combined with doxorubicin/epirubicin

Adjuvant/Neo-adjuvant Trials with Taxanes

The investigation of the taxanes in an adjuvant setting is reproducing the same scenario as seen in their testing in metastatic breast cancer. The first exploratory studies have been conducted with paclitaxel. At Memorial Sloan Kettering the feasibility of single-agent paclitaxel after single-agent doxorubicin and before single agent cyclophosphamide in a program of sequential adjuvant therapy was tested (Hudis et al. 1996) and is now the reference study for a major program conducted by the CALGB (Cancer and Acute Leukemias Group B). Results of a CALGB study randomizing patients to paclitaxel versus no therapy after doxorubicin plus cyclophosphamide (AC) at different doses of doxorubicin are pending, as well as data from an NSABP (National Surgical Adjuvant Breast Program) non-randomized study of paclitaxel after AC adjuvant therapy. However, a preplanned interim analysis after the first 450 events in the CALGB study (Henderson et al. 1998) showed a statistically significant improvement of disease-free and overall survial with use of paclitaxel after AC chemotherapy. These data are the first evidence from a controlled study that women with early breast cancer may benefit from using a taxane and strongly support the carrying out of further evaluation.

In Milan, the National Cancer Institute has conducted a preliminary study of the combination of bolus doxorubicin and paclitaxel by 3-h infusion (AT) as primary chemotherapy in patients with locally advanced or operable breast cancer with a view to a larger comparative investigation of this combination in Europe, and showed feasibility and good cardiac safety of AT in all patients (Moliterni et al. 1997).

These exploratory studies are now being followed by a second and larger wave of trials with paclitaxel, while trials with docetaxel are rapidly catching up in number and design. Nineteen major trials of paclitaxel-containing che-

Table 3. Main characteristics of ongoing or planned adjuvant/neo-adjuvant studies with taxanes

Paclitaxel	Docetaxel
19 Studies	4 studies
9 adjuvant	3 adjuvant
9 neo-adjuvant	
1 adjuvant vs neo-adjuvant	1 adjuvant vs neo-adjuvant
in 17, sequential use or combination	in all, sequential use or combination
with doxorubicin or epirubicin	with doxorubicin or epirubicin

motherapy are ongoing or planned in "high-risk" breast cancer patients in the USA, Canada, and Europe, and four have been announced with the use of docetaxel (Table 3). In the vast majority of these studies the taxanes are used either in sequence or in combination with an anthracycline-containing regimen. Overall, the medical and scientific community is committing 15 000–20 000 patients with operable breast cancer to be part of the most impressive clinical effort to define the role of a new class of drugs in treating the disease. An idea of the magnitude of the human and economical resources required by these studies can be given by the projection that taxane studies will involve about a third of the total number of cases taken into account by the Early Breast Cancer Trialists' Collaborative Group (1992) to assess the role of systemic treatment by hormonal, cytotoxic, or immune therapy. A detailed analysis of the design of such trials is limited by their number and by the sketchy information that is available on the majority of them. A number of very relevant questions are addressed by these trials in addition to the key one on the actual potential value of the taxanes to improve the long-term efficacy of current treatment options. However, as a general principle, all trials are empirically based and will provide mostly empirical answers. In addition, some important aspects of the use of taxanes in early breast cancer have not been taken into account by the design of ongoing trials so far they are known.

Putting Taxanes to Work: What is Missing from Ongoing Studies

The common empirical denominator of all trials on taxanes should encourage some critical thinking. After years of controversies about the respective value and indication for hormonal and cytotoxic systemic treatment, recent studies have provided evidence of the already common opinion that the two modalities should be viewed as complementing each other. In the recently published analysis of the NSABP B-20 study of tamoxifen versus tamoxifen plus chemotherapy in node-negative, estrogen-receptor-positive patients, the concluding remark of Fisher et al. (1997) was that patients with breast cancer are candidates for chemotherapy regardless of age, lymph node status, tumor size, or estrogen receptor status. The remark is the logical conclusion of an era of breast cancer research, but it should not be viewed as the unsurpassable standard for investigational medicine. Accepted and built in all adjuvant treatment programs is the awareness that for many patients the adopted systemic therapy is not indicated because the tumor has already been eradicated, or it is not sensitive to the selected drugs. The challenge for the future is to define specific indications for individual patients to keep to a minimum the risk of unnecessary therapy. Ongoing studies with taxanes may represent a unique opportunity to test selective indications for their use rather than base each treatment decision on the risk of the average patient.

Taxanes and HER2 Status

One important aspect to assess is whether amplification/overexpression of the c-erbB-2 (HER2) gene is relevant to the therapeutic results of paclitaxel and docetaxel in early breast cancer. HER2-positive tumors are associated with a poorer prognosis, but they have also been associated with a higher probability of disease-free survival after doxorubicin-based therapy (Muss et al. 1994), so that HER2 status can be redefined as a predictor of response to the drug. More recently, Seidman et al. (1996) have shown that HER2-positivity is also an independent predictor of response to paclitaxel and docetaxel. In a retrospective evaluation of patients with metastatic breast cancer at the National Cancer Institute of Milan, HER2-positivity was associated with a higher probability of complete response following chemotherapy with doxorubicin and paclitaxel (Gianni 1997). HER2 is overexpressed/amplified in 25%–40% of breast cancers. The consistent and standardized evaluation of HER2 status in all current trials of taxanes with or without anthracyclines may clarify in large and controlled studies whether it has a true positive predictive value for the long-term efficacy of this new class of drugs. If it were to be confirmed, there would be a specific indication to use paclitaxel or docetaxel in women with HER2-positive tumors. In addition, it would allow the assessment of whether there is any advantage from the use of these drugs in women whose tumors are HER2-negative. Finally, it would be a very strong support for defining ad hoc strategies with newer drugs specifically aimed at the HER2 receptor or pathway of signal transduction. On this point, it is of note that doxorubicin and paclitaxel act synergistically with anti-HER2 monoclonal antibodies in animal models (Baselga et al. 1997). Results of a phase III trial randomizing metastatic patients to receive chemotherapy containing doxorubicin or paclitaxel with or without anti-HER monoclonal antibodies indicated a significant improvement of response rate, time to treatment failure, and survival in women who also received the antibody (Slamon et al. 1998). The results show that the same synergism as observed in experimental models occurs in humans, and strongly support the need for exploring HER2 status as a predictor of response and the possibility that the use of taxanes and their combinations should be tailored to individual characteristics rather than following the usual pattern of indiscriminate application.

Taxanes, Taxane Treatment Duration, and Angiogenesis

One question that will not be answered by the current set of adjuvant/neo-adjuvant trials is the optimal duration of treatment with taxanes. In all cases, paclitaxel and docetaxel will be given for a maximum of four cycles either alone or in combination. This is in keeping with the background of adjuvant studies showing that four to six cycles of chemotherapy are enough to achieve benefit, that additional chemotherapy is not more advantageous (Early Breast Cancer Trialists' Calloborative Group 1992), and that sequential administration of non-cross-resistant drugs/regimens provides better long-term results (Hudis et al. 1996; Bonadonna et al. 1995). In addition, the neurotoxicity of paclitaxel and severe bone marrow toxicity plus fluid retention syndrome caused by docetaxel (Table 2) suggest caution in their prolonged indiscriminate administration in any adjuvant program. However, prolonged administration of paclitaxel has been used in metastatic breast cancer patients, and there is evidence of increased antitumor activity (Gianni et al. 1997) and longer survival in a comparative trial of the taxane with CMFP (Bishop et al. 1997). These results may be viewed as a consequence of the recognized antiangiogenic effect of paclitaxel, which is able to inhibit neovascularization and endothelial cell proliferation (Klauber et al. 1997; Belotti et al. 1996). Although it is difficult to propose a design for exploiting in early breast cancer the anti-angiogenic quality of paclitaxel, and possibly of docetaxel, due to their tolerability and the theoretical need for chronic administration of antiangiogenic drugs, the possibility that breast tumor angiogenetic phenotype was not only a factor of poor prognosis (Gasparini et al. 1997), but also a predictor of response to taxanes should be take into account in ongoing trials.

Paclitaxel or Docetaxel?

A final and very relevant question relates to the respective merits and limitations of paclitaxel and docetaxel. Only one, still ongoing trial in metastatic breast cancer, and none of the adjuvant/neo-adjuvant trials in early breast cancer, directly compares the two taxanes. Indirect comparison from phase II trials in metastatic patients is generating different opinions. Given the magnitude of the human and economic resources involved in the ongoing investigation of paclitaxel and docetaxel in breast cancer, the lack of comparative evaluation may become a limiting factor. An important feature of preoperative chemotherapy in breast cancer is that it affords a rapid assessment of response with pathological evaluation as the endpoint, with the additional advantage that response is also a predictor of long-term outcome, as indicated by at least two studies (Fisher et al. 1997; Bonadonna et al. 1998). With this in mind, preoperative direct comparison of paclitaxel and docetaxel using clinical and pathological response as the surrogate marker of long-term results would require relatively low numbers of patients, and would provide a rapid answer based on evidence rather than opinion about the respective value, limitations, and benefits of the two taxanes.

Summary

The taxanes paclitaxel and docetaxel are the prototype drugs of a new class of anticancer drugs that exploits a completely new mechanism of action. Their testing in metastatic breast cancer has been extensive. The results indicating very high response rate with either taxane have given rise to an unprecedented effort in the scientific community to define their optimal application in all stages of the disease. In metastatic breast cancer, initial data suggest that paclitaxel may increase the survival obtained with standard combinations such as CMFP, and similarly promising studies of docetaxel are almost complete. Significant therapeutic benefit has also been observed by the addition of sequential paclitaxel after adjuvant doxorubicin plus cyclophosphamide in operable breast cancer. Overall, more than 20 randomized studies with paclitaxel or docetaxel, either as single agents or in combination, are ongoing or planned in women with high-risk operable breast cancer. This massive effort is mainly based on empirical study designs. However, some preclinical characteristics of the taxanes, such as their increased antitumor effect in tumors overexpressing HER2/neu, the preclinical and clinical evidence of potential synergism with monoclonal antibodies directed against the HER2 receptor, and preclinical evidence of antiangiogenic properties should be pursued to test whether the use of taxanes in breast cancer could be tailored to individual tumor characteristics rather than following the usual pattern of indiscriminate application.

References

Baselga J, Seidman AD, Rosen PP et al (1997) HER2 overexpression and paclitaxel sensitivity in breast cancer: therapeutic implications. Oncology (Huntingt) 11:43–48

Belotti D, Vergani V, Drudis T et al (1996) The microtubule-affecting drug paclitaxel has antiangiogenic activity. Clin Cancer Res 2:1843–1849

Bishop JF, Dewar J, Tattersall MH et al (1997) Taxol alone is equivalent to CMFP combination chemotherapy as frontline treatment in metastatic breast cancer. Proc Am Soc Clin Oncol 16:153a (abstract 538)

Bonadonna G, Zambetti M, Valagussa P (1995) Sequential or alternating doxorubicin and CMF regimens in breast cancer with more than three positive nodes. Ten-year results. JAMA 273:542–547

Bonadonna G, Valagussa P, Brambilla C et al (1998) Primary chemotherapy in operable breast cancer: eight-year experience at the Milan Cancer Institute. J Clin Oncol 16:93–100

Bourgeois H, Gruia G, Dieras V et al (1996) Docetaxel in combination with doxorubicin as first line CT of metastatic breast cancer. Proc Am Soc Clin Oncol 15:148 (abstract 259)

Conte PF, Baldini E, Gennari A et al (1997) Dose-finding study and pharmacokinetics of epirubicin and paclitaxel over 3 hours: a regimen with high activity and low cardiotoxicity in advanced breast cancer. J Clin Oncol 15:2510–2517

Dombernowsky P, Gehl J, Boesgaard M et al (1996) Paclitaxel and doxorubicin, a highly active combination in the treatment of metastatic breast cancer. Semin Oncol 23 (Suppl 1):13–18

Early Breast Cancer Trialists' Collaborative Group (1992) Systemic treatment of early breast cancer by hormonal, cytotoxic, or immune therapy: 133 randomized trials involving 31 000 recurrences and 24 000 deaths among 75 000 women. Lancet 339 (i):71–85

Fisher B, Brown A, Mamounas E et al (1997a) Effect of preoperative therapy for primary breast cancer on local-regional disease, disease-free survival and survival: results from NSABP B-18. Proc Am Soc Clin Oncol 16:127a (abstract 449)

Fisher B, Dignam J, Wolmark N et al (1997b) Tamoxifen and chemotherapy for lymph node-negative, estrogen receptor-positive breast cancer. J Natl Cancer Inst 89:1673–1682

Frassinetti GL, Zoli W, Tienghi A et al (1996) Phase I/II study of sequential combination of paclitaxel and doxorubicin in the treatment of advanced breast cancer. Proc Am Soc Clin Oncol 15:109

Gasparini G, Toi M, Gion M et al (1997) Prognostic significance of vascular endothelial growht factor protein in node-negative breast carcinoma. J Natl Cancer Inst 89:139–147

Gianni L (1995) Theoretical and practical aspects of paclitaxel scheduling. Ann Oncol 6:861–863

Gianni L (1997) Future directions of paclitaxel-based therapy of breast cancer. Semin Oncol 24 Suppl 17:91–96

Gianni L, Capri G (1997a) Experience at the Istituto Nationale Tumori with paclitaxel in combination with doxorubicin in women with untreated breast cancer. Semin Oncol 24 Suppl 3:1–3

Gianni L, Capri G (1997b) In: Bonadonna G, Hortobagyi GN, Gianni AM (eds) Textbook of breast cancer: a clinical guide to therapy. Martin Dunitz, London, pp 253–280

Gianni L, Munzone E, Capri G et al (1995a) Paclitaxel by 3-hour infusion in combination with bolus doxorubicin in women with untreated metastatic breast cancer: high antitumor efficacy and cardiac effects in a dose-finding and sequence-finding study. J Clin Oncol 13:2688–2699

Gianni L, Munzone E, Capri G et al (1995b) Paclitaxel in metastatic breast cancer: a trial of two doses by a 3-hour infusion in patients with disease recurrence after prior therapy with anthracyclines. J Natl Cancer Inst 87:1169–1175

Henderson IC, Berry D, Demetri G et al (1998) Improved disease-free and overall survival from the addition of sequential paclitaxel but not from the escalation of doxorubicin dose-level in the adjuvant chemotherapy of patients with node-positive primary breast cancer. Proc Am Soc Clin Oncol 17:101a

Hudis CA, Seidman A, Raptis G et al (1996) Sequential adjuvant therapy: the Memorial Sloan-Kettering Cancer Center experience. Semin Oncol 23 (Suppl 1):58–64

Klauber N, Parangi S, Flynn E et al (1997) Inhibition of angiogenesis and breast cancer in mice by the microtubule inhibitors 2-methoxyestradiol and taxol. Cancer Res 57:81–86

Moliterni A, Tarenzi E, Capri G et al (1997) Pilot study of primary chemotherapy with doxorubicin plus paclitaxel in women with locally advanced or operable breast cancer. Semin Oncol 24 (Suppl 17):10–14

Muss HB, Thor AD, Berry DA et al (1994) c-erbB-2 expression and response to adjuvant therapy in women with node-positive early breast cancer. (Published erratum appears in N Engl J Med 1994::331:211). N Engl J med 330:1260–1266

Nabholtz JM, Gelmon K, Spielmann M et al (1996) Multicenter, randomized comparative study of two doses of paclitaxel in patients with metastatic breast cancer. J Clin Oncol 14:1858–1867

Ravdin PM (1995) Taxoids: effective agents in anthracycline-resistant breast cancer. Semin Oncol 22 (Suppl 13):29–34

Ravdin PM, Burris HA, Cook G et al (1995) Phase II tiral of docetaxel in advanced anthracycline-resistant or anthracenedione-resistant breast cancer. J Clin Oncol 13:2879–2885

Schwartsmann G, Menke CH, Caleffi M et al (1996) Phase II trial of taxol (T), doxorubicin (D) plus G-CSF in patients (pts) with metastatic breast cancer (MBC). Proc Am Soc Clin Oncol 15:126

Seidman AD (1995) The emerging role of paclitaxel in breast cancer therapy. Clin Cancer Res 1:247–256

Seidman AD, Reichman BS, Crown JPA et al (1995) Paclitaxel as second and subsequent therapy for metastatic breast cancer: activity independent of prior anthracycline response. J Clin Oncol 13:1152–1159

Seidman AD, Baselga J, Yao T-Y et al (1996) HER2-/*neu* over expression and clinical taxane sensitivity: a multivariate analysis in patients with metastatic breast cancer. Proc Am Soc Clin Oncol 15:104 (abstract 80)

Slamon D, Leyland-Jones B, Shak S et al (1998) Addition of Herceptin (humanized anti-HER2 antibody) to first-line chemotherapy for HER2 overexpressing metastatic breast cancer markedly increases anticancer activity: a randomized international controlled Phase III trial. Proc Am Soc Clin Oncol 17:98a

Sledge GW, Neuberg D, Ingle J et al (1997) Phase III trial of doxorubicin vs paclitaxel vs doxorubicin plus paclitaxel as first-line therapy for metastatic breast cancer: an intergroup trial. Proc Am Soc Clin Oncol 16:1a (abstract 2)

Continuous Infusional Chemotherapy for Early Breast Cancer: The Royal Marsden Hospital Experience

I. E. Smith

Department of Medicine, Royal Marsden Hospital, Downs Road, Sutton, Surrey, SM2 5PT, UK

Introduction

Continuous infusional chemotherapy is not a new concept. The clinical use of long-term infusional fluorinated pyrimidines was first described in the 1960s (Sullivan et al. 1960), but interest has been renewed in recent years as the limitations of conventional chemotherapy in common solid tumours have become increasingly clear. 5-FU has been the major drug studied.

5-FU is a cycle-specific S-phase-dependent drug with a short half-life of 10–20 min (Ensminger et al. 1978) and is therefore appropriate for use in long-term continuous infusional chemotherapy. Lokich et al. (1981) showed that surprisingly large doses of up to 300 mg/m^2 per day could be delivered by ambulatory pump and long-term indwelling central venous lines for prolonged periods. This represents a greater than five-fold increase in dose intensity over many standard conventional schedules (e.g. CMF), with plantar-palmar syndrome and mucositis replacing myelosuppression as the dose-limiting toxicity. Subsequently Lokich et al. (1989) went on to demonstrate in a randomised trial that continuous infusional 5-FU for 10 weeks or more achieved a significantly higher response rate than 5-day conventional bolus treatment (30% vs 7%) in patients with advanced colorectal cancer, with less myelosuppression.

Continuous infusional 5-FU has been used in several small phase II studies involving patients with advanced breast cancer, usually heavily pretreated. These studies have been reviewed by Cameron et al. (1994) with an overall objective response rate of 29% in a total of 199 patients, mostly treated with doses of 200–300 mg/m^2. There was considerable variation in individual response rates, including up to 54% in one study (Huan et al. 1989), and a feature of some of these patients was that they had received previous conventional 5-FU. More recently, a larger retrospective analysis of 106 consecutive patients treated with outpatient infusional 5-FU 250 mg/m^2 every 24 h for 3-week periods followed by 1-week pauses was reported by a Swiss group (Regazzoni et al. 1996). Twenty-one percent of 80 evaluable patients achieved a formal objective response, and this included a response rate of 20% for patients previously treated with conventional 5-FU. Interestingly, the authors also reported subjective symptom improvement in 44% of 104 patients evaluable for this endpoint, and in general treatment was well tolerated. These results indicate the potential value of continuous infusional 5-FU as palliative treatment. They also hint at possible high activity for infusional 5-FU as frontline treatment, although no frontline phase II data are available.

Royal Marsden Experience: Metastatic Breast Cancer

At the Royal Marsden Hospital we have evaluated infusional 5-FU 200 mg/m^2 per day continuously for up to 6 months in combination with 3-weekly bolus epirubicin 60 mg/m^2 i.v. and cisplatin 60 mg/m^2 or cyclophosphamide 600 mg/m^2 carboplatin AUC 5 (so-called infusional ECF) in a series of phase II and randomised phase III trials. In a non-randomised sequential study we showed that carboplatin could be substituted for cisplatin with no apparent loss of efficacy (Bonnefoi et al. 1996). More recently, in a randomised phase II trial, we have shown that cyclophosphamide can be substituted for cisplatin with very similar efficacy, a lower incidence of severe nausea and vomiting and no increased toxicity, with the advantages of an outpatient schedule (Eisen et al. 1998).

The combined response rates for these schedules are shown in Table 1. This shows that these schedules of infusional chemotherapy are highly active, with an overall response rate of 80%. The median survival from start of treatment was 1 year, with an 18% 5-year survival. These data encouraged us to investigate infusional ECF (using cisplatin) in early breast cancer.

One hundred and twenty-three patients with early operable breast cancer and tumour size ≥3 cm have been entered into studies of pre-operative infusional ECF (epirubicin, cisplatin, infusional 5-FU) chemotherapy at the following dosages: epirubicin 60 mg/m^2 i.v. every 21 days, cisplatin 60 mg/m^2 i.v. every 21 days, 5-FU 200 mg/m^2 i.v. by continuous infusion for 6 months. Fifty of these patients were included in an initial phase II trial whose results have already been reported (Smith et al. 1995). The remaining 73 are part of a multicentre randomised trial described below. The median tumour size in these patients is 5 cm (range 3–12 cm). The median age of the patients is 44 years (range 25–61 years). The overall objective response rate is 96%, with 57% achieving a complete clinical remission. The actuarial 5-year survival rate is 75%.

Table 1. Infusional ECF chemotherapy: response rates in metastatic breast cancer

	Response[a]			
	ECisF	ECarboF	ECycloF	Total
No. of patients	40	36	19	95
Complete response	18%	17%	6%	15%
Overall response	80%	81%	74%	80%

[a] No previous chemotherapy for metastatic breast cancer.

Table 2. Infusional ECisF toxicity

	WHO toxicity (% of patients)	
	Grade 1–2	Grade 3–4
Leucopenia	75	12
Infection	34	14
Emesis	74	22
Alopecia	48	52
Neuropathy	37	2
Stomatitis	47	12
Plantar-palmar syndrome	40	14
Hickman infection	28	14
Thrombosis	–	12

So far the survival of clinical complete responders is the same as for partial responders, with the small number of non-responders doing significantly worse. The pathological complete remission rate in this series is 16%, with a further 5% showing DCIS alone. Current data show significant survival improvement for complete pathological responders over others, but at present the difference is not significant.

In general, infusional ECisF chemotherapy is well tolerated. WHO toxicity grades for the most important side effects are given in Table 2.

Randomised Trials of Infusional Chemotherapy in Early Breast Cancer

Currently the Royal Marsden Hospital is conducting two national multicentre randomised trials of infusional chemotherapy. The first (TOPIC trial) is a trial of pre-operative chemotherapy in which patients with tumours ≥3 cm in maximum diameter are randomised to receive infusional ECisF versus conventional AC (adriamycin 60 mg/m², cyclophosphamide 600 mg/m² i.v. every 2 days×6 courses). Three hundred and seventy patients are so far entered towards a target of 400 patients.

In the second trial (TRAFIC) patients are randomised to adjuvant infusional ECisF versus standard conventional FEC (5-FU 600 mg/m², epirubicin 60 mg/m², cyclophosphamide 600 mg/m² every 21 days×6 courses). This trial started more recently and so far 164 patients have entered. Participating centres for both trials are listed in Table 3.

Conclusions

Infusional ECisF chemotherapy is a very active treatment for metastatic breast cancer and it achieves response rates and complete remission rates as pre-operative chemotherapy that are higher than those reported for other

Table 3. Centres participating in two UK national randomised trials of infusional chemotherapy

TOPIC (*Trial Of Primary Infusional Chemotherapy*):
Royal Marsden Hospital, London and Sutton
Christie Hospital, Manchester
Mayday Hospital, Croydon
Epsom Hospital, Epsom
Mid-Kent Oncology Centre, Maidstone
Royal Bournemouth Hospital, Dorset
St George's Hospital, London
Essex County Hospital, Colchester
Addenbrooke's Hospital, Cambridge
Bristol Oncology Centre, Bristol
Yorkshire Breast Group
Royal Free Hospital, London
Southend Hospital, Essex
Ipswich Hospital, Suffolk
Salisbury Hospital, Wiltshire
University College Hospital, London
St Luke's Hospital, Guildford
St Bartholomew's Hospital, London

TRAFIC (*TRial of Adjuvant 5-FU Infusional Chemotherapy*):
Royal Marsden Hospital, London and Sutton
Yorkshire Breast Group
Royal Bournemouth Hospital, Hampshire
Salisbury District Hospital, Wiltshire
Mid-Kent Oncology Centre, Maidstone
St Luke's Hospital, Guildford

major studies. The TOPIC trial and TRAFIC trial will help to determine whether this high activity can translate into significant survival improvement in patients with early breast cancer.

Summary

5-FU is a cycle-specific S-phase-dependent drug with a short half life of 10–20 min. There is therefore a rationale for its use in long-term continuous infusional therapy, with doses of up to 300 mg/m^2 per day proving feasible for prolonged periods. The schedule is active in patients with heavily pre-treated breast cancer, with responses in up to 53% (overall 29%). At the Royal Marsden Hospital we have evaluated infusional 5-FU 200 mg/m^2 per day for up to 6 months in combination with 3-weekly bolus epirubicin (E) 60 mg/m^2 and cisplatin (C) 60 mg/m^2 (infusional ECF) as pre-operative/neo-adjuvant treatment in 123 patients with operable breast cancer greater than 3 cm (median 6 cm), initially in a phase II study of 50 patients and subsequently as part of a randomised phase III trial. One hundred and eighteen (96%) have achieved objective tumour responses, with 67 (57%) achieving CR. The 5-year actuarial survival rate is 78% and the local recurrence rate without associated metastatic disease 12%. The pathological complete remission (CR) rate was 16%, with a further 5% having residual DCIS only. Pathological CR but not clinical CR is an independent predictor for disease-fee survival. The Royal Marsden is now conducting two multicentre randomised trials of infusional ECF: (i) versus conventional AC (adriamycin cyclophosphamide) as pre-operative/neo-adjuvant chemotherapy, with 376 patients so far randomised towards a target of 400; and (ii), more recently, a similar adjuvant trial versus conventional FEC (5-FU, epirubicin, cyclophosphamide), with 168 patients so far randomised. These trials will determine whether encouraging phase II activity with continuous infusional chemotherapy translates eventually into real survival benefit for patients with early breast cancer.

References

Bonnefoi H, Smith IE, O'Brien MER et al (1996) Phase II study of continuous infusional 5-fluorouracil with epirubicin and carboplatin (instead of cisplatin) in patients with metastatic/locally advanced breast cancer (infusional ECarboF): a very active and well-tolerated outpatient regimen. Br J Cancer 73:391–396

Cameron DA, Gabra H, Leonhard RCF (1994) Continuous 5-fluorouracil in the treatment of breast cancer. Br J Cancer 70:120–124

Eisen T, Smith IE, Johnston S et al (1998) A randomised phase II trial of infusional 5-fluorouracil, epirubicin and cyclophosphamide (ECycloF) versus infusional 5-fluorouracil, epirubicin and cisplatin (ECisF) in patients with advanced breast cancer. J Clin Oncol (in press)

Ensminger WD, Rosowsky A, Raso V, Levin DC, Glode M, Come S, Steele G, Frei E III (1978) A clinical pharmacologic evaluation of hepatic arterial infusion of 5-fluoro-2'-deoxyuridine and 5-fluorouracil. Cancer Res 38:3784–3792

Huan S, Pazdur R, Singhakowinta A, Samal B, Vaikevicius V (1989) Low-dose continuous infusion 5-fluorouracil: evaluation in advanced breast cancer. Cancer 63:419–422

Lokich J, Bothe A, Fine N, Perri J (1981) Phase I study of protracted venous infusion of 5-fluorouracil. Cancer 48:2565–2568

Lokich JJ, Ahlgren JD, Gullo J et al (1989) A prospective randomised comparison of continuous infusion fluorouracil with a conventional bolus schedule in metastatic colorectal carcinoma: a Mid-Atlantic Oncology Program Study. J Clin Oncol 7:425–432

Regazzoni S, Pesce G, Marini G et al (1996) Low-dose continuous intravenous infusion of 5-fluorouracil for metastatic breast cancer. Ann Oncol 7:807–813

Smith IE, Walsh G, Jones A et al (1995) High complete remission rates with primary neoadjuvant infusional chemotherapy for large early breast cancer. J Clin Oncol 13:424–429

Sullivan RD, Young CW, Miller E et al (1960) The clinical effects of the continuous administration of fluorinated pyrimidines (5-fluorouracil and 5-fluoro-5-deoxyuridine). Cancer Chemother Rep 8:77–81

Tailored Chemotherapy to Equal Toxicity: Is It Possible?

J. Bergh

Department of Oncology, University Hospital, 75185 Uppsala, Sweden

Setting the Scene: Shortcomings of Present Dosage Strategies

The intention of chemotherapy for a malignant disease can be either curative or palliative. In breast cancer the former applies to therapy of micrometastatic disease in the adjuvant setting or as a preoperative procedure, while conventionally delivered chemotherapy for metastatic disease is considered to be strictly palliative. The latter statement, however, is challenged by different dose-intensive concepts including the use of high-dose therapy supported by autologous bone marrow stem cells (Bezwoda et al. 1995). The prognosis for breast cancer has been improved by the use of early detection programmes and adjuvant therapy, while the prognosis for patients with metastatic breast cancer is still dismal (Early Breast Cancer Trialists' Collaborative Group 1992; Nyström et al. 1993; Overgaard et al. 1997; Ragaz et al. 1997).

This review will focus on present methods of calculating chemotherapy dosage and whether other complementary methods may be better because these methods may improve the anti-tumoral effects of chemotherapy while at the same time ameliorating its side effects.

Conventionally dosed chemotherapy leads to severe side effects in some patients, with grade 3 or 4 toxicity, while others have very few/minimal or even "no" side effects. In almost all clinical studies and in clinical routine the former group will most likely receive reduced doses for all remaining courses, while in almost all protocols the latter group will continue to receive an unchanged dose. This latter group may then potentially be undertreated. Furthermore, in clinical practice many clinicians round off the dose. An unproven suspicion is that many clinicians tend to *reduce* the dose to a nearby practical dose level; e.g., a calculated 5-fluorouracil dose of 1075 mg (600 mg/m^2) may tend to be rounded down to 1000 mg. This corresponds to a "weight loss" of around 11 kg for a woman weighing 69 kg. Finally, the dose close to or the maximum tolerated dose, which is recommended for phase III/IV studies and for clinical routine, is derived from studies on a very limited number of patients.

These assumptions and facts may impair the outcome for the individual patient and for groups of patients, because the effect of most cytostatics can be related to the drug concentration and exposure time (Evans and Relling

1989). A 20% reduction in dose results in a 50% reduction of curability in certain animal tumor models (Hutchison and Schmid 1973; Schabel and Simpson-Herren 1978). The situation for humans with relatively slowly proliferating cancers is far more complicated. However, almost all breast cancer studies disclose a dose-response relationship which has translated into a survival benefit in only a few studies (Bergh 1997). The reason for this discrepancy may be related to the biology of the disease, including different resistance mechanisms, but it may also be due to suboptimal dosage setting for the individual patient, as outlined above and as will be described on the following pages. This possibility is of course a general problem for all patients receiving anti-neoplastic agents. The up to ten-fold interpatient variations that have been described in systemic exposure or for different cytostatics in patients with "normal" renal and hepatic function add to the complexity (reviewed in Gurney 1996; Sandström et al. 1996). Conventional dose intensity studies may result in equivalent areas under the curves, even when one individual receives twice the dose of another (Tables 1, 2).

Conventional Phase I Studies for Selection of the Maximum Tolerated Dose

The search for the maximum tolerated dose is normally pursued in phase I studies on the basis of triplets of patients at each dose level. If one of three patients experiences severe toxicity, three to six more patients are included at this dose level. Normally the maximum tolerated dose will be found with 14–30 patients, including all dose steps (EORTC New Drug Development Committee 1985). A so far unproven assumption is that up to 50% of the pa-

Table 1. Dose intensity in four patients receiving two different dose levels is dependent on clearance (Gurney 1996)

Dose of drug Z (mg/m^2)	Patient			
	A BSA = 1.7 CL = 85	B BSA = 1.7 CL = 0.5×A	C BSA = 2.0 CL = same as A	D BSA = 2.0 CL = 2×A
50				
Dose (mg)	85	85	100	100
AUC	1.0	2.0	1.2	0.6
100				
Dose (mg)	170	170	200	200
AUC	2.0	4.0	2.4	1.2

BSA, Body surface area; CL, clearance; AUC, area under the curve.
Note: Assumptions: (1) pharmacokinetic parameters of drug Z are linear; (2) variation in drug handling is described as the CL of each patient relative to patient A; (3) BSA does not standardize for the variation in drug handling between individuals; (4) CL = dose/AUC.

Table 2. Shortcomings of setting dosage according to body surface area

1. The formula was established on the basis of just nine healthy individuals
2. No correlation has been demonstrated between body surface area and liver function
3. For the majority of the cytostatics there is no correlation between body surface area and pharmacokinetics
4. There is no compensation for variations in clearance
5 The interpatient variation in systemic exposure/clearance is by a factor of 2–11

tients in a conventional phase I study may not have reached their individual maximum tolerated dose. The "maximum tolerated dose" may accordingly represent too low a dose for some patients (Evans 1993). Individual patient tolerance to cytostatics is dependent on a number of unknown and partly known factors: concomitant diseases, previous chemo- and/or radiotherapy, and individual normal tissue sensitivity, which may vary between different organ systems. In most phase I studies many of the patients will be severely ill and many will have been exposed to previous chemotherapy, which of course may have altered renal and liver function, not reflected by conventional laboratory tests.

These potential shortcomings will later be discussed in the light of our present findings on tailored polychemotherapy, based on the haematological tolerance of each individual patient.

Conventional Dosage of Chemotherapy in Relation to Body Surface Area

Standard practice for the dosage of almost all cytostatics is related to body surface area, with the intention to deliver equivalent drug amounts to each patient. This dosage procedure causes both overtreatment and undertreatment, resulting respectively in unwarranted toxicity and suboptimal therapy results (reviewed in Gurney 1996). In the clinic, the only general exception to this dosage principle based on body surface area is the calculation of carboplatin dose according to Calvert's formula, which is based on renal function (Calvert et al. 1989).

The calculation of two-dimensional body surface area using standard nomograms was originally based on the investigation of nine healthy individuals (Table 2) (Du Bois and Du Bois 1916). The body surface area has been demonstrated to correlate with blood volume and glomerular filtration rate (reviewed in Gurney 1996). Accordingly, in a study of five cytostatics, three of them renally excreted (actinomycin, mercaptopurine and methotrexate), a correlation was described between renal function and body surface (Pinkel 1958; reviewed in Gurney 1996). By contrast, no data have so far been presented to demonstrate a correlation between liver function and body surface area. Many cytotoxic drugs are metabolised by the liver. Another concern is the marked variations between liver function in normal individuals (Lauterburg and Preisig 1991). Taken together, these facts raise major concerns because many cytostatics are metabolised and/or excreted via the liver and biliary system.

Pharmacokinetics

Pharmacokinetic monitoring is routinely performed for anti-convulsants, anti-depressants, drugs belonging to the neuroleptic group, digoxin, theophylline and certain antibiotics. The dosages of these drugs are based on pharmacokinetic monitoring together with conventional clinical and laboratory parameters. For the majority of cytostatics analysed a positive correlation with toxicity was demonstrated for different pharmacokinetic variables (reviewed in Gurney 1996). A similar correlation was demonstrated for tumor response in certain tumors, mainly chemotherapy-sensitive ones, but this question needs to be more thoroughly studied in more patients and tumour groups.

Pharmacokinetic evaluation of cytotoxic agents is only routinely performed when high-dose methotrexate schemes are used and in phase I and sometimes phase II studies when new chemotherapeutic agents are being investigated and characterised. Later in the clinical development of cytotoxic agents, and after their formal approval, this type of monitoring is only rarely performed. This is strange, especially when severe side effects are recorded or when limited toxicity is seen. Cytostatics have a narrow therapeutic index and certain tumors demonstrate a clear dose-response relationship. This should suggest an expanded use of pharmacokinetic analyses, especially in patients with marked side effects or with no side effects on standard doses. Furthermore, the use of cytotoxic agents in different combinations will most likely alter their individual pharmacokinetic profiles, whereas the initial pharmacokinetic studies on the compounds were almost invariably performed on single agents. We have previously analysed the pharmacokinetic data for 5-fluorouracil, epirubicin and cyclophosphamide (5-hydroxycyclophosphamide) in the standard FEC combination for breast cancer patients (Sandström et al. 1996) and found no correlations between the pharmacokinetics for these cytostatics for the individual patient, further underlining the complexity in dosage and direct clinical application of these findings (Sandström et al. 1996).

Pharmacokinetics and Body Surface Area

The potential relationship between body surface area and pharmacokinetic parameters has been studied. In retrospective analyses of phase II studies no correlations could be demonstrated for busulfan and paclitaxel and other less commonly used compounds (Grochow et al. 1990). Furthermore, for the investigated parameters no correlations were revealed for carboplatin, etoposide, epirubicin, ifosfamide and some further less commonly used cytostatics (reviewed in Gurney 1996). On the other hand, correlations have been claimed for docetaxel and gemcitabine (Allerheiligen et al. 1994; Bruno et al. 1995). The possible discrepancy between findings for the closely related compounds docetaxel and paclitaxel is somewhat difficult to understand.

Why Are Pharmacokinetic Analyses Not Used on Cancer Patients?

The reasons for the critical attitudes towards pharmacokinetic analyses among physicians treating cancer patients with cytostatics could be either that solid scientific evidence to support the use of pharmacokinetic monitoring is lacking, or it could be due to the practical complexity of using conventional pharmacokinetic analyses, which require multiple samples over an extended period. The most far-fetched possibility could be the combination of these two factors together with some ignorance and conservatism. The laboratory part of pharmacokinetic analyses takes a considerable time, making this procedure less adapted to the clinical management of the individual patient. All these statements are partly correct, but present data support further investigations within this area. A potential step forward in the clinical applicability of pharmacokinetics is the limited sampling procedure and bayesean methodology described by Paalzow (1990). This will allow complete pharmacokinetic calculations on the basis of data from a few plasma samples (Sandström et al. 1996).

Other Factors Which May Influence Outcome

Apart from the pharmacokinetic factors, the determinants of outcome for the individual patient of course relate mainly to the status of the different tumor-biological factors, i.e., predictive factors including cellular factors regulating apoptosis, proliferation and resistance to cytostatics and angiogenesis. These factors demonstrate heterogeneity and variability in their longitudinal expression over time, making the picture even more complex (Sjögren et al., unpublished manuscript; Lindahl et al., unpublished data). Ideally, the therapy should be tailored and modified according to all these considerations. However, this is not a realistic option for clinical routine today.

Clinical Application of Pharmacokinetically Tailored Therapy/ Therapeutic Drug Monitoring

Pharmacokinetic monitoring is routinely performed to determine the requirement for folinic acid replacement when high-dose methotrexate schemes are used, to avoid severe haematological and gastrointestinal toxicity. Pharmacokinetic monitoring is required to avoid renal and neurological toxicity when suramin is used (Mirza et al. 1997). Pharmacokinetic analyses were also used in a small randomised study of etoposide which concluded that patients should receive a fixed dose of 260 mg etoposide, because there was no correlation between pharmacokinetic variables and body surface area (Ratain et al. 1991).

Pharmacokinetics and Individual Tailoring of Therapy Based on Haematological Toxicity

We have chosen to explore haematological toxicity as a determinant of dose selection (Bergh et al. 1998). This is used as a pragmatic alternative to pharmacokinetically guided dosage or the use of fixed doses depending strictly on body surface area (Bergh et al. 1998). We use six different dose levels in our dose-escalated programmes for patients with metastatic disease and in the neo-adjuvant and adjuvant setting (Table 3) (Lindman, unpublished data; Bergh et al. 1998). The selection of dose levels and the tailoring are based on our previous pharmacokinetic results obtained by the limited sampling technique (Sandström et al. 1996). This study has demonstrated marked interpatient variability, with a clearance variation with a factor of 2–7 (Sandström et al. 1996). We have chosen to restrict the tailoring of the therapy to cyclophosphamide and epirubicin, excluding 5-fluorouracil, because the dosage is based only on haematological toxicity (Table 4). The epirubicin and cyclophosphamide doses vary from 38 to 120 mg/m^2 and from 450 to 1800 mg/m^2, respectively (Table 3). This strategy is further supported by a recent retrospective study demonstrating improved survival for stage II and III breast cancer patients experiencing the most marked leucocyte nadir values on standard chemotherapy (Saarto et al. 1997). The aim with our present tailored concept is to obtain this form of toxicity in all patients.

Based on these dose intervals, we have one ongoing multicentre adjuvant phase III study and a closed phase II study on patients with metastatic breast cancer, and an ongoing multicentre phase II study on patients with locally advanced breast cancer. At one centre, Uppsala, Sweden, we also intend

Table 3. Treatment arm A: dosages. Cycle length is 6 weeks and treatment is for nine courses. Course 1 is set at the level of step 1, courses 2–9 are set according to the dose modification schedule in Table 4

	5-FU (mg/m^2)	Epirubicin (mg/m^2)	Cyclophosphamide (mg/m^2)	Uromitexan (mg/m^2)
Step –2	300	38	450	
Step –1	600	60	600	
Step 1 (day 1)	600	75	900	
Step 2	600	90	1200	240, hours 0, 4, 8
Step 3	600	105	1500	300, hours 0, 4, 8
Step 4	600	120	1800	360, hours 0, 4, 8

Table 4. Dose modification schedule for the SBG 9401 trial, A arm, after amendments 17 Nov 1994 and 30 Nov 1995

Nadir day 8, 11/12 or 15			Day 8, 11/12 or 15 (except nadir value)			Day 22			Action
WBC ($\times 10^9$/l)	Platelets ($\times 10^9$/l)		WBC ($\times 10^9$/l)	Platelets ($\times 10^9$/l)		WBC ($\times 10^9$/l)		Platelets ($\times 10^9$/l)	
>1.0	>50	and	≥1.5	≥75	and	≥3.0	and	≥100	Dose escalation. Continue to next step
≤1.0	≤50	and/or	<1.5	<75	and	≥3.0	and	≥100	Stay on same step for next course
Any	≤15	and/or	any	any	and	any		any	Reduce 1 step and/or other treatment
>1.0	>50	and	≥1.5	≥75	and	2.5–2.9	and	≥100	Stay on same step for next course
Any	any	and	any	any	and	2.0–2.9	and/or	75–99	Reduce 1 step. if this is tolerated, escalate according to schedule again
Any	any	and	any	any	and	<2	and/or	<75	Delay 1 week. When values normal reduce 1 step, but ≥step 1

to take samples for later analyses of pharmacokinetic parameters. We will later investigate whether the pharmacokinetic data correlate with the bone marrow toxicity and the non-haematological toxicities using the NCI toxicity scoring system. The pharmacokinetic values will later be related to the primary and secondary endpoints in the adjuvant SBG 9401 study and in the phase II studies.

The major reasons at this stage not to have pharmacokinetic-guided dosage are the multicentre design and the fact that so far we have been unable to run analyses on a daily basis. However, if the upcoming pharmacokinetic analyses should add additional information and knowledge to the above-mentioned studies, this type of pharmacokinetic dosage should ideally be considered for testing in a prospective controlled study.

Practical Application of Tailored Therapy

In the ongoing and closed studies referred to above, the white blood cell and platelet counts on days 8, 11/12, 15 and 22 (next course) are decisive for the selection of the dose level for the next course (Table 4). Table 5 shows marked interindividual differences with reference to delivered doses (Bergh et al. 1998).

The major difference compared with conventional chemotherapy schemes is that we allow both dose escalations, unchanged doses and dose reductions on the basis of individual tolerance of therapy during each course. All patients have been treated to equivalent haematological toxicity (Table 5). The delivered epirubicin and cyclophosphamide doses were significantly higher than with conventional schemes (Tables 3, 5) (Bergh et al. 1998).

For some reason dose escalations are almost never used in phase II and III studies and in clinical routine, even if the patient has no side effects. This has of course to be related to the aim of the therapy. If the patients tolerate higher doses without increased toxicity, improved anti-tumoral effects and possible survival effects may theoretically be considered. Reductions, on the other hand, are frequently implemented in both clinical studies and clinical routine. Furthermore, once a patient has had a dose reduction, standard procedure is to continue at the reduced dose level for the remaining planned courses. This may be acceptable in the palliative situation, whenever a higher dose level is associated with more toxicity, but individual tolerance is variable, making this relationship far more complex. Dose reductions may theoretically be detrimental to the outcome of the individual patient, because although the majority of breast cancer studies have shown a dose-response relationship, most have found it difficult to demonstrate a survival gain (Bergh 1997). One possibility for the negative dose escalation studies could be that the conventional schemes have investigated fixed escalations to 50% of the study population, irrespective of clearance/pharmacokinetic factors (Table 1). Based on the above-mentioned facts relating to pharmacokinetic and clinical data, patients in both the conventional and the escalated arm

Table 5. Patient numbers treated at the different dose steps (−2 to 4) for courses 1–9

Dose step	Course number								
	1	2	3	4	5	6	7	8	9
−2	–	1	–	1	4	7	6	7	8
−1	–	1	2	4	7	8	9	14	19
1	88	14	10	13	9	10	12	16	20
2	–	71	32	26	27	22	25	17	17
3	–	–	43	28	23	23	19	25	17
4	–	–	–	15	17	16	14	6	2
Total	88[a]	87	87	87	87	86	85	85	83

[a] One patient never started therapy; there were 89 patients overall.

will then be both over- and undertreated (Bergh et al. 1998; Sandström et al. 1996). Against this background, the study sizes have most likely been too small for investigating a higher dose to *all* patients compared with a standard dose to *all* patients. The ideal study would compare conventional-dose chemotherapy with therapy tailored to the individual patient.

Toxicity in Tailored Therapy

In the ongoing randomised adjuvant study SBG 9401 we have analysed the non-haematological NCI toxicity criteria for the first 89 patients in the A arm consisting of the six dose levels of the tailored FEC arm (Tables 6, 7). It was possible to perform this analysis because it does not interfere with the primary and secondary endpoints of the study. For 73%–94% of the courses there were no differences in the toxicity profiles, irrespective of whether the patients had been treated on the highest two dose levels compared with the lower dose levels, if all courses were analysed together (Bergh et al. 1998). Despite this, a statistical difference was found for a higher toxicity profile in the patients treated at the highest two dose levels (Bergh et al. 1998). It may be concluded that for one patient or less of four treated, depending on the toxicity parameters analysed, we have failed to achieve optimal tailoring, while for the rest we accomplished our intentions. The relatively mild acute toxicity profile even in patients treated at the highest two dose levels in our study is interesting and may be explained by the fact that they had more rapid clearance of the drugs. Our toxicity data should be compared with the likely toxicity profile to be seen by escalating epirubicin and cyclophosphamide in the range 105–120 mg/m^2 and 1500–1800 mg/m^2, respectively, to *all* patients.

On the negative side, we are greatly concerned about the fact that 4 among the first 89 patients in the B arm of the SBG 9401 study have developed acute myeloid leukaemia. The two-armed study had recruited 503 patients by 31 December 1997. The induction period was 10–15 months after the last FEC course for three of them (Bergh et al. 1998), and around 2.5 years for the last patient.

Table 6. Infectious complications (NCI toxicity grading) in relation to the six dose steps after course 6

Dose step	NCI toxicity					Total number of patients
	0	1	2	3	4	
-2	6	0	0	0	0	6
-1	6	2	0	0	1	9
1	10	0	0	1	0	11
2	17	2	0	1	1	21
3	15	2	4	1	1	23
4	14	1	1	0	0	16
Total	68	7	5	3	3	86

Table 7. Dichotomized NCI toxicity grading in relation to high and low dose levels after course 6

Dose steps	Grouped NCI toxicity grades		Total patient number
	0, 1	2–4	
Anorexia			
–2, –1, 1, 2	46	1	47
3, 4	34	5	39
Total	80	6	86
Fisher's exact test 0.087 (two-tailed)			
Diarrhea			
–2, –1, 1, 2	44	3	47
3, 4	36	3	39
Total	80	6	86
Fisher's exact test 1.000 (two-tailed)			
Nausea			
–2, –1, 1, 2	43	4	47
3, 4	35	4	39
Total	78	8	86
Fisher's exact test 1.000 (two-tailed)			
Vomiting			
–2, –1, 1, 2	41	6	47
3, 4	29	10	39
Total	70	16	86
Fisher's exact test 0.167 (two-tailed)			
Stomatitis			
–2, –1, 1, 2	42	5	47
3, 4	33	6	39
Total	75	11	86
Fisher's exact test 0.536 (two-tailed)			
Infection			
–2, –1, 1, 2	43	4	47
3, 4	32	7	39
Total	75	11	86
Fisher's exact test 0.214 (two-tailed)			

Future Considerations

Therapy tailored on the basis of haematological toxicity is currently being investigated for the epirubicin and docetaxel combination as first-line therapy in patients with metastatic breast cancer. Unlike tailored FEC therapy, G-CSF is not used up-front at the first dose step in this phase II study of epirubicin combined with docetaxel. Whether G-CSF is a requirement for the tailoring of the therapy into the six different dose levels as outlined above is not known. The use of G-CSF will most likely permit higher doses, but its eventual impact on survival must be regarded as uncertain (Ardizzoni et al. 1994; Bergh et al. 1998; Lalisang et al. 1997; Muhonen et al. 1996).

It would also be tempting to explore the tailored concept in patients receiving pulsative chemotherapy combined with very long-term infusions of 5-fluorouracil, which has so far resulted in very impressive response figures (Smith et al. 1995). This long-term infusion concept demonstrates that altering the scheduling of the cytotoxic agents will change the objective response rate, most likely due to altered pharmacokinetics. The use of tailoring, including the delivery, will be essential in the further exploration of the available cytostatics. We all look forward to new and better drugs, but we must learn how to use the present drugs better and to adapt our concepts and procedures to the critical tumor-biological factors, which together with the pharmacokinetic factors are probably the most important determinants of the prognosis and outcome of the individual patient.

Summary

Conventional dosage of chemotherapy based on body surface area in patients with normal organ functions will result in marked interindividual variations in systemic exposure to the cytostatics used. This will result in over- and undertreatment of the individual patient associated with unwarranted toxicity and suboptimal outcome. The intention to modify dosage is motivated by a possible correlation between toxicity and outcome. New dosage strategies with individual tailoring of the therapy should be investigated with the aim of increasing the efficacy of therapy without increasing its toxicity. Pharmacokinetic monitoring using the limited sampling procedure could be one alternative, another toxicity-guided dosage. The dosage scheme used for tailored FEC polychemotherapy (six dose levels), based on therapy to equivalent haematological toxicity, has been clinically applicable in the multicentre setting for both adjuvant and preoperative therapy. In the adjuvant setting it has resulted in the delivery of significantly higher epirubicin and cyclophosphamide doses without increasing acute toxicity to the same extent; in two out of three patients no difference in acute toxicity could be verified for the highest two dose levels compared with the lower dose levels. In short, we could obtain better results with our present arsenal of cytostatics if we used them better.

Acknowledgements. Financial support has been obtained from the Swedish Cancer Society and the Nordic Cancer Union for exploring alternative dosage methods and for running clinical studies. For the latter we have also obtained support from Roche/Amgen and Pharmacia-Upjohn. The regional Oncological Centre in Uppsala, Sweden, is gratefully acknowledged for data management, together with the data centres in Oslo, Helsinki and Copenhagen. Special thanks to my co-investigator Dr Nils Wilking and all investigators and monitors (Rita Grönberg, Camilla Eriksson, Monica Ericson, Ulla Meirik) within the framework of the adjuvant SBG 9401 study, together with Marléne Forslund for excellent administrative assistance, and the pharmacokinetic (Drs Mats Karlsson, Agneta Freijs and Marie Sandström) and drug resistance teams (Drs Rolf Larsson and Peter Nygren) for adding a further dimension to chemotherapy.

References

Allerheiligen S, Johnson R, Hatcher B et al (1994) Gemcitabine pharmacokinetics are influenced by gender, body surface area (BSA) and duration of infusion. Proc Am Soc Clin Oncol 13:136

Ardizzoni A, Venturini M, Sertoli M et al (1994) Granulocyte-macrophage colony-stimulating factor (GM-CSF) allows acceleration and dose intensity increase of CEF chemotherapy: a randomised study in patients with advanced breast cancer. Br J Cancer 69:385–391

Bergh J (1997) Dose intensity in patients with metastatic breast cancer – time for novel thoughts? Ann Oncol 8:109–110

Bergh J, Wiklund T, Erikstein B et al (1998) Dosage of adjuvant G-CSF (filgrastim) supported FEC polychemotherapy based on equivalent hematological toxicity to high risk breast cancer patients. Ann Oncol 9:403–411

Bezwoda W, Seymour L, Dansey R (1995) High-dose chemotherapy with hematopoietic rescue as primary treatment for metastatic breast cancer: a randomized trial. J Clin Oncol 13:2483–2489

Bruno R, Hille D, Thomas L et al (1995) Population pharmacokinetics/pharmacodynamics (PK/PD) of docetaxel (Taxotere) in phase II studies. Proc Am Soc Clin Oncol 14:457

Calvert A, Newell D, Gumbrell L et al (1989) Carboplatin dosage: prospective evaluation of a simple formula based on renal function. J Clin Oncol 7:1748–1756

Du Bois D, Du Bois E (1916) A formula to estimate the approximate surface area if height and weight be known. Arch Intern Med 17:863–871

Early Breast Cancer Trialist Collaborative Group (1992) Systemic treatment of early breast cancer by hormonal, cytotoxic, or immune therapy. Lancet 339:1–15, 71–85

EORTC New Drug Development Committee (1985) EORTC guidelines for phase I trials with single agents in adults. Eur J Cancer Clin Oncol 21:1005–1007

Evans W (1993) Alternative approaches for phase I studies of anticancer drugs: a role for therapeutic drug monitoring. Ther Drug Monit 15:492–497

Evans W, Relling M (1989) Clinical pharmacokinetics-pharmacodynamics of anticancer drugs. Clin Pharmacokinet 16:327–336

Grochow L, Baraldi C, Noe D et al (1990) Is dose normalization to weight or body surface area useful in adults? J Natl Cancer Inst 82:323–325

Gurney H (1996) Dose calculation of anticancer drugs: a review of the current practice and introduction of an alternative. J Clin Oncol 14:2590–2611

Hutchison D, Schmid F (1973) Cross-resistance and collateral sensitivity. In: Mihich E (ed) Drug-resistance and selectivity: biochemical and cellular basis. Academic, New York, pp 73–126

Lalisang R, Wils J, Nortier H et al (1997) Comparative study of dose escalation versus interval reduction to obtain dose-intensification of epirubicin and cyclophosphamide with granulocyte colony-stimulating factor in advanced breast cancer. J Clin Oncol 15:1367–1376

Lauterburg B, Preisig R (1991) Quantitation of liver function. In: McIntyre N, Bircher J et al (eds) Oxford textbook of clinical hepatology. Oxford University Press, Oxford, pp 309–314

Mirza M, Jakobsen E, Pfeiffer P et al (1997) Suramin in non-small cell lung cancer and advanced breast cancer – two parallel phase II studies. Acta Oncol 36:171–174

Muhonen T, Jantunen I, Pertovaara H et al (1996) Prophylactic filgrastim (G-CSF) during mutimycin-C, mitoxantrone, and methotrexate (MMM) treatment for metastatic breast cancer. Am J Clin Oncol 19:232–234

Nyström L, Rutqvist L, Wall S et al (1993) Breast cancer screening with mammography: overview of Swedish randomised trials. Lancet 341:973–978

Overgaard M, Hansen P, Overgaard J et al (1997) Postoperative radiotherapy in high-risk premenopausal women with breast cancer who receive adjuvant chemotherapy. N Engl J Med 337:949–955

Paalzow L (1990) Therapeutical drug monitoring of anticancer drugs. In: Domellöf L (ed). Drug delivery in cancer treatment III. Springer, Berlin Heidelberg New York, pp 85–96

Pinkel D (1958) The use of body surface area as a criterion of drug dosage in cancer chemotherapy. Cancer Res 18:853–856

Ragaz J, Jackson S, Le N et al (1997) Adjuvant radiotherapy and chemotherapy in node-positive premenopausal women with breast cancer. N Engl J Med 337:956–962

Ratain M, Mick R, Schilsky R et al (1991) Pharmacologically based dosing of etoposide: a means of safely increasing dose intensity. J Clin Oncol 9:1480–1486

Saarto T, Blomqvist C, Rissanen P et al (1997) Haematological toxicity: a marker of adjuvant chemotherapy efficacy in stage II and III breast cancer. Br J Cancer 75:301–305

Sandström M, Freijs A, Larsson R et al (1996) Lack of relationship between systemic exposure for the component drugs of the fluorouracil, epirubicin, and 4-hydroxycyclophosphamide regimen in breast cancer patients. J Clin Oncol 14:1581–1588

Schabel FJ, Simpson-Herren L (1978) Some variables in experimental tumor systems which complicate interpretation of data from in vivo kinetic and pharmacologic studies with anticancer drugs. Antibiot Chemother 23:113–127

Smith I, Walsh G, Jones A et al (1995) High complete remission rates with primary neoadjuvant infusional chemotherapy for large early breast cancer. J Clin Oncol 13:424–429

Anti-angiogenesis Therapy and Strategies for Integrating It with Adjuvant Therapy

A. L. Harris

ICRF Molecular Oncology Laboratory, John Radcliffe Hospital, Oxford OX3 9DS, UK

Introduction

The growth of tumors above about 1 mm in diameter requires angiogenesis, the development of a new blood supply, from pre-existing vasculature (Folkman 1990). This applies to both the primary and secondary lesions. Angiogenesis is also essential for systemic metastasis, and it has recently been shown that it is essential for local invasion (Skobe et al. 1997). Normal vasculature is quiescent and each endothelial cell divides only once in 10 years, apart from the endometrial and ovarian angiogenesis during the menstrual cycle and during wound healing. In human tumors the number of dividing endothelial cells may be 50 times greater than in normal tissue. These vessels are leaky, have upregulated vascular growth factor receptors and cell adhesion molecules and are in a procoagulant state. Thus they provide a new therapeutic target with many factors differently expressed between tumor and normal endothelium. This review describes some of the angiogenic pathways and discusses how emerging anti-angiogenic drugs can be integrated into adjuvant trials.

Angiogenesis and Anti-angiogenesis

Many agniogenic factors have been described (Pluda 1997; Teicher 1995) that stimulate proliferation and migration of endothelial cells. Mobility and remodelling from pre-existing vasculature is an important component of angiogenesis. Amongst the most potent and specific factors for vascular growth is vascular endothelial cell growth factor (VEGF) (Claffey and Robinson 1996; Zhang et al. 1995). This exists in several isoforms produced from one gene. It binds to VEGF receptors of which there are two, VEGFR1 (flt1) and VEGFR2 (kdr). It is generally thought that VEGFR2 is the most important for angiogenesis while VEGFR1 is expressed on macrophages and stimulates their migration (Jain et al. 1996). Macrophages contribute an important component to angiogenesis and produce many angiogenic factors (Zabel et al.

1996). In one study macrophage numbers correlated with vascularity of tumors and gave a poor prognosis (Leek et al. 1996). Not all studies have shown this, but macrophage numbers are associated with other poor prognosis features.

Several novel angiogenic factors including VEGF b (Olofsson et al. 1996) and receptors such as tie have been cloned recently (Wong et al. 1997). Tissue factor has a role (Carmeliet et al. 1996), and there is clear evidence of synergy between VEGF and basic FGF (Asahara et al. 1995). Thymidine phosphorylase is a novel class of angiogenesis inducer being an enzyme that produces an angiogenic sugar from thymidine (Moghaddam et al. 1995). It is upregulated by hypoxia (Griffiths et al. 1997) and overexpressed early in breast cancer (Engels et al. 1997). High expression is associated with a good response to CMF chemotherapy, possible by preventing thymidine salvage (Fox et al. 1997a). VEGF may function via upregulation of nitric oxide production, which is also angiogenic (Montrucchio et al. 1997). A range of proteases that are expressed by endothelial cells or stroma have an important role in angiogenesis, particularly urokinase (Hildenbrand et al. 1995).

In a recent study we performed, seven different angiogenic factors were studied in 64 primary breast cancers by RNAse protection assays (Relf et al. 1997). All the factors were expressed in all the tumors but with up to a 2-log range between tumors. This shows that many factors are expressed, but it is possible that some are much more important overall. One way to assess this is their importance as a prognositc factor. A few studies suggest high VEGF is a predictor of poor survival (Toi et al. 1996), and we found mRNA expression above the median was associated with poor prognosis.

Other pathways involved include cell adhesion molecules of the integrin family. $a_v\beta_3$ and $a_v\beta_5$ integrins (Friedlander et al. 1995) are upregulated on proliferating tumor vessels and inhibition of their function cause apoptosis of growing endothelial cells (Brooks et al. 1995; Brooks 1996).

It is now recognised that angiogenesis is regulated by a balance between pro-angiogenic and anti-angiogenic factors and that loss of inhibitors may be an early stage in tumor progression. Inhibitors include thrombospondin (Taraboletti et al. 1997), several cytokines (IL4, IL12) and proteolytic breakdown products of several proteins. This is a rapidly emerging field and prolactin (Clapp and Delaescalera 1997), EGF, plasminogen (Cao et al. 1997), and collagen XVIII (O'Reilly et al. 1994, 1997) can be degraded to produce inhibitory proteins. These are amongst the most potent anti-angiogenesis factors known. Endostatin and angiostatin produce regression of tumor vasculature and complete cessation of tumor growth without the development of drug resistance (Boehm et al. 1997). It is these inhibitory peptides that produce encouragement that specific inhibition of tumour angiogenesis is possible with minimal toxicity and high efficiency.

The balance between angiogenesis and apoptosis due to poor supply of oxygen to poorly vascularised tumors probably determines dormancy of secondary deposits (Holmgren et al. 1995). Thus, onset of angiogenesis – the 'angiogenic switch' – may be critical in controlling growth of primary and secondary deposits (Hanahan and Folkman 1996). Oncogene activation is critical for this step, producing up-regulation of angiogenic factors and down-regulation of inhibitors. One such factor is a basic FGF binding protein which enhances secretion of FGF from cancer cells (Czubayko et al. 1997).

Oncogenes and Angiogenesis

Although oncogenes are generally considered from the point of view of their role in stimulating tumor cell proliferation or inhibiting apoptosis, theys also have a major role in regulating angiogenesis. This is best documented for mutant ras genes which up-regulate the expression of VEGF (Mazure et al. 1996). VEGF is the angiogenic factor most clearly responsive to hypoxia and is upregulated by a hypoxia-sensing pathway (Wenger and Gassmann 1997; Maltepe et al. 1997).

The hypoxia-sensing pathway activates a transcription factor, hypoxia-inducible factor-1a, which is phosphorylated and activated under hypoxia, heterodimerises with the arylhydrocarbon nuclear translocator and is transported to the nucleus. There it binds specific DNA regulatory elements (hypoxia response elements, HREs) to induce synthesis of VEGF and glycolytic enzymes (Bunn and Payton 1996). We showed in a mouse hepatoma line that this pathway is essential for tumour growth in vivo even in a fully transformed line (Maxwell et al. 1997). Thus mutants that were defective in hypoxia signalling grew very slowly in vivo and were poorly vascularised. This shows that oncogenes may up-regulate or utilise the existing hypoxia response pathway for growth, rather than bypass it. The transcription factor AP1 which is upregulated by many oncogenes synergises with this pathway (Damert et al. 1997).

In ras transfected cells there is a much greater response of VEGF to hypoxia. Similar results have been reported for src and more recently members of the tyrosine kinase receptor family (Petit et al. 1997). *p53* mutations are associated with loss of inhibitors (thrombospondin) and up-regulation of VEGF production (Gasparini and Harris 1997). Thus stepwise tumour progression may be due to mutation of oncogenes that increase the pro-angiogenic and decrease the anti-angiogenic profile of a tumour. Similarly, inhibitors of many oncogene signalling pathways may indirectly down-regulate angiogenesis. The hypoxic micro-environment may encourage selection of mutations that activate anti-apoptotic pathways such as *p53* (Graeber et al. 1996). These oncogenes may also activate angiogenic pathways.

Post-transcriptional Regulation and Angiogenesis

Several vascular growth factors have long 5′ untranslated regions of their mRNA (basic FGF and VEGF) and they are normally inefficiently translated into protein. Up-regulation of the rate-limiting factor for initiation of protein synthesis (eIF4e) enhances the ability to translate these mRNAs (Kevil et al. 1996). Thus, for the same amount of mRNA, more protein is produced. We showed in primary breast cancer that the ratio of VEGF protein to VEGF mRNA is greatly increased compared to normal breast tissue and this was associated with many-fold up-regulation of eIF4e. eIF4e has been shown to be an oncogene and may be particularly relevant to angiogenesis as a pathway of transformation (Nathan et al. 1997). The von Hippel-Lindau gene product is involved in stabilising VEGF mRNA, showing that factors regulating angiogenic pathways can be suppressor oncogenes (Iliopoulos et al. 1996). Other factors are involved in stabilising mRNA under hypoxia but are poorly characterised (White et al. 1995).

Assessment of Angiogenesis in Human Breast Cancer

Angiogenesis has been assessed by specifically staining blood vessels with antibodies to factor VIII associated antigen (Weidner et al. 1992) or the cell adhesion molecules CD31 (Horak et al. 1992) or CD34 (Martin et al. 1997a). The number of vessels in the most vascular areas of the tumor (vascular hot spots) is then measured in three areas and this is used to derive a measure of microvascular density (MVD). This method correlates well with computerized image analysis (Fox et al. 1995). Many studies have now been published and have generally shown high vascular density is a strong independent factor predicting poor prognosis. There is controversy in this area, as in most studies of prognostic factors, but many of the negative studies are small or have median vessel counts quite different from the majority of studies. Recommendations on the assessment of vascular density have been published (Vermeulen et al. 1996). However, it has been shown that circulating cancer cells correlate with MVD (McCulloch et al. 1995), as does the presence of micrometastases in the bone marrow at presentation (Fox et al. 1997b).

There have been few studies of secondary deposits, but we have found that lung secondaries from breast cancers often have a higher vascular density than their primaries (Pezzella et al. 1996). Other in vivo methods have been used and show reasonable correlations with MVD (Fox and Harris 1997). These include colour doppler and magnetic resonance imaging. Angiograms on mastectomy specimens have also shown a good correlation with MVD (Martin et al. 1997b). Each of these methods measures a different aspect of vessel function, so the degree of agreement is encouraging for the possibility of monitoring angiogenesis in vivo. Markers of angiogenesis that could be measrued in peripheral blood samples or urine would be useful for monitoring anti-angiogenic therapy. Soluble cell adhesion molecules expressed on tumor endothelium, VEGF and basic FGF have been measured and are often elevated, but no relationship to response to therapy has yet been shown (Dirix et al. 1997).

Anti-angiogenic Drugs in Clinical Trial

There are many steps in the angiogenic process and targets include the vascular growth factors (Rak and Kerbel 1996; Saleh et al. 1996) and receptors (Strawn et al. 1996), co-factors required for the function of these factors (heparin) (Wattenberger et al. 1996), proteases (Min et al. 1996; Brown and Giavazzi 1995) released by migrating endothelial cells and several signalling pathways. Many cytokines are anti-angiogenic, and inhibitors of macrophage function and angiotensin converting enzyme inhibitors are under study. Dominant negative pleiotrophin mutants (Zhang et al. 1997), 2 methoxy oestradiol (Yue et al. 1997) and hypoxia-activated prodrugs (Wilson and Pruijn 1995) which may synergise with the above approaches are in pre-clinical development. Several are in clinical trial, including metalloprotease inhibitor, TNP470 (Konno et al. 1996), interferons, protein kinase C antagonists, ras inhibitors and calcium channel blockers. Other drugs involved have been reviewed recently (Rak and Kerbel 1996; Millauer et al. 1996).

One of the problems with these drugs is that the are not sufficiently powerful in inhibiting angiogenesis to cause tumor regression (in contrast to angiostatin and endostatin, which are not yet in clinical trials). Thus, stabilisation of disease may occur, but not often regression. Stabilisation of disease under the influence of tamoxifen is well recognised to be of therapeutic value, and a similar approach may be needed for the current generation of anti-angiogenic drugs. This is why surrogate markers and monitoring of tumor vascularity may be useful adjuncts in assessing anti-angiogenic effects. Pre-clinical studies have shown marked synergy of conventional chemotherapy agents with a range of anti-angiogenic agents and have provided the impetus to combine them in clinical trials. Furthermore, combinations of anti-angiogenic drugs inhibiting different targets may be more effective than single agents.

Vascular Targeting and Gene Therapy

Another approach to inhibiting the vasculature of tumors is to destroy the vessels acutely. This contrasts to the approaches outlined above in that anti-angiogenesis involves inhibition of the growth of new vessels, whereas vascular targeting affects the pre-existing vasculature. One of the most successful strategies has been to use coaguligands – anti-vascular antibodies that target activated procoagulant enzymes to tumor vasculature and clot off the blood supply (Huang et al. 1997). Thus, in control of micrometastasis without vasculature, vascular targeting may be ineffective, whereas continuous anti-angiogenesis therapy may prevent the development of vessels in those sites. Pre-clinical and phase I trials of vascular toxins are producing encouraging results and these substances may be complementary to anti-angiogenesis (Wamil et al. 1997). A range of antibodies are now available that specifically recognise tumor vasculature and can be used for targeting (Castellani et al. 1994; Mariani et al. 1997).

Because all tumors have areas of intermittent hypoxia, the hypoxia response elements regulated by hif1 a may be used for specific activation of genes in tumors as a method of gene therapy. Their function has been shown in vivo using multimers of HREs linked to reporter genes (Dachs et al. 1997). The areas of the tumors in which the reporters were activated were also biologically hypoxic in that they were radio-resistant and activated bioreductive drugs.

Another approach has been to use endothelial specific promoters for gene therapy (Jagger et al. 1997). A variety of methods have been used to deliver genes to tumor vasculature, including retroviruses, adenoviruses and liposomes (Chan and Harris 1996). Other ways of selectively targeting tumor endothelium include regional delivery.

Integration of Anti-angiogenesis Therapy with Existing Treatments

Several studies have shown that high angiogenesis as assessed by MVD is associated with poor prognosis even with adjuvant chemotherapy or hormone therapy. However, anti-angiogenesis drugs have improved the response to chemotherapy with a wide range of drugs (Kakeji and Teicher 1997) or radiotherapy in xenograft models. Thus, combining anti-angiogenesis with existing modalities, rather than replacing existing modalities, is the most likely way to see an enhanced outcome for patients. Similarly, combinations of endocrine therapy with anti-angiogenic therapy may have additive effects (Lindner and Borden 1997).

Strategies to Assess the Role of Anti-angiogenic Drugs

Several strategies can be envisioned to assess the role of anti-angiogenic drugs.

Neoadjuvant Strategies

Pre-operative chemotherapy for patients with large primary tumors is standard practice and many of these patients particularly with palpable nodes, have a very poor prognosis. Randomised addition of the novel agent would allow comparison of response rates clinically and pathologically and also measurement of changes in blood flow or other markers of angiogenesis. Pre-operative and serial biopsies could be used to determine the level of expression of the therapeutic target and whether it had been modified by treatment. Validation of the reliability of core biopsies and repeat biopsies would be necessary for the target being assessed. Although this would not give single-agent data, combination therapies, as discussed above, are much more likely to be of therapeutic value.

Adjuvant Therapy

This is a more difficult area to introduce anti-angiogenesis agents since we do not know how long to give them for and currently have no data on activities in phase II or III trials, either alone or in combination therapy. Some of the trial designs described below for metastatic disease need to be completed to determine the optimum strategy.

Metastatic Disease

A trial design that allows combination and single-agent data to be collected in the same study may prove an effective use of resources. Thus, randomising patients to combination of the anti-angiogenesis agent plus conventional chemotherapy versus conventional chemotherapy alone will allow assessment of any improvement in response rate, response duration and survival. The control arm can be offered the single agent alone on progression, which will allow assessment of response to the agent alone. Thus all patients have a chance of the new therapy and both questions can be answered.

There are several strategies for combining a non-toxic agent with chemotherapy and some should be assessed pre-clinically. These include whether it is better to combine the agents and administer the anti-angiogenesis agent continuously between courses, or give it only between courses, or only with chemotherapy.

Then there is the question of maintenance therapy. This should be answered in randomised trials comparing responses to therapy and seeing if remission duration can be prolonged with continuous anti-angiogenesis therapy. The outcome of these types of trial will help determine how to use such approaches in the adjuvant situation. The use of endpoints such as micrometastases in bone marrow aspirates and whether they increase in number may be helpful markers in the adjuvant situation.

Conclusion

Anti-angiogenesis strategies will be an important component of anti-cancer therapy in the near future and will produce new challenges for clinical trial design. It is essential to integrate these new approaches with optimal conventional therapy, where possible assessing whether we are affecting the relevant biochemical pathway and relating outcome to expression of the relevant target in the primary tumor. This should help select the best strategies for different types of breast cancer defined by conventional or new biological markers.

Summary

Tumor angiogenesis is critical for the growth of primary cancers above 1–2 mm in diameter. A major vascular growth factor is VEGF, and approaches to inhibit VEGF have shown encouraging results in pre-clinical studies. The mechanisms involved in switching on angiogenesis involve activation of oncogenes and up-regulation of the hypoxia-sensing pathway. These provide novel targets for therapy. Many anti-angiogenic drugs are in clinical trial currently and there are problems in assessing these types of drugs if they only cause disease stabilisation. It will be important to develop methods to assess inhibition of vascular growth in vivo. New generations of anti-angiogenesis drugs such as endostatin of angiostatin, which are more potent, may cause tumor regression, but this has not yet been studied in patients. These approaches for advanced disease should be more successful when applied early in an adjuvant situation. This will also require careful monitoring of long-term toxicity.

References

Asahara T, Bauters C, Zheng LP, Takeshita S, Bunting S, Ferrara N, Symes JF, Isner JM (1995) Synergistic effect of vascular endothelial growth-factor and basic fibroblast growth-factor on angiogenesis in vivo. Circulation 92:365–371

Boehm T, Folkman J, Browder T, O'Reilly MS (1997) Antiangiogenic therapy of experimental cancer does not induce acquired drug resistance. Nature 390:404–407

Brooks PC (1996) Cell-adhesion molecules in angiogenesis. Cancer Metastasis Rev 15:187–194

Brooks PC, Stromblad S, Klemke R, Visscher D, Sarkar FH, Cheresh DA (1995) Antiintegrin alpha-v-beta-3 blocks in human breast-cancer growth and angiogenesis in human skin. J Clin Invest 96:1815–1822

Brown PD, Giavazzi R (1995) Matrix metalloproteinase inhibition – a review of antitumor activity. Ann Oncol 6:967–974

Bunn HF, Poyton RO (1996) Oxygen sensing and molecular adaptation to hypoxia. Physiol Rev 76:839–885

Cao YH, Chen A, An SSA, Ji RWD, Davidson D, Cao YM, Llinas M (1997) Kringle-5 of plasminogen is a novel inhibitor of endothelial-cell growth. J Biol Chem 272:22924–22928

Carmeliet P, MacKman N, Moons L, Luther T, Gressens P, Vanvlaenderen I, Demunck H, Kasper M, Breier G, Evrard P, Muller M, Risau W, Edgington T, Collen D (1996) Role of tissue factor in embryonic blood-vessel development. Nature 383:73–75

Castellani P, Viale G, Dorcaratto A, Nicolo G, Kaczmarek J, Querze G, Zardi L (1994) The fibronectin isoform containing the ed-b oncofetal domain – a marker of angiogenesis. Int J Cancer 59:612–618

Chan HY, Harris AL (1996) Gene therapy targeting to tumor endothelium. In: Sobol RE, Scanlon KJ (eds) The internet book of gene therapy – cancer therapeutics. Appleton and Lange, Stamford, pp 211–227

Claffey KP, Robinson GS (1996) Regulation of vegf/vpf expression in tumor-cells – consequences for tumor-growth and metastasis. Cancer Metastasis Rev 15:165–176

Clapp C, Delaescalera GM (1997) Prolactins – novel regulators of angiogenesis. News Physiol Sci 12:231–237

Czubayko F, Liaudetcoopman EDE, Aigner A, Tuveson AT, Berchem GJ, Wellstein A (1997) A secreted FGF-binding protein can serve as the angiogenic switch in human cancer. Nat Med 3:1137–1140

Dach GU, Patterson AV, Firth JD, Ratcliffe PJ, Townsend KMS, Stratford IJ, Harris AL (1997) Targeting gene expression to hypoxic tumor cells. Nat Med 3:515–520

Damert A, Ikeda E, Risau W (1997) Activator-protein-1 binding potentiates the hypoxia-inducible factor-1-mediated hypoxia-induced transcriptional activation of vascular-endothelial growth-factor expression in c6 glioma-cells. Biochem J 327:419–423

Dirix LY, Vermeulen PB, Pawinski A, Prove A, Benoy I, Depooter C, Martin M, Vanoosterom AT (1997) Elevated levels of the angiogenic cytokines basic fibroblast growth-factor and vascular endothelial growth-factor in sera of cancer patients. Br J Cancer 76:238–243

Engels K, Fox SB, Whitehouse RM, Gatter KC, Harris AL (1997) Up-regulation of thymidine phosphorylase expression is associated with a discrete pattern of angiogenesis in ductal carcinomas in-situ of the breast. J Pathol 182:414–420

Folkman J (1990) What is the evidence that tumors are angiogenesis dependent? J Natl Cancer Inst 82:4–6

Fox SB, Harris AL (1997) Markers of tumor angiogenesis – clinical applications in prognosis and anti-angiogenic therapy. Invest New Drugs 15:15–28

Fox SB, Leek RD, Weekes MP, Whitehouse RM, Gatter KC, Harris AL (1995) Quantitation and prognostic value of breast cancer angiogenesis: comparison of microvessel density, Chalkley count and computer image analysis. J Pathol 177:275–283

Fox SB, Engels K, Comley M, Whitehouse RM, Turley H, Gatter KC, Harris AL (1997a) Relationship of elevated tumor thymidine phosphorylase in node-positive breast carcinomas to the effects of adjuvant CMF. Ann Oncol 8:271–275

Fox SB, Leek RD, Bliss J, Mansi JL, Gusterson B, Gatter KC, Harris AL (1997b) Association of tumor angiogenesis with bone-marrow micrometastases in breast-cancer patients. J Natl Cancer Inst 89:1044–1049

Friedlander M, Brooks PC, Shaffer RW, Kincaid CM, Varner JA, Cheresh DA (1995) Definition of 2 angiogenic pathways by distinct alpha(v) integrins. Science 270:1500–1502

Gasparini G, Harris AL (1997) p53 and angiogenesis in neoplasia. In: Klijn JGM (ed) Prognostic and predictive value of p53. Elsevier, Rotterdam, pp 115–130

Graeber TG, Osmanian C, Jacks T, Housman DE, Koch CJ, Lowe SW, Giaccia AJ (1996) Hypoxia-mediated selection of cells with diminished apoptotic potential in solid tumors. Nature 379:88–91

Griffiths L, Dachs G, Bicknell R, Harris AL, Stratford IJ (1997) The influence of oxygen tension and pH on the expression of platelet-derived endothelial cell growth factor/thymidine phosphorylase in human breast tumor cells grown in vitro and in vivo. Cancer Res 57:570–572

Hanahan D, Folkman J (1996) Patterns and emerging mechanisms of the angiogenic switch during tumorigenesis. Cell 86:353–364

Hildenbrand R, Dilger I, Horlin A, Stutte HJ (1995) Urokinase plasminogen-activator induces angiogenesis and tumor vessel invasion in breast cancer. Pathol Res Pract 191:403–409

Holmgren L, O'Reilly MS, Folkman J (1995) Dormancy of micrometastases – balanced proliferation and apoptosis in the presence of angiogenesis suppression. Nat Med 1:149–153

Horak ER, Leek R, Klenk N (1992) Angiogenesis, assessed by platelet/endothelial cell adhesion molecule antibodies, as indicator of node metastasis and survival in breast cancer. Lancet 340:1120–1124

Huang XM, Molema G, King S, Watkins L, Edgington TS, Thorpe PE (1997) Tumor infarction in mice by antibody-directed targeting of tissue factor to tumor vasculature. Science 275:547–550

Iliopoulos O, Levy AP, Jiang C, Kaelin WG, Goldberg MA (1996) Negative regulation of hypoxia-inducible genes by the von-Hippel-Lindau protein. Proc Natl Acad Sci USA 93:10595–10599

Jagger RT, Chan HY, Harris AL (1997) Endothelial cell-specific expression of tumor necrosis factor-alpha from the KDR or E-selectin promotors following retroviral delivery. Hum Gen Ther 8:2239–2247

Jain RK, Koenig GC, Dellian M, Fukumura D, Munn LL, Melder RJ (1996) Leukocyte-endothelial adhesion and angiogenesis in tumors. Cancer Metastasis Rev 15:195–204

Kakeji Y, Teicher BA (1997) Preclinical studies of the combination of angiogenic inhibitors with cytotoxic agents. Invest New Drugs 15:39–48

Kevil CG, Debenedetti A, Payne DK, Coe LL, Laroux FS, Alexander JS (1996) Translational regulation of vascular-permeability factor by eukaryotic initiation-factor 4e – implications for tumor angiogenesis. Int J Cancer 65:785–790

Konno H, Tanaka T, Kanai T, Maruyama K, Nakamura S, Baba S (1996) Efficacy of an angiogenesis inhibitor, tnp-470, in xenotransplanted human colorectal cancer with high metastatic potential. Cancer 77:1736–1740

Leek RD, Lewis CE, Whitehouse R, Greenall M, Clarke J, Harris AL (1996) Association of macrophage infiltration with angiogenesis and prognosis in invasive breast carcinoma. Cancer Res 56:4625–4629

Lindner DJ, Borden EC (1997) Effects of tamoxifen and interferon-beta or the combination on tumor-induced angiogenesis. Int J Cancer 71:456–461

Maltepe E, Schmidt JV, Baunoch D, Bradfield CA, Simon MC (1997) Abnormal angiogenesis and responses to glucose and oxygen deprivation in mice lacking the protein arnt. Nature 386:403–407

Mariani G, Lasku A, Balza E, Gaggero B, Motta C, Diluca L, Dorcaratto A, Viale GA, Neri D, Zardi L (1997) Tumor targeting potential of the monoclonal-antibody bc-1 against oncofetal fibronectin in nude mice bearing human tumor implants. Cancer 80:2378–2384

Martin L, Green B, Renshaw C, Lowe D, Rudland P, Leinster SJ, Winstanley J (1997a) Examining the technique of angiogenesis assessment in invasive brreast cancer. Br J Cancer 76:1046–1054

Martin L, Holcombe C, Green B, Leinster SJ, Winstanley J (1997b) Is a histological section representative of whole tumor vascularity in breast cancer? Br J Cancer 76:40–43

Maxwell PH, Dachs GU, Gleadle JM, Nicholls LG, Harris AL, Stratford IJ, Hankinson O, Pugh CW, Ratcliffe PJ (1997) Hypoxia-inducible factor-I modulates gene expression in solid tumor and influences both angiogenesis and tumor growth. Proc Natl Acad Sci USA 94:8104–8109

Mazure NM, Chen EY, Yeh P, Laderoute KR, Giaccia AJ (1996) Oncogenic transformation and hypoxia synergistically act to modulate vascular endothelial growth-factor expression. Cancer Res 56:3436–3440

McCulloch P, Choy A, Martin L (1995) Association between tumor angiogenesis and tumor-cell shedding into effluent venous blood during breast cancer surgery. Lancet 346:1334–1335

Millauer B, Longhi MP, Plate KH, Shawver LK, Risau W, Ullrich A, Strawn LM (1996) Dominant-negative inhibition of flk-1 suppresses the growth of many tumor types in vivo. Cancer Res 56:1615–1620

Min HY, Doyle LV, Vitt CR, Zandonella CL, Strattonthomas JR, Shuman MA, Rosenberg S (1996) Urokinase receptor antagonists inhibit angiogenesis and primary tumor growth in syngeneic mice. Cancer Res 56:2428–2433

Moghaddam A, Zhang H-T, Fan T-PD, Hu D-E, Lees VC, Turley H, Fox SB, Gatter KC, Harris AL, Bicknell R (1995) Thymidine phosphorylase is angiogenic and promotes tumor growth. Proc Natl Acad Sci USA 92:998–1002

Montrucchio G, Lupia E, Demartino A, Battaglia E, Arese M, Tizzani A, Bussolino F, Camussi G (1997) Nitric oxide mediates angiogenesis induced in vivo by platelet-activating-factor and tumor-necrosis-factor-alpha. Am J Pathol 151:557–563

Nathan CA, Carter P, Liu L, Li BD, Abreo F, Tudor A, Zimmer SG, Debenedetti A (1997) Elevated expression of eif4e and FGF-2 isoforms during vascularization of breast carcinomas. Oncogene 15:1087–1094

O'Reilly MS, Holmgren L, Shing Y, Chen C, Rosenthal RA, Moses M, Lane WS, Cao YH, Sage EH, Folkman J (1994) Angiostatin – a novel angiogenesis inhibitior that mediates the suppression of metastases by a Lewis lung carcinoma. Cell 79:315–328

O'Reilly MS, Boehm T, Shing T, Fukai N, Vasios G, Lane WS, Flynn E, Birkhead JR, Olsen BR, Folkman J (1997) Endostatin: an endogenous inhibitor of angiogenesis and tumor growth. Cell 88:277–285

Olofsson B, Pajusola K, Kaipainen A, Voneuler G, Joukov V, Saksela O, Orpana A, Petersson RF, Alitalo K, Eriksson U (1996) Vascular endothelial growth-factor-b, a novel growth factor for endothelial cells. Proc Natl Acad Sci USA 93:2576–2581

Petit AMV, Rak J, Hung MC, Rockwell P, Goldstein N, Fendly B, Kerbel RS (1997) Neutralizing antibodies against epidermal growth-factor and erbb-2/neu receptor tyrosine kinases down-regulate vascular endothelial growth factor production by tumor cells in vitro and in vivo – angiogenic implications for signal transduction therapy of solid tumors. Am J Pathol 151:1523–1530

Pezzella F, Dibacco A, Andreola S, Nicholson AG, Pastorino U, Harris AL (1996) Angiogenesis in primary lung cancer and lung secondaries. Eur J Cancer 32 A:2494–2500

Pluda JM (1997) Tumor-associated angiogenesis – mechanisms, clinical implications, and therapeutic strategies. Semin Oncol 24:203–218

Rak J, Kerbel RS (1996) Treating cancer by inhibiting angiogenesis – new hopes and potential pitfalls. Cancer Metastasis Rev 15:231–236

Relf M, Lejeune S, Scott PAE, Fox S, Smith K, Leek R, Moghaddam A, Whitehouse R, Bicknell R, Harris AL (1997) Expression of the angiogenic factors vascular endothelial-cell growth-factor, acidic and basic fibroblast growth-factor, tumor-growth factor-beta-1, platelet derived endothelial-cell growth factor, placenta growth factor, and pleiotrophin in human primary breast cancer and its relation to angiogenesis. Cancer Res 57:963–969

Saleh M, Vasilopoulos K, Stylli SS, Kaye AH, Wilks AF (1996) The expression of antisense vascular endothelial growth-factor (vegf) sequences inhibits intracranial c6 glioma growth in vivo by suppressing tumor angiogenesis. J Clin Neurosci 3:366–372

Skobe M, Rockwell P, Goldstein N, Vosseler S, Fusenig NE (1997) Halting angiogenesis suppresses carcinoma cell invasion. Nat Med 3:1222–1227

Strawn LM, McMahon G, App H, Schreck R, Kuchler WR, Longhi MP, Hui TH, Tang C, Levitzki A, Gazit A, Chen I, Keri G, Orfi L, Risau W, Flamme I, Ullrich A, Hirth KP, Shawver LK (1996) Flk-1 as a target for tumor-growth inhibition. Cancer Res 56:3540–3545

Taraboletti G, Belotti D, Borsotti P, Vergani V, Rusnati M, Presta M, Giavazzi R (1997) The 140-kilodalton antiangiogenic fragment of thrombospondin-1 binds to basic fibroblast growth factor. Cell Growth Differ 8:471–479

Teicher BA (1995) Angiogenesis and cancer metastases – therapeutic approaches. Crit Rev Oncol Hematol 20:9–39

Toi M, Kondo S, Suzuki H, Yamamoto Y, Inada K, Imazawa T, Taniguchi T, Tominaga T (1996) Quantitative analysis of vascular endothelial growth factor in primary breast cancer. Cancer 77:1101–1106

Vermeulen PB, Gasparini G, Fox SB, Toi M, Martin L, McCulloch P, Pezella F, Viale G, Weidner N, Harris AL, Dirix LY (1996) Qunatification of angiogenesis in solid human tumors – an international consensus on the methodology and criteria of evaluation. Eur J Cancer 32 A:2474–2484

Waltenberger J, Mayr U, Frank H, Hombach V (1996) Suramin is a potent inhibitor of vascular endothelial growth-factor – a contribution to the molecular basis of its antiangiogenic action. J Mol Cell Cardiol 28:1523–1529

Wamil BD, Thurman GB, Sundell HW, Devore RF, Wakefield G, Johnson DH, Wang YF, Helleqvist CG (1997) Soluble e-selection in cancer patients as a marker of the therapeutic efficacy of cm101, a tumor-inhibiting anti-neovascularization agent, evaluated in phase I clinical trial. J Cancer Res Clin Oncol 123:173–179

Weidner N, Folkman J, Pozza F, Bevilacqua P, Allred EN, Moore DH, Meli S, Gasparini G (1992) Tumor angiogenesis. A new significant and independent prognostic indictor in early-stage breast carcinoma. J Natl Cancer Inst 84:1875–1887

Wenger RH, Gassmann M (1997) Oxygen(es) and the hypoxia-inducible factor-i. Biol Chem 378:609–616

White FC, Carroll SM, Kamps MP (1995) Vegf messenger-RNA is reversibly stabilized by hypoxia and persistently stabilized in vegf-overexpressing human tumor-cell lines. Growth Factors 12:289–301

Wilson WR, Pruijn FB (1995) Hypoxia-activated prodrugs as antitumor agents – strategies for maximizing tumor-cell killing. Clin Exp Pharmacol Physiol 22:881–885

Wong AL, Haroon ZA, Werner S, Dewhirst MW, Greenberg CS, Peters KG (1997) Tie2 expression and phosphorylation in angiogenic and quiescent adult tissues. Circ Res 81:567–574

Yue TL, Wang XK, Louden CS, Gupta S, Pillarisetti K, Gu JL, Hart TK, Lysko PG, Feuerstein GZ (1997) 2-methoxyestradiol, an endogenous estrogen metabolite, induces apoptosis in endothelial cells and inhibits angiogenesis – possible role for stress-activated protein-kinase signaling pathway and fas expression. Mol Pharmacol 51:951–962

Zabel DD, Feng JJ, Scheuenstuhl H, Hunt TK, Hussain MZ (1996) Lactate stimulation of macrophage-derived angiogenic acitivity is associated with inhibition of poly(adp-ribose) synthesis. Lab Invest 74:644–649

Zhang H-T, Craft P, Scott PAE, Ziche M, Weich HA, Harris AL, Bicknell R (1995) Enhancement of tumor growth and vascular density by transfection of vascular endothelial cell growth factor into MCF-7 human breast carcinoma cells. J Natl Cancer Inst 87:213–219

Zhang N, Zhong R, Wang ZY, Deuel TF (1997) Human breast-cancer growth inhibited in vivo by a dominant-negative pleiotrophin mutant. J Biol Chem 272:16733–16736

X. Adjuvant Systemic Treatments: Cytotoxics and Their Dosage

New Developments in High-Dose Chemotherapy for Breast Cancer

R. L. Basser

Department of Haematology and Medical Oncology, Royal Melbourne Hospital, Parkville, Victoria, and Western Hospital, Footscray, and Ludwig Institute for Cancer Research, Parkville, Victoria, Australia

Introduction

A hint is given that escalation in chemotherapy dose might improve outcome for women with breast cancer by the results of single-arm studies of high-dose chemotherapy (HDC) with autologous stem cell rescue (Gradishar et al. 1996). Response rates, and in some instances survival rates, also appear to be superior following a single cycle of myeloablative chemotherapy with bone marrow (BM) or peripheral blood progenitor cells (PBPC) support when compared to lower-dose regimens. In addition, long-term survival (up to 8 years) has been observed in patients who would otherwise have been expected to live a relatively short time (Peters 1995). In response to these promising reports, the use of HDC for the treatment of breast cancer has grown and changed dramatically over the last decade. In the USA, the percentage of autotransplants for breast cancer has increased from 16% to 40% of all autotransplants, so that now breast cancer is the most common indication for this therapy (Antman et al. 1997). The proportion of breast cancer autotransplants for local disease has increased from 7% to about 50% (Antman et al. 1997). The impact this has had on the treatment of breast cancer worldwide is reflected in the number of publications cited in a Medline search of "high-dose chemotherapy" and "breast cancer," which yielded over 700 entries since the first report of HDC for breast cancer in 1982. Although the early mortality from breast cancer HDC procedures was as high as 22%, it is now less than 5% (Antman et al. 1997). Improved control of acute toxicities and supportive care has greatly simplified this treatment. More rapid engraftment with the use of PBPC and the use of hematopoietic growth factors (HGF) and oral prophylactic antibiotics have allowed an increase in the proportion of care given in the outpatient setting (Ayash et al. 1994, Gianni et al. 1997a), and reduced the costs substantially (Gilbert 1996). These factors in part explain the widespread adoption of HDC as a treatment for breast cancer. More than 95% of autotransplants for breast cancer in the USA have been performed outside of clinical trials (Antman et al. 1997), possibly due to due to a belief that, as stated by one US physician, "the issue is whether patients are randomly assigned to treatment we believe has no hope of cure, or to a treatment that does have a chance of cure" (Rushing 1997). A survey of oncologists conducted at the 1995 meeting of the American Society of Clinical Oncology gives additional insight into the dilemma. Besides the belief that randomized trials were no longer necessary because the phase II data had already provided sufficient data, problems cited for not putting patients on trial included the effort and time necessary and patient preferences (either wanting HDC or fearing it because of the toxicity) (Mathew 1995).

How has the field evolved so that preconceived prejudices on the benefit of HDC in the treatment of breast cancer are held? What evidence of benefit are they based on?

High-Dose Chemotherapy Approaches in Breast Cancer

Development of Single-Cycle HDC

The first reports of autotransplants for breast cancer came in the early 1980s (Stewart 1982), and were largely studies of the feasibility of high-dose single cytotoxic agents. By the late 1980s, single-cycle combinations of alkylating agents emerged as the most promising regimens (Peters et al. 1986). Responses were seen in women with breast cancer refractory to standard-dose chemotherapy, but response durations were short and relapses tended to occur at sites of previous bulky metastases (Peters et al. 1988). In an attempt to improve on the results, induction therapy with standard-dose chemotherapy was introduced to eradicate as much disease as possible prior to consolidation with myeloablative therapy (Antman et al. 1992; Kotasek et al. 1994). The hypothesis was that intensive therapy would be more effective at eradicating small volume than bulky disease. An overview comparing published studies of HDC and stem cell transplantation with conventional dose regimens in metastatic breast cancer was reported by Eddy in 1992. He noted that average overall and complete response rates, but not disease-free (DFS) or overall survival (OS), were higher in HDC studies. The longest DFS and OS were observed in patients who had responded to induction therapy, which was consistent with observations made by investigators previously.

Multicycle HDC

In contrast to the single-cycle consolidation approach, other models of dose-intensive chemotherapy for breast cancer treatment have been based on the biological properties of both solid tumors and some hematological malignancies. The relatively slow doubling times, low growth fraction, and a microenvironment that inhibits drug access suggest that maximum cell kill in these cancers requires delivery of multiple cycles of chemotherapy at the maximum possible dose intensity (De Vita 1993). Indirect clinical support for the need to deliver optimal doses from the start of therapy comes from studies in patients with small cell lung cancer (Arriagada et al. 1993) and non-Hodgkin's lymphoma (De Vita et al. 1987).

The development of techniques to mobilize and collect large numbers of stem cells from peripheral blood (To et al. 1997) have enabled support of multiple cycles of HDC. A number of groups have reported on the feasibility of delivering multiple cycles of myeloablative (Ayash et al. 1994) or nonablative intensive (Shea et al. 1992) chemotherapy.

Australian Pilot Study in Poor-Prognosis Breast Cancer

We conducted a pilot study involving 100 women designed to test the safety and feasibility of the delivery of multiple cycles of dose-intensive chemotherapy supported with filgrastim-mobilized PBPC. Eligible patients were aged between 18 and 60 years with histologically confirmed poor-prognosis breast cancer, defined as stage II disease with ten or more positive axillary nodes or an estrogen-receptor-negative tumor with at least four positive axillary nodes, or stage III disease. All patients initially had PBPC collected during administration of filgrastim (Basser et al. 1995), with or without stem cell factor (SCF) (Begley et al. 1997; Basser et al. 1998), as soon as possible after surgery. High-dose chemotherapy consisted of three cycles of epirubicin 200 mg/m^2 and cyclophosphamide 4 g/m^2 at 21- or 28-day intervals. One-third of each daily apheresis product was infused after each cycle of chemotherapy. All cycles were also supported with filgrastim and broad-spectrum antibiotics. Hematological recovery was rapid after each cycle of chemotherapy, although there was a tendency for myelosuppression to be more severe with successive cycles. There was no difference in recovery between patients given chemotherapy at 28-day intervals ($n=78$) and those treated every 21 days ($n=20$). Severe mucositis also occurred with increasing frequency with successive cycles. Other non-hematological events were mild to moderate (grade 1 or 2). There were two fatal adverse events (2% of patients). For all patients enrolled on the study, the actuarial DFS at 48 months was 62% [95% confidence interval (CI), 51%–73%], and the actuarial OS at 48 months was 66% (95% CI, 53%–78%).

High-Dose Sequential Chemotherapy

The Milan group has had an innovative approach to the intensive treatment of breast cancer (Gianni et al. 1997a) and a number of other malignancies (Gianni et al. 1991, 1994, 1997b). They have developed a chemotherapy regimen that delivers several non-cross-resistant drugs in sequence, each in very high doses. Hematopoietic growth factors are used after each cycle to enhance neutrophil recovery and to enable collection of PBPC, which are then reinfused after te final myeloablative course. The phase II reports in myeloma, Hodgkin's disease, and adjuvant therapy for high-risk breast cancer are all promising. It is noteworthy that in a randomized trial in de novo non-Hodgkin's lymphoma, this regimen resulted in significantly longer survival than a standard regimen (Gianni et al. 1997b). This is the first transplant trial in lymphoma to demonstrate such an effect.

Randomized Trials of HDC in Breast Cancer

There is widespread recognition of the need for randomized trials to assess the effectiveness of HDC in metastatic breast cancer from both proponents (Peters 1995) and skeptics (Eddy 1992). While a number of large trials are actively enrolling patients (Antman et al. 1997), recruitment has been slow because of physician and patient bias that HDC is the most effective treatment. There are currently only three published randomized studies, two in abstract form. Bezwoda et al. (1995) randomized 90 women with untreated metastatic breast cancer to two cycles of high-dose cyclophosphamide 2.4 g/m^2, mitoxantrone 35–45 mg/m^2, and etoposide 2.5 g/m^2 versus six to nine cycles of conventional-dose cyclophosphamide 600 mg/m^2, mitoxantrone 12 mg/m^2, and vincristine 1.4 mg/m^2. The high-dose regimen was supported with autologous bone marrow or progenitor cells. The high-dose regimen was associated with a significantly higher response rate, response duration, and survival. While the results of this trial were very exciting, a number of reservations have led to caution in the interpretation of the results. The number of patients in the study was very small and the regimens used in both treatment options are generally not given outside of South Africa. These limitations necessitate confirmatory studies elsewhere and have prevented widespread adoption of the approach.

Peters et al. (1997) enrolled 422 women with metastatic breast cancer to receive four cycles of doxorubicin, 5-fluorouracil, and methotrexate. Those who achieved a complete remission ($n=98$) were randomized to HDC with cyclophosphamide 5 625 g/m^2, cisplatin 165 mg/m^2, and carmustine 600 mg/m^2 immediately or at the time of progression of disease. DFS was better in those having the immediate transplant (1.85 vs 0.32 years, $p<0.01$), but OS was significantly longer in women having the delayed treatment (1.7 vs 3.2 years, $p=0.04$). This raises intriguing biological questions, but does not address the value of high-dose versus standard chemotherapy.

In a randomized, phase II pilot study, the Netherlands Breast Cancer Group initially treated women with high-risk breast cancer with three cycles of CEF (Rodenhuis et al. 1997). High risk was defined as tumor-positive apical axillary lymph node, a group with 5-year DFS of only 20%. Patients with at least a minimal clinical response subsequently underwent definitive surgery. They were then randomized to a further cycle of CEF alone, or to a cycle of CEF with G-CSF to mobilize PBPC and followed by HDC with cyclophosphamide 6 g/m^2, thiotepa 480 mg/m^2, and carboplatin 1600 mg/m^2. Ninety-seven patients were enrolled in the study, but 16 were not randomized, 4 because they did not respond to CEF and 12 because they refused. Of the 81 patients randomized after surgery, only 35 of the 41 allocated HDC patients underwent transplantation, because of refusal by 5 and development of myelodysplasia in 1. At a median follow-up of 42 months, 38 patients had relapsed and there was no difference in DFS or OS between treatment groups. Both groups had superior OS and DFS compared with historical controls. Patients who were not randomized had a worse survival than those who were. The study had an 80% power to detect a true relapse-free survival advantage of 30%. These data indicate that the benefit of this HDC in this patient population was not great enough to be detected by such a small study (although it was only designed as a pilot for a larger phase III trial), and that patient selection is clearly an important factor when interpreting small studies.

Limitations of Currently Available Data

Results from the larger studies (>25 patients) of HDC for poor-prognosis breast cancer appear similar to each other and cannot be distinguished because of the differing study designs and variable patient eligibility. The difficulty with interpreting the available studies of HDC in poor-prognosis breast cancer is that they are small and the patients carefully selected. In an intersting analysis, Garcia-Carboneri et al. (1997) assessed with ten nodes or more and treated with standard therapy according to whether or not they would have been eligible for HDC by their institutional selection criteria. These were compared with patients treated with HDC at their institution. Of the patients treated with conventional therapy, those meeting the criteria for HDC had a more favorable DFS and OS than those not eligible and similar to patients treated with HDC. The extent of evaluation may also compound interpretation of small single-arm studies. Crump et al. (1996) found 7 of 30 women (23%) screened for an HDC trial had metastatic disease on CT scan or bone marrow biopsy that was not detected on routine screening. Such biases exclude patients from phase II studies that might be included in historical data, therefore making comparisons invalid. Finally, the selective nature of small studies is emphasized by reports of long-term survivors in a single-institution experience of better-than-published outcome of poor-prognosis, early-stage breast cancer treated with standard multimodality therapy (Ung et al. 1995).

In conclusion, HDC for breast cancer shows much promise but remains an experimental treatment until the results of phase III trials are available.

Tumor Contamination of Stem Cell Collections

Background

The increased use of HDC with PBPC support for breast cancer has raised as an issue the relevance of tumor contamination of BM harvests and apheresis collections. Circulating cancer cells in patients with solid tumors were reported as early as 1869 (Ashworth 1869). Reports in the early 1980s from the Ludwig Institute for Cancer Research in London showed that a polyclonal rabbit serum raised against human milk fat globule membrane [epithelial membrane antigen (EMA)] could stain solitary breast carcinoma cells in BM (Sloane et al. 1980). The cells of interest were isolated by density centrifugation, and counterstained with a goat anti-rabbit alkaline-phosphatase conjugate and Brentamine fast-red substrate. This allowed easy identification of positive (red) cells on smears without obscuring their morphology. In a study of 110 patients with breast cancer and no evidence of distant metastases, tumor cells were detected in the BM aspirates of 31 (28%) patients, whereas no tumor cells were detected in conventionally stained smears (Redding et al. 1983). The presence of EMA-positive cells in the BM correlated with tumor size and histological vascular invasion (Berger et al. 1988). These investigators were also able to show that women with contaminated BM developed distant metastases more rapidly than those without (Berger et al. 1988), particularly in the bones (Mansi et al. 1987).

Monoclonal antibodies to other markers of epithelial cells, such as cytokeratin, were later found to be more sensitive and specific for the identification of neoplasms of epithelial origin than those to EMA (Thomas and Battifora 1987). Other targets have included the 17-1A epithelial antigen (Schlimok et al. 1987), cassein (Gugliotta et al. 1990), estrogen receptors (Berger, et al. 1987), and other membrane glycoproteins or glycolipids (Osborne and Rosen 1994).

Methods of Detection of Micrometastases

Immunohistochemistry

Morphological examination of BM by light microscopy detects very few metastases and is less sensitive than isotope bone scan (Ceci et al. 1988). Monoclonal antibodies are remarkably sensitive in the detection of single cancer cells and clumps of cells. One line of current research is attempting to reduce nonspecific staining by the use of Fc-free- Fab-antibody fragments that are directly conjugated to trhe preferred marker enzyme (i.e., alkaline phosphatase) (Pantel and Moss 1996). Other techniques that show promise involve the enrichment of breast cancer cells. One report suggests linking monoclonal antibodies to immunomagnetic beads can detect micrometastases with greater sensitivity and specificity than more standard approaches (Naume et al. 1997).

Reverse-Transcriptase Polymerase Chain Reaction

The adjavent of the highly sensitive polymerase chain reaction (PCR) has allowed detection of tissue-specific or tumor-specific mRNA by amplification by the reverse transcriptase technique (RT-PCR). Early reports using RT-PCR for cytokeratin suggested that this was an effective and specific way to detect breast cancer cells (Schoenfeld et al. 1994). Datta et al. (1994) showed that detection of mRNA for cytokeratin 19 in BM of patients with breast cancer was rapid and not detectable in 39 controls. Other investigators have reported the potential use of mRNA for hormone receptors (Chevillard et al. 1996) and mapsin (Luppi et al. 1996). One group combined enrichment with immunomagnetic beads coated with a cytokeratin monoclonal antibody and examined by PCR (Eaton et al. 1997). However, the power of PCR is also possibly its greatest limitation, and cytokeratin mRNA can be detected in nonepithelial tissues (Traweek et al. 1993). A high rate of detection of cytokeratin mRNA has been reported in the blood (Krismann et al. 1995), and BM (Zippelius et al. 1997) of controls. This might be overcome with careful selection of the target cytokeratin (perhaps cytokeratin 20) (Burchill et al. 1995), but at present PCR has not fulfilled the promise of a more rapid and effective method for detection of micrometastases.

Clinical Relevance

Contamination of Bone Marrow Harvests

In patient with early breast cancer, occult micrometastases in the BM have been detected at the rate of 5%–67%. The variation in detection results from the lack of a standardized methodology and differences in the patient populations tested. While these reports have included patients either prior to or after adjuvant systemic therapy, it is difficult to identify a difference in the frequency of micrometastases between the groups.

A recent meta-analysis has assessed the prognostic significance of the presence of BM micrometastases in breast cancer (Funke and Schraut 1998). This report suggested a possible increased risk of relapse in patients with BM micrometastases, but concluded that the prognostic impact of epithelial cells in BM remains to be substantiated by further studies using standardized protocols before its entrance into the TNM classification.

Contamination of Apheresis Collections

A number of studies have documented tumor contamination of autologous hematopoietic grafts from patients with breast cancer. Ross et al. (1993) analyzed paired samples of BM and PBPC collections from 48 women with metastatic breast cancer after prior chemotherapy. They detected immunostained tumor cells in 10% (13/133) of apheresis samples from 19% (9/48) of patients after chemotherapy and G-CSF or GM-CSF, and in 62% (38/61) BM specimens from 67% (32/48) of patients. It was concluded that PBPC collections contained fewer tumor cells than paired BM specimens, and that these cells appear, based on a clonogenic assay, to be capable of clonogenic tumor growth. In a study of 240 patients, Franklin et al. (1996) found tumor cells in

30% of BM and 17% of PBPC harvests, although these specimens were not paired. While others have also reported less frequent tumor cell contamination of apheresis samples than BM, it is difficult to compare the frequency of detection of cancer cells between reports because of the different assays used and variation in the patient populations studied.

At present it is not known whether the presence of circulating tumor cells is influenced by different cytokine regimens. Franklin et al. (1997) found no difference in the incidence of contamination of apheresis collections obtained after G-CSF alone and those collected after G-CSF and SCF.

It is interesting to note that the above studies describe the presence of contaminating tumor cells after standard-dose chemotherapy, suggesting that in vivo "purging" (i.e., reduction in contamination) by cytotoxics is either incomplete or does not occur. The impact of the mobilizing regimen on the incidence and load of contamination is unclear. Brügger et al. (1994) described a study in which a small number of patients with a variety of metastatic solid tumors were assessed. The observed an increase is numbers of circulating tumor cells after administration of a single cycle of chemotherapy followed by G-CSF. Furthermore, tumor cells appeared in the circulation of patients who had no detectable cells prior to treatment. Clearance of circulating tumor cells was observed after an additional cycle of chemotherapy, although tumor cells were still detectable in a number of patients with breast cancer. In contrast, Passos-Coelho et al. (1995) observed no increase in circulating breast cancer cells in women with metastatic disease receiving cyclophosphamide and GM-CSF.

Conclusions

The phenomenon of circulating tumor cells has not been described in a number of solid malignancies. These observations give insight into the biological behavior of cancer, but as yet there are insufficient data to indicate the clinical relevance of micrometastatic disease. The detection of micrometastatic cells probably portends a poor prognosis not only in diseases that commonly metastasize to the BM, but also those that rarely do so. Furthermore, micrometastatic cells have phenotypic characteristics, such as loss of HLA-class 1 antigens and high incidence of erbB2 oncogene expression, that distinguish them from nonmetastatic cells (Pantel et al. 1993), and may be associated with more aggressive behavior. The escape of these cancer cells to the BM appears to be indicated by the degree of tumor angiogenesis and vascular invasion in the primary cancer (Fox et al. 1997), suggesting that these processes contribute to metastases.

A major impediment to the interpretation of published data is the lack of standardization of methods for detection of hematogenous micrometastases. There are conflicting data regarding the specificity of PCR and it appear to be no more sensitive than immunohistochemistry. Moreover, a recent report suggested that monoclonal antibodies might nonspecifically label BM cells that simulate metastases. On closer morphological examination the labeled cells were nonmalignant and could be found in the BM of normal controls (Lagrange et al. 1997). Before this assay can be used to enhance clinical management of breast and other cancers, there needs to be broad agreement regarding methodology for detection, and prospective clinical studies of interventions based on the detection of micrometastatic cells need to be conducted.

New Directions

Whatever role HDC finds in the management of breast cancer, it is apparent that additional strategies will be required to optimize patient outcome. Emerging technologies hold exciting prospects. Monoclonal antibodies to cellular oncogenes, such as HER 2/*neu*, have already been demonstrated to possess clinical activity (Basetga et al. 1996) and are currently being evaluated in conjunction with standard-dose chemotherapy. Oncostatin M has recently been shown to inhibit hormone-receptor-negative breast cancer cell growth in vitro (Douglas et al. 1997, 1998), and is currently being assessed in preclinical in vivo models. Finally, agents that prevent the growth of cancer through inhibition of angiogenesis (Boehm et al. 1997) or tumor stroma raise the hope of treatments that circumvent the problems associated with chemotherapy resistance.

Summary

High-dose chemotherapy with autologous stem cell support as applied to the treatment of breast cancer has shown promise for over 15 years. Three main approaches have been used: (1) standard-dose induction chemotherapy followed by one or two cycles of myeloablative therapy, (2) multicycle nonablative combination chemotherapy, and (3) high-dose sequential chemotherapy using single agents at the maximum tolerated doses in rapid sequence. Each of these approaches has a strong biological rationale and is being pursued in randomized trials. Unfortunately, comparative data are limited and there is only one fully published randomized trial of the use of high-dose chemotherapy in metastatic breast cancer. This small study from South Africa showed a significant improvement in response rate and survival for women receiving high-dose chemotherapy compared to those given standard dose treatment. It is anticipated that results from larger studies in the USA and Europe evaluating the use of high-dose chemotherapy in metastatic breast cancer and in adjuvant treatment of poor-prognosis early-stage disease will be available within the next 2–3 years. A potentially important and related issue is that of tumor contamination of bone marrow and apheresis collections. Current data suggest that finding epithelial tumor cells with sensitive techniques (such as immunohistochemistry or polymerase chain reaction) gives prognostic information. However, it is not clear whether reinfusion of these cells after high-dose chemotherapy contributes to relapse of breast cancer. Unfortunately, understanding of the data is marred by a lack of standardization of assay methodology. Further work is needed to develop a widely accepted method for the detection of circulating tumor cells before the clinical relevance of such a finding can be meaningfully interpreted.

References

Antman K, Ayash L, Elias A, Wheeler C, Hunt M, Eder JP, Teicher BA, Critchlow J, Bibbo J, Schnipper LE et al (1992) A phase II study of high-dose cyclophosphamide, thiotepa, and carboplatin with autologous marrow support in women with measurable advanced breast cancer responding to standard-dose therapy [see comments]. J Clin Oncol 10:102–110

Antman KH, Rowlings PA, Vaughan WP, Pelz CJ, Fay JW, Fields KK, Freytes CO, Gale RP, Hillner BE, Holland HK, Kennedy MJ, Klein JP, Lazarus HM, McCarthy PL Jr, Saez R, Spitzer G, Stadtmauer EA, Williams SF, Wolff S, Sobocinski KA, Armitage JO, Horowitz MM (1997) High-dose chemotherapy with autologous hematopoietic stem-cell support for breast cancer in North America. J Clin Oncol 15:1870–1879

Arriagada R, Le Chevalier T, Pignon JP, Riviere A, Monnet I, Chomy P, Tuchais C, Tarayre M, Ruffie P (1993) Initial chemotherapeutic doses and survival in patients with limited small-cell lung cancer. N Engl J Med 329:1848–1852

Ashworth TR (1869) A case of cancer in which cells similar to those in the tumours were seen in the blood after death. Aust Med J 14:146

Ayash LJ, Elias A, Wheeler C, Reich E, Schwartz G, Mazanet R, Tepler I, Warren D, Lynch C, Gonin R, Schnipper L, Frei E III, Antman K (1994) Double dose-intensive chemotherapy with autologous marrow and peripheral-blood progenitor-cell support for metastatic breast cancer: a feasibility study. J Clin Oncol 12:37–44

Baselga J, Tripathy D, Mendelsohn J, Baughman S, Benz CC, Dantis L, Sklenar I, Seidman AD, Hudis CA, Moore J, Rosen PP, Twaddell T, Henderson IC, Norton L (1996) Phase II study of weekly intravenous recombinant humanized anti-p185HER2 monoclonal antibody in patients with HER2/neu-overexpressing metastatic breast cancer. J Clin Oncol 14:737–744

Basser RL, To BL, Begley CG, Juttner CA, Maher DW, Szer J, Cebon J, Collins JP, Russell I, Olver I, Gill PG, Fox RM, Sheridan WP, Green MD (1995) Adjuvant treatment of high-risk breast cancer using multi-cycle high-dose chemotherapy and filgrastim-mobilized peripheral blood progenitor cells. Clin Cancer Res 1:715–721

Basser RL, To LB, Begley CG, Maher D, Juttner C, Cebon J, Mansfield R, Olver I, Duggan G, Szer J, Collins J, Schwartz B, Marty J, Menchaca D, Sheridan WP, Fox RM, Green MD (1998) Rapid hematopoietic recovery after multicycle high-dose chemotherapy: enhancement of filgrastim-induced progenitor cell mobilization by recombinant human stem cell factor. J Clin Oncol (in press)

Begley CG, Basser R, Mansfield R, Thomson B, Parker W, Layton J, To B, Sheridan WP, Fox RM, Green MD (1997) Enhanced levels and clonogenic capacity of blood progenitor cells following administration of stem cell factor and filgrastim to humans. Blood 90:3378–3389

Berger U, Mansi JL, Wilson P, Coombes RC (1987) Detection of estrogen receptor in bone marrow from patients with metastatic breast cancer. J Clin Oncol 5:1779–1782

Berger U, Bettelheim R, Mansi JL, Easton D, Coombes RC, Neville AM (1988) The relationship between micrometastases in the bone marrow, histopathologic features of the primary tumor in breast cancer and prognosis. Am J Clin Pathol 90:1–6

Bezwoda WR, Seymour L, Dansey RD (1995) High-dose chemotherapy with hematopoietic rescue as primary treatment for metastatic breast cancer: a randomized trial. J Clin Oncol 13:2483–2489

Boehm T, Folkman J, Browder T, O'Reilly MS (1997) Antiangiogenic therapy of experimental cancer does not induce acquired drug resistance. Nature 390:404–407

Brügger W, Bross KJ, Glatt M, Weber F, Mertelsmann R, Kanz L (1994) Mobilization of tumor cells and hematopoietic progenitor cells into peripheral blood of patients with solid tumors [see comments]. Blood 83:636–640

Burchill SA, Bradbury MF, Pittman K, Southgate J, Smith B, Selby P (1995) Detection of epithelial cancer cells in peripheral blood by reverse transcriptase-polymerase chain reaction. Br J Cancer 71:278–281

Ceci G, Franciosi V, Nizzoli R, De Lisi V, Lottici R, Boni C, Di Blasio B, Passalacqua R, Guazzi A, Cocconi G (1988) The value of bone marrow biopsy in breast cancer at time of diagnosis. A prospective study. Cancer 61:96–98

Chevillard S, Muller A, Levalois C, Laine-Bidron C, Viehl P, Magdelenat H, (1996) Reverse transcription-polymerase chain reaction (RT-PCR) assays of estrogen and progesterone receptors in breast cancer. Breast Cancer Res Treat 41:81–89

Crump M, Goss PE, Prince M, Girouard C (1996) Outcome of extensive evaluation before adjuvant therapy in women with breast cancer and 10 or more positive axillary lymph nodes. J Clin Oncol 14:66–69

Datta YH, Adams PT, Drobyski WR, Ethier SP, Terry VH, Roth MS (1994) Sensitive detection of occult breast cancer by the reverse-transcriptase polymerase chain reaction. J Clin Oncol 12:475–482

De Vita VT Jr (1993) Principles of chemotherapy. In: De Vita VT Jr, Hellman S, Rosenberg SA (eds) Cancer: principles and practice of oncology. Lippincott, Philadelphia, pp 276–292

De Vita VT Jr, Hubbard SM, Longo DL (1987) The chemotherapy of lymphomas: looking back, moving forward – the Richard and Hinda Rosenthal Foundation Award lecture. Cancer Res 47:5810–5824

To LB, Haylock DN, Simmons PJ, Juttner CA (1997) The biology and clinical uses of blood stem cells. Blood 89:2233–2258

Douglas AM, Goss GA, Sutherland RL, Hilton DJ, Berndt MC, Nicola NA, Begley CG (1997) Expression and function of members of the cytokine receptor superfamily on breast cancer cells. Oncogene 14:661–669

Douglas AM, Grant SL, Goss GA, Clouston DR, Sutherland RL, Begley CG (1998) Oncostatin M induces the differentiation of breast cancer cells. Int J Cancer 75:64–73

Eaton MC, Hardingham JE, Kotasek D, Dobrovic A (1997) Immunobead RT-PCR: a sensitive method for detection of circulating tumor cells. Biotechniques 22:100–105

Eddy DM (1992) High-dose chemotherapy with autologous bone marrow transplantation for the treatment of metastatic breast cancer [see comments]. J Clin Oncol 10:657–670 (Erratum in J Clin Oncol 10:1655–1658)

Fox SB, Leek RD, Bliss J, Mansi JL, Gusterson B, Gatter KC, Harris AL (1997) Association of tumor angiogenesis with bone marrow micrometastases in breast cancer patients. J Natl Cancer Inst 89:1044–1049

Franklin WA, Shpall EJ, Archer P, Johnston CS, Garza-Williams S, Hami L, Bitter MA, Bast RC, Jones RB (1996) Immunocytochemical detection of breast cancer cells in marrow and peripheral blood of patients undergoing high dose chemotherapy with autologous stem cell support. Breast Cancer Res Treat 41:1–13

Franklin WA, Pflaumer SM, Jones RB, Hami L, Garza-Williams S, Turner SA, Davis HW, Martinez C, Bearman S, Cagnoni P, Ross M, Shpall EJ (1997) The addition of stem cell factor (SCF) to filgrastim (r-metHuG-CSF) for mobilization of PBPC does not enhance mobilization of tumor cells into the peripheral blood of breast cancer patients. Proc Am Soc Clin Oncol 16:118 a

Funke I, Schraut W (1998) Meta-analyses of studies on bone marrow micrometastases: an independent prognostic impact remains to be substantiated. J Clin Oncol 16:557–566

Garcia-Carbonero R, Hidalgo M, Paz-Ares L, Calzas J, Gomez H, Guerra JA, Hitt R, Hornedo J, Colmer R, Cortes-Funes H (1997) Patient selection in high-dose chemotherapy trials: relevance in high-risk breast cancer. J Clin Oncol 15:3178–3184

Gianni AM, Siena S, Bregni M, Lombardi F, Gandola L, Valagussa P, Bonadonna G (1991) Prolonged disease-free survival after high-dose sequential chemo-radiotherapy and haemopoietic autologous transplantation in poor prognosis Hodgkin's disease. Ann Oncol 2:645–653

Gianni AM, Tarella C, Bregni M, Siena S, Lombardi F, Gandola L, Caracciolo D, Bonadonna G, Boccadoro M, Pileri A (1994) High-dose sequential chemoradiotherapy, a widely applicable regimen, confers survival benefit to patients with high-risk multiple myeloma. J Clin Oncol 12:503–509

Gianni AM, Siena S, Bregni M, Di Nicola M, Orefice S, Cusumano F, Salvadori B, Luini A, Greco M, Zucali R, Rilke F, Zambetti M, Valagussa P, Bonadonna G (1997a) Efficacy, toxicity, and applicability of high-dose sequential chemotherapy as adjuvant treatment in operable breast cancer with 10 or more involved axillary nodes: five-year results. J Clin Oncol 15:2312–2321

Gianni AM, Bregni M, Siena S, Brambilla C, Di Nicola M, Lombardi F, Gandola L, Tarella C, Pileri A, Ravagnani F, Valagussa P, Bonadonna G, Stern AC, Magni M, Caracciolo D (1997b) High-dose chemotherapy and autologous bone marrow transplantation compared with MACOP-B in aggressive B-cell lymphoma. N Engl J Med 336:1290–1297

Gilbert CJ (1996) Peripheral blood progenitor cell transplantation for breast cancer: pharmacoeconomic considerations. Pharmacotherapy 16:101S–108S

Gradishar WJ, Tallman MS, Abrams JS (1996) High-dose chemotherapy for breast cancer. Ann Intern Med 125:599–604

Gugliotta P, Botta G, Bussolati G (1990) Immunocytochemical detection of tumour markers in bone metastases from carcinoma of the breast. Histochem J 13:953–959

Kotasek D, Sage RE, Dale BM, Norman JE, Bolton A (1994) Dose intensive therapy with autologous blood stem cell transplantation in breast cancer. Aust N Z J Med 24:288–295

Krismann M, Todt B, Schröder J, Gareis D, Müller KM, Seeber S, Schütte J (1995) Low specificity of cytokeratin 19 reverse transcriptase-polymerase chain reaction analyses for detection of hematogenous lung cancer dissemination. J Clin Oncol 13:2769–2775

Lagrange M, Ferrero JM, Lagrange JL, Machiavello JC, Monticelli J, Bayle C, Creisson A, Namer M, Thyss A, Bourcier C, Gioanni J, Schneider M (1997) Non-specifically labelled cells that simulate bone marrow metastases in patients with non-metastatic breast cancer. J Clin Pathol 50:206–211

Luppi M, Morselli M, Bandieri E, Federico M, Marasca R, Barozzi P, Ferrari MG, Savarino M, Frassoldati A, Torelli G (1996) Sensitive detection of circulating breast cancer cells by reverse-transcriptase polymerase chain reaction of maspin gene. Ann Oncol 7:619–624

Mansi JL, Berger U, Easton D, McDonnell T, Redding WH, Gazet JC, McKinna A, Powles TJ, Coombes RC (1987) Micrometastases in bone marrow in patients with primary breast cancer: evaluation as an early predictor of bone metastases. Br Med J [Clin Res] 295:1093–1096

Mathew J (1995) NCI survey explores the M.D.'s perspective on ABMT trials. J Natl Cancer Inst 87:1510–1511

Naume B, Borgen E, Beiske K, Herstad TK, Ravnas G, Renolen A, Funderud S, Kvalheim G (1997) Immunomagnetic techniques for the enrichment and detection of isolated breast carcinoma cells in bone marrow and peripheral blood. J Hematother 6:103–114

Osborne MP, Rosen PP (1994) Detection and management of bone marrow micrometastases in breast cancer. Oncology 8:25–31

Pantel K, Moss TJ (1996) First international ISHAGE symposium on minimal residual cancer. J Hematother 5:511–517

Pantel K, Schlimok G, Braun S, Kutter D, Lindemann F, Schaller G, Funke I, Izbicki JR, Riethmuller G (1993) Differential expression of proliferation-associated molecules in individual micrometastic carcinoma cells. J Natl Cancer Inst 85:1419–1424

Passos-Coelho JL, Ross AA, Moss TJ, Davis JM, Huelskamp A-M, Noga SJ, Davidson NE, Kennedy MJ (1995) Absence of breast cancer cells in a single-day peripheral blood progenitor cell collection after priming with cyclophosphamide and granulocyte-macrophage colony-stimulating factor. Blood 85:1138–1143

Peters WP (1995) High-dose chemotherapy with autologous bone marrow transplantation for the treatment of breast cancer: yes (Review) Important Adv Oncol 215–230

Peters WP, Eder JP, Henner WD, Schryber S, Wilmore D, Finberg R, Scoenfeld D, Bast R, Gargone B, Antman K, Anderson J, Anderson K, Kruskall MS, Schnipper L, Frei E III (1986) High-dose combination alkylating agents with autologous bone marrow support: a phase I trial. J Clin Oncol 4:646–654

Peters WP, Shpall EJ, Jones RB, Olsen GA, Bast RC, Gockerman JP, Moore JO (1988) High-dose combination alkylating agents with bone marrow support as initial treatment for metastatic breast cancer. J Clin Oncol 6:1368–1376

Peters WP, Jones RB, Vredenburgh J, Shpall EJ, Hussein A, Elkordy M, Rubin P, Ross M, Berry D (1997) A large, prospective, randomized trial of high-dose combination alkylating agents (CPB) with autologous cellular support (ABMS) as consolidation for patients with metastatic breast cancer achieving complete remission after intensive doxorubicin-based induction therapy (AFM) (Abstr.) Proc Am Soc Clin Oncol 15:121

Redding WH, Coombes RC, Monaghan P, Clink HM, Imrie SF, Dearnaley DP, Ormerod MG, Sloane JP, Gazet JC, Powles TJ et al (1983) Detection of micrometastases in patients with primary breast cancer. Lancet 2:1271–1274

Rodenhuis S, Richel DJ, Baars JW, van der Wall E, Schornagel JH, Schaake-Koning C, Rutgers E (1997) A randomized phase II study of high-dose chemotherapy in high-risk breast cancer. Proceedings of 2nd International Symposium: Changes in the treatment of breast cancer, June 1–2, Madrid, pp 101–105

Ross AA, Cooper BW, Lazarus HM, Mackay W, Moss TJ, Ciobanu N, Tallman MS, Kennedy MJ, Davidson NE, Sweet D et al (1993) Detection and viability of tumor cells in peripheral blood stem cell collections from breast cancer patients using immunocytochemical and clonogenic assay techniques. Blood 82:2605–2610

Rushing DA (1997) High-dose chemotherapy for breast cancer (Letter). Ann Intern med 126:917

Schlimok G, Funke I, Holzmann B, Gottlinger G, Schmidt G, Hauser H, Swierkot S, Warnecke HH, Schneider B, Koprowski H et al (1987) Micrometastatic cancer cells in bone marrow: in vitro detection with anti-cytokeratin and in vivo labeling with anti-17-1A monoclonal antibodies. Proc Natl Acad Sci USA 84:8672–8676

Schoenfeld A, Luqmani Y, Smith D, O'Reilly S, Shousha S, Sinnett HD, Coombes RC (1994) Detection of breast cancer micrometastases in axillary lymph nodes by using polymerase chain reaction. Cancer Res 54:2986–2990

Shea TC, Mason JR, Storniolo AM, Newton B, Breslin M, Mullen M, Ward DM, Miller L, Christian M, Taetle R (1992) Sequential cycles of high-dose carboplatin administered with recombinant human granulocyte-macrophage colony-stimulating factor and repeated infusions of autologous peripheral blood progenitor cells: a novel and effective method for delivering multiple courses of dose-intensive therapy. J Clin Oncol 10:464–473

Sloane JP, Ormerod MG, Neville AM (1980) Potential pathological application of immunocytochemical methods to the detection of micrometastases. Cancer Res 40:3079–3082

Stewart PS (1982) Autologous bone marrow transplantation in metastatic breast cancer. Breast Cancer Res Treat 2:85–92

Thomas P, Battifora H (1987) Keratins versus epithelial membrane antigen in tumor diagnosis: an immunohistochemical comparison of five monoclonal antibodies. Hum Pathol 18:728–734

Traweek ST, Liu J, Battifora H (1993) Keratin gene expression in non-epithelial tissues. Detection with polymerase chain reaction. Am J Pathol 142:1111–1118

Ung O, Langlands AO, Barraclough B, Boyages J (1995) Combined chemotherapy and radiotherapy for patients with breast cancer and extensive nodal involvement. J Clin Oncol 13:435–443

Zippelius A, Kufer P, Honold G, Köllermann MW, Oberneder R, Schlimok G, Rithmüller G, Pantel K (1997) Limitations of reverse-transcriptase polymerase chain reaction analyses for detection of micrometastic epithelial cancer cells in bone marrow. J Clin Oncol 15:2701–2708

Summary

N. E. Davidson[1] and P. Valagussa[2]

[1] The Johns Hopkins Oncology Center, Baltimore, Maryland, USA
[2] Istituto Nazionale Tumori, Milan, Italy

Despite several decades of clinical research, a variety of questions about how to administer optimal adjuvant chemotherapy remain. One lingering question is the importance of dose as a determinant of outcome in both early and advanced stage breast cancer. The possibility that the dose of chemotherapy actually received by the patient might influence clinical outcome was first raised by Bonadonna and colleagues in their retrospective analysis of the seminal trial of cyclophosphamide, methotrexate, and 5-fluorouracil chemotherapy versus observation for treatment of women with node-positive breast cancer. The concepts of dose intensity, dose density, total dose, dose size, etc., have gradually evolved from this initial work. Technological developments such as the advent of colony-stimulating factors and the ability to harvest autologous bone marrow or peripheral blood progenitor cells have permitted substantial dose escalation of cytotoxics like the alkylating agents whose primary toxicity is myelosuppression. In addition, the administration of cytotoxics more frequently or at high doses repetitively has become feasible. However, few trials that explicitly test the value of these approaches have been reported as yet. In addition, those trials reported have not been uniformly positive. For example, two sequential trials of dose escalation of cyclophosphamide with a fixed dose of doxorubicin for women with node-positive breast cancer have thus far failed to show a major advantage of a fourfold escalation in cyclophosphamide dose from 600 mg/m^2 to 2400 mg/m^2 per cycle. Early follow-up of a trial of dose escalation of doxorubicin from 60 mg/m^2 to 90 mg/m^2 per cycle with a fixed dose of cyclophosphamide in the same group of women also shows no benefit. Thus, though supported by preclinical models, regimens with greatly increased dose, dose intensity, or dose density cannot be regarded as standard at present in the absence of clear proof of superiority. However, the area remains an active area of clinical investigation, as exemplified by two presentations during the session on cytotoxics and their dose.

A comprehensive analysis of dose density and intensity was presented by Martine Piccart from the Jules Bordet Institute in Belgium. Piccart reviewed various strategies by which dose intensity and density may theoretically be modulated. She identified at least five models which vary the dose per course of therapy, time interval between courses, and/or the cumulative dose of therapy in order to permit delivery of a higher dose of cytotoxic drug per unit time. Design of and results from completed and ongoing anthracycline-based trials which addressed each of these strategies were also reviewed. In Piccart's view three major lessons may be drawn from these studies thus far. First, administration of low doses in each course can lead to inferior clinical outcome as exemplified by results from CALGB 8541, a trial of low- versus moderate- versus high-dose cyclophosphamide, doxorubicin, and 5-fluorouracil as adjuvant therapy for women with node-positive breast cancer. Second, an increase in dose per course and cumulative dose may be beneficial in certain high-risk patients. Finally, dose densification with hematopoietic growth factor support is feasible but has not been shown to offer any advantage in trials reported to date.

This discussion was continued in the presentation on new developments in the area of high-dose chemotherapy by Russell Basser from the Royal Melbourne and Western Hospitals in Australia. Two general approaches, standard-dose therapy followed by a single myeloablative course of chemotherapy with autologous hematopoietic support and administration of multiple cycles of nonmyeloablative chemotherapy with stem cell support, have been utilized in numerous phase I and II trials. The feasibility of such approaches with acceptable toxicity has been well established. However, unequivocal evidence of additional benefit over that seen with standard-dose approaches is not yet available. To date, results from three randomized trials of high-dose chemotherapy have been presented from South Africa, the United States, and the Netherlands. None of these trials has demonstrated conclusively that high-dose approaches provide superior clinical results. Several large randomized trials are ongoing around the world and should ultimately define the role for this approach in patients with high-risk stage II and stage IV disease. However, there is no consensus currently about what level of benefit will be required in these trials in order to recommend these therapies as standard practice.

In the meantime, numerous pilot trials continue as part of efforts to improve the efficacy of high-dose approaches. Basser described one such approach utilized in a pilot trial of about 100 women with newly diagnosed breast cancer involving more than nine axillary lymph nodes. Administration of three cycles of epirubicin (200 mg/m^2) and cyclophosphamide (4 g/m^2) with peripheral blood stem cell reinfusion after each cycle was shown to be feasible and long-term toxicity was apparently low. Testing of this strategy against a more standard regimen is ongoing in the International Breast Cancer Study Group. In addition, other issues related to autologous transplantation were discussed. These include our uncertainty about what role, if any, tumor cell contamination of reinfused bone marrow or stem cell preparations may play in relapse as well as the possibility that transplant recipients might be excellent candidates for inclusion in trials of more biologically based therapies such as inhibitors of angiogenesis or matrix metalloproteinase activity, antibodies directed against critical determinants such as the HER-2/ neu gene product, or novel molecules such as oncostatin M.

Another vexing issue, the role of anthracyclines in the adjuvant setting, was addressed in the presentation by Mark Levine for the National Cancer Institute of Canada. It is generally accepted that anthracycline-based regimens improve response rate and progression-free survival over those results obtained with non-anthracycline-containing regimens in the setting of stage IV breast cancer. However, these findings have not readily translated into improved outcome in the adjuvant setting. Indeed, a number of clinical trials examining anthracycline vs non-anthracycline-containing adjuvant chemotherapy have not shown any additional benefit. Against this background, Levine presented updated information on a randomized trial of cyclophosphamide, epirubicin, and 5-fluorouracil (CEF) versus cyclophosphamide, methotrexate, and 5-fluorouracil (CMF) in premenopausal women with node-positive breast cancer. With a median follow-up of nearly 5 years, the 5-year relapse-free survivals for CMF and CEF were 53% and 63% respectively while corresponding 5-year survivals were 70% and 77%. Cardiotoxicity was minimal but acute leukemia was noted in 5 of the 351 CEF patients. Nonetheless CEF resulted in a significant improvement in relapse-free and overall survival in the trial. Although the trial was not strictly a comparison of methotrexate and epirubicin, as dose of cyclophosphamide and 5-fluorouracil differed between the CMF and CEF regimens, it does represent one of the largest and best-designed trials of this question. It is not clear why this trial was positive whereas a number of other studies testing the same question were not. Levine speculates that the dose intensity of the CEF regimen may be higher than that utilized in other trials. In addition, this trial was limited to premenopausal women with node-positive breast cancer, a group found in a number of studies to have the greatest absolute benefit from adjuvant chemotherapy; this group may therefore be the most revealing for studies examining relative benefits of different chemotherapy regimens. In any case, the results of this positive trial must be viewed in the context of the many completed trials addressing this question, several of which show little or no advantage for the anthracycline-containing combinations. In the near future, information from the Oxford overview analysis about this issue should be available. In addition initial results from a large trial of CMF versus CAF (cyclophosphamide, doxorubicin, and 5-fluorouracil) in women with high-risk node-negative breast cancer should be available this year.

In sum this session on cytotoxics and their dose provided an excellent overview of the current state of knowledge about dose intensity and density and reviewed the multiple unanswered questions in this field. Also the value of anthracycline-based chemotherapy in the adjuvant setting was assessed with specific attention to the outcome of a recent positive randomized clinical trial. It is hoped that these issues will be more fully resolved within the next several years.

XI. Integrated Treatments: Quality of Life

Quality of Life Assessment in the Adjuvant Setting: Is It Relevant?

R. D. Gelber [1,2,4], M. Bonetti [1,2], B. F. Cole [3], S. Gelber [4],
and A. Goldhirsch [5] for the International Breast Cancer Study Group *

[1] Department of Biostatistical Science, Dana-Farber Cancer Institute, Boston,
   MA 02115, USA
[2] Department of Biostatistics, Harvard School of Public Health, Boston,
   Massachusetts, USA
[3] Department of Community and Family Medicine,
   Dartmouth-Hitchcock Medical Center, Lebanon, New Hampshire, USA
[4] Frontier Science and Technology Research Foundation, Brookline,
   Massachusetts, USA
[5] Department of Medical Oncology and Radiation Oncology,
   European Institute of Oncology, Milan, Italy,
   and Department of Medical Oncology, Ospedale Civico, Lugano, Switzerland,
   and International Breast Cancer Study Group, Bern, Switzerland

Introduction

In this paper we address a question concerning quality-of-life assessment in
the adjuvant setting: is it relevant? Like the science of quality-of-life evaluation itself, the answer to this question is multifaceted. The most direct answer is yes, but only if there is a well-defined question of importance for patient care. This requires a specific hypothesis and an appropriate methodology to test it.

The assessment of quality of life in cancer patients was first introduced by
Karnofsky et al. in 1948. Initial considerations were given to the patients
with advanced disease. Clearly the disease process as well as the treatments
had an influence on the patients' quality of life in this setting.

The situation in the setting of postsurgical adjuvant therapy is different.
Following local treatment, patients are otherwise well as they begin on the
road to recovery from the shock of the diagnosis and initial therapy. Patients' adaptation to their situation substantially influences the reported quality of life as the disease-free survival interval increases. A critical question
also concerns the impact of adjuvant therapy on quality of life.

One perspective could be that patients simply want to live as long as possible, with only secondary consideration given to the quality of life. This is
supported by evidence from patients who would be willing to repeat a previously completed course of toxic adjuvant therapy even if they would gain
relatively little additional survival time (Simes et al. 1989; Lindley et al.
1998).

---

* See Appendix for participants and authors.

However, the current evidence concerning the effectiveness of adjuvant therapies (Early Breast Cancer Trialists' Collaborative Group 1992) is sufficient to routinely prescribe chemotherapy and tamoxifen for all patients, if these therapies could be given free of charge and were not associated with any toxic side effects. Given that cost considerations are not overwhelming factors in determining oncology therapies, one must presume that the concern for side effects is the main reason physicians are reluctant to prescribe chemoendocrine therapy for all patients. Therefore, despite the evidence that survival is of primary concern, aspects of quality of life remain important for treatment decision-making.

In this paper we discuss several reasons why the assessment of quality of life in the adjuvant setting is relevant. We illustrate how quality-of-life considerations can be incorporated into an overall evaluation of the quality and quantity of survival in this setting. The current controversy concerning the worth of adding adjuvant chemotherapy to tamoxifen for postmenopausal patients serves as an example.

What Is Quality-of-Life Assessment?

Quality-of-life assessment has been defined as the measurement of multiple domains including physical, mental, social, psychological dimensions using valid and reliable instruments. There are two approaches to this measurement: health status and utility assessment. The first approach describes patient experience in the major domains of health, while the second approach elicits patient preferences (utilities) for particular health states. Utilities are usually measured on an interval scale from 0.0 (death) to 1.0 (perfect health). These values can be incorporated in quality-adjusted survival and cost-effectiveness analyses.

Reasons for Quality-of-Life Assessment

There are several reasons why one might conduct quality-of-life assessments in clinical trials in the adjuvant setting. An obvious goal is to describe the subjective quality-of-life differences between treatment groups being compared. This is useful to inform patients and clinicians about what to expect with respect to quality-of-life issues. Another reason is to indicate situations in which psychosocial interventions might be useful (Ganz et al. 1998). A third reason is to provide an additional measure with prognostic significance. Coates et al. (1992) found that baseline quality-of-life measures were significant predictors of subsequent survival for patients with metastatic breast cancer. A fourth objective is to document patient adaptation to their diagnosis and treatment. A recent study by the International Breast Cancer Study Group (IBCSG) of node-positive patients reported that the initial decrease in quality of life (during adjuvant chemotherapy) was of lower magnitude than the subsequent improvement in quality of life associated with patient adaptation (Hürny et al. 1996). A fifth reason to incorporate quality-of-life considerations in the adjuvant setting is to assess the tradeoffs between quantity and quality of life. A relevant question is whether the gain in disease-free survival and overall survival balance the decreased quality of life that might be associated with the use of adjuvant therapy following local management of operable breast cancer. A quality-of-life oriented endpoint designed to address this question is the Q-TWiST method. A controversial area of treatment decision-making for which quality-of-life considerations are particularly relevant concerns the worth of chemotherapy added to tamoxifen for postmenopausal patients.

A Complementary Outcome in the Adjuvant Setting (Q-TWiST)

Q-TWiST stands for Quality-adjusted Time Without Symptoms of disease or Toxicity of treatment (Goldhirsch et al. 1989; Glasziou et al. 1990; Gelber et al. 1995). The Q-TWiST method has been previously applied to evaluate treatments for cancer and AIDS, with a number of analyses conducted to compare adjuvant therapies for breast cancer (Gelber et al. 1991, 1992). To use the Q-TWiST method to evaluate adjuvant chemotherapy for breast cancer we start by defining three clinical health states through the course of the disease: TOX is the period of time when chemotherapy patients experience toxicity, REL is the period of time after relapse, and TWiST is the period of relatively good quality of life following the completion of treatment, if given, and before a recurrence. Second, using the data from the clinical trial and Kaplan-Meier plots for disease-free survival (DFS) and overall survival (OS), we partition the overall survival time for each treatment separately into the clinical health states of TOX, TWiST, and REL. This provides estimates of the average amount of time that patients spend in each of these health states. The quality-adjusted survival relative to TWiST (Q-TWiST) is then defined as

$$Q\text{-}TWiST = u_{TOX} \times TOX + TWiST + u_{REL} \times REL,$$

where u_{TOX} and u_{REL} are weights which can take on values between zero and one, with values of one being equivalent to TWiST (i.e., no loss in quality of life) and values of zero being equivalent to death.

Finally, using a threshold utility plot, treatment groups can be compared with respect to the amount of Q-TWiST they provide for a range of possible values for u_{TOX} and u_{REL}. This plot illustrates the utility values for which each treatment provides more Q-TWiST. In this way, the relative worth of the treatments can be assessed with adjustments for possible influences on quality of life. Note that the average DFS is simply Q-TWiST with the utility for TOX set equal to one and the utility for REL set equal to zero, i.e., treatment toxicity carries no disutility, but postrelapse survival has the same quality weight as death. Similarly, average OS is obtained from the equation by setting both utilities equal to one. Thus, estimates of the average amounts of DFS and OS are obtained as specific endpoints in a Q-TWiST analysis.

International Breast Cancer Study Group (IBCSG) Trial VII

Trial Design and Analysis of Disease-Free Survival and Overall Survival

Between July 1986 and April 1993, the IBCSG enrolled 1212 postmenopausal patients with node-positive breast cancer into a two-by-two factorial clinical trial evaluating chemoendocrine treatment versus endocrine therapy alone for postmenopausal breast cancer patients. As previously reported (International Breast Cancer Study Group 1997), the patients were randomized to receive one of four adjuvant regimens: tamoxifen alone for 5 years; tamoxifen plus three early single cycles of cyclophosphamide, methotrexate, and fluorouracil (CMF) on months 1, 2, and 3; tamoxifen plus delayed single courses of CMF on months 9, 12, and 15; tamoxifen plus early and delayed CMF on months 1, 2, 3, 9, 12, and 15. Estrogen-receptor (ER) status was known for all patients and was used to stratify the randomization. Tumors with hormone receptor concentrations above or aqual to 10 fmol/mg cytosol protein were considered positive, and those with lower values negative.

The median age was 60 years. Twenty-three percent of patients had primary tumors classified as ER-negative. Twenty-four percent had surgery with breast preservation. Sixty-two percent had fewer than four axillary lymph nodes involved, and the median number of involved nodes was three. Treatment groups were balanced according to age, race, type of primary surgery, number of positive nodes, and tumor size.

Date of relapse was defined as the time when recurrent disease was diagnosed or, if confirmed later, when it was first suspected. DFS was defined as the length of the time from the date of randomization to any relapse (including ipsilateral breast recurrence), the appearance of a second primary cancer (including contralateral breast cancer), or death, whichever occurred first.

In this paper, we focus on the comparison of two of the four treatment arms: tamoxifen plus three early cycles of CMF chemotherapy (tamoxifen plus early CMF) versus tamoxifen alone. At 5 years median follow-up, there was a significant difference in DFS favoring the chemoendocrine therapy (Fig. 1A). The 5-year DFS was 64% for tamoxifen plus early CMF versus 55% for tamoxifen alone ($p = 0.02$).

This difference might be considered enough evidence to recommend that chemotherapy should be added to tamoxifen for postmenopausal, node-positive patients. However, at this analysis there was no difference in OS between the two arms (5-year OS: 74% versus 77%; $p = 0.56$; Fig. 1B).

When the treatments are compared with respect to DFS separately for the prospectively stratified subpopulations of patients defined according to ER status of the primary tumor, the magnitude of effect appears to be larger for the ER-positive cohort (Fig. 2). It is important to recall that all patients are assigned to receive 5 years of tamoxifen and the 3 cycles of early CMF are given currently with the first three months of tamoxifen. No OS differences were observed even for the ER-positive group that had the best response in terms of DFS.

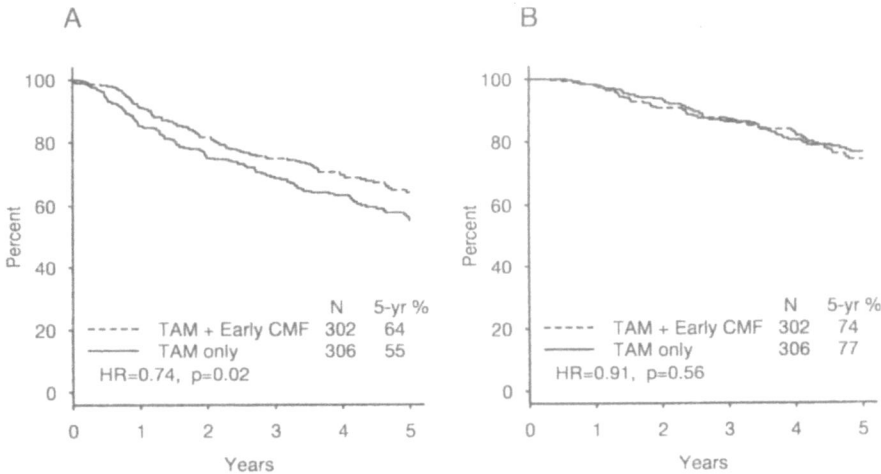

Fig. 1. Disease-free survival (**A**) and overall survival (**B**) according to treatment group (tamoxifen plus early CMF versus tamoxifen alone) for 608 postmenopausal, node-positive patients enrolled in International Breast Cancer Study Group Trial VII. Median follow-up is 5 years *HR*, Hazards ratio

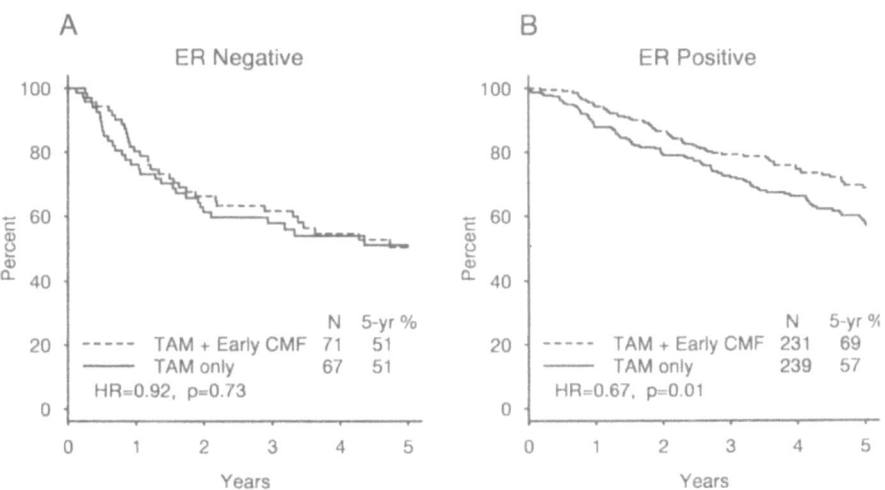

Fig. 2. Disease-free survival for 138 patients with ER-negative tumors (**A**) and for 470 patients with ER-positive tumors (**B**) according to treatment group in IBCSG Trial VII at 5 years' median follow-up. *HR*, Hazards ratio

Because OS gains are minimal at best, the treatment decision can be synthesized based on quality-of-life considerations. In fact, adding chemotherapy is beneficial because it reduces the risk of disease relapse, which has quality-of-life implications. But this benefit needs to be balanced against the reduced quality of life associated with the toxicity of the treatment. The Q-TWiST methodology allows us to explore which of the two arms is to be preferred with respect to such tradeoff between quantity and quality of life for the two treatment groups.

A Q-TWiST Analysis of IBCSG Trial VII at 5 Years of Follow-up

To be conservative in comparing the toxic effects of tamoxifen plus CMF versus tamoxifen alone, no TOX period was assigned to patients who received tamoxifen alone. Instead these patients began in TWiST at the time of randomization. For the TOX health state for patients who received tamoxifen plus CMF, only symptomatic toxicities – those that have an impact on quality of life – were considered. These were primarily nausea/vomiting, alopecia, stomatitis/mucositis, eye disorders, and diarrhea. The entire duration of CMF treatment was included in TOX for any patient who experienced any of these toxicities. An additional 3 months was added for alopecia and weight gain to allow for recovery.

Figure 3 shows the partitioned survival plots for the tamoxifen plus early CMF group and for the tamoxifen alone group separately. The average number of months patients spend in the Q-TWiST health states – the areas between the partitioning Kaplan-Meier curves in Fig. 3 – are shown in Table 1. Patients in the chemoendocrine group spend an average of 3.3 months in TOX, 44.8 months in TWiST, and 5.2 months in REL within 60 months of follow-up. This is compared with zero months, 44.7 months, and 8.9 months for tamoxifen alone, respectively. The average OS time is the sum of the times spent in each of these three health states: 53.3 months for tamoxifen + CMF and 53.6 months for tamoxifen alone, out of a possible 60 months if everyone survived for 5 years.

By varying the values of the weights (utilities), u_{TOX} and u_{REL}, one can explore how the treatment comparison changes according to the values associated to the various health states. We can compare the effect of chemoendocrine therapy relative to tamoxifen alone according to all possible values by looking at the threshold utility plot shown in Fig. 4. The vertical and horizontal axes show the utility coefficient values (ranging from 0 to 1) for TOX and REL, respectively. The solid line in the middle corresponds to utility values for which the Q-TWiST for tamoxifen + CMF is equal to the Q-TWiST for tamoxifen alone, i.e., it shows the set of the threshold values for the utilities. Utility values in the upper left region are those for which tamoxifen + CMF provides more Q-TWiST, while those in the lower right portion are those for which tamoxifen alone provides more Q-TWiST. Utility values in the extreme corners of Fig. 4A are those for which the differences in average

Q-TWiST are statistically significant. The upper left and upper right hand corners of the figure correspond to the utility values for average DFS and OS, respectively.

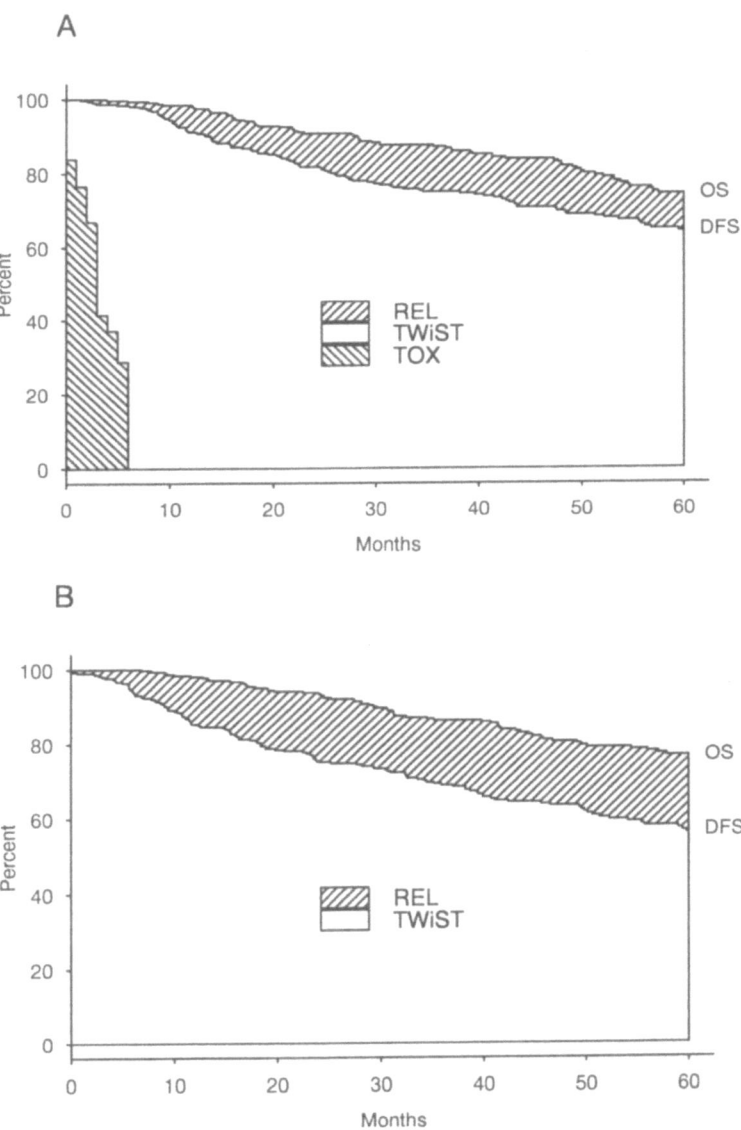

Fig. 3. Partitioned survival plots for tamoxifen plus early CMF (**A**) and for tamoxifen alone (**B**). The areas between the end of toxicity curve, the DFS curve, and the OS curve are the average amounts of time patients spend in the clinical health states TOX, TWiST, and REL within 5 years of follow-up (see Table 1 for values)

The threshold plot in Fig. 4B is the same as that in Fig. 4A, except that in addition to the bold threshold line showing utility values for which the Q-TWiST difference is zero, other lines are included to show utility values for which other specific average increases (decreases) in Q-TWiST occur between the two arms. This plot allows one to identify the amount of Q-TWiST gained or lost as the utility values change within the range of their possible values. The two $\times$'s shown in Fig. 4B indicate the two scenarios ($u_{TOX} = 0.9$, $u_{REL} = 0.5$) and ($u_{TOX} = 0.5$, $u_{REL} = 0.9$) illustrated in Table 1. These correspond to two situations in which the impact of toxicity is either not as severe as or worse than the impact of relapse. For instance, in the first scenario a woman would value time spent after a relapse as half as much as time in good health, while only assigning a slight decrement to time spent in TOX. In the second scenario a woman would value time spent with toxicity as half as much as time in good health, but would only give time after a relapse a slight disutility. The use of chemotherapy

Table 1. Average months spent in the Q-TWiST clinical health states (within 60 months of follow-up) for patients assigned to tamoxifen plus early CMF versus tamoxifen alone in IBCSG Trial VII

	Tamoxifen +early CMF	Tamoxifen alone	Months gained[a]	95% Confidence interval
For all 608 patients				
TOX	3.3	0.0	3.3	(3.1, 3.6)
TWiST	44.8	44.7	0.1	(−3.1, 3.3)
REL	5.2	8.9	−3.7	(−5.8, −1.6)
OS	53.3	53.6	−0.3	(−2.5, 2.0)
DFS	48.1	44.7	3.4	(0.2, 6.7)
Q-TWiST				
($u_{TOX} = 0.9$; $u_{REL} = 0.5$)	50.4	49.2	1.2	(−1.3, 3.8)
($u_{TOX} = 0.5$; $u_{REL} = 0.9$)	51.1	52.7	−1.6	(−3.9, 0.7)
For 138 patients with ER-negative tumors				
TOX	3.2	0.0	3.2	(2.7, 3.7)
TWiST	37.4	39.0	−1.6	(−9.2, 6.1)
REL	6.3	8.3	−2.0	(−6.2, 2.2)
OS	46.9	47.3	−0.4	(−6.5, 5.9)
DFS	40.6	39.0	1.6	(−6.0, 9.3)
Q-TWiST				
($u_{TOX} = 0.9$; $u_{REL} = 0.5$)	43.4	43.1	0.3	(−6.3, 7.0)
($u_{TOX} = 0.5$; $u_{REL} = 0.9$)	44.7	46.5	−1.8	(−7.9, 4.5)
For 470 patients with ER-positive tumors				
TOX	3.4	0.0	3.4	(3.1, 3.7)
TWiST	47.1	46.4	0.7	(−2.6, 4.0)
REL	4.9	9.1	−4.2	(−6.6, −1.8)
OS	55.4	55.5	−0.1	(−2.3, 2.0)
DFS	50.5	46.4	4.1	(0.8, 7.4)
Q-TWiST				
($u_{TOX} = 0.9$; $u_{REL} = 0.5$)	52.6	50.9	1.7	(−0.9, 4.1)
($u_{TOX} = 0.5$; $u_{REL} = 0.9$)	53.2	54.6	− 1.4	(−3.6, 0.7)

[a] Months in the tamoxifen plus early CMF group minus months in the tamoxifen alone group.

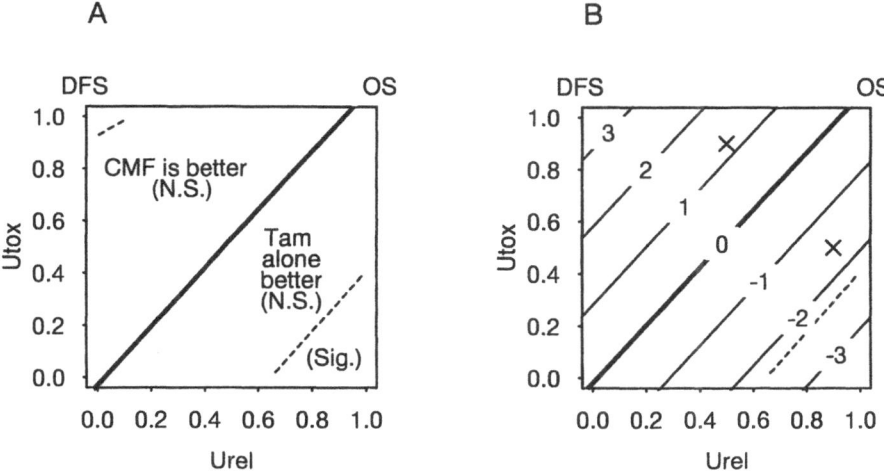

Fig. 4. Threshold utility plots comparing the amount of Q-TWiST gained for tamoxifen plus early CMF versus tamoxifen alone. Panel **A** shows the utility values for which one treatment is better than the other, with some differences reaching statistical significance (e.g., average DFS as shown in the *upper left* corner). Panel **B** shows the number of months of Q-TWiST gained within 5 years of follow-up for different pairs of utility values. The x-marks on panel B indicate the two scenarios described in the text

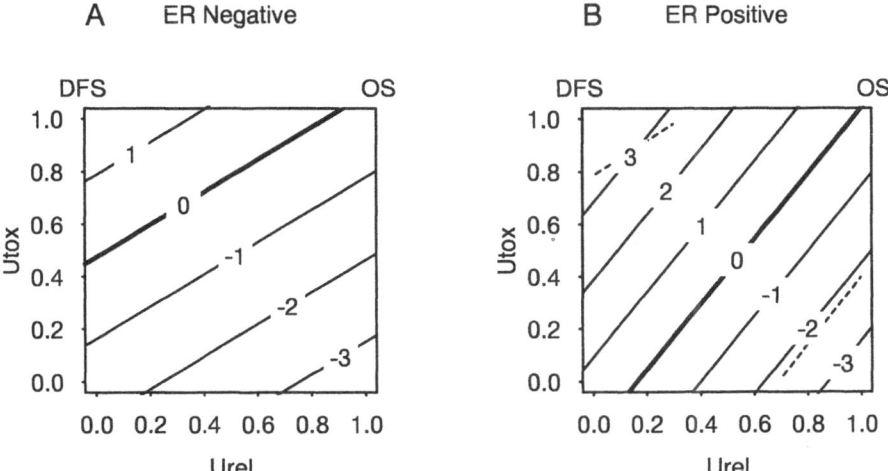

Fig. 5. Threshold utility plots comparing tamoxifen plus early CMF versus tamoxifen alone for patients with ER-negative tumors (**A**) and for patients with ER-positive tumors (**B**)

produced a gain of 1.2 months of Q-TWiST in the first scenario, and it was associated with a loss of 1.6 months of Q-TWiST in the second. Thus, the first patient described above should consider having chemoendocrine therapy, while the second might prefer tamoxifen alone.

The Q-TWiST analysis can be repeated separately for the ER-negative and ER-positive subgroups (see Table 1). Figure 5 shows the two corresponding threshold utility plots for these analyses. There is a wider range of utility coefficients for which adding chemotherapy is preferred for the ER-positive cohort than for the ER-negative group. In addition, the amount of time gained is larger for the ER-positive group.

How Do We Get the Utilities?

As with the majority of other Q-TWiST analyses conducted to date, the analysis reported above is summarized using the threshold utility plots without relying on specific values for the utility coefficients. The analysis highlights the extent to which different utility values between zero and 1 might influence the choice of therapy based on the amount of Q-TWiST gained for one treatment compared with another. Defining appropriate utility values to reflect patient preferences is complicated by adaptation of patients to their condition over time and differences in perspective concerning whose utilities to use.

Utilities measure the value of health states using standards such as time, money, or risk of death. There are four methods that can be used to obtain utility assessments from patients. The standard gamble and the time-tradeoff methods involve an iterative series of questions, which must be administered to the patient by an interviewer or conducted with the aid of a computer. The third method, the rating scale, is a single-item global health question presented on a 0 to 100 scale. The final method for eliciting utilities is based on the principles of multiattribute utility theory; it maintains the ease of administration of a traditional health status questionnaire, while also producing utility estimates appropriate for use in clinical and economic decision-making (Torrance et al. 1995). This system consists of two components: a simple patient-completed questionnaire and a formula that assigns a utility to each patient's set of responses to that questionnaire. Examples of multiattribute systems are the McMaster Health Utility Index (Feeny et al. 1995), the Euroqol (EuroQol Group 1990), and the Q-tility Index (Weeks et al. 1994). Several ongoing clinical trials that include a prospectively planned Q-TWiST analysis are collecting patient-derived utility values obtained from multiattribute utility systems.

Discussion

Assessment of quality of life can be very relevant for treatment decision-making in the adjuvant setting. The assessments must be made only when there are clear hypotheses to be tested and a well-defined methodology to evaluate the results. In this paper, we have described several specific purposes for such assessments. In addition, we presented an application of the Q-TWiST method to address questions involving tradeoffs between quality and quantity of life. We reported results from an analysis of the IBCSG Trial VII comparing 3 months of CMF chemotherapy plus tamoxifen versus tamoxifen alone for postmenopausal patients with node-positive breast cancer. This analysis indicated that the choice of whether or not to add chemotherapy should depend upon the relative utility weights or patient preferences assigned to periods of toxicity and periods of postrelapse survival.

In addition to the IBCSG trial, the National Surgical Adjuvant Breast and Bowel Project (NSABP) Trial B-20 recently reported a significant DFS and OS advantage for chemotherapy (MF or CMF for 6 months) given with tamoxifen compared with tamoxifen alone for patients with node-negative, estrogen-receptor-positive breast cancer (Fisher et al. 1997). The effects of chemotherapy were positive, but not statistically significant for patients aged 50 years of age or older. It would be interesting to conduct a Q-TWiST analysis to determine the extent to which patient preference might influence selection of 6 months of chemotherapy based on the B-20 data, which yielded 85% 5-year DFS and 94% 5-year OS for the tamoxifen alone group.

Some recently reported studies have demonstrated improved efficacy in terms of DFS and OS for more intensive (and more toxic) chemotherapy regimens compared with standard regimens. For example, Levine et al. (1998) reported a Canadian study showing that cyclophosphamide, 4-epidoxorubicin, and 5-fluorouracil (CEF) given in a CMF-like schedule (4-epidoxorubicin, and 5-fluorouracil given on days 1 and 8 every 4 weeks and cyclophosphamide given orally on days 1-14) was more effective than a "classical" CMF regimen. CEF had to be given together with antibiotics, which successfully reduced the incidence of febrile neutropenia. An ECOG/Intergroup trial showed that an intensive 16-week regimen provided more efficacy than standard CAF (Fetting et al. 1995), and a CALGB/Intergroup trial showed that adding taxol after completion of CA improved efficacy compared with CA alone (Henderson et al. 1998). For each of these randomized comparisons, a quality-of-life oriented question can be asked concerning the tradeoff between improved disease control on one hand and decreased quality of life due to treatment intensity and duration on the other. By summarizing treatment outcomes in terms of the amounts of time patients spend in the relevant clinical health states, the Q-TWiST approach provides a proper assessment of tradeoffs with respect to quality-of-life implications of more intensive therapies. For adjuvant therapy decision-making, quality-of-life assessment and evaluation of tradeoffs are indeed relevant.

Summary

In the breast cancer adjuvant therapy setting, the critical issue to consider in treatment decision-making is the tradeoff between quality and quantity of life. The toxicities of adjuvant therapies, both acute and late, must be balanced against the potential benefits of delayed recurrence and improved survival. The question should be addressed concerning when quality-of-life assessment is relevant in the adjuvant setting. Such assessments can inform patients about what to expect from their treatment, describe quality-of-life differences between treatments, provide an additional baseline measure with potential prognostic significance, inform clinicians about their patients' experiences with toxicities, indicate situations in which psychosocial interventions might be useful, and document patient adaptation to diagnosis and treatment. The relevance of quality-of-life assessment in the adjuvant setting can be illustrated by investigating one of the most controversial questions of today: When should chemotherapy be added to tamoxifen for postmenopausal patients? Data from the International Breast Cancer Study Group (IBCSG) Trial VII showed that adding 3 months of CMF (cyclophosphamide 100 mg/m^2 orally days 1-14; methotrexate 40 mg/m^2 i.v. days 1, 8; fluorouracil 600 mg/m^2 i.v. days 1, 8; repeated every 28 days) to tamoxifen significantly improved disease-free survival compared with tamoxifen alone. The Quality-adjusted Time Without Symptoms of disease or Toxicity of treatment (Q-TWiST) method was used to compare the adjuvant therapies with respect to quality-adjusted survival. The analysis indicated that the decision to use adjuvant chemotherapy in this setting should be based on patient preferences concerning the relative importance of treatment toxicity versus disease recurrence.

Acknowledgements. This work was partially supported by grants from the American Cancer Society (RPG-90-013-08-PBP) and from the United States National Cancer Institute (CA-75362). We thank the patients, nurses, physicians, and data managers who participated in the International Breast Cancer Study Group Trial VII and acknowledge additional support for study conduct provided by the Swiss Cancer League, Cancer League of Ticino, the Swiss Group for Clinical Cancer Research, the Australian-New Zealand Breast Cancer Trials Group, the Australian Cancer Society, Frontier Science and Technology Research Foundation, the Dana-Farber Cancer Institute, the National Health and Medical Research Council of Australia (grant numbers 910420, 920876, 940892 and 950328), the Anti-Cancer Council of Victoria, and the New South Wales Cancer Council. We also acknowledge the special contributions of Dr. Monica Castiglione-Gertsch, Ms. Mary Isley, and Ms. Karen Price to the conduct and evaluation of IBCSG Trial VII.

Appendix

International Breast Cancer Study Group
Participants and Authors, Trials VI-IX

Coordinating Center, Bern, Switzerland	M. Castiglione, A. Goldhirsch (Studies Coordinators), K. Geiser, A. Berlinger, G. Egli (Data Management), R. Maibach, R. Pedowski
Statistical Center, Harvard School of Public Health and Dana-Farber Cancer Institute, Boston, MA, USA	R. Gelber (Group Statistician), K. Price, H. Peterson, M. Zelen, S. Gelber, A. O'Neill
Quality of Life Office, Bern, Switzerland	J. Bernhard, C. Hürny, H. Gusset
Pathology Office, Institute of Cancer Research, Royal Cancer Hospital, Sutton, UK	B. Gusterson, R. Bettelheim, R. Reed
Data Management Center, Frontier Science & Technology Research Foundation, Amherst, NY, USA	M. Isley, R. Hinkle
Auckland Breast Cancer Study Group, Auckland, New Zealand	R.G. Kay, V.J. Harvey, C.S. Benjamin, P. Thompson, A. Bierre, M. Miller, B. Hochstein, A. Lethaby, J. Webber
Centro di Riferimento Oncologico Aviano, Italy	D. Crivellari, S. Monfardini, E. Galligioni, A. Veronesi, A. Buonadonna, S. Massarut, C. Rossi, E. Candiani, A. Carbone, R. Volpe, M. Roncadin, M. Arcicasa, G.F. Santini, F. Villalta, F. Coran, S. Morassut
Spedali Civili & Fondazione Beretta, Brescia, Italy	G. Marini, E. Simoncini, P. Marpicati, A. Barni, P. Grigolato, L. Morassi
Groote Schuur Hospital, Cape Town, Republic of South Africa	D.M. Dent, A. Gudgeon, E. Murray, P. Steynor, J. Toop
West Swedish Breast Cancer Study Group, Göteborg, Sweden	C.M. Rudenstam, A. Wallgren, S. Ottosson-Lönn, R. Hultborn, G. Colldahl-Jäderström, E. Cahlin, J. Mattsson, S. Holmberg, S. Jansson, L. Ivarsson, O. Ruusvik, L.G. Niklasson, S. Dahlin, G. Karlsson, B. Lindberg, A. Sundbäck, S. Bergegårdh, H. Salander, C. Andersson, M. Heideman,

Y. Hessman, O. Nelzén, G. Claes, T. Ramhult, J.H. Svensson, P. Liedberg

General Hospital,
Gorizia, Italy

S. Foladore, L. Foghin, G. Pamich, C. Bianchi, B. Marino, A. Murgia, V. Milan

Sandton Oncology
Center, Johannesburg,
Republic of South Africa

D. Vorobiof, M. Chasen, G. Fotheringham, G. de Muelenaere, B. Skudowitz, C. Mohammed, A. Rosengarten

The Institute of Oncology,
Ljubljana, Slovenia

J. Lindtner, D. Erzen, E. Majdic, B. Stabuc, A. Plesnicar, R. Golouh, J. Lamovec, J. Jancar, I. Vrhoved, M. Kramberger

Madrid Breast Cancer Group,
Madrid, Spain

H. Cortés-Funes, D. Mendiola, C. Gravalos, Colomer, M. Mendez, F. Cruz Vigo, P. Miranda, A. Sierra, F. Martinez-Tello, A. Garzon, S. Alonso, A. Ferrero, C. Vargas

Anti-Cancer Council of Victoria,
Melbourne, Australia

J. Collins, P. Gregory, P. Kitchen, S. Hart, S. Neil, M. Henderson, I. Russell, T. Gale, M. Pitcher, R. Snyder, R. McLennan, M. Schwarz, I. Burns, M. Green, R. Basser, R. Drummond, A. Rodger, G. Richardson, J. McKendrick, M. Chipman

Royal Adelaide Hospital,
Adelaide, Australia

I. Olver, A. Robertson, P. Gill, M.L. Carter, P. Malycha, E. Yeoh, G. Ward, A.S.Y. Leong, J. Lommax-Smith, D. Hoosfall, R. D'Angelo

Sir Charles Gairdner Hospital,
Nedlands, Western Australia

M. Byrne, G. van Hazel, J. Dewar, M. Buck, D. Ingram, G. Sterret

Australian New Zealand Breast
Cancer Trials Group (ANZ BCTG),
Mater Hospital, Waratah, Newcastle,
Australia

J.F. Forbes, J. Stewart, D. Jackson, R. Gourlay, J. Bishop, C. Flower, A. Wilson, S. Cox, S. Ackland, A. Bonaventura, C. Hamilton, J. Denham, P. O'Brien, M. Back, S. Brae, A. Price, Muragasu, H. Foster, D. Clarke, R. Sillar, V. Clarke, S. Brew

University of Sydney,
Dubbo Base Hospital and
Royal Prince Alfred Hospital,
Sydney, Australia

M.H.N. Tattersall, A. Coates, F. Niesche, R. West, S. Renwick, J. Donovan, P. Duval, R. J. Simes, A. Ng, D. Glenn, R.A. North, J. Beith, RG. O'Connor, M. Rice, G. Stevens,

	J. Grassby, S. Pendlebury, C. McLeod, M. Boyer, A. Sullivan, J. Hobbs
European Institute of Oncology, Milan, Italy	A. Goldhirsch, G. Martinelli, U. Veronesi, A. Luini, R. Orecchia, G. Viale, M. Colleoni, F. Nolè, F. Peccatori, A. Costa, S. Zurrida, P. Veronesi, V. Sacchini, V. Gallimberti
Ospedale Infermi, Rimini, Italy	A. Ravaioli, D. Tassinari, G. Oliverio, F. Barbanti, P. Rinaldi, E. Pini, G. Drudi
Ospedale S. Eugenio, Rome, Italy	M. Antimi, M. Minelli, V. Bellini, R. Porzio, E. Pernazza, G. Santeusanio, L.G. Spagnoli
Ospedale S. Bortolo, Vicenza, Italy	M. Magazu, V. Fosser, P. Morandi, G. Scalco, M. Balli, M. Gion, S. Meli, G. Torsello
Toronto Sunnybrook Regional Cancer Centre, Toronto, Canada	K. Pritchard, D. Sutherland, C. Sawka, G. Taylor, R. Choo, C. Catzavelos, K. Roche

SAKK (Swiss Group for Clinical Cancer Research):

– Inselspital, Bern	M.F. Fey, E. Dreher, H. Schneider, S. Aebi, K. Buser, J. Ludin, G. Beck, H. Bürgi, A. Haenel, J.M. Lüthi, R. Markwalder, H.J. Altermatt, M. Nandedkar
– Kantonsspital, St. Gallen	H.J. Senn, B. Thürlimann, Ch. Oehlschlegel, G. Ries, M. Töpfer, U. Lorenz, O. Schiltknecht, B. Späti
– Ospedale San Giovanni, Bellinzona	F. Cavalli, O. Pagani, H. Neuenschwander, W. Müller, L. Bronz, C. Sessa, G. Martinelli, M. Ghielmini, P. Luscieti, E. Passega, T. Rusca, P. Rey, J. Bernier, S. Martinoli, E. Pedrinis, G. Losa, T. Gyr, L. Leidi, G. Pastorelli, A. Goldhirsch
– Kantonsspital, Basel	R. Hermann, J.F. Harder, O. Köchli, U. Eppenberger, J. Torhorst
– Hôpital des Cadolles, Neuchâtel	D. Piguet, P. Siegenthaler, V. Barrelet, R.P. Baumann
– Kantonsspital, Luzern	R. Joss
– Kantonsspital, Zürich	B. Pestalozzi, C. Sauter, V. Engeler, U. Haller, U. Metzger, P. Huguenin, R. Caduff

– Centre Hôpitalier Universitaire, Lausanne	L. Perey, S. Leyvraz, P. Anani, F. Gomez, D. Wellman, G. Chapuis, P. De Grandi, P. Reymond, M. Gillet, J.F. Delaloye
– Hôpital Cantonal, Geneva	P. Alberto, H. Bonnefoi, P. Schäfer, F. Krauer, M. Forni, M. Aapro, R. Egeli, R. Megevand, E. Jacot-des-Combes, A. Schindler, B. Borisch, S. Diebold
– Kantonsspital Graubünden, Chur	F. Egli, P. Forrer, A. Willi, R. Steiner, J. Allemann, T. Rüedi, A. Leutenegger, U. Dalla Torre
Swiss Cancer League, Bern, Switzerland	U. Metzger, W. Weber, G. Noseda

References

Bernhard J, Hürny C, Coates AS, Peterson HF, Castiglione-Gertsch M, Gelber RD, Goldhirsch A, Senn H-J, Rudenstam C-M for the International Breast Cancer Study Group (IBCSG) (1997) Quality of life assessment in patients receiving adjuvant therapy' for breast cancer: the IBCSG approach. Ann Oncol 8:825–835

Coates A, Gebski V, Signorini D, Murray P, McNeil D, Byrne M, Forbes JF for the Australia New Zealand Breast Cancer Study Group (1992) Prognostic value of quality-of-life scores during chemotherapy for advanced breast cancer. J Clin Oncol 10:1833–1838

Early Breast Cancer Trialists' Collaborative Group (1992) Systemic treatment of early breast cancer by hormonal, cytotoxic or immune therapy: 133 randomized trials involving 31,000 recurrences and 24,000 deaths among 75,000 women. Lancet 339:1–15, 71–85

EuroQol Group (1990) EuroQol: a new facility for the measurement of health-related quality of life. Health Policy 16:199–208

Feeny D, Furlong W, Boyle M, Torrance GW (1995) Multi-attribute health status classification systems. Pharmacoeconomics 7:490–503

Fetting J, Gray R, Abeloff MD, Fowble B, Smith T, Vail S et al (1995) CAF vs. a 16 week multidrug regimen as adjuvant therapy for receptor-negative, node-positive breast cancer: an Intergroup study. Proc Am Soc Clin Oncol 114:96

Fisher B, Dignam J, Wolmark N, DeCillis A, Emir B, Wickerham DL, Bryant J, Dimitrov NV, Abramson N, Atkins JN, Shibata H, Deschenes L, Margolese RG (1997) Tamoxifen and chemotherapy for lymph node-negative, estrogen receptor-positive breast cancer. J Natl Cancer Inst 89:1673–1682

Ganz PA, Rowland JH, Desmond K, Meyerowitz BE, Wyatt GE (1998) Life after breast cancer: understanding women's health-related quality of life and sexual functioning. J Clin Oncol 16:501–514

Gelber RD, Goldhirsch A, Cavalli F for the International Breast Cancer Study Group (1991) Quality-of-life-adjusted evaluation of a randomized trial comparing adjuvant therapies for operable breast cancer. Ann Intern Med 114:621–628

Gelber RD, Goldhirsch A, Hürny C, Bernhard J, Simes RJ for the International Breast Cancer Study Group (1992) Quality of life in clinical trials of adjuvant therapies. J Natl Cancer Inst Monogr 11:127–135

Gelber RD, Cole BF, Gelber S, Goldhirsch A (1995) The Q-TWiST method. In: Spilker B (ed) Quality of life and pharmacoeconomics in clinical trials, 2nd ed). Raven, New York; pp 427–435

Glasziou PP, Simes RJ, Gelber RD (1990) Quality adjusted survival analysis. Stat Med 9:1259–1276

Goldhirsch A, Gelber RD, Simes RJ, Glasziou P, Coates A for the Ludwig Breast Cancer Study Group (1989) Costs and benefits of adjuvant therapy in breast cancer: a quality-adjusted survival analysis. J Clin Oncol 7:36–44

Goldhirsch A, Coates AS, Colleoni M, Castiglione-Gertsch M, Gelber RD for the International Breast Cancer Study Group (1998) Adjuvant chemoendocrine therapy in postmenopausal breast cancer: cyclophosphamide, methotrexate, and fluorouracil dose and schedule may make a difference. J Clin Oncol 16:1358–1362

Henderson IC, Berry D, Demetri G, Cirrincione C, Goldstein L, Martino S et al (1998) Improved disease-free (DFS) and overall survival (OS) from the addition of sequential paclitaxel (T) but not from the escalation of doxorubicin (A) dose level in the adjuvant chemotherapy of patients (pts) with node-positive primary breast cancer (bc). Proc Am Soc Clin Oncol 17:101a

Hürny C, Bernhard J, Coates AS, Castiglione-Gertsch M, Peterson HF, Gelber RD, Forbes JF, Rudenstam C-M, Simoncini E, Crivellari D, Goldhirsch A, Senn H-J for the International Breast Cancer Study Group (1996) Impact of adjuvant therapy on quality of life in women with node-positive operable breast cancer. Lancet 347:1279–1284

International Breast Cancer Study Group (1997) Effectiveness of adjuvant chemotherapy in combination with tamoxifen for node-positive postmenopausal breast cancer patients. J Clin Oncol 15:1385–1394

Karnofsky DA, Abelmann WH, Craver LF, Burchenal JH (1948) The use of nitrogen mustards in the palliative treatment of carcinoma. Cancer 1:634

Levine M, Bramwell V, Pritchard KI et al (1998) A randomized trial of cyclophosphamide, epirubicin, fluorouracil chemotherapy compared with cyclophosphamide, methotrexate, fluorouracil in premenopausal women with node positive breast cancer. J Clin Oncol (in press).

Lindley C, Vasa S, Sawyer WT, Winer ET (1998) Quality of life and preferences for treatment following systemic adjuvant therapy for early-stage breast cancer. Cancer 16:1380–1387

Simes RJ, Cocker K, Glasziou P et al (1989) Costs and benefits of adjuvant chemotherapy for breast cancer: an assessment of patient preferences. Proc Am Soc Clin Oncol 8:52A

Torrance GW, Furlong W, Boyle M, Torrance EW (1995) Multi-attribute preference functions. Pharmacoeconomics 7:503–520

Weeks J, O'Leary J, Fairclough D, Paltiel D, Weinstein M (1994) The "Q-tility Index": a new tool for assessing health-related quality of life and utilities in clinical trials and clinical practice. Proc Am Soc Clin Oncol 13:426

Quality of Life Assessment in the International Breast Cancer Study Group: Past, Present, and Future

C. Hürny[1], J. Bernhard[2], and A. Coates[3] for the IBCSG

[1] Bürgerspital, Rorschacherstrasse 94, 9000 St. Gallen, Switzerland
[2] IBCSG Coordinating Center, Effingerstrasse 40, 3008 Bern, Switzerland
[3] Department of Medical Oncology, Royal Prince Alfred Hospital, Missenden Road, Camperdown NSW 2050, Australia

Introduction

The IBCSG is a large multinational, multilingual cooperative group that has been devoted to the study and improvement of adjuvant therapy in breast cancer patients for more than 20 years (International Breast Cancer Study Group 1997). Since 1986, patients, quality of life (QL) has been assessed in all the trials with the aim to establish QL as a complementary outcome in randomized clinical trials. The IBCSG approach to QL assessment in patients receiving adjuvant therapy for breast cancer has recently been reported in detail (Bernhard et al. 1997). Rather than repeat what already has been said in this paper, we will comment on some selected issues from a personal viewpoint.

As clinicians and QL researchers we have the privilege of having been part of the development of QL research within the IBCSG from the beginning. The fact that we have been asked to comment on past, present and future means that QL research already has a history. It is not only the history of the development of a new field in oncology and medicine in general, it is also a history of the value and position of this field within the medical community.

The Past

Surprisingly, QL research in cancer medicine was born in Europe and in Australia, not in the United States. Since in many treatment situations in cancer patients prolongation of survival was not possible, i.e., treatments basically had a palliative intention, oncologists were asking the question whether toxic treatments were justified – whether they would improve patiens' well-being. This meant that the subjective experience of the patient, his or her QL, had to be assessed. In the 1970s, lengthy conceptual discussions aiming to reach a definition of QL were going on. This problem of definition has now been solved; there is a consensus among involved researchers that QL is a multi-dimensional construct involving physical, psychological, social, cultural and eventually spiritual and economic dimensions. There is also a consensus that the concept of QL has to be adapted to the research question.

In these pioneer times oncological clinicians were very skeptical about the assessment of QL. There was widespread opinion that QL was not measurable, and that if it was measured it would yield soft data.

In the 1980 s, the main issue was the development of assessment instruments. Most researchers in most cooperative groups had toxicity and disease symptoms as a main focus in their mind while developing instruments like the FLIC (Schipper et al. 1984) and the FACT (Cella et al. 1993). The QLQ-C30 of the EORTC, for instance, assesses all major toxicities of chemotherapy and major disease symptoms (Aaronson et al. 1993). Even if global components of QL are also assessed, they are not within the main focus of the investigator. In the particular situation of adjuvant treatment, however, QL measures need to be sensitive to changes both under cytotoxic therapy and follow-up periods with relatively minor symptoms of disease and toxicity of treatment.

In the IBCSG we developed mainly global indicators of components of QL such as physical well-being, mood and coping (Bernhard et al. 1997; Butow et al. 1991). These global indicators are assessed with single items in the Linear Analogue Self-Assessment (LASA) format (Priestman et al. 1976). When estimating their global physical well-being, for instance, patients intuitively take into account their experience of chemotherapy and disease symptoms as well as their experience of cancer diagnosis and surgery and automatically give a weight to these factors relating to their pyhsical well-being. Since the goal of clinical trials is to compare different treatments, a global assessment of QL components is more appropriate than a detailed assessment of toxicity and disease symptoms. Furthermore, global indicators may have more commonality cross-culturally (Bernhard et al. 1996).

While QL researchers were testing and reporting on their new instruments, more clinicians were becoming interested in the problem; the medical community became somewhat less skeptical and started to accept QL research tentatively as a true scientific endeavour. The IBCSG has contributed to this shift of opinion through thorough methodological studies concerning cross-cultural validation of global indicators (Hürny et al. 1992, 1993, 1996 a), feasibility and compliance (Hürny et al. 1992), impact of timing of assessments (Bernhard et al. 1998 a), practical and statistical issues of missing data (Hürny et al. 1994), baseline covariates (Bernhard et al. 1986) and clinically meaningful differences, e.g. changes between pre- and post-failure timepoints (Hürny et al. 1996 b).

The Present

We have recently published the QL results of the first two large-scale clinical trials (IBCSG VI and VII) including QL assessments (Hürny et al. 1996 b). We have shown that adjuvant chemotherapy (CMF) had a measurable adverse effect on health-related QL but, contrary to expectation, this effect was transient and minor compared with patient adjustment to cancer diagnosis and surgery. Overall, patients' QL, especially coping, improves over the first 18 months.

At first glance these results seem to be trivial. However, the fact that adaptation to diagnosis and surgery is more important than treatment toxicity forces us to change our focus of attention. If we want to improve patients' QL it is less important to mitigate treatment side effects, which are transient, than it is to help them to adjust. Furthermore, these findings have direct clinical implications. They should encourage patients and doctors to choose appropriate adjuvant therapy with less concern for its initial toxicity.

In the 1990 s, with the results of the IBCSG and other groups, QL research in oncology has finally reached one of its goals, namely to contribute to evidence-based medicine.

Another intriguing finding meriting the attention of the scientific community is the fact that baseline QL scores predict survival in metastatic disease independently of other prognostic factors (Coates et al. 1992). Whether this is also true for the adjuvant setting is currently under investigation.

The Future

Now that we have shown that we are able to reliably assess QL in cancer clinical trials, the next logical step will be to try to improve patients' QL. Since we know now that adjusting to diagnosis and the sequelae of surgery is the most important determinant of QL for breast cancer patients in the adjuvant setting, we will have to aim at fostering adjusting. Psychosocial interventions may improve patient well-being (Anderson 1992; Mey et al. 1995; Greer et al. 1992; Fawzy et al. 1995; Fallowfield 1995; Worden and Weisman 1984) and even survival (Fawzy et al. 1993; Spiegel et al. 1989), but are not uniformly implemented in the care of patients with early breast cancer. If we want to implement psychosocial intervention within the framework of an international adjuvant breast cancer trial it has to be feasible; in other words, simple and affordable but nevertheless effective. We are currently studying ways to implement and test a simple psychosocial intervention in our group.

Since resources are more and more limited, another way to improve the QL at least of those patients who are obviously adjusting poorly might be psychosocial screening that could be carried out with the QL instruments we use currently. Intervention could be offered to those patients with „maladaptive" coping. However, the sensitivity and specificity of our indicator approach for screening purposes would need to be investigated.

Another possible way to improve patients' QL is to train medical professionals (nurses, data managers, physicians) in psychosocial skills. It has been shown that patient-centred consultations lead to improved satisfaction and psychological adjustment of the patients (Butow et al. 1995).

In addition, our group's approach to the integration of patients' subjective experience into the evaluation of our trials has followed two different lines: assessment of health-related QL and estimation of utility. The concept of QL has its roots in psychosocial science and includes physical, emotional, social and sometimes also cultural and spiritual components of subjective experience. As stated above, multi-dimensional scales have been developed to allow patient self-assessment of QL. In contrast, the concept of utility is derived from economic science in the framework of cost-benefit considerations. Utilities may be defined as patient-stated preferences for various health states under conditions of uncertainty. Utility values are more easily integrated than QL scores with the conventional endpoints to allow weighted comparison of time spent in different health states.

The Q-TWiST model developed by Gelber and Goldhirsch since 1986 (Goldhirsch et al. 1989) is a utility-based assessment that divides the lifespan of the patients from the beginning of adjuvant treatment until death into three time segments corresponding to distinct health states: TOX (time with toxicity from treatment), TWiST (time without symptoms of treatment or disease) and REL (time from relapse until death). TOX and REL are weighted by arbitrary utility coefficients and added to TWiST to reach an overall assessment of different treatment groups.

So far the shortcoming of the Q-TWiST method is that utility coefficients for the different health states have been assigned arbitrarily. We have developed a simple single-item measure to assess subjective health estimations as an adapted utility concept for clinical trials (Hürny et al. 1998). In our second generation of clinical trials with QL assessments this item will allow us to gather direct utility assessments from the patients which can be fed into the TWiST model. In this way the two different approaches can be integrated.

Conclusions

I have reviewed the attempts and efforts of the IBCSG over the last 10 years to integrate patients' subjective experience into the scientific evaluation of adjuvant therapy in breast cancer. Through these efforts the IBCSG has contributed to the notion that the subjective experience of patients is important, scientifically evaluable and meaningful for clinical decision making. By accepting QL research as a truly scientific endeavour, the medical community documents that physicians are willing to restore patients' subjective experience to the position it lost during the enormous scientific and technical progress of this century.

Summary

The past: Since 1986, the IBCSG has been accruing a comprehensive longitudinal health-related quality of life (QL) database in addition to biomedical data of patients with early breast cancer who are receiving or have received adjuvant treatment. Our aim is to establish QL as a complementary outcome in randomized clinical trials and to gain new insight in biopsychosocial interactions. In regard to methodology, the IBCSG has made major contributions to the field through the development of global indicators, cross-cultural validation, impact of timing of assessments and working on practical and statistical issues relating to missing data. *The present:* In two large-scale clinical trials (IBCSG VI and VII) adjuvant chemotherapy (CMF) had a measurable effect on health-related QL, but contrary to expectations this effect was transient and minor compared with the effect of patients' adjustment and coping after diagnosis and surgery. *The future:* In addition to the assessment of health-related QL, the IBCSG is currently developing and applying a global indicator for a patient-derived adapted utility concept in order to better assess the cost-benefit ratio of adjuvant treatment. However, the real challenge for the immediate future is the question how patients' adjustment can be fostered within primary care.

References

Aaronson NK, Ahmedzai S, Bergman B et al (1993) The European Organization for Research and Treatment of Cancer QLQ-C30: a quality-of-life instrument for use in international clinical trials in oncology. J Natl Cancer Inst 85:365–376

Andersen BL (1992) Psychological interventions for cancer patients to enhance the quality of life. J Consult Clin Psychol 60:552–568

Bernhard J, Hürny C, Coates A, Gelber RD (1996) Applying quality of life principles in international cancer clinical trials. In: Spilker B (ed) Quality of life and pharmacoeconomics in clinical trials. Lippincott-Raven, Philadelphia, pp 693–705

Bernhard J, Hürny C, Coates AS et al for the International Breast Cancer Study Group (IBCSG) (1997) Quality of life assessment in patients receiving adjuvant therapy for breast cancer: the IBCSG approach. Ann Oncol 8:825–835

Bernhard J, Peterson H, Coates A et al for the International Breast Cancer Study Group (IBCSG) (1998a) Quality of life assessment in international breast cancer study group (IBCSG) trials: practical issues and factors associated with missing data. Stat Med (in press)

Bernhard J, Hürny C, Coates AS et al for the International Breast Cancer Study Group (1998b) Factors affecting baseline quality of life in two international adjuvant breast cancer trials. Br J Cancer (in press)

Butow PN, Coates A, Dunn S, Bernhard J, Hürny C (1991) On the receiving end IV: validation of quality of life indicators. Ann Oncol 2:597–603

Butow PN, Dunn SM, Tattersall MH, Jones QJ (1995) Computer-based interaction analysis of the cancer consultation. Br J Cancer 71:1115–1121

Cella DF, Tulsky DS, Gray G et al (1993) The functional assessment of cancer therapy scale: development and validation of the general measure. J Clin Oncol 11:570–579

Coates A, Gebski V, Signorini D et al for the Australian New Zealand Breast Cancer Trials Group (1992) Prognostic value of quality-of-live scores during chemotherapy for advanced breast cancer. J Clin Oncol 10:1833–1838

Fallowfield LJ (1995) Psychosocial interventions for cancer. Br Med J 311:1316–1317

Fawzy FI, Fawzy NW, Hyun CS et al (1993) Malignant melanoma. Effects of an early structured psychiatric intervention, coping and affective state on recurrence and survival 6 years later. Arch Gen Psychiatry 50:681–689

Fawzy FI, Fawzy NW, Arndt LA et al (1995) Critical review of psychosocial interventions in cancer care. Arch Gen Psychiatry 52:100–103

Goldhirsch A, Gelber RD, Simes RJ, Glasziou P, Coates AS for the Ludwig Breast Cancer Study Group (1989) Costs and benefits of adjuvant therapy in breast cancer: a quality-adjusted survival analysis. J Clin Oncol 7:36–44

Greer S, Moorey S, Baruch JD et al (1992) Adjuvant psychological therapy for patients with cancer: a prospective randomised trial. Br Med J 304:675–680

Hürny C, Bernhard J, Gelber RD et al (1992) Quality of life measures for patients receiving adjuvant therapy for breast cancer: an international trial. The International Breast Cancer Study Group. Eur J Cancer 28:118–124

Hürny C, Bernhard J, Bacchi M et al (1993) The perceived adjustment to chronic illness scale (PACIS): a global indicator of coping for operable breast cancer patients in clinical trials. Swiss Group for Clinical Cancer Research (SAKK) and the International Breast Cancer Study Group (IBCSG). Support Care Cancer 1:200–208

Hürny C, Bernhard J, Coates A et al for the International Breast Cancer Study Group (1994) Timing of baseline quality of life assessment in an international adjuvant breast cancer trial: its effect on patient self-estimation. Ann Oncol 5:65–74

Hürny C, Bernhard J, Coates AS et al (1996a) Responsiveness of a single-item indicator versus a multi-item scale: assessment of emotional well-being in an international breast cancer trial. Med Care 34:234–248

Hürny C, Bernhard J, Coates AS et al (1996b) Impact of adjuvant therapy on quality of life in women with node-positive operable breast cancer. International Breast Cancer Study Group. Lancet 347:1279–1284

Hürny C, von Wegberg B, Bacchi M et al (1998) Subjective health estimations (SHE) in patients with advanced breast cancer: an adapted utility concept for clinical trials. Br J Cancer 77:985–991

International Breast Cancer Study Group (1997) IBCSG celebrates its 20th anniversary. IBCSG Coordinating Center, Bern

Meyer TJ, Mark MM (1995) Effects of psychosocial interventions with adult cancer patients: a meta-analysis of randomized experiments. Health Psychol 14:101–108

Priestman T, Baum M (1976) Evaluation of quality of life in patients receiving treatment for advanced breast cancer. Lancet 1:899–900

Schipper H, Clinch J, McMurray A, Levitt M (1984) Measuring the quality of life of cancer patients: the functional living index-cancer: development and validation. J Clin Oncol 2:472–483

Spiegel D, Bloom JR, Kraemer HC et al (1989) The effect of psychosocial treatment on survival of patients with metastatic breast cancer. Lancet 2:888–891

Worden JW, Weisman AD (1984) Preventive psychosocial intervention with newly diagnosed cancer patients. Gen Hosp Psychiatry 6:243–249

Impact of Different Adjuvant Therapy Strategies on Quality of Life in Breast Cancer Survivors

P. A. Ganz[1], J. H. Rowland[2], B. E. Meyerowitz[3], and K. A. Desmond[4]

[1] Jonsson Comprehensive Cancer Center and UCLA Schools of Medicine and Public Health, Los Angeles, California, USA
[2] Lombardi Cancer Center and Department of Psychiatry, Georgetown University Medical Center, Washington, DC, USA
[3] Department of Psychology, University of Southern California, Los Angeles, California, USA
[4] Jonsson Comprehensive Cancer Center and the UCLA School of Public Health, Los Angeles, California, USA

Introduction

Primary breast cancer treatment includes various combinations of surgery, radiation therapy, chemotherapy, and/or hormone therapy (Harris et al. 1992). The multimodal treatment of breast cancer improves survival outcome (Early Breast Cancer Trialists' Collaborative Group 1992), but it also contributes to a prolonged period of medical intervention with associated physical and emotional sequelae. The literature describes a wide range of disruptions in day-to-day living because of a breast cancer diagnosis and treatment (Meyerowitz et al. 1983, 1998; Ganz et al. 1987; Schag et al. 1993; Rowland and Massie 1996). Many treatment-related physical and psychosocial problems resolve during the first year of follow-up (Schag et al. 1993; Ganz et al. 1992a; Wolberg et al. 1989; Maunsell et al. 1989; Vinokur et al. 1990; Tasmuth et al. 1996; Hürny et al. 1996). However, in one study, sexual problems did not resolve during the year after breast cancer diagnosis (Ganz et al. 1992a), and were noted to worsen during further follow-up (Ganz et al. 1996).

Relatively little is known about the health-related quality of life (HRQL) of long-term breast cancer survivors (Ganz et al. 1996; Omne-Pontén et al. 1994; Dow et al. 1996; Ganz et al. 1998), and few studies have examined the long-term effects of adjuvant therapy on HRQL or sexual functioning in breast cancer survivors. In a recently completed survey study of 864 early stage breast cancer survivors (Ganz et al. 1998), on standardized measures we observed high levels of quality of life. Sexual functioning in the survivors was similar to age-matched controls. However, there was somewhat more disruption in sexual functioning in younger women who had been made prematurely menopausal as a result of adjuvant chemotherapy, and all women who had received chemotherapy experienced worse sexual functioning than those who had not received this treatment (Ganz et al. 1998). Between January 1996 and June 1997, we conducted a second mailed survey of an additional 1098 breast cancer survivors who had been diagnosed with early stage disease between 1 and 5 years earlier. The second survey was also very comprehensive and focused on the assessment of HRQL, intimate relationships, and sexuality. In this paper, we describe the impact of the type of adjuvant therapy received and the comparative effects of each treatment (or no treatment) on HRQL, symptoms, and sexual functioning.

Materials and Methods

Subject Eligibility and Recruitment

This research was conducted in two large metropolitan centers (Los Angeles, and Washington, DC). Women eligible for study: (1) had a past diagnosis of breast cancer (stage 0, I or II at diagnosis); (2) were between 1 and 5 years after initial breast cancer diagnosis; (3) had completed local and/or systemic adjuvant cancer therapy a minimum of 4 months earlier; (4) were currently considered disease-free and were not receiving cancer therapy other than tamoxifen; (5) had no prior history of treatment of other cancers, with the exception of noninvasive skin cancer and cervical cancer; (6) could read and write English; (7) could provide informed consent; and (8) had no other major disabling medical or psychiatric conditions that would confound evaluation of health-related quality of life.

Subjects were identified and recruited through a variety of mechanisms, including tumor registry listings, the offices of surgeons, medical or radiation oncologists, and from hospital or clinic logs from a variety of clinical environments (NCI-designated Cancer Centers, staff model health maintenance organizations, private community hospitals, or office practices). Once the list of potential subjects was determined, a recruitment letter was sent to each breast cancer survivor (BCS) including a response form to indicate her willingness to participate. Women who responded affirmatively were contacted by telephone and were screened for eligibility. The eligible BCS were given more detailed information about the study, including the personal nature of the survey content. If the BCS still wanted to participate, she was mailed a questionnaire and written consent form. Institutional review board approval to conduct this study was obtained at all institutions participating in the study. BCS who were recruited from the practices of community physicians signed consent forms from either of the primary research sites, or in some cases signed an institution-specific consent form.

Conceptualization and Measurement of Health-Related Quality of Llife

Health-related quality of life (HRQL) is the subjectively evaluated health and well-being of a breast cancer survivor as rated by the survivor herself (Aaronson 1988; Ware 1984). HRQL is a multidimensional construct that generally includes functional status, disease and treatment-related symptoms, psychological functioning/emotional well-being, and social functioning. Sexual functioning and body image were identified as additional important dimensions in this study population.

The survey battery for this study was 47 pages in length and included standardized measures of HRQL, with an emphasis on instruments that had been used in healthy populations of middle-aged and elderly women. Also included were several reliable and valid cancer-specific instruments or scales, as well as new questions that were designed for the study population. This report will focus on results from the following instruments:

Global Quality of Life

Overall quality of life was measured with a single item measure that is widely used in epidemiological studies (Kilpatrick and Cantril 1960). On this quality of life measure, the "ladder of life," patients provide single-item subjective ratings of their own quality of life at the present time. Ratings are made on a ten-point scale ranging from a score of 10 or the "best possible life" to 1 or the "worst possible life."

The RAND 36-Item Health Survey 1.0, Alternatively Known as Medical Outcomes Study (MOS) SF-36

The RAND 36-Item Health Survey contains eight individual subscales that are part of the three general areas of HRQL (Hays et al. 1993; Ware and Sherbourne 1992). Each subscale is scored from 0 to 100, with 100 being the most favorable score. The subscales are physical functioning, role function-physical, bodily pain, social functioning, emotional well-being, role function-emotional, energy/fatigue, and general health perceptions (Ware and Sherbourne 1992). General population norms are available for this instrument (McHorney et al. 1994)[1]. The instrument can also be scored as two composite scales – one for physical functioning and a second for mental health (Ware et al. 1994). The data for these composite scores are presented as T-scores with a normal healthy population mean score set at 50 and a score of 60 or 40 representing one standard deviation above or below the mean, respectively.

Center for Epidemiologic Studies-Depression Scale (CES-D)

The CES-D is a 20-Item self-report scale developed for the general population to measure depressive symptomatology over the past week (Radloff 1977). Normative data are available from community-based samples (Roberts

---

[1] The RAND 36-Item Health Survey includes the same items as those in the MOS-SF-36, but the recommended scoring algorithm is somewhat different (Hays et al. 1993). Scoring differences between the two methods are noted for the pain and general health scales only; however, despite these differences, correlations of 0.99 are found between the two methods using the MOS panel sample (Hays et al. 1993). In this study we scored the instrument using the RAND method (Hays et al. 1993).

and Vernon 1983; Myers and Weissman 1980). The instrument has excellent reliability and validity, including use with multi-ethnic samples (Radloff 1977). Responses to the CES-D are rated on a 4-point scale, and the instrument total score ranges from a minimum score of 0 to a maximum score of 60. A higher score on the CES-D indicates a greater risk of depression, with scores greater than or equal to 16 indicating potentially significant levels of depression (Radloff 1977). The expected frequency of scores 16 or greater in the general population ranges from 21% in community samples (Radloff 1977) to as high as 35% in some primary care settings (Coyne et al. 1994). The CES-D has been used in recent studies of healthy women participating in large clinical trials (Ganz et al. 1995; Greendale et al. 1996).

Breast Cancer Prevention Trial (BCPT) Symptom Checklist

This is a 43-item list of commonly reported physical and psychological symptoms, as well as symptoms that have been associated with the menopause and tamoxifen use. This checklist was developed specifically for the BCPT (Ganz et al. 1995). In this survey, we used 16 items that were found to be commonly reported in breast cancer survivors (Ganz et al. 1998); these included vasomotor symptoms, urinary symptoms, vaginal symptoms, body image and weight problems, and cognitive problems. The respondent was asked whether she was bothered by any of the symptoms during the past 4 weeks, with responses ranging from 0 ("not at all") to 4 ("extremely"). For the purposes of this analysis, all responses with a severity of 0 were categorized as no and those that were 1–4 were categorized as yes.

Cancer Rehabilitation Evaluation System (CARES)

The CARES is a self-administered survey instrument that assesses the quality of life and rehabilitation needs of cancer patients (Schag et al. 1983; Ganz et al. 1990). The CARES has excellent reliability, validity, and psychometric properties (Schag et al. 1990). Although the CARES is a generic, cancer-specific quality-of-life measure (Ganz et al. 1992b), extensive normative data are available in breast cancer patients (Schag et al. 1993; Ganz et al. 1992a, 1996, 1998). In this paper we report on data from the body image subscale and the sexual functioning summary score. The subscale and summary scale scores range from 0 to 4 and represent the average severity score for the 3 or 8 items contained within each scale, respectively. Because the CARES detects the severity of problems, a higher score indicates more difficulty or severity of problems in that area.

Statistical Methods

Descriptive statistics were used to examine the characteristics of the samples from the two sites (Los Angeles and Washington) prior to combining them for subsequent analyses. All hypotheses tested in the combined file were with regard to the equality of specific measures across the four adjuvant treatment categories. Standard appropriate tests were performed for continuous and categorical variables. χ^2 tests were used for comparisons of categorical measures; one-way analysis of variance was used to compare means of continuous measures among the four groups; analysis of covariance was used in comparing means of continuous measures between groups, adjusting for covariates; and likelihood ratio χ^2 tests based on logistic regression were used in comparing dichotomous measures between groups, adjusting for covariates. Statistical testing was performed only for a limited number of pre-specified hypotheses. Fewer than 50 significance tests were performed. Therefore, p-values of 0.001 or less can be viewed as satisfying the most rigorous standards in yielding an experiment-wise error rate of 0.05 or less.

Results

Subjects

Between January 1996 and June 1997, we received completed surveys from 1098 eligible breast cancer survivors (Los Angeles, $n = 611$; Washington, $n = 487$). Recruitment letters were mailed to 2212 potential subjects in Los Angeles and 1474 in Washington (total $n = 3686$ letters mailed). About 6.5% of the subjects ($n = 240$) were identified as inaccessible (dead, returned mail), and thus were not available for the study. More women may have fallen into this category, but no further information was available to identify them as such. A second mailing was routinely sent to nonrespondents, but telephone contact was not performed if there was no response to the mailings. The two sites had similar response rates and the recruitment results are combined and shown in Fig. 1.

Overall, about 59% of the BCS responded to the mailed letter of invitation ($n = 2019$) (see Fig. 1). Of those who responded to the letter of invitation, 83% were willing to consider participation in the study ($n = 1671$). At each phase of recruitment, older women were significantly less likely to participate, yielding a final study sample that was younger than the general population of breast cancer patients. In addition, those who were screened out as ineligible were also significantly older than the final study participants. Non-white and unmarried women were less likely to respond to the initial study invitation; however, among those who returned the invitation response form, there were fewer differences between participants and nonparticipants on these characteristics. Among those BCS who were sent the survey booklet, there were no differences in ethnicity, marital status, or age between those who returned a questionnaire and those who did not (data not shown). The final sample of 1098 eligible subjects represents a yield of 54% of those who responded to the mailed letter of invitation. Two women did not answer questionnaire items relating to adjuvant therapy, leaving 1096 subjects for

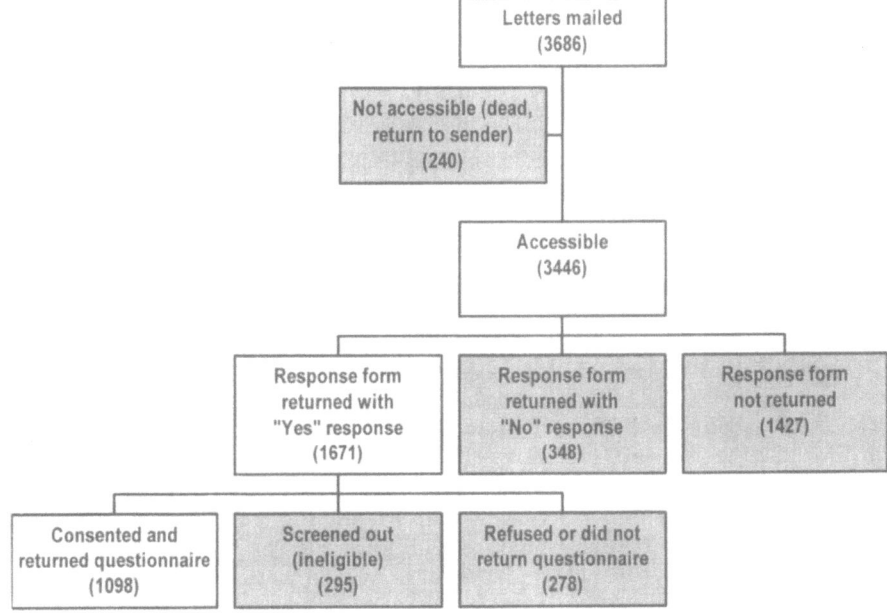

Fig. 1. Summary of recruitment results for the study

these analyses related to the impact of adjuvant therapy. The pattern of response in this survey study was similar to an earlier study conducted by these investigators between 1994 and 1995 (Ganz et al. 1998).

Demographic and Medical Characteristics of the Sample

Prior to combining the Los Angeles and Washington samples, the demographic and medical characteristics of each sample were examined through cross-tabulations, means, and range scores. The two samples had similar proportions of white and nonwhite BCS; however, the nonwhite populations differed between sites. In Los Angeles, the sample included 8.7% African Americans versus 12.7% in Washington. In Los Angeles, the other ethnic groups included 5.9% Hispanics, 6.1% Asian-Pacific Islanders, and 0.3% others, as compared to Washington which had 1.6% Hispanics, 1.2% Asian-Pacific Islanders, and 1.0% others. Respondents from both sites were equally likely to be married or in a relationship. Los Angeles respondents were on average older (56.8 years vs 54.3 years in Washington, $p = 0.0001$). Correspondingly, the Los Angeles respondents had also been with their current partner for a longer time (25.4 years vs 23.7 years, $p = 0.075$). Subjects from Washington were better educated ($p = 0.001$), more likely to be employed ($p = 0.011$), and had significantly higher household incomes ($p = 0.001$). In terms of medical characteristics, there were few differences between the two samples. Breast-conserving surgery was done with the same frequency in both geographic regions, but for women undergoing mastectomy, more women in Washington DC had reconstructive surgery ($p=0.001$). Participants from Washington DC were surveyed at a longer time since diagnosis (3.02 years vs 2.68 years, $p=0.0001$), and were more likely to be taking tamoxifen at the time of the survey (52% versus 46%, $p=0.022$). Similar numbers of survivors had received chemotherapy or radiation therapy in the past at the two sites. As few significant medical or demographic differences were noted, the two site samples were combined for all further analyses.

Demographic and Medical Characteristics of the Sample

The demographic and medical characteristics of the sample, according to adjuvant treatment group, are shown in Table 1. About one-fourth of the sample had not received any adjuvant therapy (NO RX), and therefore this group can serve as a control or reference group for the impact of breast cancer that has been treated with surgery alone (with or without radiation therapy). The study sample ranged in age from 29 to 90 years. As can be seen in Table 1, there are significant and expected differences in age among the NO RX and

Table 1. Medical and demographic characteristics of the sample by adjuvant therapy status

	NO RX ($n=265$)	TAM ($n=356$)	CHEM ($n=180$)	TAM+CHEM ($n=295$)	p-value[a]
Age (year, mean&SD)	55.5 (11.7)	62.6 (9.8)	46.8 (8.6)	52.8 (8.6)	0.0001
Time since diagnosis (years, mean&SD)	2.7 (1.1)	2.7 (1.1)	2.7 (1.1)	3.1 (1.1)	0.0001
Education					
High school or less	15.5%	23.3%	11.7%	12.5%	0.002
College or less	47.9%	48.3%	52.2%	54.6%	
Postgraduate	36.6%	28.4%	36.1%	32.9%	
Ethnicity					
Non-Hispanic white	84.5%	84.0%	73.3%	79.3%	0.054
African American	9.1%	9.0%	15.0%	10.5%	
Other	6.4%	7.0%	11.7%	10.2%	
Marital status					
Partner	72.0%	69.9%	78.3%	77.1%	0.079
No Partner	28.0%	30.1%	21.7%	22.9%	
Type of surgery					
Lumpectomy	67.9%	66.0%	63.9%	49.8%	0.001
Mastectomy with recon	17.4%	10.7%	14.4%	22.0%	
Mastectomy	14.7%	23.3%	21.7%	28.1%	

NO RX, No adjuvant therapy; TAM, tamoxifen; CHEM, chemotherapy.
[a] Age and time since diagnosis tested with ANOVA. All other tests were χ^2.

adjuvant therapy samples ($p = 0.0001$), with the tamoxifen alone group (TAM) being the oldest (mean age 62.6 years) and the chemotherapy alone (CHEM) being the youngest (mean age 46.8 years). The TAM+CHEM group is intermediate in age (mean age 52.8 years). There is also a significant difference in time since diagnosis that is not readily explained. The differences observed in educational attainment correspond to the differing ages of the four study groups, as does the marital status of each group, with the oldest women most likely to be without a partner. There are significantly more nonwhite women in the two CHEM groups, which likely reflects the lower rate of estrogen-receptor-positive tumors in African American breast cancer patients (Trock 1996; Roach et al. 1997; Simon and Severson 1997). We also observed significant differences in the rate of breast conserving surgery among the four treatment groups ($p = 0.001$), with a lower rate in the TAM+CHEM group. This could well reflect more advanced clinical disease in this patient group. As a result of the significant differences in age and time since diagnosis among the four treatment groups, these variables were controlled for in all subsequent statistical comparisons. Since estrogen receptor status and advanced clinical stage of disease are intrinsically related to choice of adjuvant therapy, ethnicity and type of surgery were not controlled for.

Health-Related Quality of Life

Results of the HRQL scales are reported in Table 2. There were no significant differences in global quality of life among the four treatment groups. Similarly, the subscales of the MOS-SF-36, when adjusted for age and time since diagnosis, showed few treatment group differences. The exception was the physical functioning subscale ($p = 0.0002$), where the NO RX group showed the highest level of functioning in comparison to the adjuvant therapy treatment groups. Importantly, there are no significant differences among the groups with regard to emotional functioning ($p = 0.96$) or energy/fatigue ($p = 0.16$). This is further supported by scores on the CES-D, for which there are no significant differences in the mean scores for each group, or the percentage of each group who might be considered at risk for depression. The percentage of women in each group scoring at or above 16 is within the range reported in noncancer outpatient samples (Radloff 1977; Coyne et al. 1994).

We also summarized the subscales of the MOS-SF-36 into the two composite scales for physical functioning and mental health (Fig. 2). The NO RX group had a physical functioning composite score that was at the mean for a normal healthy population sample of women, while those in the adjuvant treatment groups scored slightly lower ($p = 0.0101$). The mental health composite score approximated the normal healthy population sample of women, and there was no significant difference among the four treatment groups ($p = 0.7553$).

Table 2. Measures of quality of life according to adjuvant therapy status. Scale scores reported are unadjusted, with presentation of the mean and one standard deviation in parentheses

	NO RX (n = 265)	TAM (n = 356)	CHEM (n = 180)	TAM+CHEM (n = 295)	p-value[a]
Global quality of life[b]	7.6 (1.9)	7.8 (1.8)	7.5 (1.7)	7.5 (1.9)	0.7484
MOS-SF-36[c]					
Physical functioning	84.8 (19.0)	76.1 (23.4)	82.6 (21.9)	81.4 (19.1)	0.0002
Role function, physical	81.3 (30.4)	71.2 (37.8)	76.8 (33.1)	76.0 (35.8)	0.0330
Emotional functioning	75.3 (16.2)	76.3 (17.5)	72.6 (18.1)	74.0 (18.6)	0.9591
Role function, emotional	81.4 (30.4)	76.6 (34.6)	71.9 (37.4)	75.8 (35.8)	0.0679
Social functioning	86.7 (20.1)	86.1 (20.3)	81.9 (22.6)	85.5 (20.8)	0.1954
Pain	79.9 (20.3)	78.3 (21.8)	78.7 (21.5)	78.4 (20.4)	0.5689
Energy/fatigue	61.7 (21.3)	60.7 (20.8)	56.5 (20.9)	58.0 (22.2)	0.1639
General health perceptions	75.4 (18.6)	71.0 (21.1)	72.3 (20.2)	71.7 (20.2)	0.0692
CES-D[d]					
Mean score	10.4 (9.2)	10.7 (9.2)	12.3 (10.8)	11.2 (10.3)	0.5558
Percentage with score ≥16	24.8%	26.8%	30.2%	24.9%	0.4694
CARES scales[e]					
Body Image	0.86 (1.07)	0.94 (1.21)	0.91 (1.12)	1.06 (1.16)	0.1662
Sexual functioning	0.98 (0.88)	1.08 (0.87)	1.20 (0.96)	1.28 (0.93)	0.0078

[a] All statistical comparisons adjusted for age and time since diagnosis; all tests done using analysis of covariance with the exception of the %CES-D score, which used a likelihood ratio χ^2 test based on logistic regressions with and without treatment indicators.
[b] Measured by the Ladder of Life scale with 1 being the lowest and 10 the highest score.
[c] Scales are scored from 0 to 100 with higher scores being better.
[d] Subjects with scores at or above 16 are considered to be potentially depressed.
[e] Scales range from 0 to 4 with a higher score indicating more problems and poorer functioning.

Body Image and Sexual Functioning

There were no significant differences in self-reported body image among the four treatment groups (Table 2), suggesting that, unlike type of surgery (Ganz et al. 1992a), adjuvant therapy does not contribute significantly to this aspect of quality of life after breast cancer. However, in contrast, sexual functioning is affected by therapy ($p = 0.0078$).

Symptoms

A variety of symptoms have been reported in healthy middle-aged women (Ganz et al. 1995) and in BCS (Ganz et al. 1998). We were interested in exploring the relationship between these common symptoms and the type of adjuvant therapy. In Table 3 we present the results from this study sample. Across all treatment groups, the NO RX sample has the lowest rate of symptoms for all but difficulty with bladder control (a problem that increases with age). Hot flashes, night sweats, bladder control problems, and vaginal

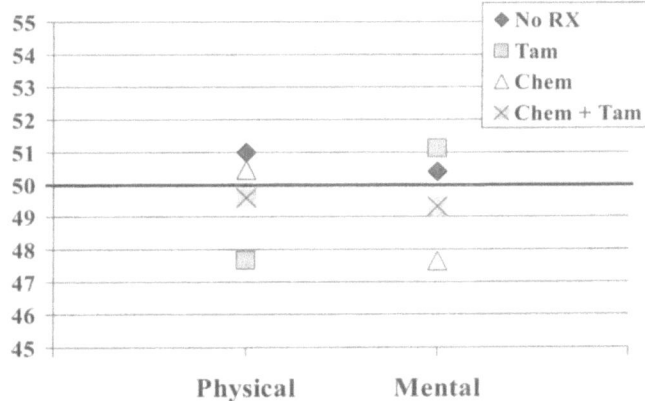

Fig. 2. Results of MOS-SF-36 composite scale scores. The scores of the breast cancer survivors are near the mean for healthy women (score=50). There are no significant differences among the treatment groups for the physical score ($p=0.0101$) or the mental health score ($p=0.7553$)

Table 3. Percentages of breast cancer survivors reporting symptoms, according to adjuvant therapy status. Frequencies presented are unadjusted for age and time since diagnosis

	NO RX (n=265) %	TAM (n=356) %	CHEM (n=180) %	TAM+CHEM (n=295) %	p-value[a]
Hot flashes	40.0	60.7	51.1	72.0	<0.0001
Night sweats	33.3	47.2	43.9	53.4	<0.0001
Difficulty with bladder control	34.7	43.1	30.0	37.4	0.3924
Vaginal dryness	38.5	47.6	51.1	57.4	0.0002
Pain with intercourse	25.8	27.0	36.5	42.0	0.0076
Vaginal discharge	24.2	34.2	29.4	42.5	<0.0001
Weight gain	47.2	54.1	59.4	59.3	0.0443
Difficulty concentrating	49.8	48.6	59.4	56.8	0.6349
Forgetfulness	66.4	67.1	72.8	71.4	0.0691

[a] All statistical comparisons adjusted for age and time since diagnosis; all tests done using likelihood ratio chi-square tests based on logistic regressions with and without treatment indicators.

dryness are all symptoms associated with the menopause and decreased levels of estrogen. All but bladder control problems differed significantly by adjuvant treatment group. Vaginal discharge also differed significantly by adjuvant therapy ($p=0.0001$) and was most frequent among those receiving TAM therapy. Pain with intercourse showed differences ($p=0.0076$), and was reported more frequently in the two CHEM groups, which may well contribute to the sexual dysfunction described earlier. Self-reported weight gain, a problem that has been frequently attributed to adjuvant chemotherapy (Knobf et al. 1983; Camoriano et al. 1990; Demark-Wahnefried et al. 1993, 1997), was not significantly different among the treatment groups ($p=0.04$). Forgetfulness and problems with concentration were not significantly different among the four groups.

Discussion

In this paper we describe the results of a cross-sectional survey of 1096 breast cancer survivors who completed an extensive quality-of-life questionnaire battery about 3 years after the diagnosis of cancer. These disease-free survivors had been treated for breast cancer in a variety of medical settings, in two large metropolitan areas in the United States. The participants in this research study were fairly representative of the population with stage 0, I, and II breast cancer, with the exception of being somewhat younger than the general population with this disease. We examined the impact of the type of adjuvant therapy received on HRQL, body image, sexual functioning, and symptoms. Fortuitously, the study sample had relatively equal distributions of patients who had received no adjuvant therapy, therapy with tamoxifen alone, therapy with chemotherapy alone, or combined therapy with chemotherapy and tamoxifen. Thus, we could compare the impact of the each adjuvant therapy strategy on quality of life about 3 years after breast cancer diagnosis.

About one-quarter of the study sample received no adjuvant therapy. Although medical record review was not performed, we believe that this group is largely composed of patients with noninvasive or very small breast tumors for whom adjuvant therapy is not usually recommended. This group has the highest rate of breast conserving surgery. In contrast, patients in the chemoendocrine group (tamoxifen plus chemotherapy) have the lowest rate of breast conserving surgery. This most likely relates to more extensive clinical disease at diagnosis that was not amenable to breast conserving treatment, or to a perceived risk of more serious disease warranting the choice of mastectomy on the part of the patient and/or surgeon. The age distributions in each group, as well as biologic differences in breast cancer in African American women, explain other differences in education and ethnicity among the treatment groups. Because age and time since diagnosis could affect quality of life assessment independently, these variables were controlled in all statistical comparisons.

An important finding from this study is the limited impact of receipt of adjuvant therapy on overall quality of life, as well as the multiple dimensions of HRQL that are measured by the MOS-SF-36. Overall, these breast cancer survivors are functioning at a high level, that is comparable to or better than age-matched healthy controls (Ware 1993). The only exception is the dimension of physical functioning, where patients who have received adjuvant therapy report poorer functioning. Importantly, mental health, as measured by the MOS-SF-36 emotional functioning scale, and the CES-D depression measure, did not differ significantly among these treatment groups.

In our past research, we and others have demonstrated a significant impact of the type of surgical treatment on self-reported body image in breast cancer patients and survivors (Ganz et al. 1992a, 1998; Rowland et al. 1996; Schover et al. 1995). Although the loss of the breast contributes to this assessment, other qualitative data from breast cancer survivors suggests that they are equally upset about their body appearance in general, as well as by the effects of weight gain on their body image (Ganz et al. 1998 and unpublished qualitative data). In this paper, we were able to explore the impact of adjuvant therapy on body image. We found no significant differences among the four treatment groups, even though the women in the chemoendocrine group were less likely to receive breast conserving surgery.

In this paper we confirm our prior finding of poorer sexual functioning among women who received chemotherapy, with less impact of tamoxifen on sexual functioning (Ganz et al. 1998). In additional analyses (not shown), when we compared the NO RX group to the CHEM only group and to the TAM only group, we found a more significant effect ($p=0.0096$) in the CHEM group than in the TAM group ($p=0.0304$). This is further supported by more frequent reporting of vaginal dryness and pain with intercourse in the two chemotherapy groups as compared to the no treatment and tamoxifen alone group. Explanatory mechanisms for poorer sexual functioning after chemotherapy are uncertain (Sarrel 1990; Kaplan 1992; Schover 1991, 1997; Bines et al. 1996). Possible causes include a chemically induced oophorectomy resulting in diminished ovarian androgens (decreased libido), reduced levels of estrogen leading to vaginal atrophy and dyspareunia (especially in premenopausal women), as well as a manifestation of the poorer physical functioning reported by women who have received adjuvant chemotherapy. Future prospective studies that evaluate quality of life, hormone levels, and sexual functioning in patients receiving different adjuvant therapy strategies (compared to controls) might be helpful in elucidating the mechanisms by which sexual dysfunction occurs after chemotherapy. Strategies to treat this problem in those who are dissatisfied with their level of sexual functioning need to be developed (Ganz 1997). In this study sample, less than 5% of women were using some form of hormone replacement therapy. Studies of the safety of estrogens in this target population are urgently needed (Cobleigh et al. 1994; Roy et al. 1996), as such therapy is very effective in alleviation of vaginal dryness and dyspareunia.

We also examined a number of symptoms that are common in middle-aged women to determine the impact of adjuvant therapy on their frequency. Vasomotor symptoms (hot flashes, night sweats) are significantly more frequent in women who received tamoxifen, consistent with reports in the literature (Love et al. 1991; Fisher et al. 1989). Similarly, vaginal discharge was more common in the tamoxifen-treated patients.

Interestingly, weight gain was a perceived problem in almost half of all breast cancer survivors, independent of the type of adjuvant therapy, but was slightly more frequent in the groups receiving chemotherapy. We had also asked these women to report their current height and weight on our survey, allowing us to calculate their body mass index (BMI), which is weight in kilograms divided by the square of the height in meters. We found significant differences in BMI ($p=0.0012$), with the three adjuvant therapy groups scoring in the range of 25.4–25.6, as compared to 24.1 in the NO RX group. Recent studies suggest that adjuvant chemotherapy causes acute changes in resting metabolic rate, as well as a decline in physical activity and energy intake during treatment (Demark-Wahnefried et al. 1997). Since weight gain after breast cancer treatment may be detrimental with regard to breast cancer as well as other health problems, interventions should be developed for these survivors.

There are several limitations to this study, including the lack of detail on the specific adjuvant therapy regimens and the use of patient self-report for description of medical treatments. In addition, the use of a cross-sectional design allowed description of associations rather than determination of causal mechanisms. Nevertheless, these data are consistent with those few reports in the literature that have examined the impact of breast cancer adjuvant therapy on quality of life (Hürny et al. 1996; van Dam et al. 1998). Specifically, while there is more acute impact of chemotherapy on HRQL during treatment, over time these effects diminish. In particular, emotional functioning was similar among all treatment groups and reflects the common diagnosis of breast cancer and not the specifics of treatment. The only lasting effect of chemotherapy appears to be a modest decrement in physical functioning, compared to women who received no adjuvant therapy and to healthy women in the general population. Future prospective studies need to describe in more detail the long-term physical and symptomatic effects of adjuvant chemotherapy, especially among regimens with higher doses than were used at the time these patients were treated in the early 1990s (Ganz 1998). Sexual dysfunction is an important problem associated with adjuvant therapy, and needs to be addressed in women who have had adjuvant therapy, especially those who have become prematurely menopausal. However, overall we can reassure our breast cancer patients that they can expect to recover after their adjuvant therapy and function at levels that are only modestly different from women who do not require adjuvant therapy.

Summary

Little is known about the long-term effects of adjuvant therapy on quality of life, sexual functioning and symptoms in breast cancer survivors. Between January 1996 and June 1997, we surveyed 1098 women who had been diagnosed with early stage breast cancer between 1 and 5 years earlier. The breast cancer survivors were recruited in two large metropolitan centers in the USA. They completed a survey battery that contained standardized measures of health-related quality of life (HRQL), depression, body image, sexual functioning, and symptoms. A total of 1096 had useable responses for these analyses. In this sample, $n = 356$ had received tamoxifen (TAM) alone, $n = 180$ received chemotherapy (CHEM) alone, $n = 395$ received CHEM + TAM, and $n = 265$ received no adjuvant therapy (NO RX). There were significant differences in the mean age of each group, with the TAM group being the oldest (mean 62.6 years) and the CHEM group being the youngest (mean 46.8 years). Both age and time since diagnosis were controlled for in all statistical analyses. We found no significant differences in global quality of life among the four treatment groups. For the MOS-SF-36, there were no significant differences on the subscale scores except for the physical functioning subscale ($p = 0.0002$); the NO RX group had the highest functioning. There were no significant differences in depression scores among the four treatment groups. The MOS-SF-36 physical functioning composite score differed by treatment group ($p = 0.012$); the NO RX group had a physical functioning composite score that was at the mean for a normal healthy population of women, while those in the adjuvant treatment groups scored slightly lower. The mental health composite score was not significantly different among the four treatment groups and approximated scores from the normal population of healthy women. There were no differences in body image scores among the four treatment groups; however, sexual functioning scores did differ ($p = 0.0078$) with patients receiving chemotherapy (either alone or with tamoxifen) experiencing more problems. Hot flashes, night sweats, and vaginal discharge differed by treatment ($p = 0.0001$); all symptoms were reported more often in breast cancer survivors on tamoxifen. Vaginal dryness and pain with intercourse also differed significantly by adjuvant treatment, occurring more often in survivors treated with chemotherapy. Overall, breast cancer survivors function at a high level, similar to healthy women without cancer. However, compared to survivors with no adjuvant therapy, those who received chemotherapy have significantly more sexual problems, and those treated with tamoxifen experience more vasomotor symptoms.

Acknowledgements. The authors would like to thank the many physicians and hospitals that allowed us to approach the breast cancer survivors for this study. In addition, we owe many thanks to the breast cancer survivors who have been our partners in this research. Finally, we would like to thank the fine support of our research staff in Los Angeles (Barbara Kahn, Jane Peredo, Randy Patterson) and Washington DC (Amy Busch, Lorraine Morgan, Bridget Szymanski). This research was supported by a grant from the National Cancer Institute (USA) R01 CA 63028. Dr. Ganz is the recipient of an Avon Breast Cancer Research Leadership Award.

References

Aaronson NK (1988) Quality of life: what is it? How should it be measured. Oncology 2(5):69–74

Bines J, Oleske DM, Cobleigh MA (1996) Ovarian function in premenopausal women treated with adjuvant chemotherapy for breast cancer. J Clin Oncol 14:1718–1729

Camoriano JK, Loprinzi CL, Ingle JN, et al (1990) Weight change in women treated with adjuvant therapy or observed following mastectomy for node-positive breast cancer. J Clin Oncol 8:1327–1334

Cobleigh MA, Berris RF, Bush T et al (1994) Estrogen replacement therapy in breast cancer survivors. A time for change. JAMA 272:540–545

Coyne JC, Fechner-Bates S, Schwenk TL (1994) Prevalence, nature, and comorbidity of depressive disorders in primary care. Gen Hosp Psychiatry 16:267–276

Demark-Wahnefried W, Winer EP, Rimer BK (1993) Why women gain weight with adjuvant chemotherapy for breast cancer. J Clin Oncol 11:1418–1429

Demark-Wahnefried W, Hars V, Conaway MR, Havlin K, Rimer BK, McElveen G, Winer EP (1997) Reduced rates of metabolism and decreased physical activity in breast cancer patients receiving adjuvant chemotherapy. Am J Clin Nutr 65:1495–1501

Dow KH, Ferrell BR, Leigh S, Ly J, Gulasekaram P (1996) An evaluation of the quality of life among long-term survivors of breast cancer. Breast Cancer Res Treat 39:261–273

Early Breast Cancer Trialists' Collaborative Group (1992) Systemic treatment of early breast cancer by hormonal, cytotoxic, or immune therapy. Lancet 339:1–15, 71–85

Fisher B, Costantino J, Redmond C, et al (1989) A randomized clinical trial evaluating tamoxifen in the treatment of patients with node-negative breast cancer who have estrogen-receptor-positive tumors. N Engl J Med 320:479–484

Ganz PA (1997) Sexual functioning after breast cancer: a conceptual framework for future studies. Ann Oncol 8:105–107

Ganz PA (1998) Cognitive dysfunction following adjuvant treatment of breast cancer: a new dose-limiting toxic effect? J Nat Cancer Inst 90:182–183

Ganz PA, Schag CC, Polinsky ML, Heinrich RL, Flack VF (1987) Rehabilitation needs and breast cancer: the first month after primary therapy. Breast Cancer Res Treat 10:243–253

Ganz PA, Schag CC, Cheng H (1990) Assessing the quality of life – a study in newly-diagnosed breast cancer patients. J Clin Epidemiol 43:75–86

Ganz PA, Schag CAC, Lee JJ, Polinsky ML, Tan S-J (1992a) Breast conservation versus mastectomy: is there a difference in psychological adjustment or quality of life in the year after surgery? Cancer 69:1729–1738

Ganz PA, Schag CAC, Lee JJ, Sim M-S (1992b) The CARES: A generic measure of health-related quality of life for cancer patients. Qual Life Res 1:19–29

Ganz PA, Day R, Ware JE Jr, Redmond C, Fisher B (1995) Base-line quality-of-life assessment in the National Surgical Adjuvant Breast and Bowel Project Breast Cancer Prevention Trial. J Natl Cancer Inst 87:1372–1382

Ganz PA, Coscarelli A, Fred C, Kahn B, Polinsky ML, Petersen L (1996) Breast cancer survivors: psychosocial concerns and quality of life. Breast Cancer Res Treat 38:183–199

Ganz PA, Rowland JH, Desmond K, Meyerowitz BE, Wyatt GE (1998) Life after breast cancer: understanding women's health-related quality of life and sexual functioning. J Clin Oncol 16:501–514

Greendale GA, Hogan P, Shumaker S for the Postmenopausal Estrogen/Progestins Intervention Trial (PEPI) Investigators (1996) Sexual functioning in postmenopausal women: the Postmenopausal Estrogen/Progestins Intervention (PEPI) Trial. J Womens Health 5:445–458

Harris JR, Lippman ME, Veronesi U, Willett W (1992) Breast cancer. N Engl J Med 327(5):319–328, 327(6):390–398, 327(7):473–480

Hays RD, Sherbourne CD, Mazel RM (1993) The RAND 36-item health survey 1.0. Health Econ 2:217–227

Hürny C, Bernhard J, Coates AS, Castiglione-Gertsch M, Peterson HF, Gelber RD, Forbes JF et al (1996) Impact of adjuvant therapy on quality of life in women with node-positive operarable breast cancer. International Breast Cancer Study Group. Lancet 347:1279–1284

Kaplan HS (1992) A neglected issue: the sexual side effects of current treatments for breast cancer. J Sex Marital Ther 18(1):3–19

Kilpatrick FP, Cantril H (1960) Self-anchoring scaling: a measure of individuals' unique reality worlds. J Individ Psychol 16:158–173

Knobf MK, Mullen JC, Xistris D, Moritz DA (1983) Weight gain in women with breast cancer receiving adjuvant chemotherapy. Oncol Nurs Forum 10(2):28–33

Love RR, Cameron L, Connell BL, Leventhal H (1991) Symptoms associated with tamoxifen treatment in postmenopausal women. Arch Intern Med 151:1842–1847

Maunsell E, Brisson J, Deschennes L (1989) Psychological distress after initial treatment for breast cancer: a comparison of partial and total mastectomy. J Clin Epidemiol 42:765–771

Mc Horney CA, Kosinski M, Ware JE (1994) Comparison of the costs and quality of norms for the SF-36 health survey collected by mail versus telephone interview: results from a national survey. Med Care 32:551–567

Meyerowitz BE, Watkins IK, Sparks FC (1983) Psychosocial implications of adjuvant chemotherapy. A two-year follow-up. Cancer 52:1541–1545

Meyerowitz BE, Leedham B, Hart S (1998) Psychosocial considerations for breast cancer patients and their families. In: Kavanagh JJ, DePetrillo AZ, Einhorn N, Pecorelli S, Singletary E (eds) Cancer in women. Blackwell, Malden, MA, pp 549–564

Myers JK, Weissman MM (1980) Use of a self-report symptom scale to detect depression in a community sample. Am J Psychiatry 137:1081–1084

Omne-Pontén M, Holmberg L, Sjödén P-O (1994) Psychosocial adjustment among women with breast cancer stages I and II: six year follow-up of consecutive patients. J Clin Oncol 12:1778–1782

Radloff LS (1977) The CES-D scale: a self-report depression scale for research in the general population. Appl Psychol Measure 1:385–401

Roach M III, Cirrincione C, Budman D, Hayes D, Berry D, Younger J, Hart R, Henderson IC (1997) Race and survival from breast cancer: based on Cancer and Leukemia Group B trial 8541. Cancer J Sci Am 3(2):107–112

Roberts RE, Vernon SW (1983) The Center for Epidemiologic Studies Depression Scale: its use in a community sample. Am J Psychiatry 140:41–46

Rowland JH, Massie MJ (1996) Psychologic reactions to breast cancer diagnosis, treatment and survival. In: Harris JR, Lippman ME, Morrow M, Hellman S (eds), Diseases of the breast. Lippincott-Raven, Philadelphia, pp 919–939

Rowland J, Meyerowitz B, Ganz PA, Wyatt G, Desmond K, Honig S (1996) Body image and sexual functioning following reconstructive surgery in breast cancer survivors (BCS). Proc Am Soc Clin Oncol 15:124

Roy JA, Sawka CA, Pritchard KI (1996) Hormone replacement therapy in women with breast cancer: do the risks outweigh the benefits? J Clin Oncol 14:997–1006

Sarrel PM (1990) Sexuality and menopause. Obstet Gynecol 75:26S–30S

Schag, CC, Heinrich RL, Ganz PA (1983) Cancer inventory of problem situations: an instrument for assessing cancer patients' rehabilitation needs. J Psychosoc Oncol 1(4):11–24

Schag CC, Heinrich RL, Aadland R, Ganz PA (1990) Assessing problems of cancer patients: psychometric properties of the cancer inventory of problem situations. Health Psychol 9:83–102

Schag CAC, Ganz PA, Polinsky ML, Fred C, Hirji K, Petersen L (1993) Characteristics of women at risk for psychosocial distress in the year after breast cancer. J Clin Oncol 11:783–793

Schover LR (1991) The impact of breast cancer on sexuality, body image, and intimate relationships. CA Cancer J Clin 41(2):112–120

Schover LR (1997) Sexuality and fertility after Cancer. Wiley, New York

Schover LR, Yetman RJ, Tuason LJ, Meisler E, Esselstyn CB, Hermann RE et al (1995) Partial mastectomy and breast reconstruction. A comparison of their effects on psychosocial adjustment, body image, and sexuality. Cancer 75:54–64

Simon MS; Severson RK (1997) Racial differences in breast cancer survival: the interaction of socioeconomic status and tumor biology. Am J Obstet Gynecol 176(6):S233–S239

Tasmuth T, von Smitten K, Kalso E (1996) Pain and other symptoms during the first year after radical and conservative surgery for breast cancer. Br J Cancer 74:2024–2031

Trock BJ (1996) Breast cancer in African American women: epidemiology and tumor biology. Breast Cancer Res Treat 40(1):11–24

Van Dam FSAM, Schagen SB, Muller MJ, Boogerd W, Wall Evd, Droogleever Fortuyn ME, Rodenhuis S (1998) Impairment of cognitive function in women receiving adjuvant treatment for high-risk breast cancer: high-dose versus standard-dose chemotherapy. J Nat Cancer Inst 90:210–218

Vinokur A, Threatt B, Vinokur-Kaplan D, Satariano W (1990) The process of recovery from breast cancer for younger and older patients: changes during the first year. Cancer 65:1242–1254

Ware JE Jr (1984) Conceptualizing disease impact and treatment outcome. Cancer 53 (Suppl 10):2316–2326

Ware JE Jr (1993) SF-36 health survey. Manual and interpretation guide. The Health Institute, New England Medical Center, Boston, MA

Ware JE Jr, Sherbourne CD (1992) A 36-item short form health survey (SF-36). I. Conceptual framework and item selection. Med Care 30:473–483

Ware JE, Kosinski M, Keller SD (1994) SF-36 physical and mental health summary scales: a user's manual. The Health Institute, Boston, MA

Wolberg WH, Romsaas EP, Tanner MA, Malec JF (1989) Psychosexual adaptation to breast cancer surgery. Cancer 63:1645–1655

Summary

A. Coates[1] and L. Fallowfield[2]

[1] International Breast Cancer Study Group, University of Sydney, Sydney, Australia
[2] CRC Psychosocial Oncology Group, Department of Oncology, University College London Medical School, London, UK

No scientific meeting on adjuvant therapy for breast cancer would be complete without a session devoted to the quality of life of the patients. There is clear evidence that the diagnosis, the decision-making process and the therapy associated with early breast cancer each have an impact on patients' quality of life. In this session we are privileged to have three contributions from workers who have made major contributions to the understanding of this important topic.

Quality of Life Assessment in the Adjuvant Setting: Is It Relevant?

Integration of qualitative and quantitative outcomes in the assessment of adjuvant therapy for early breast cancer is essential if patients are to be given the best possible description of the choices they face at this difficult time. Informal summation is widely practised, but the assumptions vary widely. In the absence of systematically collected data from clinical trials, clinicians' views are polarised. Consequently, patients may receive advice which depends on the individual clinician rather than on the available evidence. A more rational, quantitative approach is provided by the Q-TWiST method pioneered by the group of Gelber et al. reporting in this paper (Gelber and Goldhirsch 1986; Goldhirsch et al. 1989). Their approach involves reducing the value assigned to time periods complicated by the adverse effects of therapy or the symptoms of cancer recurrence, then adding the time without symptoms and toxicity (TWiST) to give a quality-adjusted score for each policy being compared. The duration of each state is estimated from clinical trial data, while the coefficients used to estimate the relative value of symptomatic periods are arbitrary. In an earlier study in postmenopausal women comparing 1 year of tamoxifen and prednisone to the same treatment plus 12 cycles of chemotherapy, or to no adjuvant therapy, a benefit of combined chemo-endocrine therapy could be demonstrated for most values of the coefficients assigned to symptoms of treatment or relapse (Goldhirsch et al. 1989). The study described by Gelber et al. at this meeting also involves a comparison of endocrine therapy alone (5 years' tamoxifen) to chemoendo-crine therapy with the addition of three cycles of cyclophosphamide, metho-trexate and 5-fluorouracil (CMF) either given together at the commencement of treatment, as delayed single cycles at months 9, 12 and 15, or both initial and delayed CMF for a total of six cycles. In this trial, the effect of initial CMF was beneficial, but that of delayed CMF was less definite, and there was a tendency to an adverse impact on disease-free survival (DFS) among wom-en with estrogen-receptor (ER)-negative tumours. Gelber et al. conclude that on the basis of a Q-TWiST analysis of these data, a decision to recommend the addition of CMF should be based on each patient's preferences for the re-lative importance of treatment toxicity and disease recurrence. This is in keeping with the conclusion of a similar analysis based on the Overview data on chemo-endocrine therapy in post-menopausal women (Gelber et al. 1996).

Quality of Life Measurements in the IBCSG: Past, Present and Future

As Hürny et al. reminded us in this paper, the International Breast Cancer Study Group (IBCSG) has been including patient self-assessment of quality of life as an endpoint in all adjuvant trials since 1986. The initial linear analo-gue self-assessment instruments showed that adjuvant chemotherapy had only a transient and minor adverse impact on patient self-assessment of qual-ity of life (Hürny et al. 1996). The instruments have been modified and aug-mented in more recent studies (Bernhard et al. 1997), including a new scale which correlates closely with utility as measured by classical time trade-off methods (Hürny et al. 1998). The observation that patients report progres-sively better quality of life with time after diagnosis implies a form of adap-tation. Interventions to improve adaptation are currently being explored.

Impact of Different Adjuvant Therapy Strategies on Quality of Life in Breast Cancer Survivors

In contrast to the previous, pragmatic assessments of quality of life designed for use in large clinical trials, Patti Ganz described a retrospective cross-sec-tional study that utilised a broad range of measures of quality of life and sexual function in women who received a variety of adjuvant therapies (or no such therapy) after local therapy for early breast cancer. The non-randomised de-sign distinguishes this from the IBCSG studies, and carries the possibility of confounding between the factors which led to the choice of a particular thera-py and the outcomes observed. At an average of 2.8 years after diagnosis the authors found no differences in quality of life scores between patients receiv-ing no adjuvant therapy, tamoxifen alone, chemotherapy or combined chemo-therapy plus tamoxifen. This observation is in keeping with that of Hürny et al.

(described above) who found no significant differences in quality of life scores by 18 months after diagnosis. So too is the observation that in general the quality of life of breast cancer patients was good. However, Ganz et al. found significantly increased sexual difficulties among patients who had received chemotherapy, perhaps reflecting an adverse effect of chemotherapy on ovarian function, while patients treated with tamoxifen reported more hot flushing, night sweats and vaginal discharge, a finding in keeping with other studies of this agent (Fisher et al. 1989; Love et al. 1991). Another interesting finding was that patients who had not received adjuvant therapy experienced symptoms of weight gain and difficulties with cognitive functioning and body image. This demonstrates the need for researchers to beware of attributing all side effects to treatment – some may be related simply to age.

Overall, the studies reported underline the importance of assessment of quality of life in patients undergoing adjuvant systemic therapy for early breast cancer. Systematic evaluation has two advantages. It may help patients and their clinicians to make more informed choices between the many treatments which may have similar efficacy, and it may identify specific areas in which the development and assessment of preventative, ameliorative and supportive interventions are required.

References

Bernhard J, Hürny C, Coates AS, Peterson H, Castiglione-Gertsch M, Gelber RD, Goldhirsch A, Senn H-J, Rudenstam C-M, International Breast Cancer Study Group (1997) Quality of life assessment in patients receiving adjuvant therapy for breast cancer: the IBCSG approach. Ann Oncol 8:825–835

Fisher B, Costantino J, Redmond C, Poisson R, Bowman D, Couture J, Dimitrov NV, Wolmark N, Wickerham DL, Fisher ER et al (1989) A randomized clinical trial evaluating tamoxifen in the treatment of patients with node-negative breast cancer who have estrogen-receptor-positive tumors. N Engl J Med 320:479–484

Gelber RD, Goldhirsch A (1986) A new endpoint for the assessment of adjuvant therapy in postmenopausal women with operable breast cancer. J Clin Oncol 4:1772–1779

Gelber RD, Cole BF, Goldhirsch A, Rose C, Fisher B, Osborne CK, Boccardo F, Gray R, Gordon NH, Bengtsson NO, Sevelda P (1996) Adjuvant chemotherapy plus tamoxifen compared with tamoxifen alone for postmenopausal breast cancer: meta-analysis of quality-adjusted survival. Lancet 347:1066–1071

Goldhirsch A, Gelber RD, Simes RJ, Glasziou PP, Coates AS (1989) Costs and benefits of adjuvant therapy in breast cancer: a quality-adjusted survival analysis. J Clin Oncol 7:36–44

Hürny C, Bernhard J, Coates AS, Castiglione M, Peterson HF, Gelber RD, Forbes JF, Rudenstam C-M, Simoncini E, Crivellari D, Goldhirsch A, Senn H-J (1996) Impact of adjuvant therapy on quality of life in women with node-positive operable breast cancer. Lancet 347:1279–1284

Hürny C, van Wegberg B, Bacchi M, Bernhard J, Thürlimann B, Ral O, Perey L, Bonnefoi H, Coates AS (1998) Subjective Health Estimations (SHE) in patients with advanced breast cancer: an adapted utility concept for cancer clinical trials. Br J Cancer (in press)

Love RR, Cameron L, Connell BL, Leventhal H (1991) Symptoms associated with tamoxifen treatment in postmenopausal women. Arch Intern Med 151:1842–1847

XII. Clinical Research Around the World: Review of Cooperative Group Trials

North American Adjuvant Breast Cancer Trials

J. S. Abrams

National Cancer Institute, Clinical Investigations Branch, 6130 Executive Blvd, #741, Bethesda, MD 20892, USA

Introduction

Clinical trials in breast cancer have demonstrated convincingly that agents with systemic activity in advanced disease can improve survival when these agents are given adjuvantly to patients in early stages of the disease (Early Breast Cancer Trialist's Collaborative Group 1992). Results from controlled adjuvant trials do appear to translate into benefits for the average patient as shown by improvements in both population-based surveys of disease-specific survival (Olivotto et al. 1994) and recent US and international breast cancer mortality statistics (Chu et al. 1996). For these reasons, the National Cancer Institute (NCI) continues to rely on large, adjuvant, randomized trials as the best way to make important clinical progress against this devastating disease.

Networks of multi-institution Cooperative Groups are sponsored by the NCI to perform these trials (Table 1). The NCI gives full support to the US Cooperative Groups for their trials and offers partial funding for statistical support to several foreign Cooperative Groups. The US trialists are segregated into two main bodies which perform adjuvant trials in various stages of early breast cancer. These are the National Surgical Adjuvant Breast and Bowel Project (NSABP) and the Intergroup [composed of the Eastern Cooperative Oncology Group (ECOG), the Cancer and Leukemia Group B (CALGB), the North Central Cancer Treatment Group (NCCTG), the Southwest Oncology Group (SWOG), and the National Cancer Institute of Canada (NCIC)]. The rationale behind the NCI's funding of International Groups is twofold. These Groups complement US trials by expanding the number of new questions that can be studied and by performing confirmatory trials. In addition, sharing of specimens, data, and computer science initiatives between US and International Groups provides scientists with additional resources for discovery and innovation.

Table 1. NCI-sponsored adjuvant breast cancer trials

USA:	Cancer and Leukemia Group B (CALGB)
	Eastern Cooperative Oncology Group (ECOG)
	National Surgical Adjuvant Breast and Bowel Project (NSABP)
	North Central Cancer Treatment Group (NCCTG)
	Southwest Oncology Group (SWOG)
	Radiation Therapy Oncology Group (RTOG)
International: [a]	National Cancer Institute, Canada (NCIC)
	European Organization for Research and Treatment of Cancer (EORTC)
	International Breast Cancer Study Group (IBCSG)

[a] Limited funding.

Ductal Carcinoma In Situ

The NSABP demonstrated in trial B-17 that conservative treatment with lumpectomy and breast irradiation is an acceptable alternative for most patients with ductal carcinoma in situ (DCIS) (Fisher et al. 1993). Recently published follow-up data at 8 years continues to show that less than 2% of patients treated with lumpectomy alone or lumpectomy and breast irradiation have died from breast cancer (Fisher et al. 1998). As this outcome compares favorably with results from series of patients treated with mastectomy (Swain 1989), a trial directly comparing the two is no longer needed. Rather, current strategies are directed towards extending the indications for conservative treatment. NSABP B-24 compares lumpectomy and breast irradiation with or without tamoxifen. Unlike B-17, this trial accepted women with multifocal DCIS. Accrual of 1804 patients has been completed and initial results are anticipated this year. An Intergroup trial (ECOG 5194) is focused on whether breast irradiation is essential or if some women with DCIS can be managed with lumpectomy alone. This single-arm observational trial will enroll 1000 women with "low risk" DCIS, defined as low/intermediate grade tumors ≤2.5 cm, or high-grade tumors <1 cm, and targets local recurrence rates as its primary endpoint. In the event that the occurrence of ipsilateral breast tumors exceed an overall 5-year failure rate of 10% or an invasive cancer 5-year rate of 5%, early stopping rules will be invoked.

Occult, Invasive Breast Cancers

The subgroup of patients with tumors ≤1 cm and negative axillary nodes has been shown to have a particularly favorable prognosis with surgical resection alone in a large case series (Rosen et al. 1989). Guidelines for treatment of this subset of tumors have generally counseled against chemotherapy (Goldhirsch et al. 1995). As a consequence, most studies of systemic therapy for node-negative breast cancer have included few patients in this category. In an effort to optimize primary treatment for such patients, the NSABP developed a trial (B-21) which tests whether tamoxifen can replace breast irradiation as part of conservative primary treatment or whether the combination of breast irradiation and tamoxifen will yield better survival results compared to breast irradiation alone (Fig. 1). Despite widespread agreement about the importance of this question, accrual to this trial has been slow; the accrual goal of 1690 patients may not be reached for several more years unless new investigators can be recruited.

Node-Negative, Receptor-Positive Breast Cancer

The NSABP has performed consecutive studies in "low risk" patients characterized by negative axillary nodes and positive estrogen receptor status (Table 2). The B-14 trial demonstrated a role for 5 years of tamoxifen in this subgroup irrespective of menopausal status (Fisher et al. 1996a). In B-20, chemotherapy was found to add to tamoxifen's benefits in this population, although younger women (< 50 years old) had greater improvements in survival than did older women (Fisher et al. 1997a). Based on these results, the current trial for this patient population, NSABP B-29, has made chemotherapy optional and randomizes patients to octreotide and tamoxifen versus tamoxifen alone (Fig. 2). Octreotide is a somatostatin analoge that has shown preclinical activity in breast cancer models (Seytono-Ham et al. 1987). Potential mechanisms of action include a direct effect on somatostatin receptors found in some breast cancers and an indirect effect by lowering tumor growth factors such as insulin-like growth factor (IGF-1). Octrogtide is administered monthly by intramuscular injection (90 mg) for 2 years. The NCIC is performing a trial (MA.14) identical in design to B-29 except that octreotide will be given for 5 years. The patient population in the NCIC trial also differs from B-29 as node-positive and node-negative patients are included, only post-menopausal women are eligible, and hormone receptor status can be negative, positive, or unknown.

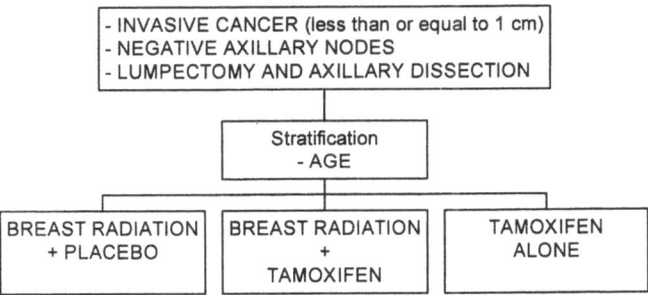

Fig. 1. Trial design of NSABP B-21

Table 2. NSABP node-negative ER-positive studies

B-14:	Tamoxifen vs placebo
B-20:	Chemotherapy (CMF or M → F) and tamoxifen vs tamoxifen alone
B-29:	Octreotide + tamoxifen vs tamoxifen alone (± AC chemotherapy)

CMF, Cyclophosphamide, methotrexate, fluorouracil; M → F, methotrexate followed by fluorouracil; AC, doxorubicin, cyclophosphamide.

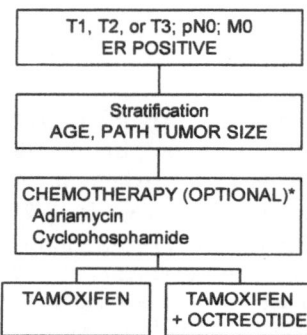

Fig. 2. Trial design of NSABP B-29. *The decision to use chemotherapy must be made before randomization

High-Risk Node-Negative Breast Cancer

In 1989, two important studies (NSABP B-13 and Intergroup 0011) were published demonstrating for the first time a role for chemotherapy in women with high-risk node-negative breast cancers (Fisher et al. 1989; Mansour et al. 1989). The designation "high risk" was determined either by negative estrogen receptors (B-13 and Intergroup 0011) or by positive receptors with a tumor size >3 cm (Intergroup 0011). Building on these findings, the Intergroup launched a trial (0102) that segregated patients into high, intermediate, and low risk categories (Table 3). Patients in the high-risk group were randomized to one of four groups: CMF alone, CMF followed by 5 years of tamoxifen, CAF alone, or CAF followed by 5 years of tamoxifen. Patients in the low-risk group were observed without systemic therapy. For patients with an intermediate-risk, flow cytometric measurement of tumor S-phase at a central site was performed. Patients with high S-phase measurements were treated as high-risk while those with low S-phase were put into the low-risk observation cohort. Results from this study are anticipated this year. The NSABP has completed a study (B-19) which tested methotrexate followed by 5-fluorouracil in node-negative, ER-negative women (Table 4). Results show an overall advantage in disease-free survival for CMF, but subset analyses revealed that this advantage retained significance only in the women below 49 years of age (Fisher et al. 1996b). The current trial, B-23, attempts to build on this result by comparing CMF alone, CMF + tamoxifen, CAF alone, and

Table 3. Treatment according to risk in Intergroup trial 0102 in patients with high-risk node-negative breast cancer

High risk (ER/PR-negative or tumor > 2 cm):
  CAF×6±Tam vs CMF×6±Tam
Uncertain risk (ER/PR-positive and tumor = 1–2 cm:
                High/unknown = high risk
S phase <
                Low = low risk
Low risk (tumor < 1 cm): Observation only

ER, Estrogen receptor; PR, progesterone receptor; C, cyclophosphamide; A, doxorubicin; F, fluorouracil; Tam, tamoxifen; M, methotrexate.

Table 4. Studies in patients with high-risk node-negative breast cancer

Intergroup 0102: CMF vs CAF±Tam
NSABP B-19: M → F vs CMF
NSABP B-23: CMF±Tam vs AC±Tam
INT 0137: A (54 mg/m^2) C (1.2 g/m^2 vs A (81 mg/m^2) → C (2.4 g/m^2)

CAF + tamoxifen. Meanwhile, the Intergroup completed accrual of 1500 women last year to INT 0137, a trial that compares combination to sequential chemotherapy. Patients with 1–3 positive nodes were eligible along with node-negative tumors that had negative hormone receptor status or were above 2 cm in diameter. This study delivered the same total cumulative dose to patients in both arms, but the dose intensity in the sequential arm was 66% higher for doxorubicin and 300% higher for cyclophosphamide.

Node-Positive Breast Cancer

In the late 1980s and early 1990s, studies in node-positive women centered around two main questions: Is combination chemo-hormonal therapy preferable to either modality alone for pre- and/or post-menopausal women? Do higher than standard doses of chemotherapy lead to improvements in survival? To answer the first of these questions, the Intergroup have completed accrual to two studies that test chemotherapy versus combined modality therapy in pre-menopausal women and hormonal therapy versus combined modality therapy in post-menopausal women (Table 5). Results from the former study are not yet available, but results from the latter indicate an advantage in disease-free survival for the bimodality arm. This trial should also eventually resolve the debate over whether it is preferable to start tamoxifen concurrently with chemotherapy or to delay it until chemotherapy is completed. The NCIC also is testing whether chemotherapy adds to tamoxifen in pre-menopausal women in their MA.12 trial (Fig. 3). In contrast to INT 0101, this study accepts high-risk node-negative patients as well as receptor-negative/unknown patients.

Table 5. Completed Intergroup trials in patients with node-positive breast cancer

Group/trial	Design	Eligibility	Accrual
INT 0101	CAF CAF + Zoladex CAF + Zoladex + Tam	Pre-menopausal Receptor-positive	1500
INT 0100	Tam CAF + Tam CAF → Tam	Post-menopausal Receptor-positive	1410

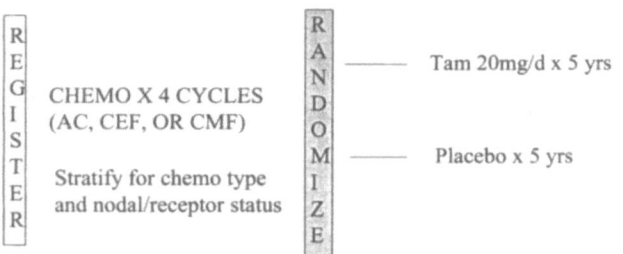

Fig. 3. NCIC trial MA.12: role of tamoxifen in pre-menopausal node-positive or high-risk node-negative breast cancer. CHEMO, Chemotherapy; A, doxorubicin; C, cyclophosphamide; E, epirubicin; F, fluorouracil; M, methotrexate; Tam, tamoxifen

As regards standard versus high-dose chemotherapy, the advent of stem cell rescue and hematopoietic growth factors permitted major dose escalation of cytotoxics in adjuvant trials by 1990. The NCI sponsored two adjuvant studies for women at high risk with ≥10 positive axillary nodes; high doses of multiple alkylating agents with stem cell support were compared to either standard therapy (INT 0121) or to the same drugs at doses not requiring stem cell support (CALGB 9082) (Table 6). Accrual to these trials should be completed this year and preliminary analyses should be available before the year 2000. A new Intergroup study (SWOG 9623) was opened recently in women with 4–9 positive axillary nodes to assess whether high-dose chemotherapy with stem cell support is superior to an intense, sequential, dose-dense regimen that appears promising based on pilot experience from Memorial Sloan-Kettering Hospital (Hudis et al. 1996) (Table 6). The NSABP has reported the results from two consecutive trials designed to assess whether dose escalation of cyclophosphamide alone was beneficial (Fisher et al. 1997b; Wolmark et al. 1997) (Table 7). These two trials did not reveal a significant dose-response effect for this agent. In conclusion, little evidence exists currently to support dose escalation beyond standard doses for adjuvant breast cancer therapy in routine practice (Zujewski et al. 1998). However, results from the aforementioned Intergroup trials will establish if dose escalation of multiple drugs with hematopoietic growth factor and/or stem cell support will become a mainstay of treatment.

Table 6. Intergroup adjuvant high-dose chemotherapy trials

Group	Eligibility	Randomized treatment	Target (no. of patients)
CALGB 9082 (SWOG, NCIC)	≥10 axillary nodes (stage II or IIIA)	High-dose CPB with stem cells vs lower-dose CPB with growth factor	815
INT 0121 (ECOG, SWOG)	≥10 axillary nodes (stage II or IIIA)	High-dose CT with stem cells vs observation	429
SWOG 9623 (CALGB, ECOG, NCCTG)	4–9 axillary nodes (stage II or IIIA)	Sequential A → Ta → Ca with growth factor vs high-dose CPB or C, CBDCA, T	1000

Table 7. Completed NSABP trials in patients with node-positive breast cancer

Group/trial	Design	Eligibility	Accrual
NSABP B-22 22 [b]	AC (60/600×4) [a] AC (60/1200×2) AC (60/1200×4)		2306
NSABP B-25 25 [c]	AC (60/1200×4) AC (60/2400×2) AC (60/2400×4)		2534

[a] AC doses are expressed in mg/m^2.
[b] No G-CSF.
[c] AU arms with G-CSF.

Integrating Taxanes Into Adjuvant Treatment

The discovery of paclitaxel (Taxol) and docetaxel (Taxotere), tubulin-stabilizing agents, has added an important new class of compounds to the breast cancer armamentarium. These agents have demonstrated activity in advanced disease that rivals or exceeds that of doxorubicin, previously the most active cytotoxic against breast cancer (Chan et al. 1997; Sledge et al. 1997). The challenge has been to integrate these agents into adjuvant regimens. Both Intergroup 0148 and NSABP B-28 utilized a sequential approach in which standard doxorubicin/cyclophosphamide for four cycles was followed by randomization to four additional cycles of paclitaxel or no further therapy. However, INT 0148 also evaluated the role of dose escalation of doxorubicin (Table 8). This trial completed accrual of 3000 women in 1997. In a follow-up trial, the Intergroup is evaluating whether the sequence of drug administration or dose intensity makes a difference in the use of doxorubicin, cyclophosphamide, and paclitaxel (Fig. 4). This study uses a 2×2 factorial design and is powered to detect a 25% improvement in median disease-free survival for either sequence or dose intensity. To follow up on the encourag-

Table 8. Integrating taxanes into adjuvant therapy

Intergroup 0148:	Taxol 175 mg/m^2, 3 h
NSABP B-28:	Taxol 200 mg/m^2, 3 h
CALGB 9741:	Taxol 200 mg/m^2, 3 h
NSABP B-27:	Taxotere 100 mg/m^2, 1 h

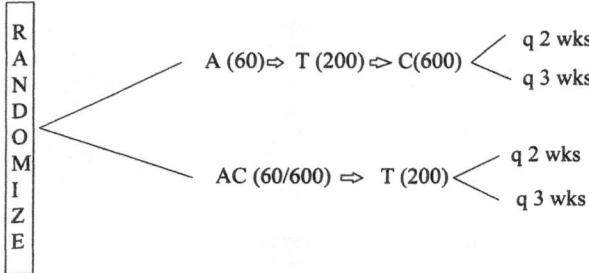

Fig. 4. Trial design of CALBG 9741, an Intergroup study. Doses are expressed in mg/m^2. A, Doxorubicin; T, taxol; C, cyclophosphamide; q, every; wks, weeks

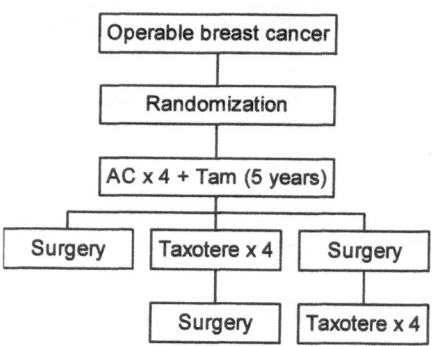

Fig. 5. Trial design of NSABP B-27. AC, Soxorubicin 60 mg/m^2 and cyclophosphamide 600 mg/m^2; Tam, tamoxifen 20 mg daily; Taxotere 100 mg/m^2

ing results from their first neoadjuvant trial (B-18) the NSABP is currently studying the role of docetaxel as part of a neoadjuvant treatment approach (Fig. 5). Results from B-18 indicated that preoperative adjuvant therapy compared to postoperative treatment can downstage tumors, permitting more women to undergo conservative treatment as primary therapy with no decrease in disease-free or overall survival at 5 years (Fisher et al. 1997c). Thus, neoadjuvant treatment offers some potential benefits for certain subsets of patients, especially those with large primary tumors, without impairing survival. It also provides investigators with a way to evaluate the activity of promising new agents in the early disease setting, which may be particularly valuable if primary tumor response rates can be shown to correlate closely with survival. In addition to evaluating the role of docetaxel in B-27, a secondary aim of this trial is to assess whether there are subsets of patients who particularly benefit from additional chemotherapy with docetaxel (i.e., those with positive axillary nodes postoperatively).

Studies in Older Women

Although there is no evidence to suggest that adjuvant treatments become less effective with advancing age, it is desirable to tailor treatment for older women. An increased likelihood of co-existing illness, an inability of some older patients to tolerate severe or even moderate toxicity, and a different risk-benefit ratio based on life expectancy place a premium on finding effective but less aggressive and easily tolerated treatments for older individuals. The Cooperative Groups have designed two trials that ask specific questions in older women with breast cancer. INT 0151 attempts to improve upon tamoxifen, the gold standard for adjuvant treatment in older women, by adding fenretinide, a synthetic vitamin A analogue that appears to complement the activity of tamoxifen in preclinical models (Ratko et al. 1989). The second trial, CALGB 9343, compares tamoxifen to breast irradiation in women 70 years or older treated with breast-conserving surgery. If tamoxifen can be shown to be an adequate substitute for breast irradiation by providing adequate local control, it is likely that more elderly women would opt for conservative surgery. The necessity for breast irradiation as part of conservative therapy can be an important disincentive in choosing this approach over mastectomy, especially in older women, where transportation for the daily treatments over 6 weeks can be problematic.

Correlative Science Studies

The Cooperative Groups have long recognized that the large, adjuvant trials provide an invaluable opportunity to perform correlative science studies. An earlier generation of studies provided the basis for much of our knowledge about the importance of nodes, tumor grade and size, histology, and hormone receptors. More recently, studies have begun to focus on using the molecular characteristics of tumors, such as S phase, c-erbB-2, bcl-2, and others, to predict the response to various treatments. This type of research requires large cohorts of patients treated in a homogeneous fashion, a resource that is unique to Cooperative Group trials. All patients on adjuvant trials sponsored by NCI's Cooperative Groups are now asked to contribute a specimen from their tumor to a central tumor bank. Methods have been instituted to make this resource accessible to all qualified scientists. The NSABP has also begun to bank serum from patients on many of its adjuvant trials. Therefore, it can be hoped that, in addition to answering clinical treatment questions for patients with breast cancer today, participation in clinical trials will provide the scientific leads to enable better therapies for patients in the future.

Future Studies

Pilot trials to plan the next generation of adjuvant studies are already underway. Promising leads that will likely be exploited fall into four major categories. These are: improved cytotoxic regimens, inclusion of agents directed at tumor vascularization and paracrine growth factors, targeted therapy with monoclonal antibodies, and organ-specific therapy that may interfere with metastatic seeding. Combinations of doxorubicin and taxanes administered concurrently, rather than sequentially, have demonstrated high response rates in metastatic disease (Gianni et al. 1995; Bozec et al. 1997) and merit evaluation in the adjuvant setting. Matrix metalloproteinase inhibitors and angiogenesis inhibitors have shown much promise preclinically (Sledge et al. 1995; O'Reilly et al. 1996) and are now being studied in patients with advanced disease. Studies with a her2/neu humanized monoclonal antibody have recently reported encouraging results in the treatment of metastatic disease and adjuvant trials are certain to follow. Finally, the bisphosphonates have demonstrated a positive effect in preventing and decreasing bone metastases, and suggest that strategies that attack the "soil" of the disease may offer substantial benefit (Body et al. 1996). Although faster progress against breast cancer is desired by all, it is likely that these new strategies will require careful testing in large clinical trials if physicians are properly to discern their role in improving the lives of people with this disease.

Summary

The National Cancer Institutes in the United States and Canada sponsor Cooperative Groups to perform randomized trials in distinct subsets of patients with early breast cancer. In women with low-risk ductal carcinoma in situ (DCIS), ongoing studies are evaluating the role of adjuvant breast irradiation. For those with low-risk, node-negative invasive tumors, efforts have been directed to improving the efficacy of tamoxifen, while in high-risk patients the focus has been on improving chemotherapy. The roles of dose intensity and dose density have been evaluated at dose levels requiring either G-CSF or stem cells. More recently, the introduction of taxanes into adjuvant regimens has been a major area of investigation. Following treatment with doxorubicin-cyclophosphamide (AC), patients have been randomized to receive paclitaxel or no further therapy in INT 0148 and NSABP B-28 and to receive docetaxel in NSABP B-27. For women with 4–9 involved nodes, sequential treatment A(doxorubicin)-T(paclitaxel)-C(cyclophosphamide) with G-CSF is being compared to AC×4 followed by high-dose chemotherapy with stem cell support. Cooperative Group trials have been critical in defining the standard of care in the past, and successful completion of these new trials is essential for further progress against breast cancer.

References

Body JJ, Coleman RE, Piccart M (1996) Use of bisphosphonates in cancer patients. Cancer Treat Rev 22:265–287

Bozec L, Nabholtz J-M, Dieras V et al (1997) Docetaxel in combination with doxorubicin and with cyclophosphamide as first-line chemotherapy in metastatic breast cancer: high activity and absence of cardiotoxicity. Proc Am Soc Clin Oncol 16:163a

Chan S, Friedrichs K, Noel D et al (1997) A phase III study of Taxotere vs doxorubicin in patients with metastatic breast cancer who have failed an alkylating containing regimen. Breast Cancer Res Treat 46:23

Chu KC, Tarone RE, Kessler LG et al (1996) Recent trends in US breast cancer incidence, survival and mortality rates. J Natl Cancer Inst 88:1571–1579

Early Breast Cancer Trialists' Collaborative Group (1992) Systemic treatment of early breast cancer by hormonal, cytotoxic, or immune therapy: 133 randomized trials involving 31,000 recurrences and 24,000 deaths among 75,000 women. Lancet 339:1–15, 71–85

Fisher B, Redmond C, Dimitrov N et al (1989) A randomized clinical trial evaluating sequential methotrexate and fluorouracil in the treatment of patients with node-negative breast cancer with estrogen receptor-negative tumors. N Engl J Med 320:473–478

Fisher B, Costantino J, Redmond C et al (1993) Lumpectomy compared with lumpectomy and radiation therapy for the treatment of intraductal breast cancer. N Engl J Med 328:1581–1586

Fisher B, Dignam J, Bryant J et al (1996a) Five versus more than five years of tamoxifen therapy for breast cancer patients with negative lymph nodes and estrogen receptor-positive tumors. J Natl Cancer Inst 88:1529–1542

Fisher B, Dignam J, Mamounas EP et al (1996b) Sequential methotrexate and fluorouracil for the treatment of node-negative breast cancer patients with estrogen receptor-negative tumors: eight-year results from NSABP-B-13 and first report of NSABP-B-19 comparing methotrexate and fluorouracil with conventional CMF. J Clin Oncol 14:1982–1992

Fisher B, Dignam J, DeCillis A et al (1997a) The worth of chemotherapy and tamoxifen over tamoxifen alone in node negative patients with estrogen-receptor positive invasive breast cancer: first results from NSABP B-20. Proc Am Soc Clin Oncol 16:1a

Fisher B, Anderson S, Wickerham DL et al (1997b) Increased intensification and total dose of cyclophosphamide in a doxorubicin-cyclophosphamide regimen for the treatment of primary breast cancer: findings from the National Surgical Adjuvant Breast and Bowel Project B-22. J Clin Oncol 15:1858–1869

Fisher B, Brown A, Mamounas E et al (1997c) Effect of preoperative therapy for primary breast cancer on local-regional disease, disease-free survival and survival: results from NSABP B-18. Proc Am Soc Clin Oncol 16:127a

Fisher B, Dignam J, Wolmark N et al (1998) Lumpectomy and radiation therapy for the treatment of intraductal breast cancer: findings from the National Surgical Adjuvant Breast and Bowel Project B-17. J Clin Oncol 16:441–452

Gianni L, Munzone E, Capri G et al (1995) Paclitaxel by 3-hour infusion in combination with bolus doxorubicin in women with untreated metastatic breast cancer: high antitumor efficacy and cardiac effects in a dose-finding and sequence-finding study. J Clin Oncol 13:2688–2699

Goldhirsch A, Wood WC, Senn H-J, Glick JH, Gelber RD (1995) Meeting highlights: International Consensus Panel on the treatment of primary breast cancer. J Natl Cancer Inst 87:1441–1445

Hudis C, Seidman G, Raptis J et al (1996) Sequential dose-dense doxorubicin (A) paclitaxel (T) cyclophosphamide (C) is less toxic than A concurrent T + C as adjuvant therapy in resected node (+) breast cancer. Proc Am Soc Clin Oncol 15:119

Mansour EG, Gray R, Shatila AH et al (1989) Efficacy of adjuvant chemotherapy in high-risk node-negative breast cancer: an Intergroup study. N Engl J Med 320:485–490

O'Reilly MS, Holmgren L, Chen C, Folkman J (1996) Angiostatin induces and sustains dormancy of human primary tumors in mice. Nat Med 2:689–692

Olivotto IA, Bajdik CD, Math M et al (1994) Adjuvant systemic therapy and survival after breast cancer. N Engl J Med 330:805–810

Ratko TA, Detrisac CJ, Dinger NM et al (1989) Chemopreventive efficacy of combined retinoid and tamoxifen treatment following surgical excision of a primary mammary cancer in female rats. Cancer Res 49:4472–4476

Rosen PP, Groshen S, Saigo PE, Kinne DW, Hellman S (1989) A long-term follow-up study of survival in stage 1 ($T_1N_0M_0$) and stage II ($T_1N_0M_0$) breast carcinoma. J Clin Oncol 7:355–366

Setyono-Ham B, Henkelman MS, Foekens JA, Klijn JGM (1987) Direct inhibitory effects of somatostatin (analogues) on the growth of human breast carcinoma. Cancer Res 47:1566–1570

Sledge GW Jr, Qulali M, Goulet R, Bone EA, Fife R (1995) Effect of matrix metalloproteinase inhibitor Batimastat on breast cancer regrowth and metastastis in athymic mice. J Natl Cancer Inst 87:1546–1550

Sledge GW Jr, Neuberg D, Ingle J et al (1997) Phase III trial of doxorubicin vs paclitaxel vs doxorubicin + paclitaxel as first-line therapy for metastatic breast cancer: an Intergroup trial. Proc Am Soc Clin Oncol 16:1a

Swain SM (1989) Ductal carcinoma in situ – incidence, presentation, guidelines to treatment. Oncology 3:25–31

Wolmark N, Fisher B, Anderson S (1997) The effect of increasing dose intensity and cumulative dose of adjuvant cyclophosphamide in node positive breast cancer: results of NSABP B-25. Breast Cancer Res Treat 46:A16

Zujewski J, Nelson A, Abrams J (1998) Much ado about not...enough data: high-dose chemotherapy with autologous stem cell rescue for breast cancer. J Natl Cancer Inst 90:200–209

International Breast Cancer Study Group Trials

A. Coates

International Breast Cancer Study Group, University of Sydney, Sydney, Australia

The International Breast Cancer Study Group (IBCSG) is the direct successor of the Ludwig Breast Cancer Study Group, which was established in 1978 within the Bern branch of the Ludwig Institute for Cancer Research (LICR). This paper will review the history and achievements of the Group, and describe the further projects currently in the accrual and planning stages.

From its inception, the Group included clinical units both inside and outside the LICR. When LICR decided to discontinue funding of clinical research, the Group established itself in 1987 as IBCSG. It has enjoyed stability both in membership and leadership over more than 20 years of continuous clinical trials research. The Group has completed seven trials in three generation groups, and has another eight trials open for accrual, with planning well advanced for another half dozen. In the process, it has generated a database of carefully documented patients, treated according to standard protocols, which allow valuable spin-off pathological and biological studies. The Group pioneered the use of the Q-TWiST method, and the direct measurement of quality of life in patients participating in adjuvant therapy trials.

Adjuvant Treatment Works

The first generation of trials was conducted between 1978 and 1981. The trials were designed in the light of the demonstrated efficacy of adjuvant systemic therapy, at least for premenopausal women with node-positive disease treated with single-agent (Fisher et al. 1975) or combination chemotherapy (Bonadonna et al. 1976). The first four Ludwig trials addressed questions of combined modality chemoendocrine therapy, and allocated patients to separate trial questions according to menopausal and risk status. These themes have continued to influence the work of the Group.

Trial I was open to premenopausal women with 1, 2 or 3 involved axillary lymph nodes, and compared the Bonadonna standard of 12 cycles of CMF chemotherapy (Bonadonna et al. 1976) to the same therapy with the addition of low-dose continuous prednisone, a therapy designed to reduce adrenal steroid hormone synthesis (Ludwig Breast Cancer Study Group 1985a). Altogether,

491 eligible patients were entered, and at 15 years' median follow-up no difference has emerged in overall survival (OS) or disease-free survival (DFS). Larger doses of CMF were administered in patients receiving prednisone, presumably because neutrophil demargination reduced the perceived need for dosage modification. In this and later studies, it was noted that women who developed amenorrhoea as a result of chemotherapy had a better outcome than those who did not (Pagani et al. 1998). In 327 premenopausal patients with higher-risk disease, defined as four or more involved axillary nodes, the companion trial II examined a more stringent endocrine therapy, surgical oophorectomy, as an addition to 12 cycles of CMF (Ludwig Breast Cancer Study Group 1985b). Again, 15 years of follow-up have not revealed significant differences in OS or DFS, though the relatively small group of 107 patients with estrogen-receptor (ER)-positive had a trend to superior survival with oophorectomy ($p = 0.14$). Because in 1978 the value of adjuvant systemic therapy for postmenopausal patients was not established, trials in older women included an untreated control group. Trial III included 463 eligible postmenopausal patients aged 65 or younger, and compared chemoendocrine therapy with 12 cycles of CMF plus tamoxifen (T) and low-dose prednisone (p) with endocrine therapy (p+T) alone, or with no adjuvant therapy (Ludwig Breast Cancer Study Group 1984). At 15 years' median follow-up, chemoendocrine therapy yielded significantly superior OS and DFS. In this period, ER determination was incomplete, and although among the 156 patients known to have ER-positive tumors endocrine therapy alone (p+T) yielded similar results to chemoendocrine therapy (CMFpT), later studies have confirmed the value of CMF in addition to tamoxifen alone in women with ER-positive tumors (International Breast Cancer Study Group 1997). In the remaining group of 320 patients aged over 65 years, chemotherapy was not tested, but endocrine therapy (p+T) yielded significantly superior OS and DFS than observation.

But Is It Worth It?

Statistical analysis of randomised clinical trials yields high-quality evidence that treatment offers an improvement in survival and DFS, and can make a good if conservative estimate of the magnitude of that benefit, but it cannot alone answer the clinically important question of whether the treatments that produce the benefits are worthwhile. The Q-TWiST model (Gelber and Goldhirsch 1986; Goldhirsch et al. 1989) allowed various assumptions about the relative value of time spent during toxic therapy (TOX), time with neither disease symptoms nor toxicity (Time Without Symptoms or Toxicity – TWiST) and the time after disease relapse (REL). The actual average periods in each state could be observed in a clinical trial, and the time in TOX and REL discounted by some arbitrary utility factor to produce an overall weighted outcome score for each therapy, known as Q-TWiST. If one therapy produced superior Q-TWiST for all plausible utility coefficients of TOX and REL, it could reasonably be assumed that the benefits of treatment were sufficient to outweigh the adverse effects. Direct measurement of the utility values associated with various health states traditionally requires labour-intensive time trade-off or standard gamble techniques (Coates and Simes 1993), but recent work has shown that useful approximations to utilities can be directly measured with appropriate linear analogue (LASA) scales (Stigglebout et al. 1996; Hürny et al. 1998). The demonstration in trial III that, for almost all values of the utilities associated with TOX and REL, chemoendocrine therapy produced superior quality-adjusted outcomes, did much to reassure clinicians about the acceptability of cytotoxic therapy. Patient self-assessment of quality of life, described below, later largely confirmed this impression.

A Second Question: Timing and Duration of Therapy

As accrual to the first four studies was completed, their results were unknown. Therefore, while waiting for information to guide future studies of chemoendocrine therapy, the Group decided to test the value of starting adjuvant therapy as early as possible after surgery. An earlier study (Kjellgren et al. 1989) had suggested the value of perioperative cyclophosphamide, and we wished to test the concept using combination chemotherapy (CMF).

Node-Negative Patients

Perioperative treatment was administered to patients so randomised before the pathology of the axillary nodes was known, and thus the trial included women whose axillary nodes were later shown to be uninvolved. In such patients no further treatment was given, and the trial for them was therefore a single cycle of perioperative CMF versus no adjuvant therapy. The initial results for the 1275 node-negative patients showed a significant benefit in DFS (Ludwig Breast Cancer Study Group 1989), but this difference has diminished with further follow-up. At 12 years' median follow-up the OS was 74% with therapy and 70% without ($p = 0.22$) while DFS was 59% and 56% respectively ($p = 0.17$). Hypothesis-generating subset analysis showed that the benefit of a single perioperative cycle of CMF appeared to be greatest in the group of 160 postmenopausal patients with ER-negative tumors (DFS 70% versus 48%, $p = 0.001$; OS 75% versus 48%, $p = 0.008$).

Node-Positive Patients

Patients with positive nodes were randomised to receive the perioperative cycle only, six conventionally timed cycles of CMF or both perioperative and conventionally timed therapy for a total of seven cycles. The single cycle was not as effective as more prolonged therapy in these patients (Ludwig Breast Cancer Study Group 1988). Tamoxifen was given during conventionally timed CMF in postmenopausal patients only. We had considered including tamoxifen in premenopausal patients, so that the therapy was the same in both groups to allow later analysis by various age divisions, but the report of an apparent adverse effect of adding tamoxifen to melphalan therapy (Fisher et al. 1981) led us to avoid tamoxifen in premenopausal patients, so that the trial is best regarded as separate questions in the two menopausal subgroups. At 12 years of follow-up, the 715 node-positive premenopausal patients showed DFS of 37%, 41% and 21% for seven, six and one cycle respectively (p <0.0001). Corresponding OS figures were 53%, 52% and 31% ($p = 0.001$). Among the 514 postmenopausal node-positive patients the DFS figures were 35%, 32% and 22% for seven, six and one cycle ($p = 0.0002$), with OS of 48%, 37% and 35% ($p = 0.05$).

Booster Chemotherapy

Resistance to adjuvant cytotoxic chemotherapy is not absolute. Patients whose tumor relapses after such therapy may still respond to the same therapy used for metastatic disease (Valagussa et al. 1989; Castiglione-Gertsch et al. 1997). This demonstrates that the tumor cells are still potentially sensitive to the regimen which "fails", and suggests that relapse might be avoided by appropriately scheduled reintroduction of the same therapy before relapse. Accordingly, the Group has been interested in schedules of timed reintroduction of cytotoxic treatment. Trial VI included 1475 eligible premenopausal node-positive patients between 1986 and 1993. It used a factorial 2×2 design to compare initial CMF with or without three single cycles of CMF given 3, 6 and 9 months after completion of the initial course, and whether the initial course should be three or six cycles of CMF. It emerged that three cycles of initial CMF was less effective than six cycles, but the effect was mainly in younger premenopausal patients. Reintroduction of late CMF cycles showed a promising trend, but remains experimental (International Breast Cancer Study Group 1996). This study and the corresponding study for postmenopausal patients represent the first trials in which the Group prospectively measured quality of life, and also allowed for local treatment by either mastectomy or breast conservation.

Chemoendocrine Therapy Revisited: Node-Positive Patients

The value of adding chemotherapy to tamoxifen had been shown in trial III, but doubt remained as to whether such treatment was worthwhile. In trial VII we therefore randomised 1212 eligible postmenopausal node-positive patients to tamoxifen alone, or to the addition of three initial cycles of CMF (given concurrently with tamoxifen) or three delayed single cycles of CMF at months 9, 12 and 15, or both initial and delayed CMF. Initial chemotherapy added to the efficacy of tamoxifen alone, especially in patients with ER positive tumors (International Breast Cancer Study Group 1997).

Ongoing Trials in Node-Negative Patients

Premenopausal Patients

There is still a lack of data directly comparing ovarian ablation with chemotherapy, and exploring the additional value of combining the two modalities. In 1990 the Group launched trial VIII which randomised premenopausal patients with node-negative disease to six cycles of CMF versus ovarian ablation using goserelin for 2 years versus the sequence of six cycles of CMF followed by goserelin for 18 months. The trial initially had a no-treatment control arm, but this was dropped in 1992 when it became apparent that in the light of evolving data from the Overview of other studies (Early Breast Cancer Trialists' Collaborative Group 1992) some clinicians were reluctant to randomise the selected node-negative patients for whom chemotherapy was deemed a reasonable option to a trial where they might receive no adjuvant therapy. At the end of 1997 the trial had accrued 983 of a planned 1200 patients, making this probably the largest trial to date of an ovarian ablation strategy. Although the choice of 2 years' goserelin was made on logistic grounds, the concept of benefit from a potentially reversible ovarian suppression is supported by the observation that patients who develop amenorrhoea on adjuvant chemotherapy retain the beneficial effect even if their menses subsequently resume (Pagani et al. 1998).

Postmenopausal Patients

The added morbidity of cytotoxic therapy in older patients at relatively low risk of relapse is a particular concern, especially since the magnitude of incremental benefit over tamoxifen alone may be less than in younger patients. Trial IX therefore compares tamoxifen alone to a sequential use of three cycles of CMF followed by tamoxifen. Quality of life is measured prospectively and is an especially important endpoint in this group of patients. At 31 December 1997 accrual was virtually complete, with 1540 of a planned 1600 patients.

Ongoing Trials in Node-Positive Patients

The current set of trials for node-positive patients was commenced in 1993. In the light of the demonstration of the efficacy of adjuvant ovarian ablation (Early Breast Cancer Trialists' Collaborative Group 1992), patients were divided into those considered potentially suitable for endocrine therapy alone, and those considered to absolutely require chemotherapy. In this and subsequent generations of trials, numbering was changed from Roman to Arabic numerals. Perimenopausal patients were included with postmenopausal for these studies, whereas in earlier studies they had been included with the premenopausal group.

Premenopausal Patients Suitable for Endocrine Therapy Alone

In this population the Group identified as the most important question the comparison of ovarian ablation alone with ablation plus chemotherapy. Trial 11–93 includes premenopausal patients with involved lymph nodes and at least one positive hormone receptor. It allows ablation by surgical oophorectomy, ovarian irradiation or prolonged LHRH analogue, and randomises patients to ablation alone or to ablation plus four cycles of intravenous anthracycline (doxorubicin or epirubicin) and cyclophosphamide (AC). All patients then receive tamoxifen for a total of 5 years. As with all studies comparing widely disparate treatments, accrual has been slow, but at 31 December 1997 the trial had accrued 157 of a revised target of 400 patients.

Premenopausal Patients Not Suitable for Endocrine Therapy Alone

Although this study was conceived as mainly for patients with receptor-negative tumors, clinicians and patients were allowed to opt for trial 13–93 if for any reason they were unwilling to contemplate endocrine therapy alone. In fact about 60% of the patients entering the study have ER-positive tumors, and this led to upward revision of the target accrual to allow for the better than expected baseline prognosis. All patients receive four cycles of AC followed by three cycles of CMF. The study revisits the question of a gap between therapy blocks, assigning patients to receive CMF either immediately after AC or at 6 months from the start of AC. The second question addressed in a factorial 2×2 design is the addition of tamoxifen after chemotherapy. The study has proved popular and at 31 December 1997 accrual was 1042 of a revised target of 1225.

Postmenopausal Patients Suitable for Endocrine Therapy Alone

Trial 12–93 compares the two anti-estrogens tamoxifen and toremifene, each given for 5 years. It initially sought to compare the addition of chemotherapy to anti-estrogen by randomising patients to anti-estrogen alone or to four cycles of AC concurrently with or before the commencement of anti-estrogen therapy. Accrual proved unacceptable, and in early 1997 the chemotherapy randomisation was dropped, leaving the trial as a simple comparison of tamoxifen versus toremifene. Prior chemotherapy is now allowable at the investigator's discretion, and is a stratification factor in the randomised portion of the trial.

Postmenopausal Patients Not Suitable for Endocrine Therapy Alone

In this population of selected high-risk postmenopausal patients, the treatment arms of trial 14–93 are similar to two of those in trial 13–93, with all patients receiving four cycles of AC and three cycles of CMF, randomised to a gap or no gap. All patients, however, receive 5 years' anti-estrogen, and the second question is the comparison of tamoxifen and toremifene, as in trial 12–93. At 31 December 1997 trial 14–93 had accrued 723 of a planned 884 patients, the target accrual again having been increased to allow for the inclusion of a greater than expected proportion (59%) of patients with ER-positive tumors.

High-Risk Patients

One of the most important unresolved questions in the adjuvant treatment of high-risk patients is the value of high-dose therapy requiring peripheral blood progenitor cell (PBPC) rescue. Trial 15–95 is testing a triple transplant regimen developed in Australia, in which premenopausal and younger postmenopausal patients with ten involved nodes (five if also ER-negative or stage T3) have stem cells harvested with G-CSF, without initial priming cytotoxic therapy, then proceed to three cycles of epirubicin 200 mg/m^2 plus cyclophosphamide 4g/m^2 with MESNA uroprotection and PBPC rescue, with further G-CSF. Cycles are repeated at 21-day intervals. This therapy is randomised against the same standard dose sequence of four cycles of AC and three cycles of CMF which is the control arm for trial 13–93. Accrual has been good, and a decision was recently taken to extend the target accrual to 300, to allow a more sensitive test of the high-dose regimen.

Quality of Life

As discussed above, quality of life has been regarded as an important endpoint in all Group trials since 1986. Sequential self-assessment of quality of life in studies VI and VII showed that, on average, patients reported a steadily improving quality of life during the first 18 months after diagnosis, and that chemotherapy during that time had a measurable, but mild and transient effect on reported quality of life scores (Hürny et al. 1996). In more recent studies, the instruments used for patient self-assessment of quality of life have been refined (Bernhard et al. 1997), and in selected studies economic analyses are also included.

New Trial Projects

Although the Group has a record of successful accrual for over 20 years, it is recognised that many currently important questions can better be addressed with more rapid accrual of very large numbers of patients. This requires inter-Group collaboration. The past year has seen great progress toward an effective model through several ad hoc arrangements, and most recently the emergence of the Breast International Group (BIG) as a forum in which established clinical trial Groups including IBCSG contribute to trials organised and led by one of the constituent Groups, supported by the BIG secretariat.

Taxanes

Paclitaxel and docetaxel have a high level of activity in the treatment of metastatic breast cancer, but the place of these agents in adjuvant therapy is unknown. The Breast European Adjuvant Studies Team (BREAST) is leading a BIG inter-Group trial which will examine sequential or combined use of docetaxel and doxorubicin, each followed by CMF, against appropriate non-taxane control therapies.

Aromatase Inhibitors

Several new agents in this class are available. A BIG trial led by IBCSG will compare 5 years of letrozole to 5 years of tamoxifen, and to the two sequences of tamoxifen followed by letrozole and vice-versa. Another study led by Charles Coombes is investigating the introduction of exemestane to patients who have received 2–3 years of tamoxifen, versus continuing the tamoxifen to 5 years. Further trials are examining the use of letrozole versus placebo in women who complete 5 years of tamoxifen, and the use of anastrozole as an alternative or in combination with tamoxifen.

Hormone Replacement Therapy

IBCSG is collaborating in the HABITS (*h*ormonal replacement therapy *a*fter *b*reast cancer: *is* *i*t *s*afe?) study led by Lars Holmberg. This trial addresses the important question of whether estrogen replacement therapy can safely be given to women who have been treated for early breast cancer.

Spin-Off Studies

The large database of IBCSG patients allows useful analysis of a number of questions not the direct subject of the particular trials. A sample of recent studies is described below.

Pregnancy After Breast Cancer

IBCSG investigators wished to evaluate the impact of subsequent pregnancy on the prognosis of patients with breast cancer. We identified 108 patients who became pregnant after diagnosis of breast cancer. Of these 22 (20%) had relapsed before the pregnancy. We selected a matched control group for the remaining 86 patients from the IBCSG database. Overall 5- and 10-year survival from the diagnosis of breast cancer was superior among patients who subsequently became pregnant (odds ratio 0.30; 95% confidence interval 0.12–0.92; $p=0.035$). It therefore appears that subsequent pregnancy does not adversely affect the prognosis of early breast cancer.

Timing of Surgery in the Menstrual Cycle

It has been suggested that the prognosis of premenopausal patients is influenced by the timing of breast surgery during the menstrual cycle. To address this issue, we examined the outcome of 1033 patients in trial VI whose surgery could be assigned to the follicular ($n=358$) or luteal ($n=675$) phase of the cycle. We found a slightly worse outcome among patients whose operation was in the follicular phase (5-year DFS 53% versus 58%; hazard ratio 1.16 (95% confidence interval 0.94–1.38; $p=0.20$). Among patients with ER-negative tumors the effect appeared more marked (hazard ratio 1.60; 1.12–2.25; $p=0.008$) (Goldhirsch et al. 1997). Less traumatic procedures such as fine needle biopsy in the follicular phase were not associated with any detectable adverse effect.

Prognostic Importance of Thymidylate Synthase

Thymidylate synthase (TS) is a target for fluoropyrimidine antimetabolites such as 5-fluorouracil. High levels might therefore be expected to confer relative resistance to these agents. TS was estimated in stored tumor tissue from 210 node-negative and 278 node-positive patients in trial V. High TS levels were associated with inferior DFS in node-positive patients only (44% versus 27% at 10 years; $p=0.03$). The additional benefit of extending CMF treatment beyond a single perioperative cycle was especially marked in patients with tumors containing high levels of TS (Pestalozzi et al. 1997).

Conclusion

The IBCSG has a record of successful adjuvant clinical trials research over more than 20 years. It has been instrumental in stressing the value of chemoendocrine therapy, maintaining scientific scrutiny of the role of ovarian ablation. It has had a leading role in incorporating the concepts of quality of life into adjuvant therapy trials and decision making, and has contributed to numerous studies of prognostic and predictive markers. It has been a great privilege and pleasure to contribute to the Group's work in the past 20 years. It is exciting to be part of its future.

Summary

The International Breast Cancer Study Group (IBCSG) was established in 1978 as the Ludwig Breast Cancer Study Group. It involved member institutions from Switzerland, Australia, New Zealand, Sweden, Italy, Slovenia, South Africa, Spain, Canada, Hong Kong and at various times from other countries. It has completed seven trials in three generations, and has a further eight trials currently open. Total accural to December 1997 exceeds 12 000, and more than 9000 of these patients are in active follow-up. Early trials established the pattern of addressing important biological questions and adapting the randomisation to the risk group of the patient. The first two generations of trials demonstrated that combined modality chemoendocrine therapy was superior to endocrine therapy alone or no therapy in node-positive postmenopausal patients; that a single perioperative cycle improved disease-free survival (DFS) in node-negative patients, but was inferior to more prolonged therapy in node-positive patients; and that six conventionally timed cycles of CMF were as effective as seven cycles commenced in the perioperative period. Recently reported trials in node-positive patients showed that three early cycles of CMF chemotherapy added to tamoxifen in postmenopausal patients, while late reintroduction of chemotherapy appeared detrimental, particularly in patients with ER-negative tumors. In premenopausal patients six initial cycles were superior to three, especially in younger patients. Current studies in node-positive patients are addressing the role of a gap between courses of different chemotherapy, and the relative value of the anti-estrogens tamoxifen and toremifene. In node-negative premenopausal patients ovarian suppression with goserelin is being tested either instead of or added to CMF, while the value of initial CMF before tamoxifen is being tested in node-negative postmenopausal patients. For high-risk patients a triple-transplant regimen is being compared with conventional dose therapy. Planning for future trials recognises the need for rapid accrual of large numbers of similar patients, and therefore the need for inter-Group collaboration. The emergence of the Breast International Group as a consortium of European, Australasian and Canadian cooperative Groups is important to the rapid evaluation of new agents and strategies.

References

Bernhard J, Hürny C, Coates AS, Peterson H, Castiglione-Gertsch M, Gelber RD, Goldhirsch A, Senn H-J, Rudenstam C-M, International Breast Cancer Study Group (1997) Quality of life assessment in patients receiving adjuvant therapy for breast cancer: the IBCSG approach. Ann Oncol 8:825–835

Bonadonna G, Brusamolino E, Valagussa P, Rossi A, Brugnatelli L, Brambilla C, De LM, Tancini G, Bajetta E, Musumeci R, Veronesi U (1976) Combination chemotherapy as an adjuvant treatment in operable breast cancer. N Engl J Med. 294:405–410

Castiglione-Gertsch M, Tattersall MH, Hacking A, Goldhirsch A, Gudgeon A, Gelber RD, Lindtner J, Coates AS, Collins J, Isley M, Senn H-J, Rudenstam C-M, International Breast Cancer Study Group (1997) Retreating recurrent breast cancer with the same CMF-containing regimen used as adjuvant therapy. Eur J Cancer 14:2321–2325

Coates AS, Simes RJ (1993) Patient assessment of adjuvant treatment in operable breast cancer. In: Williams CJ (ed) Introducing new treatments for cancer: practical, ethical and legal problems. Wiley, Chichester, pp 447–458

Early Breast Cancer Trialists' Collaborative Group (1992) Systemic treatment of early breast cancer by hormonal, cytotoxic or immune therapy. 133 randomised trials involving 31000 recurrences and 24000 deaths among 75000 women. Lancet 339:1–15, 71–85

Fisher B, Carbone P, Economou SG, Frelick R, Glass A, Lerner H, Redmond C, Zelen M, Band P, Katrych DL, Wolmark N, Fisher ER (1975) L-phenylalanine mustard (L-PAM) in the management of primary breast cancer. A report of early findings. N Engl J Med 292:117–122

Fisher B, Redmond C, Brown A, Wolmark N, Wittliff J, Fisher ER, Plotkin D, Bowman D, Sachs S, Wolter J, Frelick R, Desser R, LiCalzi N, Geggie P, Campbell T, Elias EG, Prager D, Koontz P, Volk H, Dimitrov N, Gardner B, Lerner H, Shibata H (1981) Treatment of primary breast cancer with chemotherapy and tamoxifen. N Engl J Med. 305:1–6

Gelber RD, Goldhirsch A (1986) A new endpoint for the assessment of adjuvant therapy in postmenopausal women with operable breast cancer. J Clin Oncol 4:1772–1779

Goldhirsch A, Gelber RD, Simes RJ, Glasziou PP, Coates AS (1989) Costs and benefits of adjuvant therapy in breast cancer: a quality-adjusted survival analysis. J Clin Oncol 7:36–44

Goldhirsch A, Gelber RD, Castiglione-Gertsch M, O'Neill A, Thürlimann B, Rudenstam C-M, Lindtner J, Collins J, Forbes JF, Crivellari D, Coates AS, Cavalli F, Simoncini E, Fey M, Pagani O, Price K, Senn H-J, International Breast Cancer Study Group (1997) Menstrual cycle and timing of breast surgery in premenopausal node-positive breast cancer: results of the International Breast Cancer Study Group (IBCSG) Trial VI. Ann Oncol 8:751–756

Hürny C, Bernhard J, Coates AS, Castiglione M, Peterson HF, Gelber RD, Forbes JF, Rudenstam C-M, Simoncini E, Crivellari D, Goldhirsch A, Senn H-J (1996) Impact of adjuvant therapy on quality of life in women with node-positive operable breast cancer. Lancet 347:1279–1284

Hürny C, van Wegberg B, Bacchi M, Bernhard J, Thürlimann B, Ral O, Perey L, Bonnefoi H, Coates AS (1998) Subjective health estimations (SHE) in patients with advanced breast cancer: an adapted utility concept for cancer clinical trials. Br J Cancer (in press)

International Breast Cancer Study Group (1996) Duration and reintroduction of adjuvant chemotherapy for node-positive premenopausal breast cancer patients. J Clin Oncol 14:1885–1893

International Breast Cancer Study Group (1997) Effectiveness of adjuvant chemotherapy in combination with tamoxifen for node-positive postmenopausal breast cancer patients. J Clin Oncol 15:1385–1394

Kjellgren K, Nissen-Meyer R, Norin T (1989) Perioperative adjuvant chemotherapy in breast cancer. The Scandinavian adjuvant chemotherapy study 1. Acta Oncol 28:899–901

Ludwig Breast Cancer Study Group (1984) Randomized trial of chemo-endocrine therapy, endocrine therapy and mastectomy alone in postmenopausal patients with operable breast cancer and axillary node metastasis. Lancet 1:1256–1260

Ludwig Breast Cancer Study Group (1985a) A randomized trial of adjuvant combination chemotherapy with or without prednisone in premenopausal breast cancer patients with metastases in one to three axillary nodes. Cancer Res 45:4454–4459

Ludwig Breast Cancer Study Group (1985b) Chemotherapy with or without oophorectomy in high-risk premenopausal patients with operable breast cancer. J Clin Oncol 3:1059–1067

Ludwig Breast Cancer Study Group (1988) Combination adjuvant chemotherapy for node-positive breast cancer. Inadequacy of a single perioperative cycle. N Engl J Med 319:677–683

Ludwig Breast Cancer Study Group (1989) Prolonged disease-free survival after one course of perioperative adjuvant chemotherapy for node-negative breast cancer. N Engl J Med 320:491–496

Pagani O, O'Neill A, Castiglione-Gertsch M, Gelber RD, Goldhirsch A, Rudenstam C-M, Lindtner J, Collins J, Crivellari D, Coates AS, Cavalli F, Thürlimann B, Simoncini E, Fey M, Price K, Senn H-J, International Breast Cancer Study Group (1998) Prognostic impact of amenorrhea after adjuvant chemotherapy in premenopausal breast cancer patients with axillary node involvement. Eur J Cancer (in press)

Pestalozzi BC, Peterson HF, Gelber RD, Goldhirsch A, Gusterson BA, Trihia H, Lindtner J, Cortes FH, Simmoncini E, Byrne MJ, Golouh R, Rudenstam CM, Castiglione-Gertsch M, Allegra CJ, Johnston PG (1997) Prognostic importance of thymidylate synthase expression in early breast cancer. J Clin Oncol 15:1923–1931

Stigglebout AM, Eijkemans MJC, Kiebert GM, Kievit J, Leer J-WH, de Haes JCJM (1996) The 'utility' of the visual analog scale in medical decision making and technology assessment. Is it an alternative to the time trade off? Int J Technol Assess Health Care 12:291–298

Valagussa P, Brambilla C, Zambetti M, Bonadonna G (1989) Salvage treatments in relapsing resectable breast cancer. Recent Results Cancer Res 115:69–76

Nordic Trials of Adjuvant Therapy in Primary Breast Cancer

H. T. Mouridsen

Department of Oncology 5074, Rigshospitalet, 9 Blegdamsvej, 2100 Copenhagen, Denmark

The Scandinavian (Nordic) countries are Denmark, Finland, Iceland, Norway and Sweden, with a combined total population of approximately 23 millions and an annual number of new breast cancer patients of approximately 12 000. The health care systems are very similar in the Scandinavian countries and virtually all cancer patient care occurs within the framework of the public health care system.

Scandinavian Breast Group

The Scandinavian Breast Group (SBG) was established in 1989 with members representing all the disciplines involved in the diagnosis, treatment, and research of breast cancer, i.e., surgery, histopathology, oncology, statistics, and basic research.

The group of approximately 70 nominated members, chaired by an executive committee of 4 members, meet once a year to exchange experience and ideas. The group was established with the general objectives were to improve knowledge of all aspects of breast cancer and to facilitate the interchange of information between colleagues involved in active breast cancer research, to facilitate the exchange of information on breast cancer between the Scandinavian group and those in other countries, to review critically methods used in breast cancer research, to keep a record of ongoing clinical trials and other research work in progress, to make better utilization of available biological material, and to promote research in all aspects of breast cancer.

The first analysis of ongoing trials in primary breast cancer was done 1992. Questionnaires were sent to representatives from all clinical research groups in the Scandinavian countries. The questionnaires asked questions related to current practice and research within the field of surgery, radiotherapy, and systemic therapy.

As regards the latter it appeared that approximately 20 protocols were active, analysing seven major questions of adjuvant systemic therapy. However, a substantial proportion of the individual trials recruited an insufficient number of patients to enable valid conclusions within a reasonable time, which called for closer Scandinavian cooperation.

Clinical Trials Group of the SBG

As a results of this analysis the Clinical Trials Group of the SBG was established with the major objective of coordinating and organizing trials in primary and advanced breast cancer.

The Clinical Trials Group is made up of approximately 25 representatives from all the departments in the Scandinavian countries responsible for the treatment of patients with primary and advanced breast cancer. Representatives from each of the national (Denmark, Iceland, Finland, Norway) or regional (Sweden, six oncology regions) cooperative groups form the Clinical Trials Committee which also includes two biostatisticians. The latter are nominated among the statistical committee composed of statisticians from all the Scandinavian countries.

Current Activities

The current active protocols of systemic therapy in primary breast cancer briefly to be described here are two studies initiated by the Danish Breast Cancer Cooperative Group (DBCG 89 B and DBCG 89 D), with later participation by other Scandinavian countries, and two studies initiated by the Scandinavian Clinical Trials Group.

DBCG 89 B Trial

This study enrolls premenopausal patients with operable receptor-positive invasive breast cancer, either with a tumor size greater than 5 cm or with positive axillary nodes. Patients are randomized to either castration by radiotherapy (5 Gy×3) or surgery or to chemotherapy with CMF (C 600 mg/m^2, M 40 mg/m^2, F 600 mg/m^2) administered intravenously day 1 every 3 weeks for nine cycles. Radiotherapy is recommended in patients having breast-conserving surgery and in subsets of mastectomized patients with positive nodes. Following preliminarly analysis of a previous trial (DBCG 82 B), initially radiotherapy following mastectomy was recommended in patients below 45 years of age with four or more positive nodes. However, from January 1995 radiotherapy was recommended in all patients, with avoidance of axillary irradiation if ten or more nodes had been removed (Overgaard et al. 1997).

As of January 1, 1998, 650 patients from Denmark, Iceland, and Sweden have been randomized in this study. In Denmark all eligible patients are registered, but among these 815 patients did not accept randomization. Following patient preference, 40% had castration and 60% CMF. Data from both randomized and nonrandomized patients are reported to the secretariat. The scheduled number of patients to be randomized is 750, and the study will probably be closed during 1998. Adjoining studies of cardiac and bone morbidity are been planned by linking the DBCG Register and the Hospital Discharge Register, which reports the diagnoses of patients admitted to hospital.

Rationale of the Study

Indirect comparisons indicate that similar mortality reductions can be achieved with ovarian ablation and chemotherapy in premenopausal patients (Early Breast Cancer Trialists' Collaborative Group 1992). In a randomized trial in premenopausal node-positive patients, unselected for receptor status, similar prognoses were achieved with CMF and castration (Scottish Cancer Trials Breast Cancer Group and IRCF Breast Unit 1993). Retrospective subgroup analysis according to receptor status indicated that the relative benefits of chemotherapy and ovarian ablation depend on the estrogen receptor status. The authors conclude that ovarian ablation seems more effective in patients with receptor-positive tumors whereas CMF may be more effective for patients with low or negative receptor status. These data from indirect comparisons and from retrospective subgroup analyses should be confirmed in a prospective study.

DBCG 89 D Trial

This study enrolls three groups of patients with operable breast cancer: (a) premenopausal patients with negative or unknown receptor status in a tumor more than 5 cm in size or with positive nodes, (b) postmenopausal patients with receptor-negative tumor more than 5 cm in size or with positive nodes, and (c) premenopausal patients with a node-negative tumor, malignancy grade II–III.

Patients are randomized according to a 2×2 design, into four groups receiving CMF (as in DBCG 89 B), CEF (C 600 mg/m^2, E 60 mg/m^2, F 600 mg/m^2) administered intravenously day 1 every 3 weeks for nine cycles, CMF + pamidronate (PAM, 150 mg twice daily for 4 years), and CEF+pamidronate. Postoperative radiotherapy is recommended following breast-conserving surgery and following mastectomy in premenopausal node-positive patients according to the guidelines described for DBCG 89 B.

As of January 1, 1998, 1410 patients in Denmark, Iceland, and Sweden have been randomized. Of these 1050 have been randomized to chemotherapy with or without pamidronate. That part of the study was closed for patient entry January 1996. At that time it was concluded by an independent external committee that because there was a lower rate of bone metastases (endpoint in the pamidronate part of the study) than expected, the study had either to include an additional unrealistically high number of patients or to prolong the time of observation before the first analysis was undertaken. Due to toxicity problems with oral pamidronate in patients with osteoporosis, the latter solution was chosen.

In Denmark another 1250 patients were eligible but did not agree to be randomized. Of these 90% have received CMF and 10% have received CEF. Data from both randomized and nonrandomized patients are reported to the secretariat. The scheduled number of randomized patients is 1500 so the study will close during 1998. Long term cardiac and bone morbidity will also be analyzed in the study by linking the DBCG Register and the Hospital Discharge Register.

Rationale of the Study

In the Scandinavian countries CMF remains standard adjuvant chemotherapy and the role of substituting methotrexate by an equitoxic dose of anthracycline remains to be demonstrated (Mouridsen 1996). One recent major study and several earlier smaller studies (Hortobagyi et al. 1996) have demonstrated that bone-related events can be postponed with pamidronate in advanced breast cancer. The role of pamidronate as an adjuvant treatment has not been analyzed previously.

SBG 9401 Trial

This study enrolls patients aged less than 60 years with operable breast cancer with eight or more positive axillary nodes or with five or more positive nodes if the tumor is receptor-negative and with malignancy grade II–III or with high S-phase fraction. Patients are randomized to receive dose-escalating CEF (dose levels 1–4, C 900–1800 mg/m^2, E 75–120 mg/m^2, F 600 mg/m^2) administered intravenously day on 1 every 3 weeks for nine cycles + filgrastim or to three cycles of CEF (first two cycles C 600 mg/m^2, E 60 mg/m^2, F 600 mg/m^2, third cycle C 1200 mg/m^2, E 90 mg/m^2, F 600 mg/m^2 + filgrastim) followed by high-dose chemotherapy (C 1.5 g/m^2 days –7 to –4, thiotepa 125 mg/m^2 days –7 to –4 and carboplatin 200 mg/m^2 days –7 to –4) followed by autologous stemcell support. Patients in both arms receive subsequent radiotherapy and tamoxifen for 5 years.

As of January 1998 503 patients, have been randomized. The target accrual is 600 patients, which will be reached during 1998.

Rationale of the Study

Provided high-dose chemotherapy plus stem cell support proves beneficial in primary high-risk breast cancer patients, a relevant subsequent question would be if similar results can be achieved with standard chemotherapy dose-escalated according to individual tolerability.

SBG 9701 Trial

This study enrolls patients with climacteric symptoms given previous treatment for in situ or invasive breast cancer stage I–II with four or fewer positive nodes. Patients are randomized to observation versus hormone replacement therapy (HRT) for 2 years. In the observation group patients are offered symptomatic treatment with clonidine or β-blockers. At 2 years HRT may continue according to patient preference, but patients will be informed that continued therapy is outside the framework of the scientific study. The study has recently been activated in some of the Scandinavian regions. Other groups are strongly encouraged to participate.

Rationale of the Study

The potential risks of HRT in patients previously treated for breast cancer remain under debate (Bergkvist et al. 1989; Dhodapka et al. 1995; Roy et al. 1996) and should be analyzed and balanced against the potential benefit in terms of relief of menopausal symptoms.

Future Activities

As concerns endocrine therapy, tamoxifen, for 5 years is considered standard in the Scandinavian countries. Research questions relate to the role of aromatase inhibitors in the adjuvant situation, either against tamoxifen or via sequential administration of the two agents. Studies investigating this area will also analyze potential long-term bone and cardiac morbidity.

As concerns chemotherapy, CMF is still generally considered standard. Immediate questions include the role of dose-escalating chemotherapy, the role of anthracyclines and taxanes, and the predictive values of cytogenetic markers.

Summary

The Scandinavian Breast Group (SBG), established in 1989, has members representing research, diagnosis, and treatment of breast cancer. In 1992 the SBG analyzed ongoing adjuvant trials in the Scandinavian countries. Many trials were analyzing similar questions, but a substantial proportion recruited an insufficient number of patients to enable valid conclusions within a reasonable time. As a result the SBG Clinical Trials Group was established to coordinate and organize trials in primary and advanced disease. Present activities include a study in premenopausal patients with node-positive, receptor-positive disease (CMF vs castration), a study in pre- and postmenopausal patients with node-positive, receptor-negative disease (CMF vs CEF), and a study in high-risk patients aged <60 years (dose-escalating CEF vs three cycles of CEF followed by high-dose chemotherapy and autologous stem cell support). All these studies are planned to close during 1998. Another study has recently been activated. This enrolls patients with climacteric symptoms given previous treatment for in situ or invasive breast cancer, who are randomized to observation vs hormone replacement therapy for 2 years. Other groups are strongly encouraged to participate. Potential future activities are briefly described. Some of these will be undertaken in international collaboration.

References

Bergkvist L, Adami H-O, Persson I (1989) Prognosis after breast cancer diagnosis in women exposed to estrogen and estrogen-progestin replacement therapy. Am J Epidemiol 139:221–228

Dhodapka MV, Ingle JN, Ahmann DL (1995) Estrogen replacement therapy withdrawal and regression of metastatic breast cancer. Cancer 75:43–46

Early Breast Cancer Trialists' Collaborative Group (1992) Systemic treatment of early breast cancer by hormonal, cytotoxic, or immune therapy. Lancet 339:1–15, 71–85

Hortobagyi GN, Therialt RL, Porter L, Blayney D, Lipton A, Sinoff C, Wheeler H, Simeone JF, Seaman J, Knight RD, Heffernan M, Reitsma DJ (1996) Efficacy of pamidronate in reducing skeletal complications in patients with breast cancer and lytic bone metastases. N Engl J Med 335:1785–1791

Mouridsen HT (1996) The role of anthracyclines in adjuvant chemotherapy of breast cancer: a critical appraisal. Recent Results Cancer Res 127:191–199

Overgaard M, Hansen PS, Overgaard J, Rose C, Andersson M, Bach M, Kjær M, Gadeberg CC, Mouridsen HT, Jensen M-B, Zedeler K (1997) Postoperative radiotherapy in high-risk premenopausal women with breast cancer who receive adjuvant chemotherapy. N Engl J Med 337:949–955

Roy JA, Sawka CA, Pritchard KI (1996) Hormone replacement therapy in women with breast cancer: do the risks outweigh the benefits? J Clin Oncol 14:997–1006

Scottish Cancer Trials Breast Group, ICRF Breast Unit (1993) Adjuvant ovarian ablation versus CMF chemotherapy in premenopausal women with pathological stage II breast carcinoma: the Scottish trial. Lancet 341:1294–1298

The EORTC-Breast Cancer Cooperative Group Clinical Research Programme in Early Breast Cancer

M. J. Piccart[1] and C. J. H. van de Velde[2] for the EORTC-BCCG

[1] Institut Jules Bordet, Unité de Chimiothérapie, Rue Héger-Bordet 1,
1000 Brussels, Belgium
[2] University Hospital Leiden, Department of Surgery, P.O. Box 9600,
2300 RC Leiden, The Netherlands

As many as 65 institutions belonging to 19 different countries participate in the activities of the European Organization for Research and Treatment of Cancer (EORTC) Breast Cancer Cooperative Group, which is a multidisciplinary group involving surgeons, radiotherapists, and medical oncologists.

It is therefore not surprising that the EORTC Breast Cancer Cooperative Group (EORTC-BCCG) portfolio, in the field of early breast cancer, contains clinical trials looking at optimal local therapy using surgery and radiotherapy as well as trials looking at optimal systemic therapy.

EORTC Trials Addressing Optimal Local Therapy for Early Breast Cancer

Two very large studies conducted in collaboration with the EORTC radiotherapy group were closed in the summer of 1996: the first one explored whole excision versus whole excision plus radiotherapy in patients with ductal carcinoma in situ and the second one explored the value of a radiotherapy boost in patients treated with breast conserving surgery for an invasive breast carcinoma. The first trial has been powered to detect an absolute improvement of 5% in disease-free survival at 5 years in favor of the radiotherapy arm, while the second one aims at the detection of a 5% absolute survival benefit at 10 years from the "boost" administration. Preliminary results of these two important studies should be available in the next 2 to 3 years.

A third trial was an unsuccessful attempt to look at the possibility of omitting radiotherapy for small and very "low risk" invasive tumors treated with breast-conserving surgery: it had to be closed because of very poor accrual.

Finally, an ongoing trial run in collaboration with the EORTC-radiotherapy group is questioning the need, if any, for irradiation of the internal mammary chain and the medial subclavicular nodes in node-positive breast cancer patients and in those having centrally or medially located primaries with no axillary involvement. This highly controversial issue has never been addressed in a large prospective randomized clinical trial; 5000 patients will be recruited in order to be able to detect a 7% absolute improvement in 10-year survival.

EORTC Trials Investigating Optimal Systemic Therapy for Early Breast Cancer

The results of a large trial of 2795 patients looking at the value, if any, of one perioperative chemotherapy cycle of FEC (5-fluorouracil, epirubicin, cyclophosphamide) followed by conventionally-timed chemotherapy in node-positive premenopausal patients have been published: they show that this perioperative chemotherapy decreases the rate of local recurrence and suggest that this effect is mainly confined to the node-negative premenopausal subset (Clahsen et al. 1996). No survival advantage has emerged so far.

An ongoing trial, less successful in terms of accrual rate, is investigating the potential downstaging of the primary tumor through preoperative FEC chemotherapy, leading to an increase in breast-conserving surgery; the control group undergoes the more classical sequence of surgery followed by chemotherapy.

Whether or not administration of tamoxifen after completion of adjuvant chemotherapy is of benefit to the patient is the main question of another ongoing randomized trial, allowing a flexible policy as far as adjuvant chemotherapy is concerned; this trial should complete its target accrual of 1800 patients in the next few months. It aims at the detection of a 5% absolute survival gain at 5 years for the group receiving the combined modality approach.

An interesting synergism, as far as tumor growth inhibition is concerned, between fenretinide, a retinoid acid derivative, and tamoxifen in preclinical models (Ratko et al. 1989) prompted the group to design a clinical trial investigating this combination versus the anti-estrogen alone in the adjuvant setting. Unfortunately, the trial was never able to start owing to inadequate support.

The optimal sequencing of adjuvant chemotherapy and radiotherapy remains a debatable issue in 1998, and retrospective analyses of patient outcome according to which treatment was given first are feeding the controversy. One relatively small randomized clinical trial, published in the *New England Journal of Medicine* 2 years ago, examined this issue in patients with node-positive disease who had undergone breast-conserving surgery. Chemotherapy first, delivered intensively over 3 months, was found to be the preferred option in terms of distant metastases-free survival (Recht et al. 1996). This single study, however, is not able to convince the oncology community. The EORTC-BCCG has therefore decided to run a larger study looking at immediate versus delayed radiotherapy in breast cancer patients for whom both radiation and chemotherapy are indicated; its primary endpoint will be disease-free survival and its secondary endpoints locoregional control and overall survival.

Finally, with the growing evidence that a tumor switch towards an angiogenic phenotype contributes to invasion and metastasis, and with the current clinical development of anti-angiogenic compounds, the group is hoping to initiate soon a study in which half of the patients would receive an anti-angiogenic drug, immediately following breast cancer diagnosis via a needle puncture or a tru-cut biopsy, while the other half would receive a placebo; surgery and any indicated postoperative adjuvant therapy would follow in the next 2–3 weeks, according to a predetermined center policy.

EORTC Trials Conducted in Locally Advanced Breast Cancer

Locally advanced breast cancer (LABC) is an area of successful EORTC clinical trials. The short- and long-term results of the first LABC-EORTC trial have been published (Rubens et al. 1989; Bartelink et al. 1997). This trial explored the value of adding endocrine therapy or chemotherapy or both to local management with radiotherapy in a 2×2 factorial design. The important findings of this trial were (1) a significant impact of systemic therapy on locoregional relapse and (2) a long-term survival advantage for endocrine therapy. Of note, very few patients in this study have aggressive inflammatory tumors. This is in contrast with the second EORTC-LABC randomized clinical trial, run in collaboration with the National Cancer Institute of Canada Clinical Trials Group (NCI-C CTG) and the Swiss Group for Clinical Cancer Research (SAKK), which enrolled 448 patients, half of whom had inflammatory breast cancer. The trial compared two different neoadjuvant chemotherapy regimens: an innovative one, consisting in a 3-month intensive epirubicin-cyclophosphamide (EC) regimen given in an accelerated fashion every 2 weeks with growth factor (GF) support (filgrastim) and a more or less "standard" combination consisting of the Canadian CEF regimen given over 6 months without GF support. Prophylactic antibiotics were administered in both arms. A flexible policy for local therapy was allowed and all patients received tamoxifen thereafter for 5 years or until disease progression, which was the primary trial endpoint. Other endpoints included response, toxicity, survival, quality of life, and cost effectiveness. Preliminary results, presented this year at the American Society of Clinical Oncology meeting (Therasse et al. 1998), do not show a significant improvement in progression-free survival with the doubled dose intensity planned and, indeed achieved, with the accelerated treatment. Dose-dense EC + G-CSF was, however, found to be a safe and effective alternative to CEF with far less dose reductions and dose delays. Quality-of-life and cost-effectiveness data are eagerly awaited in order to determine the potential place of such a regimen in daily practice.

The future LABC trial will most likely look at further refinements in neoadjuvant chemotherapy, using infusional schedules and/or taxoid compounds, and at optimal local therapy for responding patients.

Quality Control

Quality control is a high priority of the EORTC-BCCG. The quality of surgery, radiotherapy, and chemotherapy administration has been subjected to "on site" monitoring in the DCIS, boost, and dose-intensity LABC trials.

Translational Research

Translational research has become an important component of a number of EORTC clinical trials. Using immunocytochemistry techniques, the expression of molecular markers involved in signal transduction, cell cycle control, apoptosis, and multidrug resistance is studied in relation with clinical outcome.

In the perioperative adjuvant chemotherapy trial described previously, the primary tumor blocks of the 441 node-negative pre-menopausal patients who appeared to benefit most from the investigated therapy were retrieved and assayed for C-erbB2, Bcl2, Ki67 and p53 expression (Clahsen et al. 1998). The last two markers were found to be of predictive value, while the other two were not. Collection of tumor blocks is progressing nicely in the context of the DCIS and the dose-density LABC trial: here also, there is hope to find molecular markers linked to treatment outcome.

EORTC-BCCG: A Founding Member of BIG

"BIG" is the newly created Breast International Group (Fig. 1). It has the ambition to coordinate and accelerate clinical research in the adjuvant treatment of breast cancer across Europe, Canada, Australia, and New Zealand, as well as creating close links with the American Intergroup set up 10 years ago.

The primary goals of BIG are: (1) to avoid duplication of small clinical trials which look at the same question in slightly different ways, (2) to encourage existing cooperative groups to work together, particularly in the investigation of difficult issues such as adjuvant therapy of very young or elderly patients, or hormone-replacement therapy in breast cancer survivors, (3) to generate funds for relevant clinical trials for which external funding is unlikely, and (4) to update everyone about ongoing clinical trials for early breast cancer through the publication of a "BIG booklet" every 2 years.

Intergroup collaboration has the potential to accelerate clinical research in a tremendous way; it is an exciting and challenging enterprise which has to fight individualism, skepticism, and bureaucracy; it is presently in its infancy in Europe. Let us hope that BIG will grow successfully in the coming years and allow clinical investigators to work in the best interest of their patients, in close collaboration with the pharmaceutical industry whenever indicated, but with preservation of their scientific independence.

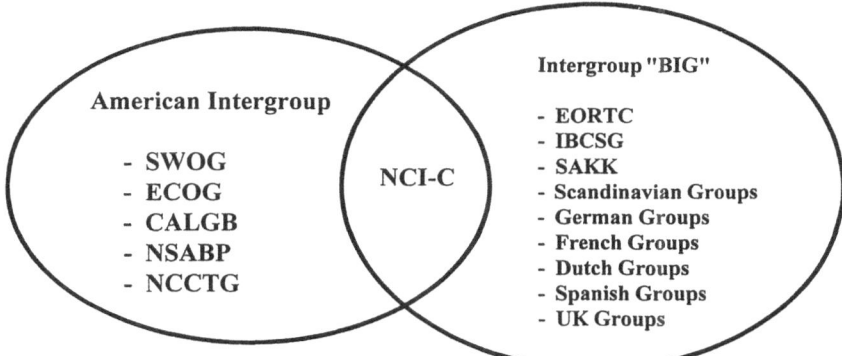

Fig. 1. Research into adjuvant treatment of breast cancer: the future

Summary

The aims of the European Organization for Research and Treatment of Cancer (EORTC) are to conduct, develop, coordinate, and stimulate research in Europe on the experimental and clinical bases of cancer treatment. Along these lines, the EORTC Breast Cancer Cooperative Group, which belongs to the EORTC treatment division, aims at improving the standard of early and advanced breast cancer treatment in Europe through the conduct of large, prospective, randomized, multicenter cancer clinical trials investigating innovative approaches as well as relevant questions regarding optimal surgery and radiotherapy or the optimal integration of these various treatment modalities. This paper reviews the current clinical research programme of this group in the field of "early" breast cancer and briefly alludes to the ongoing efforts of the group in areas such as quality control and translational research. Finally, the EORTC-BCCG has been instrumental in the foundation of the Breast International Group, "BIG", which is a large "intergroup" of existing European and Australian breast cancer research groups. It is hoped that BIG will accelerate the turnover of sufficiently large and well-designed breast cancer adjuvant clinical trials through increasing cooperation between its group members as well as collaboration, whenever indicated, with the American Breast Cancer Intergroup.

References

Bartelink H, Rubens RD, van der Schueren E, Sylvester R (1997) Hormonal therapy prolongs survival in irradiated locally advanced breast cancer: a European Organization for Research and Treatment of Cancer randomized phase III trial. J Clin Oncol 15:207–215

Clahsen PC, van de Velde CJH, Julien JP, Floiras JL, Delozier T, Mignolet FY, Sahmoud TM et al (1996) Improved local control and disease-free survival after perioperative chemotherapy for early-stage breast cancer: a European Organization for Research and Treatment of Breast Cancer Cooperative Group study. J Clin Oncol 14:745–753

Clahsen PC, van de Velde CJH, Duval C, Pallud C, Mandard AM, Delobelle-Deroide A, van den Broek L, Sahmoud TM, van de Vijver M (1998) p53 Protein accumulation and response to adjuvant chemotherapy in premenopausal women with node-negative early breast cancer. J Clin Oncol 16:470–479

Ratko TA, Detrisac CJ, Dinger NM, Thomas CF, Kelloff GJ, Moon RC (1989) Chemopreventive efficacy of combined retinoid and tamoxifen treatment following surgical excision of a primary mammary cancer in female rats. Cancer Res 49:4472–4476

Recht A, Come SE, Henderson IC, Gelman RS, Silver B, Hayes DF, Shulman LN, Harris JR (1996) The sequencing of chemotherapy and radiation therapy after conservative surgery for early breast cancer. N Engl J Med 334:1356–1361

Rubens RD, Bartelink H, Engelsman E et al (1989) Locally advanced breast cancer: the contribution of cytotoxic and endocrine treatment to radiotherapy (an EORTC Breast Cancer Co-operative Group trial 10792). Eur J Cancer Clin Oncol 25:667–678

Therasse P, Mauriac L, Welnicka M, Bruning P, Cufer T, Bonnefoi H, Tomiak E, Hamilton A, Piccart M (1998) Neo-adjuvant dose intensive chemotherapy in locally advanced breast cancer (LABC): an EORTC-NCIC-SAKK randomized phase III study comparing FEC (5FU, epirubicin, cyclophosphamide) vs high dose intensity EC + G-CSF (filgrastim). Proc Am Soc Clin Oncol 17:124a

Van Slooten HJ, Clahsen PC, van Dierendonck JH, Duval C, Pallud C, Mandard AM, Delobelle-Deroide A, van de Velde CJH, van de Vijver MJ (1996) Expression of BCL-2 in node-negative breast cancer is associated with various prognostic factors, but does not predict response to one course of perioperative chemotherapy. Br J Cancer 74:78–85

Italian Breast Cancer Adjuvant Chemo-hormone Therapy Cooperative Group Trials*

F. Boccardo[1], A. Rubagotti[2], D. Amoroso[1], M. Mesiti[3], P. Pacini[4],
L. Gallo[5], P. Sismondi[6], M. Giai[6], F. Genta[7], G. Mustacchi[8],
B. Agostara[9], A. Bolognesi[10], E. Villa[10], G. Schieppati[11],
G. P. Ausili Cefaro[12], R. Bellantone[13], A. Farris[14], M. Sassi[15], F. Patrone[16],
and other participants in the GROCTA Trials (see Appendix)

[1] Servizio di Oncologia Medica II, Istituto Nazionale per la Ricerca sul Cancro di
Genova, Geno, Italy
[2] Centro di Biostatistica, Istituto di Oncologia dell'Università, Istituto Nazionale
per la Ricerca sul Cancro di Genova, Geno, Italy
[3] Cattedra di Oncologia, Università di Messina, Messina, Italy
[4] U.O. Radioterapia, Policlinico Careggi, Florence, Italy
[5] Servizio di Oncologia Medica, Ospedali Galliera, Geno, Italy
[6] Cattedra di Ginecologia Oncologica, Università di Torino, Turin, Italy
[7] Cattedra di Ginecologia e Ostetricia 'A', Ospedale Sant'Anna, Turin, Italy
[8] Centro Oncologico 'Mario Lovenati', Trieste, Italy
[9] Divisione di Oncologia Medica II, Presidio Oncologico 'M. Ascoli',
Palermo, Italy
[10] Servizio di Oncologia – Radioterapia, Istituto Scientifico San Raffaele,
Milan, Italy
[11] Divisione Medicina I, Ospedale Generale Provinciale, Saronno, Italy
[12] Istituto di Radiologia, Università Cattolica di Roma, Rome, Italy
[13] Clinica Chirurgica, Università Cattolica di Roma, Rome, Italy
[14] Cattedra di Oncologia Clinica, Università di Sassari, Sassari, Italy
[15] Servizio di Oncologia Medica, Ospedale Spallanzani, Reggio Emilia, Italy
[16] Clinica Medica Università di Genova, Genoa, Italy

Introduction

The Adjuvant Chemo-hormone Therapy Breast Cancer Study Group (GROCTA)
was formed exactly 15 years ago with its main purpose to promote co-operation
among surgeons, clinical oncologists, clinical pathologists and basic researchers in the field of adjuvant therapy of breast cancer. This chapter will review the
main findings from the trials that have been performed since then.

Study 01

Study 01 was the first trial to be launched by GROCTA, in November 1983.
At that time chemotherapy was the usual treatment for the majority of pa-

* These studies were supported in part by Italian National Research Council, Project ACRO,
Contract nos 92.02298, 93.022275, 94.01242, 95.00473, 96.00670-PF 39.

tients with node-positive tumors, although results did not appear to be as good in post-menopausal women as they did in younger women (Bonadonna et al. 1982). Because there was preliminary evidence from Danish and British trials (Rose et al. 1983; Nolvadex Adjuvant Trial Organization 1983) that tamoxifen might also work as adjuvant therapy, at least in post-menopausal women, it was thought rational to compare chemotherapy to tamoxifen. Because tamoxifen appeared to be more effective in women with ER-positive tumors (Fisher et al. 1983), this comparison was restricted to node-positive patients with 10 fmol ER or more in their tumors. Restriction to women with ER-positive tumors also seemed appropriate from the ethical point of view. Moreover, because we had previously shown an additive effect of tamoxifen and chemotherapy in postmenopausal patients with advanced breast cancer (Boccardo et al. 1985), a third arm with concurrent administration of the same chemotherapy and of tamoxifen was included in the comparison. Details of the study design, patient eligibility, treatment of primary tumors, allocated treatments after surgery and preliminary results have been described elsewhere (Boccardo et al. 1990, 1992). In brief, 504 evaluable patients aged 35–65 years with node-positive, ER-positive tumors were entered into the trial and randomly allocated to receive either tamoxifen 30 mg daily for 5 years (group T) or ten courses of chemotherapy (six courses of CMF followed by four courses of epidoxorubicin monotherapy: all drugs given intravenously. every 3 weeks: group CT) or both treatments combined (group CTT). At the time of the present analysis (median follow-up time 144 months, range 4–170 months) 302 patients (60%) have relapsed and 248 (49%) have died. Results are summarised in Table 1 and in Figs. 1–4. The clinical outcome of patients treated with chemotherapy with respect to both disease-free and overall survival. The difference was more striking in post-menopausal women and in women with four or more involved nodes, but a trend favoured tamoxifen-treated patients in the other patient subsets as well. Following adjustment for age, menopausal status, tumor size and number of involved nodes, tamoxifen-treated patients showed risks of relapse and of death which were respectively 36% and 32% lower than those of patients treated with chemotherapy ($p = 0.001$ and $p = 0.01$ respectively). Adding ta-

Table 1. Ten-year probability of being disease-free and surviving among patients in trial 01 (percentages)

	Disease-free survival				Overall survival			
	CT	T	CTT	p	CT	T	CTT	p
All patients	32	48	49	0.000	49	65	68	0.000
Pre-menopausal patients	46	52	55	0.2	63	63	71	0.3
Post-menopausal patients	24	49	48	0.000	39	67	66	0.000
≤3 Positive nodes	46	63	60	0.002	67	84	76	0.03
>3 Positive nodes	23	31	23	0.04	33	44	49	0.007

CT, Chemotherapy arm; T, tamoxifen arm; CTT, chemotherapy plus tamoxifen arm.

moxifen to chemotherapy was able further to improve patient outcome as compared with chemotherapy alone both overall and in all the subgroups considered, although the difference with respect to chemotherapy was not significant in pre-menopausal women and was of borderline significance in women with three or fewer involved nodes. By contrast, adding chemother-

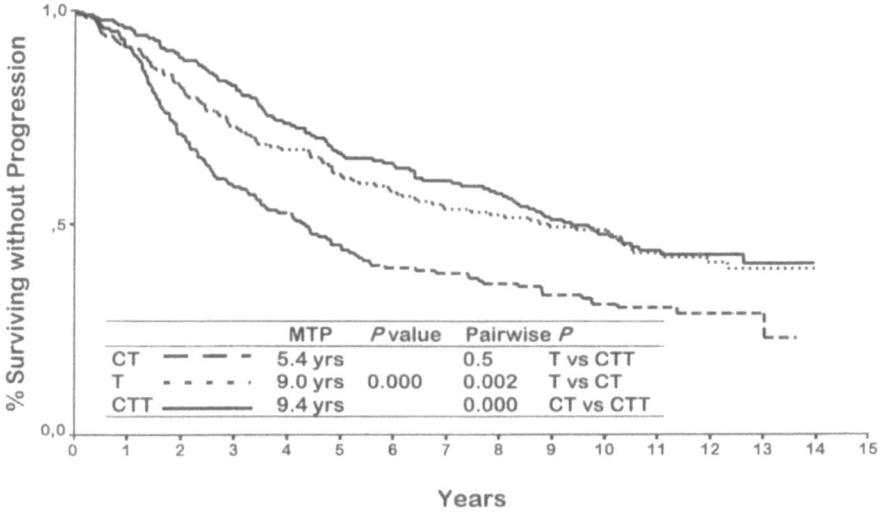

Fig. 1. Probability of surviving without progression among patients enrolled in trial 01. *MTP,* Median time to progression; *CT,* chemothrapy arm; *T,* tamoxifen arm; *CTT,* chemotherapy plus tamoxifen arm

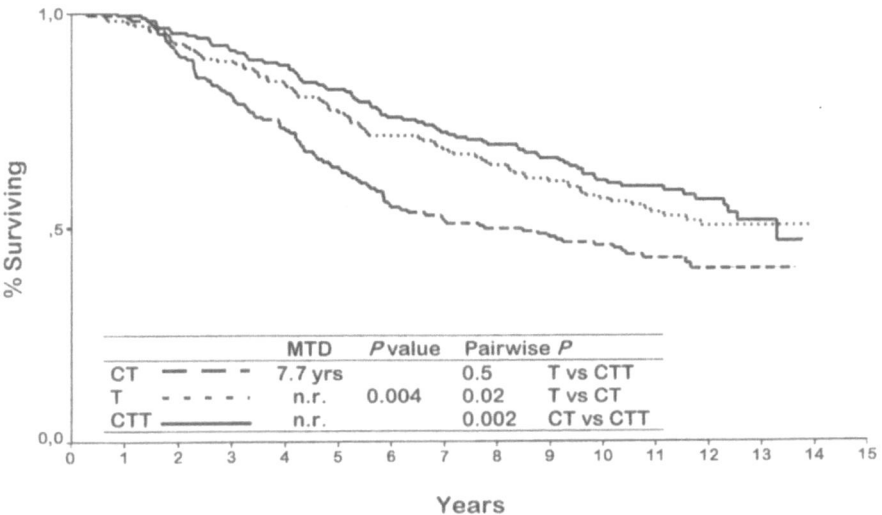

Fig. 2. Probability of surviving among patients enrolled in trial 01. *MTD,* Median time to death

apy to tamoxifen was able to produce only a limited advantage over tamoxifen alone, the difference being negligible in post-menopausal women and in women with three or fewer involved nodes. Moreover, as has been previously presented in detail (Boccardo et al. 1990), acute side effects of treatment were significantly more numerous and more severe in patients treated with

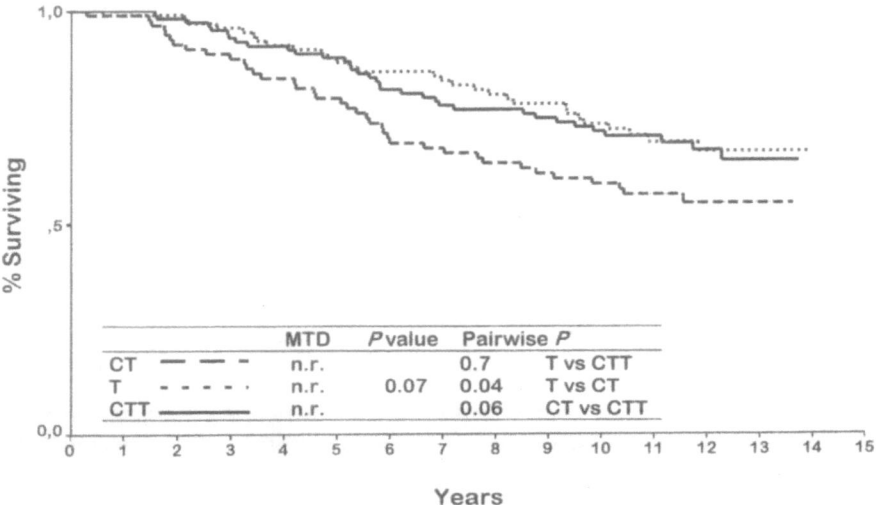

Fig. 3. Probability of surviving among patients with 1–3 involved nodes enrolled in trial 01. *n.r.*, Not reached

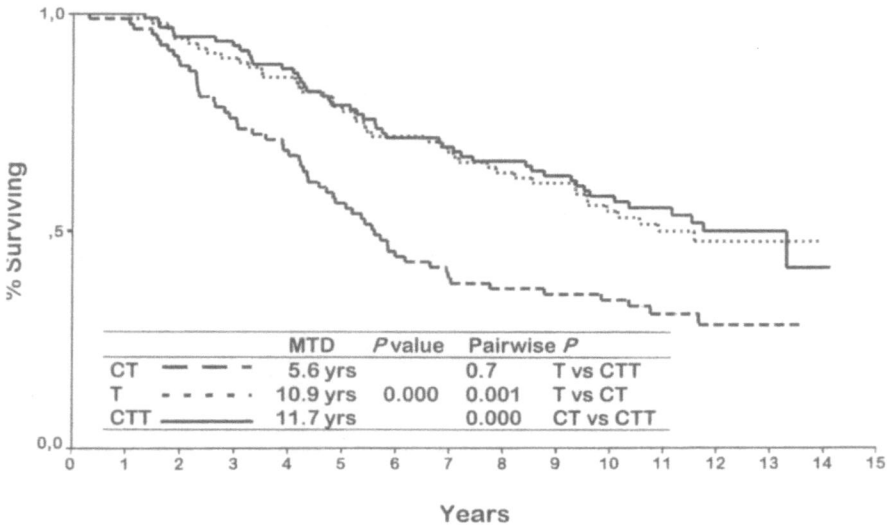

Fig. 4. Probability of surviving among post-menopausal patients enrolled in trial 01

chemotherapy. Therefore, the long-term results of this trial provide further support for our previous conclusions (Boccardo et al. 1992): that tamoxifen appears to be a safe and effective treatment for women with node-positive and ER-positive tumors, particularly those who are post-menopausal or who have three or fewer involved nodes. Moreover, chemotherapy seems to add very little to tamoxifen in these women at the cost of significantly higher acute toxicity.

Study 02

Subgroup analysis of trial 01 also showed that the efficacy of tamoxifen did not appreciably vary with patient age or menopausal status and that this treatment could achieve therapeutic results that were at least comparable to those achieved by chemotherapy even in younger women (Boccardo et al. 1992). These findings prompted us to activate a confirmatory trial with the aim of prospectively comparing the value of chemotherapy and endocrine therapy in pre-menopausal women. Such a trial was activated in January 1989 and patients recruitment ended in January 1997 with 244 patients enrolled. Again the comparison was restricted to patients with ER-positive tumors. Trial design, patient eligibility, allocated treatments after surgery and preliminary results have been also presented elsewhere (Boccardo et al. 1994a, 1997a). Following surgery, patients were randomly allocated to receive either six cycles of classical CMF or tamoxifen at a daily dose of 30 mg for 5 years in combination with goserelin, 1 depot injection every 4 weeks, usually for the first 2 years. Instead of receiving goserelin, a few patients were treated with ovarian irradiation. CMF was preferred to the chemotherapeutic regimen used by us in the previous trial because in the meanwhile the Milan group (Moliterni et al. 1991) had failed to demonstrate the superiority of sequential use of CMF followed by adriamycin over CMF alone and because the standard schedule employing oral administration of cyclophosphamide for 14 days and intravenous administration of 5-fluorouracil and methotrexate could ensure a higher dose intensity of both cyclophosphamide and the two antimetabolites as compared to the intravenous three-weekly schedule. In the other arm, the combination of tamoxifen and goserelin was preferred to tamoxifen alone because an extraincidence of uterine fibroids had been recorded in the pre-menopausal women treated with the anti-oestrogen in our previous study (Boccardo et al. 1992) and because there was some preliminary evidence from studies in advanced disease that total estrogenic deprivation might work better than gonad ablation or anti-estrogenic treatment alone (Boccardo et al. 1994b; Klijn et al. 1996). Finally, we omitted from the comparison the arm based on the combination of tamoxifen and chemotherapy, because at the time this trial was designed there was some concern about possible interference between chemotherapy and tamoxifen, especially in younger women (Fisher et al. 1986). At the time of the present analysis (median follow-up time 62 months, range 9–103 months) overall 75 patients

(32%) have relapsed and 34 patients (14%) have died. The two arms are well balanced with respect to age, menopausal status (a few patients in both groups were perimenopausal), tumor grade (the great majority of patients in both groups had well or moderately well differentiated tumors), tumor size, number of involved nodes and treatment of primary tumor. No difference has emerged so far between the groups either in terms of disease-free (Fig. 5) or overall survival (data not shown). Results are unchanged even by grouping patients according to number of involved nodes or tumor grade (data not shown). Again acute side effects were more numerous and severe in patients treated with chemotherapy (Table 2). The only relevant side effects occurring in patients treated with tamoxifen and goserelin were hot flushes and spotting, whereas most of the patients treated with CMF who achieved drug-induced amenorrhea – and this was the majority of the patients still actively menstruating when chemotherapy was started (70/106) – developed hot flushes and vaginal disorders later on. This trial is still unpowered in spite of a median follow-up time in excess of 5 years due to its small size. However, it supports the view that chemotherapy and endocrine therapy can yield equivalent results in pre-menopausal women, provided they have ER-positive tumors, with comparable long-term morbidity but with significantly more acute side effects for chemotherapy.

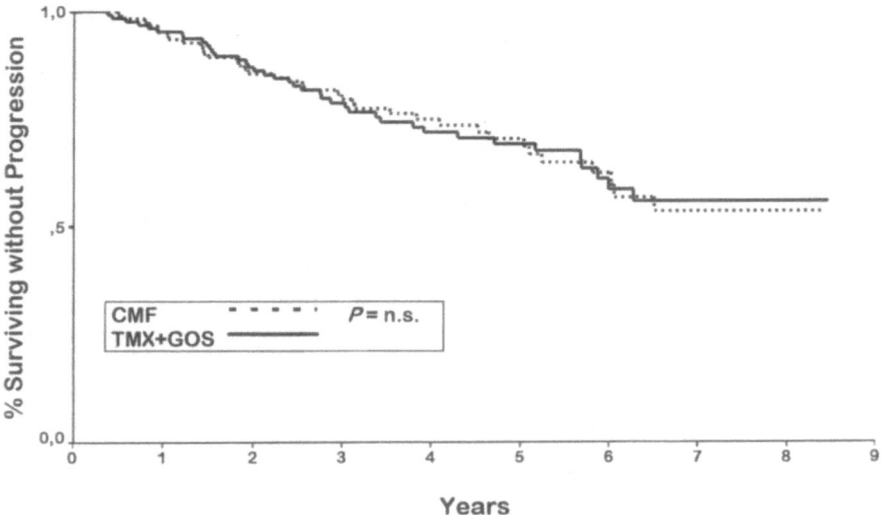

Fig. 5. Probability of surviving without progression among patients enrolled in trial 02

Table 2. Trial 02: main differences in incidence of side effects (any degree)

	CMF (n = 119) (%)	TMX+GOS (n = 124) (%)	p
Leukopenia	45.4	7.2	0.000
Thrombocytopenia	8.4	3.2	0.13
Nausea	68.1	5.6	0.000
Vomiting	52.0	1.6	0.000
Stomatitis	13.4	–	0.000
Diarrhoea	8.4	0.8	0.02
Alopecia	33.6	1.6	0.000
Hot flushes	5.1	37.1	0.000
Spotting	–	10.5	0.000

CMF, Cyclophosphamide, methotrexate and 5-fluorouracil; TMX+GOS, tamoxifen plus goserelin.

Study 04-B and ITA Study

Because in the first study chemotherapy appeared to add very little to tamoxifen in postmenopausal women, it was thought rational to develop new strategies to improve the results that could be achieved with tamoxifen alone in this menopausal subset. Looking at the annual risk of relapse of patients allocated to tamoxifen in our first study, it was evident that the protective effect of endocrine therapy on the risk of relapse declined over time, starting from the 3rd year (Boccardo et al. 1992). This might imply that a proportion of patients could develop tamoxifen resistance or even tamoxifen-dependent tumor growth, a phenomenon that had been clearly documented in animal models (Gottardis and Jordan 1988), relatively early following mastectomy. Because aromatase inhibitors had been shown to be still effective in a relevant proportion of patients relapsing in course of tamoxifen treatment (Stuart-Harris and Smith 1984), it was thought that switching tamoxifen-treated patients to an anti-aromatase drug after the first 2 or 3 years of treatment with the anti-estrogen, might help in preventing or delaying the occurrence of at least a proportion of relapses that could be expected in the same patients should they be continued on tamoxifen up to the 5th year. Aminoglutethimide was selected to be given on a random basis to a group of postmenopausal women already on treatment with tamoxifen for 3 years because at that time it was the only anti-aromatase available to us and because it had already been tested in the adjuvant setting with fairly good results (Coombes et al. 1987). However, because treatment with aminoglutethimide appeared to be quite toxic, a low dose equal to 250 mg per day without corticosteroid supplementation was selected for our study. So far 662 patients have been centrally registered and 375 have been randomly allocated either to continue with tamoxifen for further 2 years, at the same dosage they were receiving, or to be switched to treatment with aminoglutethimide, 250 mg daily, for an identical period of time: to be precise, 188 patients have been allocated to tamoxifen (TMX group) and 187 have been allocated to low-dose aminoglutethimide (AG group). All women had been previously treated for 3 years (±3 months) with tamoxifen and some of them had also been previously treated with chemotherapy. Median age was 65 years (range 45–75 years) in the TMX group and 64 years (range 43–76 years) in the AG group. All women were postmenopausal at the time of entry to the trial, mostly because of naturally occurring menopause (86% in the TMX group and 81% in the AG group). The treatment arms were also well balanced with respect to tumor size (T≤2 cm in diameter: TMX group, 35%; AG group, 42%), number of involved nodes (N0: TMX, 29%; AG, 30%; N positive 1–3: TMX, 41%; AG, 38%; N positive ≥4: TMX, 30%; AG, 30%) and treatment of primary (most patients were treated with mastectomy in both groups).

Present results, though still preliminary (median follow-up time 32 months, range 1–64 months), seem to suggest that there is no major difference between the clinical outcome of patients continuing with tamoxifen and those treated with aminoglutethimide. However, if we look at first cause of disease progression, it seems that more patients in the AG group suffered from a local recurrence (10 vs 5) while more patients in the TMX group developed distant metastases (21 vs 13). There were three new primaries (including one endometrial cancer) in each group. Moreover, six patients in the TMX group died of other causes (including two myocardial infarctions and one cerebral accident) without evidence of disease relapse ($p = 0.01$). The differences observed so far might well be due to chance. However, there is no doubt that a trend is now favouring patients in the aminoglutethimide arm (26 events recorded in 187 patients as compared to 35 events recorded in 188 patients), as was expected. However, aminoglutethimnide treatment was still more toxic than tamoxifen treatment in spite of the low dose that was employed: more patients in the aminoglutethimide group complained of gastrointestinal and skin symptoms and more patients had to suspend the treatment with this anti-aromatase (Fig. 6).

In conclusion, the results of this study seem to demonstrate the feasibility and potential superiority of sequential treatment with tamoxifen and low-dose aminoglutethimide.

These results encouraged us to activate a new study adopting a similar design to investigate the value of sequential treatment with a more selective and more potent aromatase inhibitor, anastrozole. Although results from trials in patients with advanced breast carcinoma comparing tamoxifen to anastrozole are not yet availablet, we thought it could be expected that switching to treatment with anastrozole, which has been proved to be more potent and less toxic than aminoglutethimide (Plourde et al. 1995; Buzdar et al. 1996), should produce even a greater benefit than that observed in the previous study. The new trial has been called ITA (Intergroup Tamoxifen Arimidex) trial, because other groups in addition to GROCTA will contribute to patient recruitment, and it is expected to enroll about 1000 patients in 3 years.

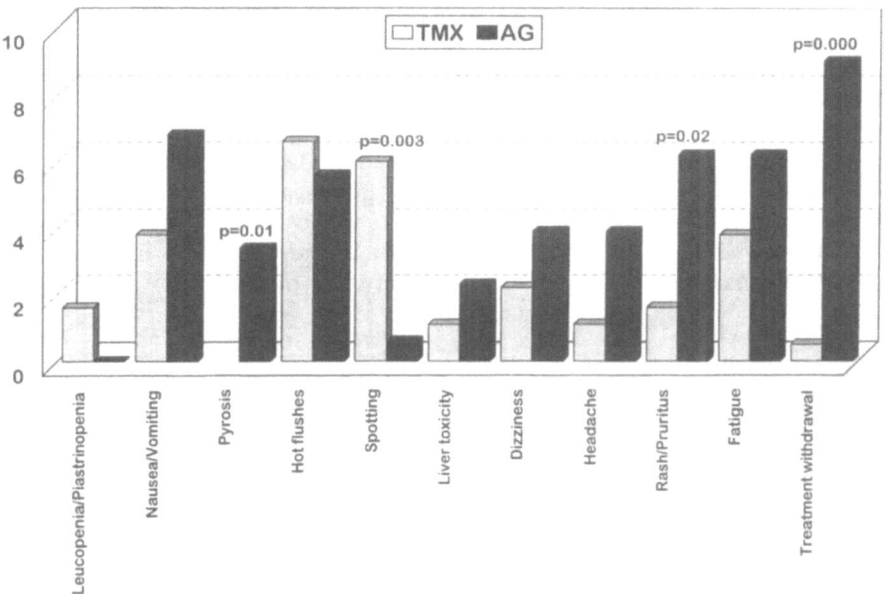

Fig. 6. Trial 04-B – Main differences in incidence of side effects. *TMX*, Tamoxifen; *AG*, aminoglutethimide

Studies 03 and 05

These trials were performed in ER-negative patients (i.e., those patients with less than 10 fmol/mg ER in their tumor cytosol) who were not suitable to be entered in previous studies. Trial 05 was restricted to post-menopausal women with node-positive tumors and was activated in 1989. At that time there was evidence that adjuvant treatment with tamoxifen might work even in patients with ER-poor tumors and that the magnitude of the benefit induced by anti-estrogenic treatment in this patient subgroup could be not dissimilar from the benefit induced by chemotherapy (Early Breast Cancer Trialists' Collaborative Group 1988). Therefore, we planned a prospective comparison between tamoxifen with or without the addition of six cycles of standard CMF. This trial was prematurely stopped both due to low recruitment and because an early trend in disease-free survival advantaged patients in the combined treatment arm.

Trial 03 was performed in pre- and perimenopausal women with node-positive, ER-negative tumors. This trial was designed to test the possible superiority of triple chemotherapy over a single chemotherapy regimen, as appeared to be suggested by the theoretical model developed by Goldie and Coldman (1984). The rationale and details of this trial have been published elsewhere (Boccardo et al. 1997b). In summary, patients were randomly allocated to receive either six cycles of standard CMF, with cyclophosphamide given per os, or two courses of a triple regimen based on the administration of one cycle of CMF, followed 21 days later by one cycle of epidoxorubicin (day 1) and vincristine (days 1, 8), in turn followed 21 days later by one cycle of mitomycin-C (day 1) and vindesine (days 1, 8), for a total of six chemotherapy cycles. This study recruited 107 patients (53 in the CMF group and 54 in the triple chemotherapy group) and was prematurely closed due to discouraging early results: there was no statistical difference in disease-free and overall survival of patients in the two groups, nor any difference in the site of first relapse. Although there was no difference in treatment-related toxicity, this study failed to show any advantage ensuing from the use of alternating chemotherapy in patients with early breast cancer.

Studies 06 and 08

Because previous studies had shown that the prognosis of patients with ten or more involved nodes was poor, irrespective of ER status and of treatment received, and because there was evidence that high-dose chemotherapy might be more effective than standard polychemotherapy in patients with disseminated disease (Eddy 1992), it was thought that our group should also be involved in this research field. Therefore, in September 1992 trial 06 was activated. This was an open study that included 53 patients. To be eligible, patients had to be aged 55 years or less and have ten or more involved nodes and no evidence of concurrent infectious disease or major bone marrow, liver or kidney impairment. Irrespective of their age or menopausal status, all patients were given three cycles of standard CEF (cyclophosphamide 600 mg/m^2, epidoxorubicin 60 mg/m^2 and 5-fluorouracil 600 mg/m^2; all drugs given by the intravenous route every 3 weeks), followed by one high-dose chemotherapy (HDC) cycle consisting of cyclophosphamide 2.5 g/m^2 days 1, 2, etoposide: 500 mg/m^2 days 1–3 and cisplatin 50 mg/m^2 days 1–3. The HDC regimen was chosen in view of the tolerability and therapeutic activity previously shown in patients with disseminated disease (Niedhart et al. 1990). While the three standard CEF cycles were given on a fully outpatient basis, patients receiving the HDC regimen were admitted into a protected environment until full recovery of blood counts, also because no form of bone marrow support was administered to them except for G-CSF (5 µg/kg/day), which was begun on day 5 and continued until a WBC count of 10×10^9/l was reached. When indicated, radiotherapy on the residual breast was postponed until HDC had been completed and blood counts had fully recovered.

The preliminary results of this trial have been presented elsewhere (Amoroso et al. 1997a,b). Median follow-up time has now reached 36 months (range 1–50 months) and overall 25 patients have relapsed (mostly at a distant level) and 8 have died. Median duration of granulocytopenia below 500/µl was 8 days (range 5–13 days) and that of thrombocytopenia below 20 000/µl was 3 days (range 1–14 days). Recovery to an ANC count of at least 1000/µl took a median of 16 days (range 14–21 days). Median red cell transfusion requirement per patient was 1 unit (range 0–4 units) and median platelet unit requirement per patient was 2 units (range 0–5 units). No toxic death occurred, although two patients developed an acute respiratory distress syndrome requiring their admission to an intensive care unit. All patients suffered from WHO grade 3–4 nausea and vomiting and complete alopecia, and most of them developed fever higher than 38 °C. Present results have been compared to those previously achieved with CMF-based chemotherapy in a historical group of patients enrolled in the previous GROCTA studies. As is shown in Table 3, GROCTA 06 and control patients were well matched with respect to age, menopausal status, number of involved nodes and ER status. No difference has emerged so far between the two groups under study with respect either to relapse-free survival (Fig. 7) or to overall survival and results appear to be unchanged even when analysis is limited to patients with 10 to 20 positive nodes (data not shown). Therefore, though still preliminary, present results confirm that the use of HDC without stem cell support is feasible with acceptable toxicity and is effective. However, it does not seem able to achieve better results than those that can be yielded by standard chemotherapy. Our HDC study is not devoid of major criticism. Firstly, the number of induction cycles with CEF could be inadequate, just as one cycle of HD chemotherapy could be. Moreover, cisplatin and etoposide are not recognised as very active drugs in breast cancer and it may be that no major benefit can be expected by increasing the doses of these drugs.

For these reasons, a new high-dose regimen has been developed and is now being tested in another open study. This trial (study 08) includes patients aged 60 years or less with ten or more involved nodes who receive four 3-weekly cycles of Taxol (paclitaxel, 175 mg/m^2) and epidoxorubicin (75 mg/m^2) followed by one course of cyclophosphamide 6 g/m^2, which in turn is followed 28 days later by one course of thiotepa 600 mg/m^2 and mel-

Table 3. Main characteristics of trial 06 patients and of historical controls

	Trial 06	Control group
No. of patients	53	51
Median age in years (range)	46 (26–56)	47 (35–55)
Median no. of involved nodes (range)	14 (10–35)	12 (10–28)
No. of involved nodes		
10–15	32 (60.4%)	39 (76.6%)
16–20	10 (18.8%)	8 (15.7%)
>20	11 (20.8%)	4 (7.8%)
Menopausal status		
Premenopause	39 (73.6%)	41 (80.4%)
Postmenopause	10 (18.9%)	10 (19.6%)
Unknown	4 (7.5%)	–
ER status		
Positive or unknown	47 (88.7%)	33 (64.7%)
Negative	6 (11.3%)	18 (35.3%)
Therapeutic regimen	CEF→HDC	CMF-based CT
Median follow-up time in months (range)	36 (1–50)	92 (7.5–151)
No. of patients relapsed (within 24 months)	17/53 (32.1%)	18/51 (35.3%)

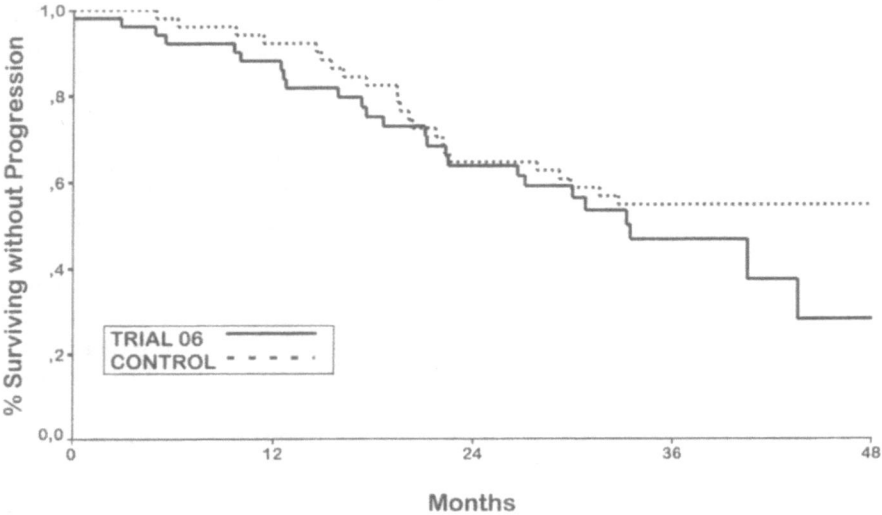

Fig. 7. Probability of surviving without disease progression among patients enrolled in trial 06 and of historical controls treated with CMF-based chemotherapy

phalan 160 mg/m². Peripheral bone marrow stem cells are collected following the third Taxol-epidoxorubicin cycle and reinfused the day after the administration of high-dose melphalan. So far 11 patients have been entered into this trial and a few of them have completed treatment without life-threatening side effects. Of course no preliminary data are available.

Study 07

Preliminary results of neoadjuvant chemotherapy studies (Bonadonna et al. 1990; Mansi et al. 1989; Mauriac et al. 1991) prompted our group also to become involved in research into this new approach. Primary chemotherapy can theoretically ensure earlier control of micrometastatic disease coupled with the possibility of substituting conservative for radical surgery in patients who would otherwise undergo mutilating procedures (Bonadonna et al. 1990). However, this approach is not devoid of major criticism, including the potential delay of local treatment. Because we had previously shown that chemotherapy could safely be combined with radiotherapy in bladder cancer (Orsatti et al. 1995), we decided to develop such a combined approach in breast cancer patients as well, in view of the possible synergism between chemotherapy and radiotherapy at tumor level and of their spatial co-operation (Vokes and Weichselbaum 1990). We were also encouraged by the preliminary results achieved in primary breast cancer with multifractionated radiotherapy in one of our centres, where nine out of ten patients, mostly with locally advanced disease, subjected to preoperative multifractionated radiotherapy achieved complete (two patients) or partial remission (seven patients) of their disease, without any prejudice to subsequent surgery. Therefore, in view of our previous experience in bladder cancer and of preliminary results achieved with preoperative multifractionated radiotherapy in breast cancer, we developed a combined chemo-radiotherapeutic neoadjuvant regimen based on the administration of two courses of CMF (all drugs given intravenously on days 1 and 8, every 4 weeks) and one course of multifractionated radiotherapy in the interval between the two courses of CMF for a total of 36 Gy (1.8 Gy twice a day, 5 days a week, for a total of 2 weeks). Surgery (quadrantectomy or lumpectomy plus axillary dissection in responding patients) was scheduled at the end of chemotherapy. Forty-four patients aged 70 or less and with tumors 3–6 cm in diameter have been entered so far into this pilot study. All of them have completed the whole therapeutic programm without major systemic or local toxicity and have been operated on, mostly using a conservative technique. Results will be available when 53 patients have been enrolled, as expected according to Simon's two-stage optimal design (Simon 1989), in view of the fact that more than 12 out of the first 19 patients enrolled achieved an objective response to treatment.

New Generation Intergroup Trials

The new generation of Intergroup trials include the so-called IBIS (Italian Breast Cancer Intergroup Studies) trials which include other groups besides GROCTA. All these studies recognise the common principle of selecting patients on the basis not only of traditional prognostic parameters (i.e., tumor size and nodal status) but also taking into account the proliferative activity of the tumor and its probability of responding to endocrine therapy. On this basis, three patient populations have been identified at increasing risk of recurrence and death, who nonetheless are candidates for some form of adjuvant treatment, according also to the guidelines of the previous St. Gallen Conference (Goldhirsh et al. 1995). Patients at the lowest risk of relapse and death include those with a tumor at least 1 cm in diameter and ER-positive (or ER status unknown if postmenopausal), and no axillary involvement or up to three involved nodes. In view of their ER status and of the low proliferative activity of their tumors (as indicated by a low tumor labelling index or a low S-phase or a high degree of differentiation), these patients are likely to derive a major benefit from the use of adjuvant therapy with tamoxifen. Therefore, tamoxifen (at a daily dose of 20 mg for 5 years) will represent the treatment in the control arm and patients will be randomized to receive in addition monotherapy with vinorelbine (30 mg/m^2 i.v. days 1, 8, every 3 weeks for a total of six cycles), a new semisynthetic vinca alkaloid that has been proven to be highly effective and moderately toxic in patients with advanced breast cancer (Canobbio et al. 1989; Goa and Faulds 1994). The expectation is to recruit 960 patients in 5 years.

Patients with tumors at least 1 cm in diameter and no or up to three involved nodes but with a high proliferative activity are expected to have an higher risk of relapse than the above patients and to be less or not responsive at all to adjuvant endocrine therapy due to the biologic aggressiveness of their tumors. Therefore, chemotherapy (CMF) will represent the treatment in the control arm. The purpose of this study will be to evaluate whether sequential use of CMF and epidoxorubicin will be superior to CMF alone in this group of patients, as could be argued on the basis of Bonadonna's previous experience (Bonadonna et al. 1995) and, especially, which of the following sequences, CMF followed by epidoxorubicin or epidoxorubicin followed by CMF, will produce the best results. The reason two different sequences are used is that, while better results have been achieved by Bonadonna with the sequence adriamycin-CMF, the tumor kinetics of patients selected for this trial could render the opposite sequence – antimetabolites first followed by the anthracycline more suitable for comparison with CMF monotherapy. About 1200 patients are expected to be recruited in 3 years.

Finally, patients with four or more involved nodes hold the worst risk of relapse and death, irrespective of tumor size or grade, ER status and the intrinsic proliferative activity of their tumors. In view of previous Milan experience (Bonadonna et al. 1995), many physicians recognise the sequential combination of four courses of an anthracycline followed by four courses of CMF as the most active regimen in these patients. The third Intergroup trial launched by GROCTA aims to assess the possible contribution of new drugs such as vinorelbine and Taxol, another drug that has been proven to be particularly effective in this disease (Hortobagyi et al. 1996; Gianni et al. 1994) to ameliorate the results of chemotherapy. Therefore, patients enrolled in this trial will be randomized to receive either the sequential Bonadonna's regimen (Bonadonna et al. 1995) with epidoxorubicin in place of adriamycin or the sequence based on the administration of four courses of Taxol monotherapy at a dose of 175 mg/m^2 followed by four courses of epidoxorubicin (75 mg/m^2 day 1) and vinorelbine (25 mg/m^2 days 1, 8), all drugs given every 3 weeks. It is expected to enter 480 patients into this trial in the next 3 years.

Acknowledgements. The authors thank Ms. A. Fossati for her skillful secretarial assistance and Mrs. G. De Stefano for her contribution in data management.

Summary

The first GROCTA trial compared 5-year tamoxifen treatment to ten chemotherapy cycles in a group of 504 pre-/post-menopausal, node-positive, ER-positive breast cancer patients. This study also included an arm combining tamoxifen with chemotherapy. Fifteen-year results showed no difference between tamoxifen and tamoxifen plus chemotherapy, while both treatments were significantly superior to chemotherapy alone. A confirmatory study (GROCTA 02) was performed in 244 pre-/perimenopausal patients by comparing 5 years of tamoxifen treatment (plus 2 years of goserelin) to six CMF cycles. No difference has emerged so far between the tamoxifen and CMF arms at a median follow-up time of 62 months. Post-menopausal women were scheduled to receive 3 years of tamoxifen treatment and then to be randomly allocated to further 2 years of tamoxifen or to 2 years of low-dose aminoglutethimide (GROCTA 04B). So far 662 patients have been entered, 375 of whom have been randomized to tamoxifen ($n=188$) or aminoglutethimide ($n=187$). Preliminary results (median follow-up time 32 months) show no major difference in patients' outcome. A new trial (ITA trial) with a similar design but employing anastrozole in place of aminoglutethimide has been activated in 1998. The GROCTA 03 study investigated the potential superiority of alternating adjuvant chemotherapy over standard CMF. This study, which included 107 node-positive ER-negative pre-menopausal women, was prematurely closed because more patients allocated to the triple alternated chemotherapy appeared to have relapsed and died at the first interim analysis. The use of high-dose chemotherapy (HDC) was explored by the GROCTA 06 trial which included 53 patients with ten or more involved nodes and a maximum age of 55 years. These patients were scheduled to receive three standard CEF cycles followed by one cycle of HDC (cyclophosphamide 5 g/m^2; etoposide 1.5 g/m^2; cisplatin 150 mg/m^2) without any form of bone marrow rescue. This HDC program proved to be feasible but was not superior to CMF-based chemotherapy we had previously employed in a comparable group of patients in previous GROCTA trials. These findings prompted us to explore new HDC programmes with the use of peripheral stem cell support and in addition the possible value of new drugs such as Taxol and vinorelbine. New-generation trials will also explore the value of new prognostic indicators such as tumor proliferative activity, which are prospectively used to allocate patients to different treatment options.

Appendix

The following investigators have contributed patients to at least one of the GROCTA trials: G.F. Porcile, Ospedale S. Lazzaro – Alba; M. Rinaldini, P. Ghezzi, Ospedale Civile – Arezzo; G. Giovaninetti, E. Piatto, Ospedale Civile – Bollate; C. Epifani, Ospedale S. Anna – Camerlata; I. Spinelli, Ospedale Civile – Carrara; S. Iacobelli, L. Irtelli, Universitá degli Studi – Chieti; P. Malacarne, D. Donati, Arcispedale S. Anna – Ferrara; M. Cappellini, P. Pacini, Policlinico Careggi – Florence; F. Patrone, F. Ferrando, A. Balestrero, Clinica Medica, N. Ragni, G. Foglia, F. Odicino, Clinica Ostetrica e Ginecologica, Università degli Studi – Genoa; F. Boccardo, D. Amoroso, Oncologia Medica II, R. Rosso, M. Venturini, Oncologia Medica I, IST – Genoa; L. Gallo, C. Caroti, Ospedale Galliera – Genoa; G. Cruciani, E. Montanari, Ospedale Umberto I – Lugo di Romagna; E. Rinaldi, Ospedale Civile – Magenta; F. Smerieri, Ospedale Civile – Mantua; G.P. Benetti, Ospedale Predabissi – Melegnano; R. Scapaticci, Ospedale Civile – Melzo; S. Banducci, Ospedale Civile – Merate; M. Mesiti, D. Romeo, Istituto di Oncologia, Universitá degli Studi – Messina; A. Scanni, S. Co-belli, Ospedale Fatebenefratelli – Milan; E. Villa, A. Bolognesi, D. Aldrighetti, Istituto S. Raffaele – Milan; M. Svanosio, Ospedale S. Croce – Moncalieri; B. Agostara, M. Cusimano, Ospedale Oncologico M. Ascoli, A. Di Carlo, A. Traina, L. Castagnetta, Universitá degli Studi – Palermo; M. Danova, IRCCS S. Matteo e Universitá degli Studi – Pavia; R. Canaletti, C. Rodinó, Ospedale Civile – Piacenza; U. Folco, Ospedale S. Corona – Pietra Ligure; P. Trompeo, Ospedale Civile – Pinerolo; M. Marangolo, Ospedale S. Maria delle Croci – Ravenna; G. Morabito, Ospedale Civile – Reggio Calabria; M. Sassi, Ospedale S. Maria Nuova – Reggio Emilia; A. Beni, Ospedale S. Giacomo – Rome; R. Bellantone, C.P. Lombardi, Clinica Chirurgica, G.P. Ausili Cefaro, L. Nardone, Istituto di Radiologia, Universitá Cattolica – Rome; G. Lelli, A. Piano, Casa Sollievo della Sofferenza – S. Giovanni Rotondo; C. Gatti, D. Guarneri, Ospedale Civile – San Remo; G. Schieppati, G. Burani, Ospedale Civile – Saronno; A. Farris, Universitá degli Studi – Sassari; L. Galletto, Ospedale Civile – Savigliano; F. Brema, Ospedale S. Paolo – Savona; F. Buzzi, Ospedale S. Maria – Terni; M. Aglietta, Ospedale Mauriziano – Turin; M. Massobrio, F. Genta, Ginecologia e Ostetricia "A", P. Sismondi, M. Giai, Ginecologia Oncologica, Università degli Studi – Turin; G. Mustacchi, P. Sandri, Centro Oncologico – Trieste; B. Marsilio, Ospedale S. Maria Misericordia – Udine.

References

Amoroso D, Boccardo F, Rubagotti A et al (1997a) Adjuvant high dose chemotherapy without bone marrow rescue in breast cancer patients with 10 or more positive nodes: preliminary results of an Italian Breast Cancer Adjuvant Study Group (GROCTA) trial. Breast 6:232

Amoroso D, Boccardo F, Rubagotti A et al (1997b) Adjuvant high-dose chemotherapy without bone marrow rescue in breast cancer patients with 10 or more positive nodes: preliminary results of an Italian Breast Cancer Adjuvant Study Group (GROCTA) trial. Proc Am Soc Clin Oncol 16:144

Boccardo F, Rubagotti A, Rosso R et al. (1985) Chemotherapy with or without tamoxifen in postmenopausal patients with late breast cancer. A randomized study. J Steroid Biochem 23:1123–1127

Boccardo F, Rubagotti A, Bruzzi P et al (1990) Chemotherapy versus tamoxifen versus chemotherapy plus tamoxifen in node-positive, estrogen receptor-positive breast cancer patients: results of a multicentric Italian study. J Clin Oncol 8:1310–1320

Boccardo F, Rubagotti A, Amoroso D et al (1992) Chemotherapy versus tamoxifen versus chemotherapy plus tamoxifen in node-positive, oestrogen-receptor positive breast cancer patients. An update at 7 years of the 1st GROCTA trial. Eur J Cancer 28:673–680

Boccardo F, Amoroso D, Rubagotti A et al (1994a) Prolonged tamoxifen treatment of early breast cancer: the experience of the Italian Cooperative Group for Chemo-Hormonal Therapy of Early Breast Cancer (GROCTA). In: Jordan VC (ed) Long-term tamoxifen therapy for breast cancer. University of Wisconsin Press, Madison, pp 159–179

Boccardo F, Rubagotti A, Perrotta A et al (1994b) Ovarian ablation versus goserelin with or without tamoxifen in pre-perimenopausal patients with advanced breast cancer: results of a multicentric Italian study. Ann Oncol 5:337–342

Boccardo F, Rubagotti A, Amoroso D et al (1997a) CMF vs tamoxifen plus goserelin as adjuvant treatment of ER positive pre-perimenopausal breast cancer patients. Preliminary results of an ongoing Italian Breast Cancer Adjuvant Study Group (GROCTA) trial. In: Salmon SE (ed) Adjuvant therapy of cancer VIII. Lippincott-Raven, Philadelphia, pp 101–108

Boccardo F, Rubagotti A, Amoroso D et al (1997b) Lack of effectiveness of adjuvant alternating chemotherapy in node positive, estrogen receptor negative premenopausal breast cancer patients. Results of a multicentric Italian study. Cancer Invest 15:505–512

Bonadonna G, Valagussa P, Rossi A et al (1982) Multimodal therapy with CMF in resectable breast cancer with positive axillary nodes. The Milan Institute experience. Recent Results Cancer Res 80:149–156

Bonadonna G, Veronesi U, Brambilla C et al (1990) Primary chemotherapy to avoid mastectomy in tumors with diameters of three centimeters or more. J Natl Cancer Inst 82:1539–1545

Bonadonna G, Zambetti M, Valagussa P (1995) Sequential or alternating doxorubicin and CMF regimens in breast cancer with more than three positive nodes. JAMA 273:542–547

Buzdar AU, Plourde PV, Hortobagyi GN (1996) Aromatase inhibitors in metastatic breast cancer. Semin Oncol 23 Suppl 9:28–32

Canobbio L, Boccardo F, Pastorino G et al (1989) Phase II study of navelbine in advanced breast cancer. Semin Oncol 16 Suppl 4:33–36

Coombes RC, Powles TJ, Easton D et al (1987) Adjuvant aminoglutethimide therapy for postmenopausal patients with primary breast cancer. Cancer Res 47:2494–2497

Early Breast Cancer Trialist's Collaborative Group (1988) Effects of adjuvant tamoxifen and of cytotoxic therapy on mortality in early breast cancer. An overview of 61 randomized trials among 28 896 women. N Engl J Med 319:1681–1692

Eddy DM (1992) High-dose chemotherapy with autologous bone marrow transplantation for the treatment of metastatic breast cancer. J Clin Oncol 10:657–670

Fisher B, Redmond C, Brown A et al (1983) Influence of tumor estrogen and progesterone receptor levels on the response to tamoxifen and chemotherapy in primary breast cancer. J Clin Oncol 1:227–241

Fisher B, Redmond C, Brown A et al (1986) Adjuvant chemotherapy with and without tamoxifen in the treatment of primary breast cancer: 5-year results from the National Surgical Adjuvant Breast and Bowel Project trial. J Clin Oncol 4:459–471

Gianni L, Capri G, Murrone E et al (1994) Paclitaxel (Taxol) efficacy in patients with advanced breast cancer resistant to anthracyclines. Semin Oncol 21:29–33

Goa KL, Faulds D (1994) Vinorelbine. A review of its pharmacological properties and clinical use in cancer chemotherapy. Drugs Aging 5:200–234

Goldhirsh A, Wood WC, Senn HJ et al (1995) Meeting highlights: International Consensus Panel on the treatment of primary breast cancer. J Natl Cancer Inst 87:1441–1445

Goldie JH, Coldman AJ (1984) The genetic origin of drug resistance in neoplasms: implications for systemic therapy. Cancer Res 44:3643–3653

Gottardis MM, Jordan VC (1988) Development of tamoxifen-stimulated growth of MCF-7 tumors in athymic mice after long-term antiestrogen administration. Cancer Res 48:5183–5187

Hortobagyi GN, Holmes FA (1996) Single-agent paclitaxel for the treatment of breast cancer: an overview. Semin Oncol 23:4–9

Klijn JGM, Seynaeve C, Beex L et al (1996) Combined treatment with buserelin and tamoxifen vs single treatment with each drug alone in premenopausal metastatic breast cancer: preliminary results of EORTC Study 10881. Proc Am Soc Clin Oncol 15:117

Mansi JL, Smith IE, Walsh G et al (1989) Primary medical therapy for operable breast cancer. Eur J Cancer Clin Oncol 25:1623–1627

Mauriac L, Durand M, Avril A et al (1991) Effects of primary chemotherapy in conservative treatment of breast cancer patients with operable tumors larger than 3 cm. Ann Oncol 2:347–354

Moliterni A, Bonadonna G, Valagussa P et al (1991) Cyclophosphamide, methotrexate, and fluorouracil with and without doxorubicin in the adjuvant treatment of resectable breast cancer with one to three positive axillary nodes. J Clin Oncol 9:1124–1130

Niedhart JA, Kohler W, Stidley C et al (1990) Phase I study of repeated cycles of high-dose cyclophosphamide, etoposide, and cisplatin administered without bone marrow transplantation. J Clin Oncol 8:1728–1738

Nolvadex Adjuvant Trial Organization (1983) Controlled trial of tamoxifen as adjuvant agent in the management of early breast cancer. Interim analysis at four years. Lancet 1:257–261

Orsatti M, Curotto A, Canobbio L et al (1995) Alternating chemo-radiotherapy in bladder cancer: a conservative approach. Int J Radiat Oncol Biol Phys 33:173–178

Plourde PV, Dyroff M, Dowsett M et al (1995) Arimidex: a new oral, once-a-day aromatase inhibitor. J Steroid Biochem Mol Biol 53:175–179

Rose C, Thorpe SM, Mouridsen HT et al (1983) Antiestrogen treatment of postmenopausal women with primary high risk breast cancer. Breast Cancer Res Treat 3 Suppl:77–84

Simon R (1989) Optimal two-stage design for the phase II clinical trials. Control Clin Trials 10:1–10

Stuart-Harris RC, Smith IE (1984) Aminoglutethimide in the treatment of advanced breast cancer. Acta Oncol 27:721–728

Vokes EE, Weichselbaum RR (1990) Concomitant chemoradiotherapy: rationale and clinical experience in solid tumors. J Clin Oncol 8:911–932

Current Trials of the German Adjuvant Breast Cancer Group (GABG)*

M. Kaufmann for the GABG

University Women's Hospital, Theodor-Stern Kai 7, 60590 Frankfurt am Main, Germany

Objectives of currently active randomised trials of the GABG in women with primary breast cancer are:
1. Risk-oriented selection of patients by tumor size, menopausal status, nodal involvement and hormonal receptor content
2. Chemo-endocrine or endocrine-endocrine sequences in pre- and post-menopausal patients
3. Chemo- or endocrine therapy in pre-menopausal patients
4. Reduction of local treatment (axillary surgery, radiotherapy)
5. Preoperative chemotherapy in operable breast cancer.

Evolution of Current GABG Trials

The German Adjuvant Breast Cancer Group (GABG) was created in 1981 by F. Kubli, M. Kaufmann, H. Maass and W. Jonat. The main aim of the group was to evaluate adjuvant systemic therapies in early breast cancer based on a risk evaluation of each patient. The history and evolution of the GABG trials is summarised in Table 1. Even in the first two trials patients were divided in two risk groups by extent of nodal involvement and hormonal receptor status. In the *GABG I trial* (Kaufmann et al. 1993) only node-positive patients were recruited. If less than four nodes were involved and the hormonal receptor content was more than 20 fmol/mg protein, patients were considered to be at low risk and randomised to either tamoxifen 30 mg for 2 years or six cycles of cyclophosphamide, methotrexate, and fluoruroacil (CMF) i. v. If the tumor was found to be receptor-negative or more than three nodes were involved patients were regarded as high-risk and randomised to either eight cycles of doxorubicin and cyclophosphamide (AC) or eight cycles AC plus tamoxifen 30 mg for 2 years. In the second trial, which first started in 1979 as a single-centre trial in Heidelberg and was later absorbed into the GABG framework, only node-negative patients with positive receptor status were re-

* These trials received financial support from ICI/Zeneca Germany, Farmitalia/Phamacia-Upjohn and the Deutsche Krebshilfe.

Table 1. History and evolution of the GABG trials

Trial	Year	Lymph nodes	No. of patients
HD 1	1976	+	124
HD 2	1979	+/−	184
GABG I	1981	+	745
GABG II	1984	−	603
GABG III	1986	+/−	1500
GABG IV	1992	+/−	1747
ZEBRA [a]	1990	+	1640
ARNO [b]	1997	+/−	
GABG V GEPARDO	1998	+/−	

[a] International.
[b] Also being performed in Austria.

cruited. These low-risk patients were randomised to either tamoxifen 30 mg for 2 years or observation. As a result of these trials it became evident that response to adjuvant therapy is dependent on the patient's age and receptor status. In the GABG I trial, which included 754 patients, chemo-endocrine treatment with AC+tamoxifen was superior to AC in patients older than 50 years and in patients with positive-receptor status but not in patients less than 50 years of age. CMF chemotherapy improved survival in patients younger than 50 years and tamoxifen did so in patients older than 50 years. In the *GABG II trial* (von Minckwitz et al. 1995), which enrolled 713 patients, response to tamoxifen was clearly dependent on age, so patients older than 70 years showed the highest benefit. Estrogen but not progesterone receptor status was also a significant predictor of response to tamoxifen.

On the basis of these results the *GABG III trials* were started in 1987. Here, for the first time patients were divided into pre- and post-menopausal, which seemed more relevant for tumor biology than patient age. Postmenopausal patients with ER-positive tumors were either treated with CMF×6+tamoxifen or with tamoxifen alone. Pre-menopausal patients irrespective of receptor status and post-menopausal patients with ER-negative tumors were randomised to either CMF×3 or to CMF×6. In a high-risk group of patients with 10+ nodes involved, an anthracycline-containing regimen (FEC) was compared to CMF. Patients with ER- and/or PR-positive tumors additionally received tamoxifen 30 mg for 2 years.

Overall no difference was found between six or three cycles of CMF (Schumacher et al. 1994). However, if one separates the patients by extent of nodal involvement it becomes obvious that CMF×6 is more effective, but only in patients with more than three involved lymph nodes. In patients with fewer positive lymph nodes the number of cycles can be reduced to three and toxicity can be spared.

Temporary Ovarian Ablation

Surgical ovarian ablation was first described by Beatson in 1898 to be an effective treatment in pre-menopausal metastatic breast cancer. During the 1960s and 1970s surgical or radiological castration was also evaluated as adjuvant treatment and was shown to significantly improve survival in pre-menopausal patients. However, irreversible castration in younger women leads to considerable long-term side effects like osteoporosis and cardiovascular disease. From the tamoxifen trials it was known that a treatment duration of 2–5 years is sufficient to eradicate micrometastasis and improve survival significantly. With the development of long-acting GnRH analogues it was possible to temporarily down-regulate ovarian function, so these compounds seemed to be ideal for an adjuvant treatment in breast cancer patients. The Zoladex Early Breast Cancer Research Association (*ZEBRA*) was founded in 1992 and included most of the GABG centres as well as trial centres in England and 13 other countries worldwide. In the trial design six cycles of CMF was compared with goserelin 3.6 mg s.c. every 4 weeks for 2 years. More than 1600 pre-menopausal patients with node-positive breast cancer had been recruited by 1996. Results of the first analysis will be presented at the ASCO conference in May 1998.

This interesting endocrine approach in pre-menopausal patients has also become part of the currently running GABG IV trials.

Currently Running Trials: GABG IV

On the basis of the St. Gallen consensus meeting in 1992 and the results of the GABG I–III trials the GABG decided to design the *GABG IV-G trials* (Fig. 1), which were started in 1993. Four main questions were addressed:

1. Does a low-toxicity endocrine treatment have the same effect as poly-chemotherapy in premenopausal patients?

This was the question of the ZEBRA trial comparing goserelin with 6×CMF. However, on the basis of previous results the GABG decided only to randomise patients with ER- and/or PR-positive tumors into this trial. A similar trial was performed in node-negative patients with hormone-receptor-positive tumors, but the number of cycles of the CMF polychemotherapy was reduced to three in line with the GABG III trial. This trial, GABG IV-A, is recruiting quite slowly as this group of patients is small, but it has nevertheless recruited 45% of the planned number of the patients so far.

2. Is the combination of chemotherapy and endocrine therapy superior to chemotherapy alone?

This question has been addressed to pre- and post-menopausal patients. Menopausal status is determined in the perimenopause by estradiol and FSH

Preoperative:

< 70 years, T size > 3 cm, N0-1, M0:   **GEPARDO:**   Preoperative chemotherapy
                                                       Doxorubicin + docetaxel

> 70 years, T size < 3 cm, N0, M0:   **GABG IV-G:** Op ± Axilla + tamoxifen 20 mg/5 years

Postoperative: (pT1-3; R0, M0, < 70 years):

	Hormone receptor status	Nodal status N0	N1-3	N4-9	N10+
Pre-meno-pausal	R+	**GABG IV-A:** Zoladex vs CMFx3	ZEBRA (closed) Zoladex vs CMFx6		**GABG IV-E:** E_{120} vs EC-CMF
	R−	**GABG IV-B:** CMFx3 ± Zoladex		**GABG IV-B*:** ECx4-CMFx3 ± Zoladex	HD chemotherapy - IMA trial
Post-meno-pausal	R+	**GBAG V** (T < 1 cm, G 1-2 Lo Ro) ± tamoxifen ± RT			- Zander
		ARNO: (T > 1 cm) Tamoxifen 2 years $\frac{1}{m}$ Arimidex 3 years vs tamoxifen 3 years			
	R−	**GABG IV-D:** CMFx3 ± tamoxifen		**GABG IV-D*:** ECx4-CMFx3 ± tamoxifen	

Fig. 1. The GABG IV/V trials. Scheme by which to identify the trial for any individual patient

levels. In the GABG-B study pre-menopausal patients with ER- and PR-negative tumors and 0–3 involved lymph nodes were treated with 3×CMF or with a sequential schedule of 3×CMF and goserelin 3.6 mg s.c. every 4 weeks for 2 years. Because of their increased risk, patients with 4–9 involved nodes received four cycles of epirubicin and cyclophosphamide (EC) before the CMF treatment and were then randomised to goserelin or observation (study GABG B*). As the ZEBRA trial was closed at the end of 1996, the hormone receptor-positive patients were from that date also included in the B studies. To date 50% of the planned number of patients have been randomised.

3. Is it possible to overcome tumor cell resistance by giving non-cross-resistant therapies in sequence?

One approach to answering this question is directed towards high-risk patients with more than nine lymph nodes involved. The comparators of the GABG IV-E study are mono-chemotherapy with an increased dose of 120 mg/m^2 epirubicin, repeated four times every 3 weeks, versus four cycles of a conventionally dosed EC regimen followed by three cycles of CMF. With hormone receptor-positive tumors, pre-menopausal patients then receive goserelin for 2 years and post-menopausal patients tamoxifen for 5 years. Due to the increased risk of recurrence or death the number of patients required is smaller, so that it will be possible to close this trial in 1998 and first results will be available in 1999.

The other approach to circumventing resistance is to combine different endocrine treatments. As the development of resistance to tamoxifen and even stimulatory effects of tamoxifen have been well described in in vitro and in vivo experiments, it is of interest to know whether total depletion of estrogen levels by highly selective aromatase inhibitors can improve the results of adjuvant tamoxifen treatment. In this trial, now called the Arimidex-Nolvadex (ARNO) trial, 5 years of tamoxifen is compared to 2 years of tamoxifen followed by 3 years of anastrozole (Arimidex). This trial design is also used in Austria; it started in 1997 and is confined to post-menopausal patients with hormone receptor-positive tumors. Treatment with tamoxifen 20 or 30 mg should have lasted for 2 years without interruption and patients need to be free of recurrent disease before they are entered in this trial.

4. What is the value of preoperative chemotherapy?

Recently the timing of chemotherapy in relation to surgery has been investigated extensively. Preoperative chemotherapy provides an "in vivo" chemosensitivity test, which is an advantage to postoperative therapy where evaluation of tumor response is very difficult. Furthermore, reduction of tumor size by preoperative chemotherapy (down staging) can improve the rate of breast-conserving surgery and the cosmetic result.

Early use of cytotoxic drugs seems to decrease the number of chemoresistant cell lines (Surbone and Norton 1993), as overall response rates using conventionally anthracycline-based chemotherapy are generally very high (Bonadonna et al. 1990, 1991; Bonadonna 1992). In patients with tumors >3 cm in diameter this can lead to breast-conserving surgery in 91% of cases. However, complete remissions can be confirmed histologically only in 4%–8% (Feldmann et al. 1986; Hortobagyi et al. 1988).

This concept was first evaluated in feasibility phase II study GABG IV-F using four cycles of EC after confirmation of diagnosis by core-cut biopsy. Patients needed to have an initial tumor size of >3 cm and no fixed or internal mammary lymph nodes. Surgery was performed according to the decision of the surgeon. If tumorectomy could be performed, postoperative irradiation of the breast followed, while if mastectomy had to be performed, only adjuvant systemic treatment was carried out. Adjuvant postoperative systemic therapy was dependent on menopausal status and receptor expression. All patients without expression of hormonal receptors received a further three cycles of CMF. Patients with receptor-positive tumors received goserelin if premenopausal and tamoxifen if postmenopausal.

The impact of preoperative chemotherapy on survival was addressed in a recently published study of the NSABP with 1523 patients (Fisher et al. 1997). In this randomised trial no difference in time to recurrence and time to death was found when preoperative and postoperative chemotherapy with four cycles of AC were compared. Small tumors, younger patients and node-negative disease were predictive of a better response to preoperative chemotherapy. The response rate has been 80%, and the tumor progressed in only 4% of the patients. The rate of breast conservation could be increased significantly from 60% to 68%, and the proportion of patients with node-positive disease was reduced to 40% (in comparison to 58% in the postoperative group).

Another randomised trial was published by Scholl et al. (1994) with 414 pre-menopausal patients with T2-3 tumors. After a follow-up period of 54 months, preoperative treatment with four cycles of CAF was superior in terms of disease-free survival to postoperative treatment with the same schedule ($p = 0.04$).

Docetaxel has shown to be highly active in metastatic breast cancer, with a response rate of 61% in first-line therapy. The effectivity has also been demonstrated in anthracycline-resistant patients (von Minckwitz and Costa 1997'). Median time to remission was 9 weeks in a 3-week schedule of 100 mg/m^2.

In a recently published trial docetaxel 100 mg/m^2 was compared with adriamycin 75 mg/m^2 in patients resistant to alkylating agents. Response rates were significantly higher in the docetaxel group, but due to the short follow-up period only a trend towards prolonged disease-free survival could be identified (Chan et al. 1997). Docetaxel is therefore considered the most active agent in the treatment of breast cancer.

A French group has combined the adriamycin and docetaxel as first-line therapy in a phase I study in 42 patients with metastatic breast cancer. For this 3-week schedule a dosage of adriamycin 60 mg/m^2 and docetaxel 60 mg/m^2 or adriamycin 50 mg/m^2 and docetaxel 75 mg/m^2 was recommended. Leukopenia with subsequent infection was dose limiting (grade IV neutropenia in 93% of the patients without G-CSF). In the schedule with adriamycin 50 mg/m^2 and docetaxel 75 mg/m^2 the nadir was observed on day 9 (range 4–13 days) with a neutrophil count of 100–1300. Anaemia and thrombocytopenia were seen occasionally (grade III: 9.5% and 7.1% respectively). In three patients grade III infections were observed. Up to a dosage of 360 mg/m^2 adriamycin no reduction in cardiac function could be documented (Bourgeois et al. 1996; Kalla et al. 1996). The complete and partial response rate was 90%; in patients with liver involvement it was 88%. This represents the highest response rate reached with a combination chemotherapy without bone marrow rescue.

In a second feasibility study of primary chemotherapy with adriamycin and docetaxel we were able to show that it can also be applied as a dose-intensified 14-day schedule. All patients except one were able to receive the full dose intensity and undergo surgery directly after the end of the fourth cycle. The remission rate was approximately 83% (Costa et al. 1998, submitted).

We concluded that:

- preoperative chemotherapy can improve operability
- preoperative chemotherapy achieves identical or even better survival rates than postoperative chemotherapy.
- response to preoperative chemotherapy can be predictive for the prognosis of the patient.

We also stated the hypothesis that if the response of the primary tumor to preoperative chemotherapy is a marker of the chemosensitivity of micrometastatic distant disease, and histological confirmation of a complete response predicts cure from breast cancer, improvement in the response rates to preoperative chemotherapy should improve the survival of breast cancer patients.

Response rates can be improved by:
- combining the most active substances (adriamycin and docetaxel)
- combining chemotherapy with endocrine therapy (adriamycin, docetaxel and tamoxifen)
- dose intensification (14-day schedule)
- modulation of drug resistance (tamoxifen modulates GP 170 activity).

This led to the next generation of *GABG V* trials, the German Preoperative Adriamycin Docetaxel (*GEPARDO*) trial. The primary objective of this trial is to determine the activity of preoperative dose-intensified therapy with adriamycin and docetaxel in patients with operable carcinoma of the breast with or without tamoxifen treatment. The primary endpoint of the trial is the rate of histologically confirmed complete remissions.

Appendix

Scientific board members of the GABG are: A. von der Assen, Cloppenburg; B. Conrad, Kassel; W. Eiermann, Munich; B. Gerber, Rostock; J. Hilfrich, Hannover; W. Jonat*, Kiel; M. Kaufmann*, Frankfurt; R. Kreienberg*, Ulm; H. Maass*, Hamburg; H. Massinger-Biebl, Eggenfelden; G. von Minckwitz, Frankfurt; M. Schuhmacher*, Freiburg; D. Wallwiener, Heidelberg.

The address of the study coordinating centre is: GABG (German Adjuvant Breast Cancer Group), c/o C. Diehl, Trial coordinator, University Women's Hospital, Theodor-Stern-Kai 7, 60590 Frankfurt am Main, Germany, tel. (+49) (0) 69 6301 7438.

Summary

Since 1981 the German Adjuvant Breast Cancer Study Group (GABG) has recruited approximately 5000 patients with primary breast caner in randomized trials to evaluate systemic therapies. More than 70 hospitals all over Germany are participating in this group. Allocation to the different trials is based on a risk-oriented selection of patients (menopausal status, nodal involvement and hormonal receptor content). In the currently running trials chemo-endocrine or endocrine-endocrine sequences are investigated. In premenopausal patients the value of GnRH analogues are compared with conventional CMF chemotherapy. The aim of two further trials is to reduce local surgery or radiotherapy in patients with low risk for locoregional relapse. In a recently started study dose-intensified preoperative chemotherapy in combination with or without tamoxifen is evaluated in patients with operable breast tumors ≥3 cm.

---

* Members of the advisory board.

References

Bonadonna G (1992) Evolving concepts in the systemic adjuvant treatment of breast cancer. Cancer Res 52:2127–2137

Bonadonna G, Veronesi U, Brambilla C, Ferrari L, Luini A, Greco M, Bartolo C, deYoldi G, Zucali R, Rilke F, Andreola S, Silvestrini R, DiFronzo G, Valgussa P (1990) Primary chemotherapy to avoid mastectomy in tumors with diameters of three centimeters or more. J Natl Cancer Inst 82:1539–1541

Bonadonna G, Valagussa P, Brambilla C (1991) Adjuvant and primary treatment of breast cancer with chemotherapy and/or endocrine therapy. Semin Oncol 18:515

Bourgeois H, Gruia G, Dieras V, Kalla S, Giaccetti S, Cvitkovic E, Aussel JP, Azli N, Riva A, Pouillart P, Misset JL (1996) Docetaxel in combination with doxorubicin as 1st line CT of metastatic breast cancer (MBC): a phase I dose finding study. Proc Am Soc Clin Oncol 15:148

Chan S, Friedrichs K, Noel D, Duarte R et al (1997) A randomized phase III study of Taxotere (T) versus doxorubicin (D) in patients (pts) with metastatic breast cancer (MBC) who have failed an alkylating containing regimen: preliminary results. Proc Am Soc Clin Oncol 16:540

Feldmann L, Hortobagyi G, Buzdar A, Ames F, Blumenstein GR (1986) Pathological assessment of response to induction chemotherapy in breast cancer. Cancer Res 46:2578–2581

Fisher B, Brown A, Mamounas E, Wieland S, Robidoux A, Margolese RG, Cruz AB Jr, Fisher ER, Wickerham DL, Wolmark N, DeCillis A, Hoehn JL, Lees AW, Dimitrov NV (1997) Effect of preoperative chemotherapy on local-regional disease in women with operable breast cancer: findings from National Surgical Adjuvant Breast and Bowel Project B-18. J Clin Oncol 15:2483–2493

Hortobagyi GN, Ames FC, Buzdar AU, Kau SW, McNeese MD, Paulus D, Hug V, Holmes FA, Romsdahl MM, Fraschini G, McBride CM, Martin RG, Montague E (1988) Management of stage III primary breast cancer with primary chemotherapy, surgery, and radiation therapy. Cancer 62:2507–2516

Kalla S, Bourgeois H, Gruia G, Dieras V, Giacchetti S, Cvitkovic E, Aussel JP, Azli N, Riva A, Pouillart P, Misset JL (1996) Docetaxel in combination with doxorubicin as first line chemotherapy of metastatic breast cancer: a phase I dose finding study. Final results. Ann Oncol 7 Suppl 5:124–125

Kaufmann M, Jonat W, Abel U, Hilfrich J, Caffier H, Kreienberg R, Trams G, Brunnert K, Schermann J, Kleine W et al (1993) Adjuvant randomized trials of doxorubicin/cyclophosphamide versus doxorubicin/cyclophosphamide/tamoxifen and CMF chemotherapy versus tamoxifen in women with node-positive breast cancer. J Clin Oncol 11(3):454–460

Scholl SM, Fouquet A, Asselain B, Pierga JA, Vilcoq JR, Durand JC, Dorval T, Palangie T, Jouve M, Beuzeboc P (1994) Primary versus adjuvant chemotherapy in premenopausal patients with tumors considered too large for breast conserving surgery: preliminary results of a randomised trial: S6. Eur J Cancer 30A(5):645–652

Schumacher M, Bastert G, Bojar H, Hubner K, Olschewski M, Sauerbrei W, Schmoor C, Beyerle C, Neumann RL, Rauschecker HF (1994) Randomized 2×2 trial evaluating hormonal treatment and the duration of chemotherapy in node-positive breast cancer patients. German Breast Cancer Study Group. J Clin Oncol 12(10):2086–2093

Surbone A, Norton L (1993) Kinetic concepts in the treatment of breast cancer. Ann NY Acad Sci 698

Von Minckwitz G, Costa SD (1997) Docetaxel (Taxotere/-E) zur Therapie des Mammakarzinoms – Höchste Wirksamkeit bei moderaten Nebenwirkungen. Med Klin 92 Suppl 4:4–9

Von Minckwitz G, Kaufmann M, Schmid H, Kleine W, Brunnert K, Ulmer MU, Stosiek U, Mahlke M, Mehrpohl HG, Neises M, Baltzer J (1995) Tamoxifen in patients with node-negative and receptor-positive breast cancer: the Heidelberg II and GABG II experience. 5th International Conference on Adjuvant Therapy of Primary Breast Cancer, St. Gallen, Abstract book, p 80

XII. International Consensus Conference on Primary Treatment of the Breast: Update 1998

International Consensus Panel on the Treatment of Primary Breast Cancer V: Update 1998*

Aron Goldhirsch [1], John H. Glick [2], Richard D. Gelber [3] and Hans-Jörg Senn [4]

[1] A. Goldhirsch, International Breast Cancer Study Group, Lugano, Switzerland, and European Institute of Oncology, I-20141 Milan, Italy
[2] J. H. Glick, University of Pennsylvania Cancer Center, Philadelphia
[3] R. D. Gelber, Department of Biostatistical Science, Dana-Farber Cancer Institute, Boston, MA
[4] H.-J. Senn, Center for Tumordetection and Prevention, CH-9006 St. Gallen, Switzerland

Providing effective care for patients with early-stage breast cancer and designing appropriate recommendations for women at high risk of developing the disease are important public health goals. More than ever, progress requires integrated understanding based on the continuous interaction among several scientific and clinical disciplines. In February 1998, the 6th International Conference on Adjuvant Therapy of Primary Breast Cancer was held in St. Gallen, Switzerland. Knowledge of breast cancer genetics, diagnosis, and treatment has evolved since the 5th International Conference that was held in March 1995. At that time, a fundamental theme was to distinguish the role of prognostic factors used in the definition of risk from predictive factors used for the selection of adjuvant treatments according to therapeutic responsiveness (Goldhirsch et al. 1995). Also, at that time, the findings from the 1992 overview publication (Early Breast Cancer Trialists' Collaborative Group 1992) that reported results on ovarian ablation, tamoxifen, and chemotherapy effects were being increasingly applied to justify adjuvant treatment for a wider spectrum of indications.

Since 1995, several specific areas have accumulated important new information and were highlighted at this year's conference. These include the following: genetic testing of women at risk; the availability of chemopreventive agents for high-risk and post-menopausal women; changes in diagnostic procedures with an intent to reduce axillary dissection by introducing sentinel-node biopsy; results from trials of preoperative chemotherapy; initiatives to evaluate preoperative endocrine therapies; and debates on the role of increased local control by postmastectomy radiation therapy, its safety, and its effectiveness.

At the conclusion of the conference, a consensus panel of experts was asked – as at the previous conference (Goldhirsch et al. 1995) – to develop a series of guidelines and recommendations for selection of adjuvant systemic treatments in specific patient populations. The panel reviewed and modified

* First published in: Journal of the National Cancer Institute, 1998, 90 (Nov. 4, 1998).

its previous guidelines and recommendations based on new evidence that has emerged from clinical research.

During the past 3 years, several new fields of interest have emerged and a variety of treatment strategies have been tested. Some of these strategies can be added to the repertoire of treatments available for patients today, while others are still undergoing clinical investigation for a better assessment of their potential usefulness in the future. Table 1 describes some examples of these recent findings and their implications for or status relative to patient care. In this commentary, we describe some areas of ongoing research and update the adjuvant treatment recommendations presented 3 years ago.

Prognosis and Prediction of Response

Several factors have been identified that define those patients who should not receive any form of adjuvant systemic therapy. The panel agreed that a population of patients who have less than a 10% chance of relapse within 10 years would not be candidates for receiving routine adjuvant systemic therapy. This represents a change from the conclusions of the previous panel, which recommended that such exclusion be based on a 10-year *mortality rate* of 10% or less. The modification reflects the panel's consensus that patient's preference to avoid relapse might be used for consideration of adjuvant chemotherapy, even when the risk of death from breast cancer is quite low. Data from cohorts followed for less than 10 years were felt to be insufficient to define a group at minimal risk.

The most relevant factors for the estimation of risk remain the nodal status and the number of nodes involved. For patients with node-negative disease, tumor size, histologic and nuclear grade, steroid hormone receptor status, lymphatic and/or vascular invasion, and age are factors considered by the panel to define groups with differential prognosis for use in treatment selection (Table 2). Additional considerations about a low relative risk of relapse within a risk category, toxic effects, socioeconomic implications, and information on patient's preference might also contribute to treatment decision-making.

Two new strategies were discussed as having great potential for altering the estimation of risk; both require validation by future studies before they are ready for routine use outside of clinical research. First, staging of the axilla might change if sentinel lymph node biopsy and workup, a limited staging procedure, replaces complete axillary dissection as the source of information on axillary nodes (Veronesi et al. 1997). Second, the use of preoperative systemic therapy will influence the prognostic information available. The assessment of pathologic features of the primary tumor will have to rely on limited material obtained from a core biopsy. The characteristics of the primary tumor and axillary lymph nodes observed in samples obtained after preoperative systemic therapy may be modified from those that would have been observed following primary surgery alone. On the other hand, the use of primary systemic therapy contributes additional prognostic features, speci-

Table 1. Recent research findings presented at the 6th International Conference on Adjuvant Therapy of Primary Breast Cancer and their implications for patient care

Field or treatment	Status of research/implications for patient care
Epidemiology	Recognition of risk factors (markers of risk that cannot be changed, e.g., sex, age, or height) and risk determinants (factors that, if changed, would alter the frequency or characteristics of the disease, e.g., exposure to ionizing irradiation, estrogen replacement therapy, alcohol consumption, body mass, and perhaps diet)
Genetics	Availability of testing for mutations in the BRCA 1 and BRCA 2 genes has led to the definition of new subpopulations of women with a substantially increased risk of developing breast (and ovarian) cancer. The lack of effective preventive modalities for these women complicates recommendations for testing and follow-up (Burke et al. 1997). Screening to define individual risk is thus not ready for routine use and presents challenges for the management of major personal, ethical, and therapeutic dilemmas. Ongoing and future chemoprevention trials might have an important impact upon the use of genetic information
Chemoprevention	Trials to test tamoxifen as a chemopreventive agent (motivated by a 40% reduction in the risk of contralateral breast cancer observed in randomized adjuvant therapy trials) have accrued about 20 000 women. (After the conference on April 5th, the NSABP released the first results for 13 388 women in the NSABP Breast Cancer Prevention Trial which showed, after about 4 years' median follow-up, a similar reduction in invasive cancer and ductal carcinoma in situ [DCIS] in the tamoxifen-treated group). Another anti-estrogen, raloxifene, tested for reduction of osteoporosis (Delmas et al. 1997), was shown after a short treatment and follow-up duration to reduce breast cancer incidence in women over 60 years of age. Fenretinide (4-HPR), a retinoid tested in patients with node-negative disease, showed some effect on reducing the incidence of contralateral breast cancer in premenopausal women
Treatment of DCIS	Incidence of DCIS has increased substantially in recent years as a result of refined and intensified diagnostic procedures, mainly mammography. Although the spread of tumor cells in these lesions is intraductal, the principles guiding the surgical management of these lesions are the same as those for invasive cancer – localization and total removal of the primary tumor with clear resection margins. Conservation of the breast, if possible and desired, should be attempted. If there is no invasive component, no additional prognostic information is obtained by removal of the axillary lymph nodes. Therefore, axillary dissection is not indicated. Radiation therapy to the conserved breast after a complete surgical removal of a DCIS lesion showed a statistically significant relative reduction (four fold) in subsequent invasive tumor growth in the breast (Fisher et al. 1998). This issue is still under investigation in Europe. Additional research is directed toward determining whether tamoxifen is effective in preventing relapse and invasion following treatment of DCIS

Table 1 (continued)

Field or treatment	Status of research implications for patient care
Extent of surgery to the breast and to the axilla	Breast-conserving surgery (and planned radiation therapy to the conserved breast) is the treatment of choice for unifocal, invasive breast cancer that can be excised with clear margins. The importance of clear margins (defined as normal tissue of about 1 cm surrounding the tumor) has been demonstrated, although clear margins do not guarantee freedom from local recurrence. Axillary staging through the pathologic evaluation of the first lymph node that drains the tumor area (sentinel-node biopsy) was tested to avoid extensive surgery on a negative axilla (Veronesi et al. 1997). The proper technique to use, extent of the pathology workup, and training required for an accurate and reproducible result have yet to be determined: thus the method remains investigational. While axillary dissection is considered the proper staging procedure for breast cancer, its impact on the curability of the disease is unclear, especially in patients with clinically N0 disease who are given adjuvant therapy
Biologic therapies, immunotoxins, antibodies, and gene therapy	Treatments with monoclonal antibodies, especially in combination with cytotoxic drugs, still await demonstration of relevant clinical effect. Vaccines against breast cancer cell components are being tested (Miles 1997). Modulation of growth factors (e.g., insulin-like growth factor 1; Bontenbal et al. 1998) and inhibition of angiogenesis (Kerbel 1997) are being evaluated in the clinical setting
Factors for prediction of treatment responsiveness	The steroid hormone receptor status of the primary tumor is the only marker of treatment response that has unequivocal clinical utility. There is some uncertainty about the level of receptor expression to use as the threshold responsiveness to endocrine therapies. Standardization of the assay procedure is desirable. Measurement of C-*erb*B 2 expression for prediction of response to anthracycline-containing chemotherapy and for resistance to treatment with tamoxifen or CMF requires further prospective verification, because currently available information is exclusively from retrospective studies (Sjogren et al. 1998)
Preoperative (primary) systemic therapy	Preoperative chemotherapy has been shown to be safe, yielding similar results in terms of disease-free survival and overall survival as did the same regimen when used following surgery. Patients who received preoperative chemotherapy were more likely to become eligible for breast conservation (Fisher et al. 1997a). Clinical and pathologic response to primary chemotherapy was associated with prolonged disease-free survival. Primary endocrine therapy with new aromatase inhibitors or pure antiestrogens is being investigated; however, primary treatment with tamoxifen appears less effective than surgery followed by tamoxifen in terms of control of disease

Table 1 (continued)

Field or treatment	Status of research implications for patient care
Radiation therapy after mastectomy	Breast irradiation is clearly indicated after breast-conserving surgery. Recent trials in postmastectomy patients (Overgaard et al. 1997; Ragaz et al. 1997) indicated that some patients at very high risk of local recurrence might benefit, even with increased survival, from local and regional postoperative radiation therapy (50 Gy comprehensive treatment, appropriately planned and delivered). Controversies exist, however, concerning the adequacy of surgery and systemic treatment delivered in these trials (Goldhirsch et al. 1998a). Nevertheless, the approximately fourfold decrease in the risk of local-regional recurrence is likely to provide a non-negligible benefit in terms of systemic disease control and survival for patients at high risk of such recurrence. Postmastectomy radiation is thus to be considered for patients who, despite proper surgery and adjuvant systemic therapy, are at high risk of local recurrence (a risk of 20% or more, e.g., those presenting with four or more metastatic axillary lymph nodes). The components of the radiation plan (chest wall, internal mammary nodes and axilla) were not separately investigated and are under investigation in clinical trials. The safety of local and regional radiation therapy given following anthracycline and/or taxane therapy has not been elucidated
High-dose chemotherapy and taxanes	High-dose chemotherapy in the adjuvant setting that uses a four- to tenfold increase in dose with autologous bone marrow or peripheral blood progenitor cell support (with the aid of hematopoietic growth factors) is a promising approach for patients at high risk of relapse but remains investigational (Zujewski et al. 1998), since definitive results from clinical trials are not yet available. Also, the use of taxanes in the adjuvant setting – either in concurrent or sequential combination with other cytotoxic drugs – is under intensive investigation

fically the clinical and pathologic responses of the primary tumor to preoperative therapy (Ellis et al. 1998; Fisher et al. 1997a).

Expression of steroid hormone receptors in tumor cells is the most relevant factor predicting treatment response to endocrine therapy (Table 1). However, the methods used to assess estrogen receptor and progesterone receptor status have changed rapidly in recent years. Cutoff points based on immunohistochemical assay results to define endocrine-therapy responsiveness are still being evaluated. This is especially true for tumors with no or a low percentage of cells that stain for steroid hormone receptors (Clark et al. 1997). In particular, the decision to avoid the use of endocrine therapies might require that no expression of such receptors be observed, whereas if 10% or more of the tumor cells are stained for these receptors, an unequivocal response to endocrine therapy is likely.

The accurate definition of node-negative status requires that proper surgical dissection (to levels I and II) be performed and a sufficient number of axillary lymph nodes be examined. For routine use, axillary staging should be based on a sufficient number of examined lymph nodes (usually at least ten) to obtain the proper prognostic information (Axelsson et al. 1992). Methods that investigate proliferative features of the primary tumor, its inva-

Table 2. Risk categories for patients with node-negative breast cancer

Factors[a]	Minimal/low risk (has all listed factors)	Intermediate risk (risk classified between the other two categories)	High risk (has at least one listed factor)
Tumor size[b]	≤1 cm	>1–2 cm	>2 cm
Grade[d]	Grade 1 (uncertain relevance for tumors ≤1 cm)	Grade 1–2	Grade 2–3
Estrogen receptor (ER) and/or progesterone receptor (PgR) status[c]	Positive	Positive	Negative
Age (years)[e]	≥35		<35

[a] Some panel members also recognize lymphatic and/or vascular invasion as an important feature that indicates an increased risk.
[b] It was generally agreed by the panel members that pathologic tumor size (i.e., size of the invasive component) was the most important prognostic factor for defining the additional risk of relapse.
[c] ER and Pg status are important biologic characteristics that identify responsiveness to endocrine therapies.
[d] Histologic and/or nuclear grade.
[e] Patients who develop breast cancer at a young age are considered to be at high risk of relapse, although an exact age threshold for this increased risk has not been defined.

sive, metastatic, and angiogenic potential, require prospective studies and assessment with respect to specific treatment programes.

Consensus Panel Recommendations and Guidelines

Tables 3 and 4 summarize the recommendations and guidelines for postoperative adjuvant systemic therapy for early breast cancer proposed by the International Consensus Panel during the St. Gallen Conference in 1998. The panel emphasized that these guidelines are based on evidence from clinical trials demonstrating that various adjuvant therapies can reduce the risk of relapse and increase survival duration. They are not intended to be used to define required treatment for all patients, since individual circumstances and attitudes toward treatment and resources may vary in different parts of the world.

The format used to construct Tables 3 and 4 reflects the four issues that are considered during treatment decision-making outside of the framework of clinical trials: prognosis, prediction of treatment response, extrapolation of results on treatment effects obtained from randomized trials, and consideration of patient's preference concerning risks and benefits of effective therapies.

Four patient populations have been defined, based on the risk for relapse (prognosis) as described in the columns in Table 3 (node negative with minimal/low risk, with intermediate risk, or with high risk) and Table 4 (node pos-

Table 3. Adjuvant treatment for patients with node-negative breast cancer

Patient group	Risk group		
	Minimal/low risk	Intermediate risk	High risk
Pre-menopausal, ER or PgR positive	None or tamoxifen	Tamoxifen ± chemo-therapy[b] Ovarian ablation[c] GnRH analogue[c]	Chemotherapy ± amoxifen[b] Ovarian ablation[c] GnRH analogue[c]
Pre-menopausal, ER and PgR positive	Not applicable	Not applicable	Chemotherapy
Post-menopausal, ER or PgR positive	None or tamoxifen	Tamoxifen ± chemo-therapy[b]	Tamoxifen+chemo-therapy[b]
Post-menopausal, ER or PgR negative	Not applicable	Not applicable	Chemotherapy[d]
Elderly	None or tamoxifen	Tamoxifen ± chemo-therapy[b]	Tamoxifen If no ER and PgR expression: chemo-therapy

ER, estrogen receptor; PgR, progesterone receptor; GnRH, gonadotropin-releasing hormone.
[a] Treatment accepted for routine use or baseline in clinical trials.
[b] The addition of chemotherapy is considered an acceptable option based on evidence from clinical trials. Considerations about a low relative risk of relapse, age, toxic effects, socioeconomic implications, and information on patient's preference might justify the use of tamoxifen alone.
[c] Still being tested in randomized trials.
[d] The addition of tamoxifen following chemotherapy might be considered for patients whose tumors are classified as ER and PgR negative, but which exhibit minimal/trace levels of either ER or PgR.

itive). The rows represent different treatment-response (or predictive) factors, including steroid hormone receptor status of the primary tumor and whether ovarian function suppression can be added as a therapeutic modality (pre-menopausal versus post-menopausal status). Also, elderly patients are listed separately, since specific considerations are required concerning tradeoffs between burdens of treatment, risks of relapse, and competing causes of morbidity and mortality.

Within the body of Tables 3 and 4, we distinguish between therapies for which direct evidence is available that have demonstrated treatment effects based on the results of randomized, controlled clinical trials and those therapies that are still investigational. Finally, footnotes indicate specific areas in which patient preference should be taken into consideration when defining appropriate treatment. Physicians should elicit the preferences of their patients concerning aversion to side effects and attitudes toward disease recurrence and weigh these preferences against the uncertainty of prognosis and of treatment effectiveness (i.e., uncertainty of the absolute magnitude of the benefit to be achieved). The recommendation to take patient preference into consideration in planning treatment does not mean that, when a physician is uncertain about what to do, he or she should invite the patient to decide.

Rather, the panel emphasizes in the Table 3 footnotes that physician judgment based on patient preference is an acceptable way to select adjuvant treatment.

Node-Negative Breast Cancer

Treatment for patients with node-negative disease varies substantially according to the prognosis, based on patient and tumor characteristics. For patients considered at high risk of recurrence, the treatment choice follows an algorithm similar to that for node-positive disease, which has a similar prognosis. For high-risk patients, the use of chemotherapy alone was considered to be appropriate when steroid hormone receptors are absent in the primary tumor. For patients with tumors that express estrogen or progesterone receptors, combined chemotherapy and tamoxifen was shown in a clinical trial (Fisher et al. 1997b) to be more effective than endocrine therapy alone, irrespective of menopausal status. This trial tested, in combination with tamoxifen, the "classical" CMF-based regimen with oral cyclophosphamide on days 1–14 and intravenous methotrexate and 5-fluorouracil on days 1 and 8, repeated every 28 days. The use of anthracyclines for these patients is currently undergoing investigation, and it is anticipated that their use might result in a small, but statistically significant, improvement in treatment outcome.

For patients with minimal/low-risk disease, the question of whether or not to treat with tamoxifen depends on a risk-benefit analysis, which should take into account both the low relapse rate within the first 10 years in these patients and the potential reduction by tamoxifen of the incidence of contralateral breast cancer. Patients classified as intermediate risk may be assigned to receive the same chemoendocrine treatment as the high-risk group, although considerations about a lower relative risk of relapse, age, toxicity, socioeconomic implications, and information on patient's preference might justify the use of tamoxifen alone as an endocrine treatment (e.g., a 65-year-old patient with a tumor expressing estrogen and progesterone receptors might be offered treatment with tamoxifen alone). For pre-menopausal women in this category, the use of hormonal manipulations other than tamoxifen, including ovarian ablation (either surgical or with gonadotropin-releasing hormone [GnRH] analogues), remains investigational, especially considering long-term side effects of these treatments.

Node-Positive Breast Cancer

Additional information became available since the last conference on the treatment of patients with node-positive presentation. For patients who had their tumors classified as estrogen or progesterone receptor positive, tamoxifen and chemotherapy with an anthracycline-based regimen (Albain et al.

Table 4. Adjuvant treatment for patients with node-positive breast cancer

Patient group	Treatments
Pre-menopausal, ER or PgR positive	Chemotherapy + tamoxifen Ovarian ablation (or GnRH analogue) ± tamoxifen[c] Chemotherapy ± ovarian ablation or (GnRH analogue) ± tamoxifen[c]
Pre-menopausal, ER or PgR negative	Chemotherapy[d]
Post-menopausal, ER or PgR positive	Tamoxifen + chemotherapy[b]
Post-menopausal, ER or PgR negative	Chemotherapy[d]
Elderly	Tamoxifen If no ER and PgR expression: chemotherapy

ER, estrogen receptor; PgR, progesterone receptor; GnRH, gonadotropin-releasing hormone.
[a] Treatment accepted for routine use or baseline in clinical trials.
[b] The addition of chemotherapy is considered an acceptable option based on evidence from clinical trials. Considerations about a low relative risk of relapse, age, toxic effects, socioconomic implications, and information on patient's preference might justify the use of tamoxifen alone.
[c] Still being tested in randomized trials.
[d] The addition of tamoxifen following chemotherapy might be considered for patients whose tumors are classified as ER and PgR negative, but which exhibit minimal/trace levels of either ER or PgR.

1997; Wils et al. 1996) or with the "classical" CMF regimen (International Breast Cancer Study Group 1997) were shown to yield a significant prolongation of disease-free survival as compared with tamoxifen alone. The use of tamoxifen alone in women of post-menopausal age may, however, be justified based on individual considerations related to risk of relapse, age, and assessment of the patient's preference (Gelber et al. 1996). Investigations on the type of regimen to be used in patients with node-positive disease take into account the cytotoxic agents to be used, dose intensification, increased frequency of chemotherapy administration, and the use of taxanes in sequential and concomitant combination (mainly with anthracyclines). The use of anthracyclines is usually accepted as a standard, based on interpretation of clinical trial information (Bonadonna et al. 1995; Levine et al. 1998). As yet unpublished overview data indicate a very modest, albeit statistically significant, difference favoring anthracycline-based regimens compared with CMF-like treatments. Treatment options for this population of patients are shown in Table 4.

Specific Aspects of Treatment

Preoperative Systemic Therapy

Starting the therapy for patients with breast cancer with a systemic treatment immediately after diagnosis represents a strategy aimed theoretically at influencing tumor growth, avoiding development of resistance, reducing the number of positive axillary lymph nodes and/or the size of the tumor (i.e., downstaging), and improving control of local and potentially also of systemic disease – thereby increasing the number of patients who are candidates for breast conservation (Bonadonna et al. 1998; Ellis et al. 1998; Fisher et al. 1997b, c). Similar results in terms of disease-free and overall survival were obtained in a randomized trial comparing the same systemic chemotherapy regimen given preoperatively or postoperatively (Fisher et al. 1997c). It is interesting to note that the histologic features that are assessed postoperatively, such as the extent of axillary lymph node involvement and – especially – the degree of response by the tumor to primary chemotherapy, were found to be the features with the most significant association with prognosis. Some current clinical research is directed toward increasing the efficacy of the preoperative treatment regimen to try to obtain more complete tumor regression. The regimens being tested as primary systemic treatment are typically those used as postoperative adjuvant therapies as well as regimens developed for locally advanced disease that include continuous infusion of 5-fluorouracil. The use of the latter agent has led to a relatively large number of complete pathologic remissions (Eisen et al. 1998; Smith et al. 1995).

Surgical Treatment of the Axilla

It has become axiomatic that the histopathologic evaluation of the axilla is the most important tool for estimation of risk of relapse. It has also been observed that node-positive and some node-negative disease presentations currently tend to receive similar treatments, thus making the determination of nodal status potentially irrelevant for treatment selection. Furthermore, it is unclear whether patients with nonpalpable axillary lymph nodes but with microscopic evidence of metastatic involvement benefit from surgical removal of these lymph nodes. Finally, it is clear that patients found not to have axillary lymph node involvement have had their lymph nodes removed at a cost of subsequent discomfort in return for having received reassuring information about the absence of tumor spread to the lymph nodes. Two new lines of research may change clinicians' attitudes toward whether performing axillary dissection should be part of a proper workup at diagnosis. One area of research is the use of primary systemic therapy (*see above*), which leads to some downstaging of axillary involvement, especially in tumors that are particularly responsive to treatment. The other is the study of the sentinel lymph node (Table 1). This procedure may be investigated most usefully in patients who present with a localized, unicentric breast tumor (Veronesi et al. 1997). In addition to whether use of the procedure is feasible and whether a negative histopathologic finding by this procedure has clinical relevance, one of the most important open questions about the procedure remains whether finding a positive sentinel node means that further axillary dissection is needed.

Radiation Therapy After Breast-Conserving Surgery and Mastectomy

Women who undergo breast conservation should be advised to have postoperative breast irradiation, mainly because its omission increases the risk of in-breast recurrence. Some impediments to breast irradiation include previous radiotherapy to the breast (for other malignant disorders), pregnancy, and anatomic hindrance to properly conduct the treatment. Autoimmune disorders are relative contraindications. Local breast irradiation should be started as soon as possible after surgery, usually within 12 weeks, except for patients in whom radiotherapy is preceded by chemotherapy. Selected chemotherapy regimens are sometimes used concurrently with radiotherapy, although there is an increased chance of toxic effects, especially when patients are given anthracycline-containing regimens.

On the basis of two recently published trials, patients at increased risk for local-regional recurrence after mastectomy (defined as at least a 20% cumulative risk of local-regional recurrence in spite of proper surgery and proper adjuvant systemic therapy) are considered to be candidates for postmastectomy irradiation (Overgaard et al. 1997; Ragaz et al. 1997; Table 1). The Danish Trial 82b (Overgaard et al. 1997) confirms the observation that 50 Gy comprehensive local-regional radiotherapy, appropriately planned and delivered, reduces the proportional risk of local-regional recurrence after total mastectomy and (partial) axillary dissection by a factor of about 4. In this premenopausal patient population, the group that received radiation therapy in addition to a chemotherapy regimen had improved overall survival as compared with the group treated with the chemotherapy regimen alone. The British Columbia Trial (Ragaz et al. 1997), although small, showed similar results. The benefit and safety associated with the combination of radiation therapy and different chemotherapy regimens, especially anthracyclines (and taxanes), remain subjects for investigation (Chen et al. 1997). The panel concluded that postmastectomy radiation therapy was clearly to be considered for patients with an increased risk of local-regional recurrence following adequate surgery and adjuvant systemic therapy.

Ovarian Ablation

The overview results (Early Breast Cancer Trialists' Collaborative Group 1996) indicated that ovarian ablation can have beneficial effects in women with primary breast cancer. This treatment significantly improved the long-term survival for women under 50 years old, at least in the absence of chemotherapy. The report called for further evidence from randomized clinical trials to define the additional effects of ovarian ablation in the presence of other adjuvant treatments, especially in relationship with hormone receptor status. The occurrence and severity of long-term side effects are still significant issues when this treatment is given to younger women, especially because the safety of treatments for the resulting menopausal symptoms is unknown for this cohort of patients.

At least four randomized trials include a GnRH analogue to suppress ovarian function. In these trials, the duration of treatment varies from 2 to 5 years. The shorter treatments are justified by data showing that the amenorrhea induced by chemotherapy is associated with improved disease-free survival, even if the patients resume menses after a cessation of at least 9 months (Pagani et al. 1998). In advanced disease, a direct comparison between surgical ovarian ablation and the use of a GnRH analogue (goserelin) resulted in similar failure-free and overall survival (Taylor et al. 1998). However, the routine use of GnRH analogues in the adjuvant setting must await results of clinical trials.

Tamoxifen

Tamoxifen continues to be an important component of adjuvant treatment for patients with tumors that express steroid hormone receptors. Recently published overview results (Early Breast Cancer Trialists' Collaborative Group 1998) show that, for women with estrogen receptor-positive tumors, the magnitude of the treatment effect of tamoxifen was similar for all age cohorts – even extending to the youngest patients. Many of the panelists noted that the magnitude of treatment effects for younger patients demonstrated in the tamoxifen overview was even larger than that shown in the chemotherapy overview without regard to estrogen receptor status. Unfortunately, these observations based on indirect evidence are being used to argue that tamoxifen rather than chemotherapy should be the treatment of choice for younger women. In fact, such an argument contradicts the results of randomized trials that directly compare tamoxifen (for 2 years only) versus chemotherapy in young patients (Kaufmann et al. 1993). It is likely that 5 years of tamoxifen would have yielded a larger effect, thus providing the proper test to identify the "best available" among the single modalities of adjuvant systemic treatments. It should be stressed that the tamoxifen overview results excluded patients with estrogen receptor-poor tumors and thus was restricted to an endocrine treatment-responsive population. In addition, several issues with respect to the use of this compound still need answers from clinical trials. Although evidence exists that tamoxifen treatment of 5 years' duration yielded an improved disease-free survival as compared with a 2-year duration (Swedish Breast Cancer Cooperative Group 1996), the evidence from trials of longer tamoxifen exposure is not entirely conclusive (Fisher et al. 1996), especially for patients with node-positive disease. For patients with node-negative breast cancer, 5 years is the standard duration of tamoxifen treatment. Also, the optimal way to administer the drug – either concomitant with or sequential to chemotherapy – is still unsettled, and a trial that was specifically designed to answer this question is still awaiting evaluation of this specific comparison (Albain et al. 1997).

Chemotherapy Regimen and Dose

Anthracycline-based regimens have been increasingly introduced into clinical practice, primarily motivated by the shorter duration of treatment that they permit. This was based on the large National Surgical Adjuvant Breast and Bowel Project (NSABP) trial, in which four courses of doxorubicin and cyclophosphamide given every 3 weeks provided similar results compared with six courses of cyclophosphamide, methotrexate, and 5-fluorouracil ("classical" CMF) repeated every 4 weeks (Fisher et al. 1990). As yet unpublished overview data on all trials begun before 1990 that compared anthracycline-containing regimens with CMF-like regimens indicate a very modest, although statistically significant, difference in favor of anthracycline use. Individual studies have shown a more toxic anthracycline-containing combination to be superior to a less toxic CMF. Such a regimen was used in the Canadian trial of cyclophosphamide, 4-epidoxorubicin, and 5-fluorouracil (CEF) given on a CMF-like schedule (4-epidoxorubicin and 5-fluorouracil given on days 1 and 8 every 4 weeks and cyclophosphamide given orally on days 1–14). To successfully reduce the incidence of febrile neutropenia (Levine et al. 1998), this regimen was given together with antibiotics. Another anthracycline-based regimen that used a low-dose doxorubicin on day 1, but a daily 5-fluorouracil administration on days 3–6 each 28-day course, was found to yield a disease-free survival advantage when compared with CMF in a small, randomized trial (Misset et al. 1996). These observations indicate that a more toxic anthracycline regimen might represent the most effective *conventional* adjuvant regimen.

Many trials of adjuvant therapy used altered forms of CMF, although no trial directly compares "classical" and "altered" CMF in the adjuvant setting. However, several randomized trials have shown that departure from the "classical" CMF regimen compromises its efficacy for patients with metastatic breast cancer (Goldhirsch et al. 1998a). Further indirect evidence of the inferiority of "altered" CMF regimens comes from the seven adjuvant therapy trials that have compared CMF regimens plus tamoxifen with tamoxifen alone. A benefit of adding CMF was seen in all three trials that used "classical" CMF but in none of the four trials using CMF schedules given on day 1 every 3 or 4 weeks or at a low continuous dosage (Goldhirsch et al. 1998b).

Chemoendocrine Therapies

Combined chemotherapy and tamoxifen was associated with a better therapeutic outcome when compared with tamoxifen alone in all trials investigating this comparison, especially if the tested cytotoxic regimens contained anthracyclines (such as doxorubicin with or without cyclophosphamide or 4-epidoxorubicin) (Albain et al. 1997; Fisher et al. 1990; Nils et al. 1996). Trials that used CMF-like regimens in combination with tamoxifen showed a benefit in terms of disease-free survival only when the chemotherapy regimen used was "classical" (Fisher et al. 1997a; International Breast Cancer Study Group 1997); no advantage in favor of the chemoendocrine therapy was detected when "altered" CMF regimens were used (Boccardo et al. 1993; Pritchard et al. 1997; Rivkin et al. 1994; Rose et al. 1992). Evidence of an interaction between the effects of tamoxifen and chemotherapy is available both from laboratory (Osborne 1994) and from clinical (International Breast Cancer Study Group 1997) studies.

High-Dose Chemotherapy with Peripheral Blood Progenitor Cell or Bone Marrow Support

This procedure continues to be experimental because evidence from reliable, large-scale clinical trials is not yet available to indicate a more favorable treatment outcome for patients treated with high-dose chemotherapy (Zujewski et al. 1998), either for patients with ten or more metastatic axillary lymph nodes or with advanced disease.

Panelists' Additional Comments

The international panel attempted to answer many questions related to the best use of treatments investigated in randomized clinical trials. The panel members were more convinced than ever that participation in clinical trials must become more acceptable to the public as well as to the medical community for much more to be achieved that increases knowledge about the disease and improves patient care. The members of the panel expressed their concern that excessive extrapolation of results from existing clinical trials and reliance upon indirect evidence might be detrimental to the development of well-established treatments.

Acknowledgements. We thank the participants of the 6th International Conference on Adjuvant Therapy of Primary Breast Cancer for their many useful remarks and Professor Umberto Veronesi, Dr. Monica Castiglione-Gertsch, Dr. Marco Colleoni, Mrs. Karen Price, and Mrs. Shari Gelber for their thoughtful contributions. The other members of the panel are listed below. All had a significant input to the discussion and the manuscript: J. S. Abrams, National Cancer Institute, Bethesda, MD; M. Baum, University College – London, U.K.; F. Boccardo, National Institute for Cancer Research, Genoa, Italy; A. S. Coates, Australian Cancer Society, Sydney, Australia; B. Fisher, University of Pittsburgh, PA; A. Howell, Christie Hospital, Manchester, U.K.; M. Kaufmann, Klinikum der Wolfgang Goethe Universität, Frankfurt am Main, Germany; J. Kurtz, University Hospital, Geneva, Switzerland; H. Mouridsen, Finseninstitutet, Copenhagen, Denmark; M. Piccart, Institut Jules Bordet, Brussels, Belgium; K. Pritchard, Toronto-Sunnybrook Regional Cancer Center, North York, Ontario, Canada; and W. C. Wood, Emory University School of Medicine, Atlanta, GA.

References

Albain K, Green S, Osborne K, Cobau C, Levine E, Ingle J for SWOG, ECOG, CALGB, NCCTG, and NCI-Canada (1997) Tamoxifen (T) versus cyclophosphamide, Adriamycin® and 5-FU plus either concurrent or sequential T in postmenopausal, receptor(+), node(+) breast cancer: a Southwest Oncology Group phase III Intergroup trial (SWOG-8814, INT-0100) [abstract 450]. Proc ASCO 16:128a

Axelsson CK, Mouridsen HT, Zedeler K (1992) Axillary dissection of level I and II lymph nodes is important in breast cancer classification. The Danish Breast Cancer Cooperative Group (DBCG). Eur J Cancer 28A:1415-1418

Boccardo F, Amoroso D, Rubagotti A, Castagnetta L, Delia P, De Sanctis C et al for the GROCTA (1993) Chemotherapy versus tamoxifen versus chemotherapy plus tamoxifen in node-positive, estrogen receptor-positive breast cancer patients: an update at 8 years of the first GROCTA trial. In: Salmon SE (ed) Adjuvant therapy of cancer VII. Lippincott, Philadelphia, pp 181–192

Bonadonna G, Zambetti M, Valagussa P (1995) Sequential or alternating doxorubicin and CMF regimens in breast cancer with more than three positive nodes. Ten-year results. JAMA 273:542–547

Bonadonna G, Valagussa P, Brambilla C, Ferrari L, Moliterni A, Terenziani M et al (1998) Primary chemotherapy in operable breast cancer: eight-year experience at the Milan Cancer Institute. J Clin Oncol 16:93–100

Bontenbal M, Foekens JA, Lamberts SW, de Jong FH, van Putten WL, Braun HJ et al (1998) Feasibility, endocrine and anti-tumour effects of a triple endocrine therapy with tamoxifen, a somatostatin analogue and an antiprolactin in post-menopausal metastatic breast cancer: a randomized study with long-term follow-up. Br J Cancer 77:115–122

Burke W, Daly M, Garber J, Botkin J, Kahn MJ, Lynch P et al (1997) Recommendations for follow-up care of individuals with an inherited predisposition to cancer. II BRCA1 and BRCA2. Cancer Genetics Studies Consortium. JAMA 277:997–1003

Chen MH, Chuang ML, Bornstein BA, Gelman R, Harris JR, Manning WJ (1997) Impact of respiratory maneuvers on cardiac volume within left-breast radiation portals. Circulation 96:3269–3272

Clark GM, Harvey JM, Osborne CK, Allred DC (1997) Estrogen receptor status (ER) determined by immunohistochemistry (IHC) is superior to biochemical ligand-binding (LB) assay for evaluating breast cancer patients. Proc ASCO 16 (abstr 454)

Delmas PD, Bjarnason NH, Mitlak BH, Ravoux AC, Shah AS, Huster WJ et al (1997) Effects of raloxifene on bone mineral density, serum cholesterol concentrations, and uterine endometrium in postmenopausal women. N Engl J Med 337:1641–1647

Early Breast Cancer Trialists' Collaborative Group (1992) Systemic treatment of early breast cancer by hormonal, cytotoxic, or immune therapy. 133 Randomised trials involving 31000 recurrences and 24000 deaths among 75000 women. Lancet 339:71–85

Early Breast Cancer Trialists' Collaborative Group (1996) Ovarian ablation in early breast cancer: overview of the randomised trials. Lancet 348:1189–1196

Early Breast Cancer Trialists' Collaborative Group (1998) Tamoxifen for early breast cancer: an overview of the randomised trials. Lancet 351:1451–1467

Eisen T, Smith IE, Johnston S, Ellis PA, Prendiville J, Seymour MT et al (1998) Randomized phase II trial of infusional fluorouracil, epirubicin, and cyclophosphamide versus infusional fluorouracil, epirubicin, and cisplatin in patients with advanced breast cancer. J Clin Oncol 16:1350–1357

Ellis P, Smith I, Ashley S, Walsh G, Ebbs S, Baum M et al (1998) Clinical prognostic and predictive factors for primary chemotherapy in operable breast cancer. J Clin Oncol 16:107–114

Fisher B, Redmond C, Legault-Poisson S, Dimitrov NV, Brown AM, Wickerham DL et al (1990) Postoperative chemotherapy and tamoxifen compared with tamoxifen alone in the treatment of positive-node breast cancer patients aged 50 years and older with tumors responsive to tamoxifen: results from the National Surgical Adjuvant Breast & Bowel Projekt B-16. J Clin Oncol 8:1005–1018

Fisher B, Dignam J, Bryant J, DeCillis A, Wickerham DL, Wolmark N et al (1996) Five versus more than five years of tamoxifen therapy for breast cancer patients with negative lymph nodes and estrogen receptor-positive tumors. Natl Cancer Inst 88:1529–1542

Fisher B, Brown A, Mamounas E, Wieand S, Robidoux A, Margolese RG et al (1997a) Effect of preoperative chemotherapy on local-regional disease in women with operable breast cancer: findings from National Surgical Adjuvant Breast and Bowel Project B-18. J Clin Oncol 15:2483–2493

Fisher B, Dignam J, Wolmark N, DeCillis A, Emir B, Wickerham DL et al (1997b) Tamoxifen and chemotherapy for lymph node-negative, estrogen receptor-positive breast cancer. J Natl Cancer Inst 89:1673–1682

Fisher B, Brown A, Mamounas E, Wieand S, Fisher E, Robidoux A et al (1997c) Effect of preoperative therapy for primary breast cancer (BC) on local-regional disease, disease-free survival (DFS) and survival (S): results from NSABP B-18. Proc ASCO 16:127A (abstr 449)

Fisher B, Dignam J, Wolmark N, Mamounas E, Costantino J, Poller W et al (1998) Lumpectomy and radiation therapy for the treatment of intraductal breast cancer: findings from National Surgical Adjuvant Breast and Bowel Project B-17. J Clin Oncol 16:441–452

Gelber RD, Cole BH, Goldhirsch A, Rose C, Fisher B, Osborne CK et al (1996) Adjuvant chemotherapy plus tamoxifen compared with tamoxifen alone for postmenopausal breast cancer: meta-analysis of quality-adjusted survival. Lancet 347:1066–1071

Goldhirsch A, Wood WC, Senn HJ, Glick JH, Gelber RD (1995) Meeting highlights: International Consensus Panel on the treatment of primary breast cancer. J Natl Cancer Inst 87:1441–1445

Goldhirsch A, Coates AS, Colleoni M, Gelber RD (1998a) Radiotherapy and chemotherapy in high-risk breast cancer (letter). N Engl J Med 338:330–331

Goldhirsch A, Coates AS, Colleoni M, Castiglione-Gertsch M, Gelber RD (1998b) Adjuvant chemoendocrine therapy in postmenopausal breast cancer: cyclophosphamide, methotrexate, and fluorouracil dose and schedule may make a difference. International Breast Cancer Study Group. J Clin Oncol 16:1358–1362

International Breast Cancer Study Group (1997) Effectiveness of adjuvant chemotherapy in combination with tamoxifen for node-positive postmenopausal breast cancer patients. J Clin Oncol 15:1385–1394

Kaufmann M, Jonat W, Abel U, Hilfrich J, Caffler H, Kreienberg R et al (1993) Adjuvant randomized trials of doxorubicin/cyclophosphamide versus doxorubicin/cyclophosphamide/tamoxifen and CMF chemotherapy versus tamoxifen in women with node-positive breast cancer. J Clin Oncol 11:454–460

Kerbel RS (1997) A cancer therapy resistant to resistance. Nature 390:335–336

Levine MN, Bramwell VH, Pritchard KI, Norris GD, Shepherd LE, Abu-Zahra H et al for the National Cancer Institute of Canada Clinical Trials Group (1998) Randomized trial of intensive cyclophosphamide, epirubicin, and fluorouracil chemotherapy in premenopausal women with node-positive breast cancer. National Cancer Institute of Canada Clinical Trials Group. J Clin Oncol 16:2651–2658

Miles D (1997) Breast cancer tumour vaccines. Cancer Treat Rev Suppl 1:S77–S85

Misset JL, di Palma M, Delgado M, Plagne R, Chollet P, Fumoleau P et al (1996) Adjuvant treatment of node-positive breast cancer with cyclophosphamide, doxorubicin, fluorouracil, and vincristine versus cyclophosphamide, methotrexate, and fluorouracil: final report after 16-year median follow-up duration. J Clin Oncol 14:1136–1145

Osborne CK (1994) Interactions of tamoxifen with cytotoxic chemotherapy for breast cancer. In: Jordan VC (ed) Long term tamoxifen for breast cancer. University of Wisconsin Press, Madison, pp 181–198

Overgaard M, Hansen PS, Overgaard J, Rose C, Andersson M, Bach F et al (1997) Postoperative radiotherapy in high-risk premenopausal women with breast cancer who receive adjuvant chemotherapy. N Engl J Med 337:949–955

Pagani O, O'Neill A, Castiglione M, Gelber RD, Goldhirsch A, Rudenstam CM et al (1998) Prognostic impact of amenorrhea after adjuvant chemotherapy in premenopausal breast cancer patients with axillary node involvement: results of the International Breast Cancer Study Group (IBCSG) Trial VI. Eur J Cancer 34:632–640

Pritchard KI, Paterson AH, Fine S, Paul NA, Zee B, Shepherd LE et al (1997) Randomized trial of cyclophosphamide, methotrexate, and fluorouracil chemotherapy added to tamoxifen as adjuvant therapy in postmenopausal women with node-positive estrogen and/or progesterone receptor-positive breast cancer: a report of the National Cancer Institute of Canada Clinical Trials Group. Breast Cancer Site Group. J Clin Oncol 15:2302–2311

Ragaz J, Jackson SM, Le N, Plenderleith IH, Spinelli JJ, Basco VE et al (1997) Adjuvant radiotherapy and chemotherapy in node-positive premenopausal women with breast cancer. N Engl J Med 337:956–962

Rivkin SE, Green S, Metch B, Cruz AB, Abeloff MD, Jewell WR et al (1994) Adjuvant CMFVP versus tamoxifen versus concurrent CMFVP and tamoxifen for postmenopausal, node-positive, and estrogen receptor-positive breast cancer patients: a Southwest Oncology Group study. J Clin Oncol 12:2078–2085

Rose C, Andersen J, Axelsson C, Blichert-Tort M, Dombernowsky P, Hansen C et al. (1992) A randomized DBCG trial of adjuvant (adj) tamoxifen (TAM)+radiotherapy (RT) vs TAM alone vs TAM+CMF in postmenopausal breast cancer patients (pts) with high risk of recurrence (meeting abstract). Proc ASCO 11:58 (abstr 57)

Sjogren S, Inganas M, Lindgren A, Holmberg L, Bergh J (1998) Prognostic and predictive value of c-erbB-2 overexpression in primary breast cancer, alone and in combination with other prognostic markers. J Clin Oncol 16:462–469

Smith IE, Walsh G, Jones A, Prendiville J, Johnston S, Gusterson B et al (1995) High complete remission rates with primary neoadjuvant infusional chemotherapy for large early breast cancer. J Clin Oncol 13:424–429

Swedish Breast Cancer Cooperative Group (1996) Randomized trial of two versus five years of adjuvant tamoxifen for postmenopausal early stage breast cancer. J Natl Cancer Inst 88:1543–1549

Taylor CW, Green S, Dalton WS, Martino S, Rector D, Ingle JN et al (1998) Multicenter randomized clinical trial of goserelin versus surgical ovariectomy in premenopausal patients with receptor-positive metastatic breast cancer: an intergroup study. J Clin Oncol 16:994–999

Veronesi U, Paganelli G, Galimberti V, Viale G, Zurrida S, Bedoni M et al (1997) Sentinel-node biopsy to avoid axillary dissection in breast cancer with clinically negative lymph-nodes. Lancet 349:1864–1867

Wils J, Bliss JM, Coombes RC, Woods E, Coombes G, Blijham EH et al for the International Collaborative Cancer Group (ICCG) (1996) A multicentre randomized trial of tamoxifen vs. tamoxifen plus epirubicin in postmenopausal women with node-positive breast cancer. Proc ASCO 15:109 (abstr 101)

Zujewski J, Nelson A, Abrams J (1998) Much ado about not enough data; high-dose chemotherapy with autologous stem cell rescue for breast cancer. J Natl Cancer Inst 90:200–209

Subject Index

Recent Results in Cancer Research
Volumes published since Vol. 146

Springer
and the
environment

At Springer we firmly believe that an international science publisher has a special obligation to the environment, and our corporate policies consistently reflect this conviction.
We also expect our business partners – paper mills, printers, packaging manufacturers, etc. – to commit themselves to using materials and production processes that do not harm the environment. The paper in this book is made from low- or no-chlorine pulp and is acid free, in conformance with international standards for paper permanency.

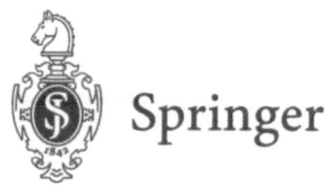 Springer